Principles and Practice of

# ASSISTED REPRODUCTIVE TECHNOLOGY

# Principles and Practice of ASSISTED REPRODUCTIVE TECHNOLOGY

## VOLUME 2

# LABORATORY ASPECTS OF IVF AND ANDROLOGY

**Third Edition**

*Editor*

**Kamini A Rao**
MBBS DGO MCh FRCOG FNAMS FICOG PGDMLE
Chief Mentor
Former Founder and Medical Director
Milann Group of Fertility Centers
Bengaluru, Karnataka, India

*Co-Editor*

**Mohammed Ashraf C** PhD
Associate Director and Senior Embryologist
Milann Fertility Centre
Bengaluru, Karnataka, India

*Foreword*

**Geeta Nargund**

JAYPEE BROTHERS MEDICAL PUBLISHERS
*The Health Sciences Publisher*
**New Delhi | London**

**Jaypee Brothers Medical Publishers (P) Ltd.**

**Headquarters**
EMCA House, 23/23-B
Ansari Road, Daryaganj
New Delhi 110 002, India
Landline: +91-11-23272143, +91-11-23272703
+91-11-23282021, +91-11-23245672
e-mail: jaypee@jaypeebrothers.com

**Corporate Office**
4838/24, Ansari Road, Daryaganj
New Delhi 110 002, India
Phone: +91-11-43574357
Fax: +91-11-43574314
e-mail: jaypee@jaypeebrothers.com

**Overseas Office**
JP Medical Ltd.
83, Victoria Street, London
SW1H 0HW (UK)
Phone: +44-20 3170 8910
e-mail: info@jpmedpub.com

**EU GPSR** Authorised Representative
Logos Europe, 9 rue Nicolas Poussin
17000, La Rochelle, France
Phone: +33 (0) 6 67 93 73 78
e-mail: contact@logoseurope.eu

Website: www.jaypeebrothers.com
Website: www.jaypeedigital.com



**Inquiries for bulk sales may be solicited at:** jaypee@jaypeebrothers.com

***Principles and Practice of Assisted Reproductive Technology—Vol. 2 (Laboratory Aspects of IVF and Andrology)***

*First Edition:* 2014
*Second Edition:* 2019
*Third Edition: 2023*, *Reprint: 2024, 2025,* **2026**

ISBN: 978-93-5696-037-4

*Printed at: Samrat Offset Pvt. Ltd.*

# Contents

## VOLUME 1: INFERTILITY

### SECTION 1: ANATOMY AND PHYSIOLOGY



### SECTION 2: REPRODUCTIVE ENDOCRINOLOGY

## SECTION 4: MALE INFERTILITY

## SECTION 5: FEMALE FACTOR INFERTILITY

## SECTION 7: OVARIAN STIMULATION

## SECTION 10: THIRD PARTY REPRODUCTION



## SECTION 11: OUTCOME FOLLOWING ASSISTED REPRODUCTIVE TECHNIQUE

# VOLUME 2: LABORATORY ASPECTS OF IVF AND ANDROLOGY

## SECTION 14: ANDROLOGY

SECTION

# 14

# Andrology

CHAPTER 97

# Semen Analysis in 21st Century Medicine: A Paradigm Shift

*Fahim L Rajwate, Ashish S Reddy, Vasan SS*

## INTRODUCTION

Nearly 15% of couples are unable to conceive after a year of unprotected intercourse. A male factor is solely responsible in about 20% of infertile couples and contributory in another 30–40%[1] and another study by Hull et al.[2] suggested spermatozoal defects accounting for some 30–50% of cases of subfertility. Although the semen analysis is not a test of fertility, it is the most important single indicator of the functional status in the male reproductive tract. Clinical studies of infertile patients have established "limits of adequacy" below which the chance of initiating a pregnancy becomes more difficult. A minimum of two evaluations is recommended to establish a profile of the seminal parameters.

## SEMEN ANALYSIS

Semen analysis is the cornerstone of the laboratory evaluation of the infertile male and helps to define the severity of the male factor. The first person to suggest that semen analysis should be a routine investigation in the evaluation of every case of infertility was Edward Martin.[3-5] Martin also demonstrated that there were two major causes of azoospermia and he was also the first to recognize the polymorphism of human sperm. John MacLeod then elevated semen analysis from being a simple observation into a science. He recognized that not only sperm numbers but sperm motility and morphology were also important in the evaluation of the potential fertility of semen.[6] He even tried to associate certain sperm shapes with specific clinical entities such as varicocele.[7] However, many clinicians and laboratory personnel did not follow MacLeod's lead in relation to semen analysis. In or around 1980s, it became clear that many laboratories worldwide were not even attempting to examine a number of variables within a semen sample that were important in the determination of fertility. Often only an estimation of the sperm concentration was being performed and no assessment of either motility or morphology was made by a number of pathology laboratories. Thus, information that could be obtained from the examination of semen was not being sought.[8]

By the early 1980s, however, Mortimer and colleagues were anxious to further advance the understanding of the inter-relationships between the different variables in a semen analysis[9] and also introduced the concept of quality assurance in relation to the analysis of semen.[10] It is now very clear that careful training in semen analysis, such as that set-up by the ESHRE Andrology Special Interest Group that includes both theoretical as well as practical training in semen analysis, is very effective in raising the skills of laboratory personnel in relation to semen analysis.[11]

However, it should be understood that semen analysis is a guide to fertility and not an absolute proof of fertility of an individual. Over the time it has become clear that the relationship between infertility and sperm numbers, sperm movement and sperm morphology is not a simple one. It has been known for a long time that reproductive pathology in the female partner reduces the potential fertility of a male with a normal sperm count[12] while a high sperm count such as that achieved using donated sperm can overcome female problems that could otherwise result in childlessness.[13] Thus the male-female interaction in infertility is immensely important to the outcome in relation to pregnancy, and this inter-relationship cannot in any way be incorporated into a semen analysis.

The literature in relation to the fate of the sperm once they enter the female genital tract in the human is very sparse. However, it is clear that, of the total number of sperm that enter this tract in a conception cycle, all but one is lost. Many of the sperm also drain out of the vagina after coitus in the phenomenon also known as flow back. What percentage of the ejaculate enters the cervical mucus is unclear but it is probably small. Of those sperms entering the cervical mucus, a proportion may become eliminated by their passage into the folds of the cervical epithelium and by their entry into the cervical glands.[14] Many sperms also loose or change their motility on entering the cervical mucus.[15]

The numbers of sperm that traverse the uterine cavity in the human and reach the uterotubal junctions in the human is unknown but probably only a few thousand sperm enter each Fallopian tube.[16] Those sperm that do succeed in entering the Fallopian tubes will therefore only make up a very small percentage of the total numbers seen in the whole ejaculate.

Due to the relatively vast surface area of the heaped-up epithelium of the Fallopian tubes (certainly vast in relation to the size of a spermatozoon); only a relatively small number of sperm will be able to access the oocyte. Not only must the sperm traverse the corona but they must also be able to exhibit hyperactivated movement and must not have undergone the acrosome reaction until they are close to the zona pellucida. It is thus also possible that human fertilization may depend frequently upon a sperm oocyte ratio that may be as low as 1:1.

## THE AMERICAN UROLOGICAL ASSOCIATION BEST PRACTICE POLICY AND THE AMERICAN SOCIETY FOR REPRODUCTIVE MEDICINE PRACTICE COMMITTEE REPORT

An initial screening evaluation of the male partner of an infertile couple should be done if pregnancy has not occurred within 1 year of unprotected intercourse. An earlier evaluation may be warranted if a known male or female infertility risk factor exists or if a man questions his fertility potential. The initial evaluation for male factor infertility should include a reproductive history and two properly performed semen analyses. A full evaluation by an urologist/andrologist or other specialist in male reproduction should be done if the initial screening evaluation demonstrates an abnormal male reproductive history or an abnormal semen analysis. Further evaluation of the male partner should also be considered in couples with unexplained infertility and in couples in whom there is a treated female factor and persistent infertility.[3,4]

## THE PROBABILISTIC NATURE OF HUMAN FERTILITY

The very term infertility is not helpful because it implies a complete incapacity to conceive, whereas most couples who fail to conceive within a year are capable of conception, just with a decreased probability of doing so in a given time. The clinician must decide which of these couples is likely to conceive in an acceptable time frame. It is no longer sensible to treat fertility as a binary categorical variable.

This differs from distinguishing between fertile and infertile populations because most (but not all) couples with a high chance of conception per cycle will conceive in the first year and never reach the clinic.

Among couples who stopped contraception and ultimately conceived, about 30% did so in the first cycle of unprotected intercourse. After 12 months, the conception rate per cycle had declined to 10%, and the average success rate per cycle in the second year of trying was about 5%. Consequently, among couples attending infertility clinics after 1 year of unprotected intercourse, even those likely to conceive will have an average spontaneous conception rate of only about 5% per cycle.

### WHO Standardization of Semen Testing

With the aim in providing standardization worldwide, WHO has published its first manual in 1980 and subsequently five editions have been released over the last four decades. The latest 6th Edition was published in July 2021 with the aim of making semen analysis worldwide more robust via extensive research and by considering the criticism and drawbacks of previous versions, thereby making it efficient to practice in clinical andrology and reproductive medicine.

### The Need for the New 6th Edition

The WHO 2010 5th Edition, aimed to facilitate the standardization of semen analysis procedures via a detailed step-by-step approach to various basic and optional semen tests. The percentile values proposed in the 5th Edition were derived from fertile men whose partners had a time to pregnancy ≤12 months (1,959 men from 8 countries representing 4 continents (Europe, Americas and Oceania).

### The 5th Edition Received the Following Criticism

1. Inadequacy to represent the general population , this can be attributed to
   a. Over- and under-representation of some areas of the world and their respective population. (8 countries and 4 continents: Oceania, Americas, Europe were included)
   b. Percentile values which represented lowest limit of fertility could be used as a fertility cut-off and these men could be classified as infertile leading to a denial of proper male fertility evaluation and may be pushed to Assisted Reproductive Technology (ART).

### WHO 6th Manual

1. Commended the importance of SA as a tool to:
   a. Assist fertility/infertility diagnosis,
   b. Assess male reproductive health and function to guide management
   c. Guide the choice of ART procedure
   d. Monitor response to treatment
   e. Measure the efficacy of male contraception.
2. Optimized SA procedures by including detailed steps and a methodological sequence for test execution.
3. Described new sperm tests for the assessment of Sperm DNA Fragmentation (SDF) and seminal Oxidative

Stress (OS), while abandoning obsolete tests such as human cervical mucus.

4. Addressed the drawback of the 5th Edition related to the demographic under-representation of some geographical regions.

The new 6th Edition served the following advantages/strengths:

1. Abandoned the "percentile values "which was construed as reference values of semen parameters.
   The 6th Edition clearly specified that the 5th centile values are only one way to interpret but not sufficient enough to diagnose male infertility and has introduced the concept of "Decision Limits".
2. The editors of the manual have been voluntarily removed the terms "Normozoospermia" "Asthenozoospermia", "Necrozoospermia", "Teratozoospermia" on the basis that reference thresholds alone are meaningless and that multiple criteria must be applied to establish a diagnosis of male infertility.
3. Combined data of the previous 5th Edition and additional new data of fertile men, whose partners had a time to pregnancy ≤12 months of last decade (2010–2020). Thus, the 6th Edition contains results of semen samples of 3,589 fertile men (1,800 subjects from 5th Edition and 1,789 new, total 3,589 subjects) providing greater statistical power to new reference range.
4. The newly added data was an analysis of semen samples of 3,589 participants, originating from 13 countries and 2 continents, two countries in Southern Europe, along with two countries from Asia and one country from Africa.
5. Recommended extended semen test namely, SDF, fluorescence in situ hybridization (FISH) in certain clinical scenarios.
6. Gives future scope to update guidelines for extended semen test namely, SDF, FISH
7. Provides scope to incorporate epigenetic and seminal OS into clinical practice.
8. More precise evaluation and reporting at low sperm concentration ($<2 \times 10^6$/mL)
9. Systematic based approach for Sperm morphology assessment with multiple and better-quality micrographs of spermatozoa from unprocessed semen samples that are considered normal, borderline, or abnormal (anomalies of the head, intermediate piece and tail) with detailed explanations, rendering the manual helpful.
10. The significance of recording the presence of large cytoplasmic droplets is emphasized.

## Why the Need to Change?

Identifying a semen problem in the early stages of infertility can help begin an appropriate treatment program more expediently or if you discover that there is a serious untreatable sperm problem, you are apprised of this early on. Also tests and investigations and possible treatment directed at the cause can be developed.

The new guidelines from the WHO as per the 6th manual have redefined the new "Decision Limits" values for semen analysis which aids the clinician in understanding the significance of the male factor more accurately as a range.

**TABLE 1:** WHO 5th, 2010 and WHO 6th, 2021 edition of semen parameters.

| *Semen parameters* | *WHO 2010* | *WHO 2021* |
|---|---|---|
| Volume (mL) | 1.5 (1.4–1.7) | 1.4 (1.3–1.5) |
| Total number ($10^6$/ejaculate) | 39 (33–46) | 39 (35–40) |
| Total motility (%) | 40 (38–42) | 42 (40–43) |
| Progressive motility (%) | 32 (31–34) | 30 (29–31) |
| Nonprogressive motility (%) | 1 | 1 (1–1) |
| Immotile (%) | 22 | 20 (19–20) |
| Vitality (%) | 58 (55–63) | 54 (50–56) |
| Normal forms (%) | 4 (3–4) | 4 (3.9–4) |

(WHO: World Health Organization).

## Comparison of the 5th and 6th WHO Manual

Thresholds of basic semen parameters used in the 5th Edition "reference values" and those described as "useful values" in the 6th Edition are shown in **Table 1.**

Important changes from the 5th manual:

1. The categorization of sperm motility has reverted to fast or rapid progressively motile, slow progressively motile, nonprogressively motile and immotile (grade a, b, c, or d, respectively)
2. The assessment of sperm vitality is recommended when total sperm motility is below 40%
3. The significance of recording the presence of large cytoplasmic droplets is emphasized
4. SDF testing "could represent an important addition in the work-up of male infertility.

# MORPHOLOGY OF SPERMATOZOA

*Morphologically normal:* Now 4% (5th centile value).

Previously 15%, this value refers to the number of sperm with normal shape and structure, 4% is considered the new bottom line of normalcy although the average percentage of morphologically normal sperm in the best fertile group was over 9%. Morphology values between 0 and 4% denote greatly impaired fertility possibly requiring intracytoplasmic sperm injection (ICSI).[17,18]

Why the decline in morphology numbers over the years:

- The implementation of strict evaluation criteria with the unfortunate result that sperm morphology evaluation became overcritical with regard to normality

- The fact that over the years more criteria for sperm morphological abnormalities were identified and introduced into the evaluation system
- True decline because of negative environmental factors.

*Other measures of sperm health include:* viscosity, fructose levels, pH to determine the level of acidity/alkalinity and tests for agglutination, antisperm antibodies, sperm penetration and "round cells" which can indicate infection.

### What are We Trying to Achieve?

The new 6th manual injects science and probability chance into reporting instead of reporting a single binary number as was done for years and also provides clarity to the physician.

During the examination of an infertile couple, the underlying problem should be diagnosed so that it can be corrected or appropriate tests ordered to understand the problem so that appropriate treatment can be suggested or we can identify problems which are not correctable and suggest the right modality of treatment.

### Sperm Functional Testing

Routine semen analysis provides useful information concerning sperm production by the testis, sperm motility and viability, the patency of the male genital tract, the secretions of the accessory organs, as well as ejaculation and emission **(Fig. 1)**. The new reporting **(Fig. 1)** shows evaluational of seminal plasmas and sperm abnormalities which aids clinicians to detect specific abnormality and plan management accordingly. Although the information revealed by this assay is obviously useful for the initial evaluation of the infertile male, it is not a test of fertility, and it provides no insights into the functional potential of the spermatozoon to fertilize an ovum or to undergo the subsequent maturation processes that are required to achieve fertilization.[19,20]

Accordingly, tests have been developed to define sperm function abnormalities in the infertile male. In the broadest sense, sperm function may simply be thought of as the ability of one spermatozoon to deliver the correct complement of chromosomes to an ovum. To do this, spermatozoa must be produced in sufficient numbers, and exhibit normal motility and shape (and these parameters generally are assessed in routine semen analysis). In addition, spermatozoa must be capable of penetrating and passing through the cervical mucus, and through the uterus to the ampulla of the oviducts, in addition to undergoing capacitation, AR, binding and penetration of the zona pellucida, and ultimately the ovum. Once the spermatozoon penetrates the ovum, it must then undergo nuclear decondensation to deliver the appropriate haploid chromosome complement; it then undergoes additional, but poorly understood, events required for fertilization and early embryonic development. Defects in any of these complex events can result in male infertility. Over the last 25 years, tests have been developed to identify abnormalities in these processes.

Often it is asked why the evaluation of the infertile male requires advanced, specialized andrology assessment of parameters, such as genetics or sperm function; all that is needed is a single spermatozoon to achieve a pregnancy with ICSI (the logic being that if fertilization can occur, a healthy baby is likely to have been conceived). Yet, we know this logic is flawed, as even healthy fertile couples may conceive a child with significant genetic or birth defects. Certainly, some of the tests of sperm function described above can provide important information to infertile couples to aid in their reproductive decision making. In some cases, sperm function testing may indicate that less expensive technologies may help a couple seeking to conceive a child; ICSI-in vitro fertilization (IVF) may not always be required. In other cases, such as men who fail the hamster Sperm Penetration Assay (SPA) test, donor spermatozoa or other options must be considered. The real strength of sperm function testing lies in its ability to identify men with normal semen parameters but who have functionally deficient spermatozoa that will fail to fertilize in routine IVF. These functional deficiencies will never be observed on a routine semen analysis. As they provide a unique insight into sperm physiology, sperm function tests may also aid in the design of improved treatment that are provided to infertile couples.

The results of such testing may allow for the use of more cost-efficient treatment or even provide the basis for a couple to cease treatment. Ultimately, it is the couple's decision to seek to achieve a pregnancy; infertile couples, however, deserve the right to decide whether this is a realistic goal with a reasonable likelihood of success. Thus, sperm function testing, as well as other genetic and andrology tests now available, allows couple to make a more informed decision.

## CONCLUSION

The long march of semen analysis to join other rigorously standardized chemical pathology tests is well underway. However, the uncritical acceptance of WHO reference values and the widespread reporting of WHO standards as a "gold standard" for all situations has led to the values being used for completely unsuitable purposes lacking specific evidence which hopefully will get streamlined with the 6th manual.[21,22]

Not surprisingly, when values are taken out of context and/or uncritically, irrelevant information may be produced. The new manual attempts to dispel this unhealthy attitude. First, it provides choices of tests that depend on the needs of the laboratory, do you need to measure very low sperm numbers accurately? If not, do not. Do you need to assess normal morphological forms only for ART? If not, examine abnormal forms as well. Do you need a quick screen of sperm antibodies

## ADVANCED SEMEN ASSESSMENT (ASA) REPORT

As per WHO 6th manual

| *Name* | *Mr.* | *Age* | *YRS* | *Hosp No* | |
|---|---|---|---|---|---|
| *Wife* | *Mrs.* | *Date* | | *Lab No* | - |
| *Ref. by* | *Dr.* | | | *Bill no* | |

### SEMINAL PLASMA – MACROSCOPIC

| *Abstinence days* | | *Volume →* | *Time of Collection* | | *Time of Evaluation* | | *Spillage:* | *No* |
|---|---|---|---|---|---|---|---|---|
| *Fructose → POSITIVE* | | *Pus cells →/ hpf* | *Ph →* | *Liquefied : YES* | | *Live →* | *Dead →* | |
| *RBC: NIL* | | *Round cells: NIL* | *Bacteria: NIL* | *Agglutination: NIL* | *Cellular debris: NO* | | *QC: DONE* | |

### IMPRESSION:

### SPERM - MICROSCOPIC
### CONCENTRATION ASSESSMENT (5th percentile value)

| Sperm Concentration per ml | mill/ml |
|---|---|
| Total Ejaculate | millions |

**SPERM CONCENTRATION: mill /ml**
(Decision Limit)Pathological/Borderline/Normal

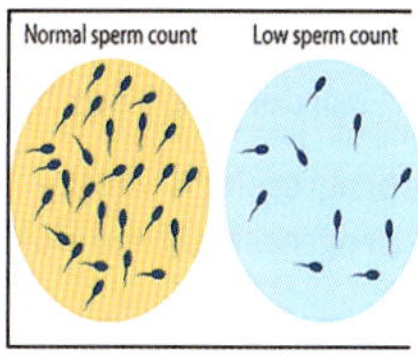


| 2.5TH | 5TH | 10TH | 25TH | 50TH |
|---|---|---|---|---|
| 11 | 16 | 22 | 36 | 66 |

### MOTILITY ASSESSMENT (5th percentile value)

| Type | 1 Hour |
|---|---|
| Rapid Progressive | % |
| Slow Progressive | % |
| Non Progressive | % |
| Immotile | % |

**TOTAL MOTILITY: %**
(Decision Limit) Pathological/Borderline/Normal

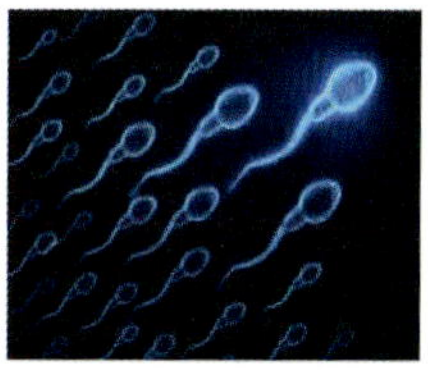

| 2.5TH | 5TH | 10TH | 25TH | 50TH |
|---|---|---|---|---|
| 35 | 42 | 47 | 55 | 64 |

### MORPHOLOGY ASESSMENT (TYGERBERG KRUGER)

| Morphology | |
|---|---|
| Normal Forms | % |
| Over all Defects | % |

| Head Defects | % |
|---|---|
| Mid Piece and Neck Defects | % |
| Tail Defects | % |

**SPERM MORPHOLOGY: %**
(Decision Limit) Pathological/Borderline/Normal

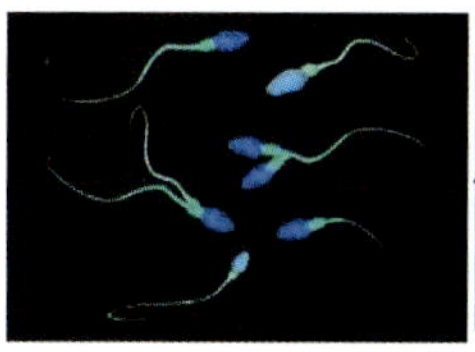

| 2.5TH | 5TH | 10TH | 25TH | 50TH |
|---|---|---|---|---|
| 3 | 4 | 5 | 8 | 14 |

| Excessive residual cytoplasma (ERC) | |
|---|---|

**EX.RESIDUAL CYTOPLASMA: 10**

**Flagellar Integrity - Hypo Osmotic Swelling Test:**

| RESULT: % (Abnormal) | NORMAL RANGE: > 60 % spermatozoa with tail coiling. |
|---|---|

**Spermiation defects – Acrosome Reaction after Ionophore Challenge:**

| RESULT: | % | NORMAL RANGE: > 15% spermatozoa with halos mean diameter of 10μm. |
|---|---|---|

**Fig. 1:** *(Contd...)*

## ADVANCED SEMEN ASSESSMENT (ASA) REPORT

As per WHO 6th manual

### FINAL IMPRESSION

**Seminal fluid abnormality:** NONE

**Sperm abnormality Decision limits:**

| | | |
|---|---|---|
| **Sperm Concentration:** | mill/ml | Pathological/Borderline/Normal |
| **Total Motility:** | % | Pathological/Borderline/Normal |
| **Morphology:** | % | Pathological/Borderline/Normal |

The "normal" reference values of the 5th edition have been replaced by "decision limits" in the WHO 6th edition.
**These are classified as "normal", "border-line", and "pathological".**

A "normal" concentration is ≥20×10 6/mL, " **border line " lies between 10 to 20×106/mL**, and **"pathological" is <10×106/Ml.**

For motility "normal" is defined as ≥50% progressively motile sperm, **"border-line" is 35% to 49% progressively motile, while a "pathological" sample is defined as <35% progressively motile sperm.**

Morphology has been categorized as "normal" when typical forms are ≥14%, **"borderline" is between 4% and 13%** and "**pathological" morphology is below 4%.**

Decision limits" concept is an attempt to emphasize that the purpose of the semen examination is not to label a man as fertile or infertile, but rather to decide next steps in terms of further evaluation and treatment. Those in borderline decision limit will may be improved and will need further evaluation.

| | 2.5 th | 5 th | 10 th | 25 th | 50 th | 75 th | 90 th | 95 th | 97.5 th |
|---|---|---|---|---|---|---|---|---|---|
| Semen volume (ml) | 1 | 1.4 | 1.8 | 2.3 | 3 | 4.2 | 5.5 | 6.2 | 6.9 |
| Sperm concentration (106 per ml) | 11 | 16 | 22 | 36 | 66 | 110 | 166 | 208 | 254 |
| Total sperm number (106 per ejaculate) | 29 | 39 | 58 | 108 | 210 | 363 | 561 | 701 | 865 |
| Total motility (PR + NP, %) | 35 | 42 | 47 | 55 | 64 | 73 | 83 | 90 | 92 |
| Progressive motility (PR, %) | 24 | 30 | 36 | 45 | 55 | 63 | 71 | 77 | 81 |
| Non-progressive motility (NP, %) | 1 | 1 | 2 | 4 | 8 | 15 | 26 | 32 | 38 |
| Immotile spermatozoa (IM, %) | 15 | 20 | 23 | 30 | 37 | 45 | 53 | 58 | 65 |
| Vitality (%) | 45 | 54 | 60 | 69 | 78 | 88 | 95 | 97 | 98 |
| Normal forms (%) | 3 | 4 | 5 | 8 | 14 | 23 | 32 | 39 | 45 |

DNA Fragmentation Index (DFI) by Flow cytometry
Reactive Oxygen Species (ROS)
Annexin V Binding,
Acrosin Proteolytic activity

| Team Andrology | Computer generated report does not require signature |
|---|---|

**Fig. 1:** Evaluational of seminal plasmas and sperm abnormalities.

on seminal spermatozoa or a more detailed examination of seminal plasma-free spermatozoa? Your choice. Quoting WHO 2021 "will no longer suffice as a method, the particular method (chamber, stain) used, has to be added."

## REFERENCES


1. Thonneau P, Marchand S, Tallec A, Ferial ML, Ducot B, Lansac J, et al. Incidence and main causes of infertility in a resident population (1,850,000) of three French regions (1988-1989). Hum Reprod. 1991;6(6):811-6.
2. Hull MG, Eddowes HA, Fahy U, Abuzeid MI, Mills MS, Cahill DJ, et al. Expectations of assisted conception for infertility. BMJ. 1992;304(6840):1465-9.
3. Jarow JP, Sharlip ID, Belker AM, Lipshultz LI, Sigman M, Thomas AJ, et al. Best practice policies for male infertility. J Urol. 167(5):2138-44.
4. Report on the optimal evaluation of the infertile male fertility and sterility (Vol. 82). An AUA Best Practice Policy and ASRM Practice Committee Report. Fertil Steril. 2006;86(5 Suppl 1):S202-9.
5. Jequier AM. Edward Martin (1859-1938). The founding father of modern clinical andrology. Int J Androl. 1991; 14(1):1-10.
6. MacLeod J. Human semen. Fertil Steril. 1956;7(4):368-86.
7. MacLeod J. Seminal cytology in the presence of varicocele. Fertil Steril. 1965;16(6):735-57.
8. Jequier AM, Ukombe EB. Errors inherent in the performance of a routine semen analysis. Br J Urol. 1983;55(4):434-6.
9. Mortimer D, Templeton AA, Lenton EA, Coleman RA. Semen analysis parameters and their interrelationships in suspected infertile men. Arch Androl. 1982;8(3):165-71.
10. Mortimer D, Shu MA, Tan R. Standardization and quality control of sperm concentration and sperm motility counts in semen analysis. Hum Reprod. 1986;1(5):299-303.
11. Björndahl L, Barrett CL, Fraser LR, Kvist U, Mortimer D. ESHRE basic semen analysis courses 1995-1999: immediate beneficial effects of standardized training. Hum Reprod. 2002;17(5):1299-305.
12. Arumugam K. Sperm dysfunction in partners of infertile patients with minimal or mild endometriosis. Clin Exp Obstet Gynaecol. 1993;20(1):43-7.
13. Hammond MG, Jordan S, Sloan CS. Factors affecting pregnancy rates in a donor insemination program using frozen semen. Am J Obstet Gynecol. 1986;155(3):480-5.
14. Kenemans P, Hafez ES. Clinical application of scanning electron microscopy in human reproduction. Scan Electron Microsc. 1984;(Pt 1):215-42.
15. Katz DF, Mills RN, Pritchett TR. The movement of human spermatozoa in cervical mucus. J Reprod Fertil. 1978;53(2): 259-65.
16. Mortimer D, Templeton AA. Sperm transport in the human female reproductive tract in relation to semen analysis characteristics and time of ovulation. J Reprod Fertil. 1982;64(2):401-8.
17. Kruger TF, Acosta AA, Simmons KF, Swanson RJ, Matta JF, Oehninger S. Predictive value of abnormal sperm morphology in *in vitro* fertilization. Fertil Steril. 1988;49(1):112-7.
18. Guzick DS, Overstreet JW, Factor-Litvak P, Brazil CK, Nakajima ST, Coutifaris C, et al. Sperm morphology, motility and concentration in fertile and infertile men. New Eng J Med. 2001;345(19):1388.
19. Lamb DJ. Semen analysis in 21st century medicine: the need for sperm function testing. Asian J Androl. 2010;12(1):64-70.
20. Björndahl L. The usefulness and significance of assessing rapidly progressive spermatozoa. Asian J Androl. 2010;12(1): 33-5.
21. World Health Organization. WHO Laboratory Manual for the Examination and Processing of Human Semen, 5th edition. Geneva: World Health Organization; 2010.
22. Handelsman DJ, CooperTG. Afterword to Semen Analysis in 21st Century Medicine special issue in Asian Journal of Andrology. Asian J Androl. 2010;12(1):118-23.

CHAPTER

# 98 Sperm Function Tests

*Anupama Deenadayal Mettler, Roopini Sathiasai Kumar*

## INTRODUCTION

The process of fertilization involves a series of complex interactions between the ejaculated sperm and the female genital tract. Starting from the exposure of the sperm to the hostile vaginal environment to the obstacle course that the sperms have to endure before they finally reach the oocyte to perform a series of orchestrated chemical reactions to fertilize the oocyte, this is what sperm function tests aim to quantify. With the progress in assisted reproductive technologies (ARTs) over decades, we are now faced with a situation where we endeavor to identify the functional defects in sperm to explain possible causes of fertilization failure, poor fertilization rate, recurrent implantation failure, or repeated miscarriages. The various sperm function tests available today are listed in **Box 1** and the rationale behind these tests is briefly explained in **Figure 1**.

Routine semen analysis parameters (sperm concentration, motility, progressive motility, and sperm morphology) used in daily practice have limited value in discriminating the fertile male from the subfertile male.[1] While, sperm functional tests are regarded as research tools[2] and not part of the routine semen testing. In this chapter, you will find a brief concept of all the tests that can be performed with special attention given to those tests, which can be used in daily practice and have influence on clinical decisions. Data shows that certain sperm function assays are highly predictive of ART results and can help in decision-making, especially for patients with repeated failed intrauterine insemination (IUI).[3] Eventually, sperm function tests will help clinicians to optimize male infertility diagnosis and management.[3]

## FRUCTOSE ESTIMATION

Fructose secreted by the seminal vesicles provides energy dependent marker of seminal vesicle function and its absence from the ejaculate will result in almost complete ranges from 63 to 500 mg/dL (3.5–28 mmol/L) and falls as the sample ages. Fructose level should be determined in men with azoospermia as a value <13 µmol suggests low androgen-specific contribution of vascular fluid.[4] An ejaculate volume <1 mL, a low pH, and very low fructose content are suggestive of partial retrograde ejaculation, androgen deficiency, or obstructive azoospermia due to ejaculatory duct obstruction or congenital bilateral absence of the vas deferens.[5-7]

**BOX 1:** Classification of sperm function tests.

- Fructose estimation
- Morphology and teratozoospermia index (TZI)
- *Tests for reactive oxygen species (ROS)*:
  - Leukocyte detection test
  - Luminol or lucigenin
  - Luminol and horseradish peroxidase
- *Sperm vitality tests*:
  - Hypoosmotic swelling (HOS) test
  - Eosin staining
  - Eosin–nigrosin staining
- *Sperm–mucus interaction tests*:
  - In vivo postcoital test
  - In vitro sperm–mucus interaction
  - In vitro capillary test (Kremer test)
- Antisperm antibody tests
- Mitochondrial activity index test
- *Test for capacitation*:
  - Incubation in albumin-containing culture
  - Using CASA
  - Chlortetracycline staining
- Tests for acrosome reaction
- Hyaluronan binding assay
- *Zona binding assays*:
  - Hemizona assay
  - Competitive intact zona sperm binding test
- Sperm penetration assay
- Nuclear chromatin decondensation test
- *Sperm DNA fragmentation index*:
  - Comet assay
  - Tunnel
  - In situ nick translation
  - Acridine orange test
  - SCSA

(CASA: computer-assisted sperm analysis; SCSA: sperm chromatin structure assay)

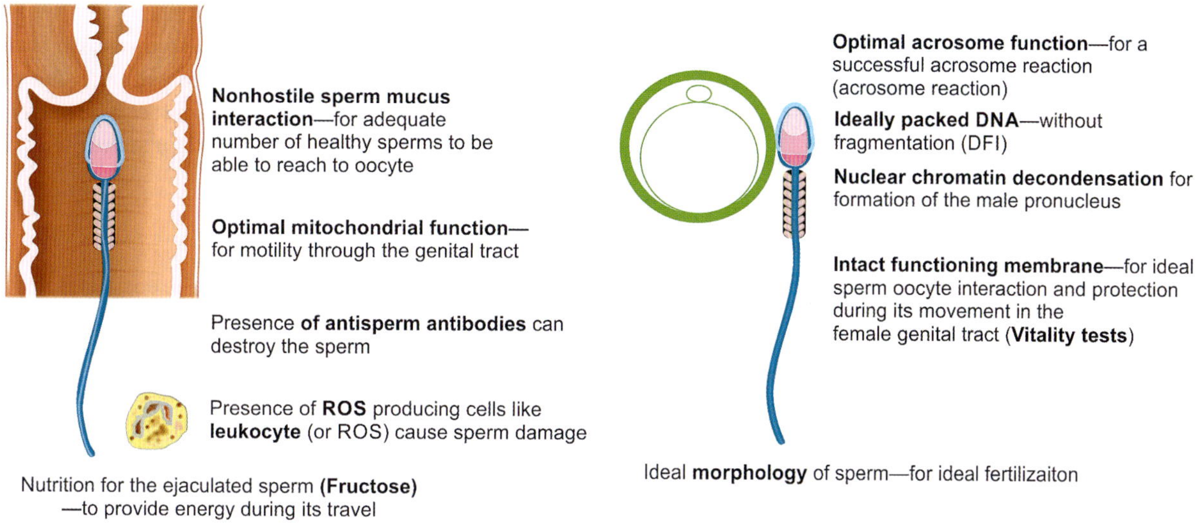


**Fig. 1:** Rationale behind sperm function tests—to test the sperm's various normal mechanisms and their interactions in the female genital tract leading to successful fertilization. (DFI: DNA fragmentation index; ROS: reactive oxygen species)

## INDICES FOR ABNORMAL MORPHOLOGY CALCULATION

Multiple abnormalities may exist in abnormal spermatozoa, and the World Health Organization (WHO) handbook for 2021 offers three indices for this multiple entry system: Teratozoospermia index (TZI), multiple anomalies index (MAI), and sperm deformity index (SDI) (WHO andrology manual, 2021).

A strong correlation was reported between the morphology (strict Kruger criteria) and fertilization rate: Morphology of <4%, 4–14%, and >14% having a fertilization rate of 7.6%, 63.9%, and >70%, respectively. Hence, teratozoospermia is a biomarker of severe gamete dysfunction and altered oocyte interaction.[8]

Teratozoospermia index is calculated by dividing the total number of defects determined by the number of abnormal spermatozoa.[9,10] It is a good predictor of fertilization and pregnancy rate. A TZI <1.6 is normal, whereas, if the TZI is >1.8, irrespective of the count of motility, intracytoplasmic sperm injection (ICSI) is advised.

Multiple anomalies index is based on the mean number of anomalies per abnormal spermatozoan.

Sperm deformity index is the number of defects divided by the total number of spermatozoa. Specific head, midpiece, and tail sperm abnormalities were strongly correlated with particular stages of embryonic development, from the observation of pronuclei to the hatched blastocyst.[11]

## TESTS FOR REACTIVE OXYGEN SPECIES

Spermatozoa require oxygen for metabolism which, in turn, damage cellular lipids, proteins, and DNA[12,13] due to the relatively large quantities of polyunsaturated fatty acids in the sperm membrane and low concentration of scavenging enzymes in the cytoplasm. Reactive oxygen species (ROS) in spermatozoa originate as a result of the monovalent reduction of molecular oxygen during oxidative phosphorylation in the mitochondria.[14-19] Presence of a varicocele, infections, or occupational exposure to toxins such as lead or cadmium causes oxidative stress and, in turn, excessive free radicles in the semen.[20-22] ROS include superoxide anions, hydrogen peroxidase, hydroxyl radicals, nitric oxide, and others. Although seminal plasma contains antioxidant enzymes, oxidative stress develops when there is an imbalance between ROS-generating and scavenging activities.

### Chemiluminescence

Reactive oxygen species concentration in semen is commonly measured by using probes such as luminol and lucigenin or a mixture of luminol and horseradish peroxidase.[23,24] While luminol measures intra- and extracellular ROS by reacting with ROS such as $H_2O_2$ and OH, lucigenin is more specific to superoxide anions released extracellularly. The reaction produces photons which are converted to electrical signals which can be measured by a luminometer.[24] The lucigenin probe is diagnostically more useful as it measures extracellular ROS, which identifies the sperm at risk for peroxidative damage.

Cellular debris and leukocytes, which can generate 100 times greater ROS than spermatozoa, have a major influence on the chemiluminescent signals generated and the results.[25]

### Nitroblue Tetrazolium Test

The test is an inexpensive, easily available test with high sensitivity.[26] It reacts with cellular superoxide ions to form a formazan derivative that can be quantitatively measured by a spectrophotometer.[27,28]

### Flow Cytometry

It uses an expensive flow cytometer and special software.

### Electron Spin Resonance or Electron Paramagnetic Resonance

It detects only selective oxidants and is the most direct and rapid test.[27-30]

### ROS-TAC Score

Total antioxidant capacity (TAC), the total amount of enzymatic and nonenzymatic antioxidants, can reduce excessive ROS concentrations in semen.[8] According to several studies, there is a positive correlation between normal semen parameters and TAC levels. When ROS production exceeds TAC, the balance between the two could shift, leading to oxidative stress (OS). Seminal ROS level and seminal plasma TAC values are used to produce the ROS-TAC score, which serves as a marker of seminal OS. Therefore, ROS-TAC score calculation is advised for predicting male reproductive potential and differentiating between fertile and infertile patients rather than using just ROS or TAC. It was demonstrated that Asthenozoospermic men had a higher ROS levels and high DNA damage compared to the normozoospermic men. ROS-TAC score improved in men with varicocelectomy.[31]

## LEUKOCYTE DETECTION TEST

Leukocytospermia (>1 × $10^6$ $mL^{-1}$ leukocytes) is currently detected by the peroxidase test, although enzyme-linked immunosorbent assay (ELISA), monoclonal antibodies against leukocyte-specific antigens (CD45), flow cytometry, and immunocytochemistry could be used. Another technique is the direct count of round cells in a wet preparation and differentiating them from immature germ cells by special differential staining.

## SPERM VITALITY TESTS

Sperm vitality testing is important when <40% of the spermatozoa are progressively motile to know if the immotile spermatozoa are dead or alive. It should be performed as soon as liquefaction is complete and preferably within 1 hour of ejaculation to prevent bias due to dehydration or temperature variability. Structural flagellar defects (immotile cilia syndrome) result in numerous vital but immotile spermatozoa.[32] Whereas, numerous nonviable immotile spermatozoa may indicate epididymal pathology.[33,34] Vitality is identified by testing the membrane integrity of the spermatozoa for dye exclusion (eosin-nigrosin) or hypotonic swelling as damaged plasma membranes will allow entry of the dye into the cell and only live cells will swell in hypotonic solutions **(Fig. 2)**.

### Eosin Staining

After exposure of the spermatozoa to the eosin stain, the unstained sperm are counted as live, whereas the pink or red spermatozoa are considered dead. It can be used for wet smears and can be theoretically used for sperm selection for ICSI.

### Eosin–nigrosin Staining

The advantage of adding nigrosin to the eosin staining is that it provides a dark background for easy assessment, and the slides could be preserved for future records and assessment.

### Hypoosmotic Swelling Test

After a 30-minute exposure to a hypoosmotic solution, the dead spermatozoa retain a normal tail shape due to a leaky membrane, while the intact spermatozoa show swelling of their tails into various sizes and shapes.[35] After counting 200 sperms, if <50% of them show tail curling, it is considered abnormal. A score between 50% and 58% is intermediate, and above 58% is considered normal. A correlation was seen between the grade of tail curling **(Fig. 3)** and DNA fragmentation with grades D, E, and F spermatozoa having lesser DNA fragmentation than grades A, B, and C. The hypoosmotic swelling (HOS) test can be used in extreme cases for the selection of sperm for ICSI by aspirating the sperm head first into the pipette and then exposing only the tail to the hypoosmotic solution while the head remains in the pipette.

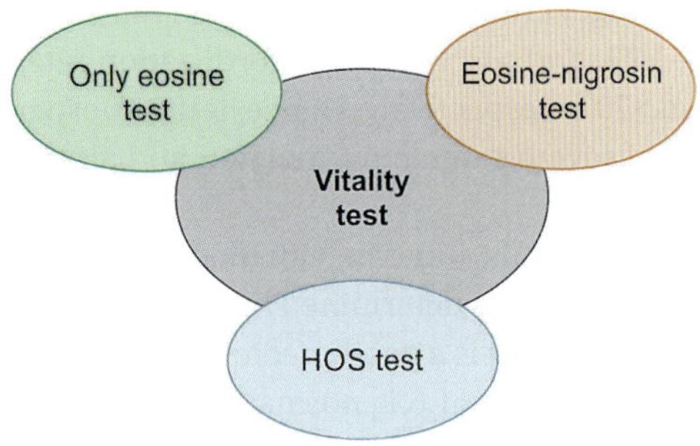


**Fig. 2:** Sperm vitality test.

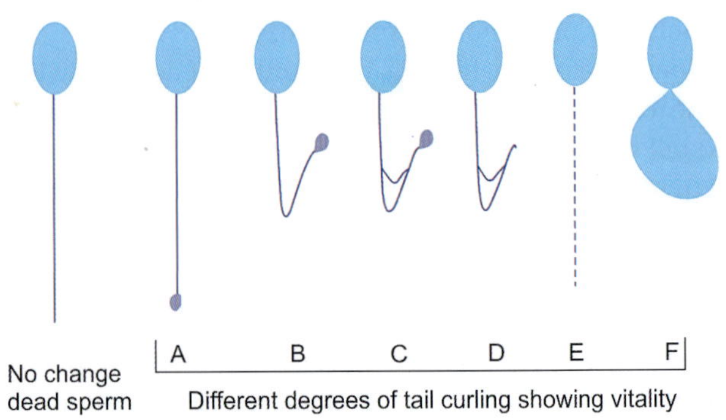


**Fig. 3:** Line diagram of morphological changes in the human sperm tail exposed to hypoosmotic stress.

Once a change in the shape of the tail is noticed, the sperm can be used for ICSI.

### Motility Activators

The majority of the sperm population is motile following ejaculation because the spermatozoa are activated during their passage through the epididymis. The gradual switch from phosphatase to kinase activity, and consequently the gradual phosphorylation of proteins, are related to the induction of motility in the epididymis. This fundamental kind of motility is characterized by low-amplitude symmetrical tail motions that allow spermatozoa to move linearly; but, once entering the uterus, spermatozoa must undergo hyperactivation through capacitation in order to successfully fertilize an egg. The process of sperm capacitation, which entails a number of physiological changes. When signalling pathways that control sperm motility are activated in spermatozoa, calcium ions [Ca2+]i functions as a secondary messenger. The majority of the cyclic adenosine monophosphate (cAMP) produced by spermatozoa is produced by soluble adenyl cyclases (sAC), which are one of them. Serine/threonine protein kinase A (PKA), which is activated by cyclic AMP, sets off a series of protein phosphorylation events that induce sperm motility.[36] Dimethylxanthine theophylline is a phosphodiesterase inhibitor that promotes a rise in intracellular cyclic adenosine monophosphate (AMP) levels, which enhances sperm motility. It works well for sperm motility recovery after thawing, enabling the injection of live sperm, and making laboratory handling easier.[37]

## SPERM–MUCUS INTERACTION TESTS

While the cervical mucus is viscous throughout the menstrual cycle, it is penetrable only during the preovulatory days, where it forms the first barrier for sperm migration. The quality of mucus is important as it tests the strength and effectiveness of sperm motility and the surface characteristics of sperm that allow them to interact appropriately with cervical mucus. However, when the sperm-mucus interaction tests are abnormal, usually the other semen characteristics are also deficient, suggesting the need of IUI, in vitro fertilization (IVF), or ICSI **(Flowchart 1)**.

**Flowchart 1:** Sperm–mucus interaction.

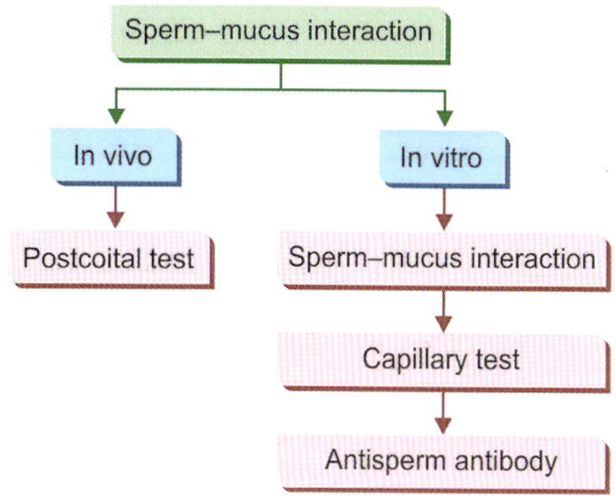


### In vivo (Postcoital) Test

After determining the time of ovulation, the man is asked to have intercourse after 2 days of abstinence. The woman is asked to report to the clinic within 9–14 hours after coitus avoiding vaginal lubricants or vaginal douching. A nonlubricated vaginal speculum is inserted, and a tuberculin syringe is used to aspirate the seminal pool from the posterior fornix. Another syringe is used to aspirate cervical mucus, which is placed on a slide and fixed with a coverslip and silicone grease. The preparation is examined under 400× magnification with phase-contrast optics. Presence of sperm in the first syringe ensures that semen was deposited in the vagina. The presence of progressive spermatozoa in the cervical aspirate is the most important indicator of normal cervical function arguing against sperm autoimmunity in the male or female[38] and evaluating the reservoir role of cervical mucus.[39] Sperm antibodies should be suspected if nonprogressive spermatozoa exhibiting a shaking phenomenon are seen. If no sperm are seen or if the test is abnormal, it is advisable to repeat it. If the man cannot provide a sample for semen analysis, a simple postcoital test can help in assessing the sperm.

### In Vitro Sperm–Mucus Interaction

A detailed sperm–cervical mucus interaction test is performed with crossover testing using donor semen and donor cervical mucus as controls. A normozoospermic sample and good quality, midcycle cervical mucus with a pH between 7 and 8.5 are taken as donor controls. Acidic mucus immobilizes sperm, whereas alkaline mucus increases motility giving a false result. The test should be performed within 1 hour of collection of the patient's semen sample and cervical mucus. After comparing the results of the interactions of the patient specimens with each other and with the donors, a conclusion can be reached regarding the significance of a positive sperm antibody test in the male or female partner.

In the in vitro simplified slide test, a mucus drop is placed in the center of slide and covered with a coverslip with silicone grease. A drop of semen is placed on each side in contact with its edges. After 30 minutes of incubation at 37°C in a humid chamber, the migration of the sperm is studied under 400× magnification with phase contrast optics. When the spermatozoa penetrate into the mucus phase and >90% are motile, it is considered normal. When there is penetration but only for about 10 sperm lengths (500 Pm), it is a poor result suggesting a problem. When there is no penetration or penetration with rapid immobilization, it suggests the presence of antisperm antibodies (AsAb) **(Flowchart 2)**.

**Flowchart 2:** In vitro simplified slide test.

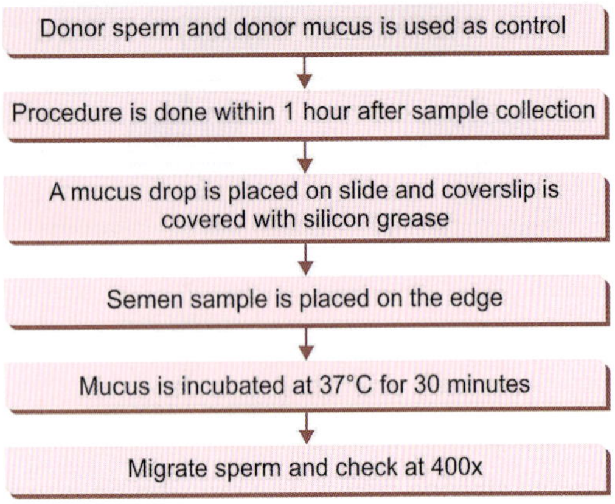


### In vitro Capillary Test (Kremer Test)

Various modifications were proposed for the original capillary tube test designed by Kremer in 1965. A flat capillary tube, 5 cm long with a 0.3 mm internal diameter, is recommended. Cervical mucus is aspirated into the tube, after which it is sealed at one end. The open end is placed in a reservoir containing the semen sample and incubated for 2 hours at 37°C in a humid chamber. It is then examined at 100× magnification with phase contrast optics. The migration distance, penetration density, migration reduction, and presence of spermatozoa with forward motility are assessed. The results are interpreted using an interpretation table. The hyaluronate migration test can be used instead without the need for relatively large quantities of midcycle cervical mucus.[40]

### Antisperm Antibody Tests

While 3–12% of infertile men have AsAb, their clinical significance and treatment are controversial since some fertile men can have high levels of AsAb. AsAb interfere with fertility by causing excessive sperm agglutination, having abnormal cervical mucus penetration, and interfering with sperm–oocyte interaction. AsAb may be generated from the breakdown of the blood–testis barrier, inoculation of the host with sperm antigens, failure of immunosuppression, or acute and chronic prostatitis.[41] Head-bound AsAb is found especially in men after a vasovasostomy,[42] while immunoglobulin M (IgM) antibodies suggest cancer or recent trauma to the male reproductive tract. Immunoglobulin G (IgG) AsAb can be present in the serum or secreted in the cervical mucus of females due to repeated exposure to sperms. The evaluation is preferably performed by immunobead (IB) **(Flowchart 3)**.

Immunoglobulin A (IgA) and IgG are the two main immunoglobulins found in the semen. IgM found in large numbers is correlated with cancer and acute infection. Antisperm antibody test can be done by direct and indirect tests.

**Flowchart 3:** Antisperm antibody tests.

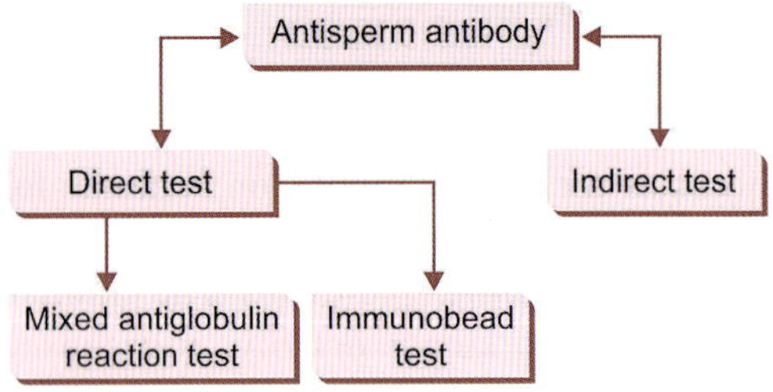


Direct test can be further divided into two types: Mixed antiglobulin reaction (MAR) test, it mainly includes unwashed spermatozoa in semen with antibody-coated beads. It is an easy, quick, and sensitive test. Direct IB includes the washed semen, which binds beads coated with covalently bound antihuman immunoglobulins. This is time-consuming, and reagents need to be prepared in the laboratory.

Indirect test includes checking of seminal plasma, cervical mucus, or blood serum. Sperm fluids should be heat inactivated before the procedure, and donor sperm is selected, which is completely washed free from seminal fluids. During the procedure, sperm-free fluids are incubated with the donor sperm which has been washed. AsAb is found binding to the donor sperm and is further assessed using direct IB test. Testing patient's sperm by *direct assay* or by *indirect assay* using male or female serum or seminal plasma can be performed by MAR (Coombs) or ELISA estimation of antibodies can also be performed.

## MITOCHONDRIAL ACTIVITY INDEX TEST

The long passage of the spermatozoa through the female tract requires energy for flagellar activity, which is supplied in the form of adenosine triphosphate (ATP) by the mitochondria in the midpiece of the spermatozoa. The evaluation of the function of the mitochondrial oxidoreductive enzyme apparatus can be done using indicators such as nitro blue tetrazolium, where the good sperms get stained while the poor or nonmotile sperms are stained poorly.

## TEST FOR CAPACITATION

The molecular and physiological events that occur in the female genital tract resulting in more fluid and pliable membranes that enable sperm to fertilize are known as capacitation.[43-46] The most significant changes experienced by sperm are loss of extrinsic proteins along with loss of membrane cholesterol leading to plasma membrane changes, an increase in certain intracellular messengers, and increased phosphorylation of a set of proteins by different kinases.[43-48] Hyperactivated sperm motility and a rapid spiraling movement that can be identified by computer-assisted sperm analysis (CASA) are commonly associated with sperm capacitation. Sperm capacitation can be assessed by stimulating an acrosome reaction in vitro.[46] It can also be tested by incubating sperm in an albumin-containing culture.

### Using Computer-assisted Sperm Analysis

With regard to sperm function tests, within 30 seconds, CASA performs an automated analysis of sperm concentration, motility, and morphology followed by a manual assessment of white blood cell (WBC) and immature germ cells. Around 200 moving objects (sperm) can be simultaneously tracked for several seconds. Hyperactivated sperm can be distinguished from nonhyperactivated by the high curvilinear velocity, low linearity, and large value of the amplitude of lateral head displacement of the former. CASAnova, a web-based program, was designed to compute and classify sperms based on their kinematic parameters. Vigorous sperm were classified as progressive, intermediate, or hyperactivated, and nonvigorous sperm as slow or weakly motile. The capacitated sperm showed vigorous patterns, including hyperactivated motility, while there was a loss of intermediate and hyperactivated motility patterns when sperm were exposed to noncapacitating medium.[49] Hence, proving that CASA can be used to confirm capacitation and, in the future, as an advanced sperm selection method.

### Chlortetracycline Staining

Using fluorescence microscopy and antibiotic chlortetracycline, the actual capacitation process can be visualized as distinct fluorescence patterns depending on the capacitation and the acrosomal status of the sperm.[50]

## TESTS FOR ACROSOME REACTION

In order to pass through the zona pellucida (ZP), the acrosomal reaction takes place where the binding of the sperm to ZP triggers fusion of the outer acrosomal membrane and the plasma membrane to discharge hydrolyzing enzymes.[51] The acrosomal status can be assessed by microscopy, flow cytometry, or fluorescently labeled lectins such as *Pisum sativum* agglutinin[52,53] after induction of the acrosome reaction either by exposing the spermatozoa to human ZP or ZP proteins.

### Triple-stain Technique

This is for evaluating normal acrosome reactions of human sperm and uses trypan blue to differentiate live from dead sperm in the sperm suspension after swim-up processing. Bismarck brown and Rose Bengal staining of the postacrosomal region and the acrosome is then done.[54] The slides are examined at 1,000× with bright-field microscopy to assess the percentage of live sperm that had undergone a normal acrosome reaction.

### Gelatin Assay Test

In this test, sperm are placed on a gelatin precoated glass slide where after being exposed to the proteolytic enzymes from the acrosome, a halo is formed around the sperm head. Acrosomal activity is calculated by counting the sperm with a positive and negative halo.

Additionally, the acrosome reaction of the motile sperm population exposed to a solubilized solution of a single human oocyte zona is calculated using a fluorescent stain. A 15% cutoff value was suggested as the difference between the zona-induced acrosome reaction (ZIAR) (stimulated) and the spontaneous (unstimulated) acrosome reaction.[23,25]

Reports show that 25% of normozoospermic subfertile men have a defective ZP-induced acrosomal reaction.[19] There appears to be a strong correlation between the percentage of acrosome-reacted sperm and sperm morphology: 13.4%, 16.1%, and 22.8% for sperm morphology groups <4%, 5–14%, and >14%.[55] Induced acrosome reaction tests have a high positive predictive value (PPV) and sensitivity, and can be used for prediction of fertilization[56] and referring a patient for ICSI early in their treatment.

## HYALURONAN BINDING ASSAY

Hyaluronan is a major component of the cumulus complex surrounding the oocyte. The hyaluronan binding assay (HBA) is a convenient and reproducible test to identify the percentage of sperm that bind to hyaluronan through specific receptors indicating the successful completion of spermiogenic events mediated by the heat shock protein A2 (HSPA2) chaperone protein.[57-59]

The test is performed by placing 7–10 μL of the liquefied semen sample within 3 hours of collection in the center of the hyaluronan-coated assay chamber of an HBA slide. Count the number of bound motile and unbound motile sperm in the same number of grid squares after 10–20 minutes of applying the coverslip. For good assay precession, at least 100 sperm or 100 grid squares need to be counted. For acceptable results, at least 30 total motile sperm need to be counted. The more sperm counted, the lower the variance. Percent-bound sperm is calculated by dividing the bound sperm with the total (bound and unbound) motile sperm multiplied by 100. A score of ≥80% is interpreted as normal maturity with normal physiological function.

When the hemoglobin (HB) is abnormal, the patient can be counseled for ICSI rather than an IVF[60] as the HBA scores have a significant association with fertilization rates and biochemical pregnancies.[61] A physiological intracytoplasmic sperm injection (PICSI) sperm selection device has three hyaluronan microdots that select sperm similar to natural fertilization based on their ability to bind to hyaluronan hydrogel. To use the PICSI dish, a 10 μL drop of media is placed on each microdot followed by flooding of the dish with mineral oil on a surface at room temperature. Some embryologists prefer placing a polyvinylpyrrolidone (PVP) drop in the same dish for convenience. Approximately 1,000–2,000 total sperm is added to the drop. The sperm begin to bind within 5 minutes. If binding is not seen, wait for 30 minutes or more for the microdot to hydrate to reach full binding capacity. Bound sperm should be selected from the interior of the microdot, especially those sperm with a helicopter rotor movement. The tip of the ICSI micropipette is lowered down next to the head of the sperm, and the sperm is gently sucked into the pipette. Continue collecting until 20–50 sperm and then expel the captured sperm into a PVP drop to process them for ICSI.

While some studies show an improvement in clinical pregnancy rate and a fall in miscarriage rate, others are not so promising. Worrilow et al. showed that 15% of all ICSI patients had an HBA score of ≤65%, and when a PICSI was used in these patients, there was a significant increase in pregnancy rate and a fall in the miscarriage rate.[62]

## COMPETITIVE BINDING ASSAY

Hemizona assay (HZA) and competitive intact zona sperm binding test are used to assess the binding of the sperm to the ZP, in turn conforming completion of capacitation and ability to undergo acrosome reaction **(Flowchart 4)**.[63-67]

As HZA has a high predictive value for the outcome of fertilization in vitro[65,68,69] and IUI in male factor infertility, it is indicated in cases with repeated poor or no fertilization. The matching halves of human ZP (hand-sectioned hemizona or oocytes bisected by a manipulator) are exposed to populations of proven fertile and patient spermatozoa, respectively. The hemizona index (HZI) is calculated by dividing the number of bound sperm in the patient divided by the number bound in control multiplied by 100.[70,71] An HZI <30 had significantly lower pregnancy rates than an HZI >30 in patients undergoing IUI.[72] While an HZI <35% was predictive of IVF outcome.[73,74]

With a high sensitivity and negative predictive value (NPV) with low false negative rates, HZA is a useful tool in investigating and counseling couples in allocating them to different treatments (IUI vs. IVF vs. ICSI).[75-78]

**Flowchart 4:** Competitive binding assay.

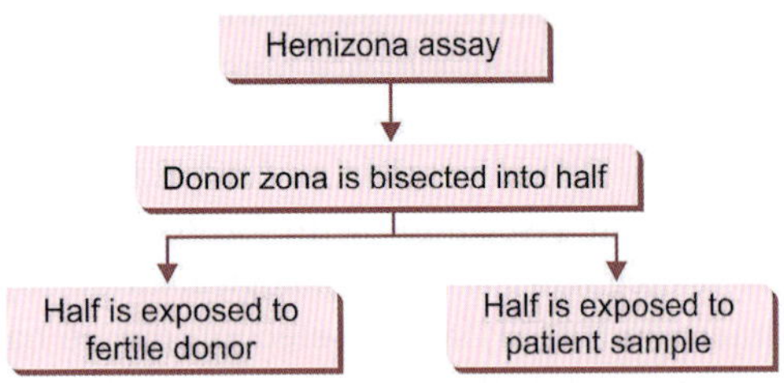


$$\text{Calculation} = \frac{\text{Number of bound sperm from patient sample}}{\text{Number of bound sperm from fertile donor}} \times 100$$

## SPERM PENETRATION ASSAY

Used widely in the pre-ICSI days, sperm penetration assay (SPA) measures sperm capacitation, spontaneous acrosome reaction (due to absence of ZP), fusion and penetration through the oolemma, and decondensation within the cytoplasm of hamster oocytes.[79] Hamster cumulus-oocyte complexes are denuded to remove the cumulus and zona by hyaluronidase and trypsin, respectively. The denuded oocytes are then incubated for around 3 hours with 1 million motile human spermatozoa. The sperm plasma membrane overlying the equatorial region initiates fusion with the hamster oocyte. The percentages for hamster oocytes penetrated are documented. Ionophore A23187 can be used as it causes an influx of calcium and cytoplasmic alkalinization to artificially induce the acrosome reaction.[26]

In spite of confounding limitations, information on the fusogenic nature of the capacitated sperm can be deducted. While the assay has poor standardization methods and reproducibility, it has good sensitivity with high false positive rates, i.e., spermatozoa of men who failed the SPA successfully fertilized human oocytes in vitro.[80] As SPA is time-consuming and relatively expensive, it should not be used till its validity and reproducibility have been established.[3]

## NUCLEAR CHROMATIN DECONDENSATION TEST

The highly condensed chromatin in spermatozoa due to the S-S cross-links between its histone units undergoes decondensation prior to formation of the male pronucleus. Hence, decondensation is a predictor of the fertilizing ability of the spermatozoa. This can be induced in vitro by sodium dodecyl sulfate (SDS) and ethylenediaminetetraacetic acid (EDTA). Fertilization was found to be normal when the decondensation percent of the sperm nuclear chromatin was beyond 70%. The combined test scores of sperm penetration assay and sperm chromatin decondensation significantly predicted failed ICSI outcomes.

## SPERM DNA FRAGMENTATION INDEX

In today's day and age, the sperm DNA fragmentation index is one of the sperm function tests that play an important role in clinical decisions in treatment of a patient undergoing ART. It will be dealt with in detail in another chapter.

## BIOCHEMICAL ASSAY

### Zinc

Concentration of Zn is high in seminal vesicle, it mainly helps in lipid flexibility and acrosome reaction during capacitation, which is essential during zona binding in vivo. During the assessment, the Zn binds with

2-(5-bromo-2-pyridylazo)-5-(N-propyl-N-sulfopropyl-amino)-phenol (5-Br-PAPS) to give a color change and absorbs maximum of 552 wavelengths in flow cytometry **(Table 1 and Box 2)**.

$$5\text{-Br-PAPS} + Zn^{2+} \rightarrow 5\text{-Br-PAPS-Zn complex}$$

## Neutral Alpha-glucosidase

It is mainly found in two forms: Neutral α-glucosidase and acidic α-glucosidase. Major forms are produced from epididymis as neutral α-glucosidase, and minor forms are produced in the prostate as acidic α-glucosidase. Low range of α-glucosidase is related to poor function of epididymis, which may lead to defective sperm maturation.

Function of acidic α-glucosidase can be inhibited by using SDS during the measurement of neutral α-glucosidase. The principle behind is α-glucosidase with the addition of glucosidase converts the synthetic glucopyranoside

**TABLE 1:** Biochemical assay for accessory sex gland.

| | |
|---|---|
| Prostate gland | Zinc, citric acid, or acid phosphatase |
| Seminal vesicle | Fructose |
| Epididymis | L-carnitine, GPC, and neutral α-glucosidase |

(GPC: glycerophosphocholine)

**BOX 2:** Biochemical assay for detection of Zinc in seminal plasma.

- Centrifuge the sample for 10-15 minutes at 3,000 g; store the sperm-free plasma at –20°C until procedure
- Thaw the sample during the procedure along with the internal quality control
- Mix the seminal plasma in a vortex mixture
- Dilution 1: Dilute the seminal plasma at 1:40 dilution using purified $H_2O$
- Dilution 2: Dilute the sample once again at 1:4 dilution
- Add 40 µL of dilution 2 sample to 96-well + 40 µL as blank purified $H_2O$ + 40 µL internal quality control
- Add 200 µL of color reagent to each well and mix for 5 minutes
- Read the plate at 550 nm wavelength

**TABLE 2:** Overview of the sperm function test performed and the reason for the test.

| ***Physiological process*** | ***Test*** | ***Reason to perform the test*** |
|---|---|---|
| Energy supply for the sperm in the ejaculate | Fructose estimation | Absence of fructose causes immotility of sperm |
| Optimal sperm shape for swift movement of the sperm through the female genital tract | Morphology and teratozoospermia index | Morphology is significantly associated with fertilization rate |
| Minimal quantities of reactive oxygen species (ROS) are required for normal sperm function | Tests for ROS | Excessive ROS produced by sperm or leukocytes causes damage to the sperm membrane, proteins, and DNA |
| A functional cell membrane of a live sperm plays an important role in fertilization | Sperm vitality tests | Helps distinguish between dead and live sperms to diagnose different syndromes |
| Cervical mucus acts as a reservoir of sperm | Sperm–mucus interaction tests | Any abnormality in this interaction leads to a block to the sperm entering the uterus to finally reach the oocyte |
| Antisperm antibodies hinder the motility and travel of the sperm in the reproductive tract | Antisperm antibody tests | Detection of the presence of antibodies helps in deciding the treatment options for the patient |
| Energy (ATP) produced by the mitochondria is necessary for the motility of the sperm | Mitochondrial activity index test | Decrease in mitochondrial activity hinders sperm motility |
| Capacitation prepares the sperm for fertilization | Test for capacitation | A problem identified in capacitation can explain fertilization failure |
| Initiates the process of cumulus cell dispersion | Hyaluronan binding assay | It identifies the percentage of mature sperm with DNA integrity and patients at risk of failed fertilization in IVF |
| Acrosome reaction initiates fertilization with fusion of the plasma membranes | Tests for acrosome reaction | A poor acrosome reaction can explain poor fertilization in a normozoospermic male |
| Binding of the sperm to the zona | Zona binding assays | Predictive of IUI and IVF outcome |
| Entry of sperm nucleus in the oocyte | Sperm penetration assay | Information on the fusogenic nature of the capacitated sperm can be deducted |
| Prior to formation of the male pronucleus | Nuclear chromatin decondensation test | Abnormal tests predicted failed ICSI |
| Intact sperm DNA for successful fertilization and development of a healthy embryo | Sperm DNA fragmentation index | Abnormal tests predicted decreased pregnancy rates and increased miscarriage rates with ART |

(ART: assisted reproductive technology; ATP: adenosine triphosphate; ICSI: intracytoplasmic sperm injection; IUI: intrauterine insemination; IVF: in vitro fertilization) substrate to p-nitrophenol, which turns yellow (wavelength 405 nm) in addition to sodium carbonate.

## SPERM SELECTION USING ARTIFICIAL INTELLIGENCE

Computer-assisted sperm analysis brought a level of automation and standardization to the field, wide persists in how sperm cells are assessed. New methods are needed to standardize, automate, and accelerate the sperm classification process. Artificial intelligence is gaining interest in the field of reproductive medicine. It involves image and object processing. The machine learning model will train with the images fed into the system and generate accurate results. There are AI-based smartphone apps that enable home testing of semen parameters (web- and artificial intelligence-based image recognition for sperm motility analysis: verification study). Recently developed computer software SiD uses artificial vision-based software that computes the progressive motility parameters, straight-line velocity (VSL), and linearity of the curvilinear path (LIN) of each sperm trajectory, along with a quantitative value and head movement pattern (HMP), which is an indicator of the characteristics of the sperm HMPs.[84]

## CONCLUSION

The diagnostic evaluation of the male partner, particularly in the event of unexplained infertility, has found the value of sperm function testing. Understanding the effects of infertility and improving prognosis can be achieved by performing testing for additional seminal parameters in addition to the usual semen analysis.

## KEY POINTS

- Many independent studies have demonstrated that a routine semen analysis lacks in providing information about the functional competence of the spermatozoa. While fructose is routinely performed for azoospermic samples, vitality tests are advised for samples with a decreased percentage of progressively motile sperm.
- The use of CASA, HBA, measurement of ROS, and DNA fragmentation have been shown to be useful in patients with fertilization failure, poor fertilization rate, recurrent implantation failure, or repeated miscarriages.
- Although, a number of sperm function tests **(Table 2)** have been invented to fill this gap, due to absence of high-quality clinical data, no standardization of methodologies, cumbersome nature of some of the assays, and the need for human material, they cannot be advised for routine use.[81,83]
- On the contrary, sperm function tests can potentially assist in important clinical decisions decreasing the time to pregnancy, expenses borne, and eliminating the physical and psychological burden the couple has to experience.
- Today, we have a strong foundation on which future research can be based[78] to develop valid and more predictive tests based on multicentric trials with strong predictive value for pregnancy outcome and have little overlap between fertile and infertile samples.

## REFERENCES

1. Weber RFA, Dohle GR, Romijn, JC. Clinical laboratory evaluation of male subfertility. Adv Clin Chem. 2005;40:317-64.
2. Aitken J, Auger J, Gordon Baker HW, Barratt CLR, Behre HM, Björndahl L, et al. Sperm preparation techniques. In: WHO Laboratory Manual for the Examination and Processing of Human Semen, 5th edition. 2010.
3. Oehninger S, Franken DR, Ombelet W. Sperm functional tests. Fertil Steril. 2014;102(6):1528-33.
4. Sikka SC, Hellstrom WJ. Current updates on laboratory techniques for the diagnosis of male reproductive failure. Asian J Androl. 2016;18(3):392-401.
5. de la Taille A, Rigot JM, Mahe P, Gervais R, Dumur V, Lemaitre L, et al. Correlation of genitourinary abnormalities, spermiogram and CFTR genotype in patients with bilateral agenesis of the vas deferens. Prog Urol. 1998;8(3):370-6.
6. Daudin M, Bieth E, Bujan L, Massat G, Pontonnier F, Mieusset R. Congenital bilateral absence of the vas deferens: clinical characteristics, biological parameters, cystic fibrosis transmembrane conductance regulator gene mutations, and implications for genetic counseling. Fertil Steril. 2000; 74(6):1164-74.
7. von Eckardstein S, Cooper TG, Rutscha K, Meschede D, Horst J, Nieschlag E. Seminal plasma characteristics as indicators of cystic fibrosis transmembrane conductance regulator (CFTR) gene mutations in men with obstructive azoospermia. Fertil Steril. 2000;73(6):1226-31.
8. Kruger TF, Acosta AA, Simmons KF, Swanson RJ, Matta JF, Oehninger S. Predictive value of abnormal sperm morphology in in vitro fertilization. Fertil Steril. 1988;49(1):112-7.
9. Menkveld R, Kruger TF. Evaluation of sperm morphology by light microscopy. In: Acosta AA, Kruger TF (Eds). Human Spermatozoa in Assisted Reproduction, 2nd edition. London: Parthenon Publishing; 1996. pp. 89-107.
10. Menkveld R, Wong WY, Lombard CJ, Wetzels AM, Thomas CM, Merkus HM, et al. Semen parameters, including WHO and strict criteria morphology, in a fertile and subfertile population: an effort towards standardization of in-vivo thresholds. Hum Reprod. 2001;16(6):1165-71.
11. Nikolova S, Parvanov D, Georgieva V, Ivanova I, Ganeva R, Stamenov G. Impact of sperm characteristics on time-lapse embryo morphokinetic parameters and clinical outcome of conventional in vitro fertilization. Andrology. 2020;8: 1107-16.
12. Aitken RJ, Baker MA, Sawyer D. Oxidative stress in the male germ line and its role in the aetiology of male infertility and genetic disease. Reprod Biomed Online. 2003;7(1):65-70.
13. Henkel R, Hajimohammad M, Stalf T, Hoogendijk C, Mehnert C, Menkveld R, et al. Influence of deoxyribonucleic acid damage on fertilization and pregnancy. Fertil Steril. 2004;81(4):965-72.

14. Holland MK, Alvarez JG, Storey BT. Production of superoxide and activity of superoxide dismutase in rabbit epididymal spermatozoa. Biol Reprod. 1982;27(5):1109-18.
15. Fraga CG, Motchnik PA, Shigenaga MK, Helbock HJ, Jacob RA, Ames BN. Ascorbic acid protects against endogenous oxidative DNA damage in human sperm. Proc Natl Acad Sci U S A. 1991;88(24):11003-6.
16. Sikka SC, Rajasekaran M, Hellstrom WJ. Role of oxidative stress and antioxidants in male infertility. J Androl. 1995;16(6):464-8.
17. Alvarez JG, Storey BT. Differential incorporation of fatty acids into and peroxidative loss of fatty acids from phospholipids of human spermatozoa. Mol Reprod Dev. 1995;42(3):334-46.
18. Aitken RJ, Baker HW. Seminal leukocytes: passengers, terrorists or good samaritans? Hum Reprod. 1995;10:1736-9.
19. Aitken RJ, West K, Buckingham D. Leukocytic infiltration into the human ejaculate and its association with semen quality, oxidative stress, and sperm function. J Androl. 1994;15(4):343-52.
20. Aitken RJ. A free radical theory of male infertility. Reprod Fertil Dev. 1994;6(1):19-23.
21. Agarwal A, Ikemoto I, Loughlin KR. Relationship of sperm parameters with levels of reactive oxygen species in semen specimens. J Urol. 1994;152(1):107-10.
22. Aitken RJ, Clarkson JS, Fishel S. Generation of reactive oxygen species, lipid peroxidation, and human sperm function. Biol Reprod. 1989;41(1):183-97.
23. Sharma RK, Agarwal A. Role of reactive oxygen species in male infertility. Urology. 1996;48(6):835-50.
24. Kobayashi H, Gil-Guzman E, Mahran AM, Rakesh, Nelson DR, Thomas Jr AJ, et al. Quality control of reactive oxygen species measurement by luminol-dependent chemiluminescence assay. J Androl. 2001;22(4):568-74.
25. Aitken RJ, Baker MA, O'Bryan M. Shedding light on chemiluminescence: the application of chemiluminescence in diagnostic andrology. J Androl. 2004;25(4):455-65.
26. Aitken RJ, Buckingham DW, Fang HG. Analysis of the responses of human spermatozoa to A23187 employing a novel technique for assessing the acrosome reaction. J Androl. 1993;14:132-41.
27. Armstrong JS, Bivalacqua TJ, Chamulitrat W, Sikka S, Hellstrom WJ. A comparison of the NADPH oxidase in human sperm and white blood cells. Int J Androl. 2002;25(4):223-9.
28. Baehner RL, Boxer LA, Davis J. The biochemical basis of nitroblue tetrazolium reduction in normal human and chronic granulomatous disease polymorphonuclear leukocytes. Blood. 1976;48(2):309-13.
29. Jones R, Mann T, Sherins R. Peroxidative breakdown of phospholipids in human spermatozoa, spermicidal properties of fatty acid peroxides, and protective action of seminal plasma. Fertil Steril. 1979;31:531-7.
30. de Lamirande E, Gagnon C. Impact of reactive oxygen species on spermatozoa: a balancing act between beneficial and detrimental effects. Hum Reprod. 1995;10(Suppl. 1):15-21.
31. Vatannejad A, Tavilani H, Sadeghi MR, Amanpour S, Shapourizadeh S, Doosti M. Evaluation of ROS-TAC Score and DNA Damage in Fertile Normozoospermic and Infertile Asthenozoospermic Males. Urol J. 2017;14(1):2973-8.
32. Chemes EH, Rawe YV. Sperm pathology: a step beyond descriptive morphology. Origin, characterization and fertility potential of abnormal sperm phenotypes in infertile men. Hum Reprod Update. 2003;9(5):405-28.
33. Wilton LJ, Temple-Smith PD, Baker HW, de Kretser DM. Human male infertility caused by degeneration and death of sperm in the epididymis. Fertil Steril. 1988;49(6):1052-8.
34. Correa-Pérez JR, Fernández-Pelegrina R, Aslanis P, Zavos PM. Clinical management of men producing ejaculates characterized by high levels of dead sperm and altered seminal plasma factors consistent with epididymal necrospermia. Fertil Steril. 2004;81(4):1148-50.
35. Jeyendran RS, Van der Ven HH, Perez-Pelaez M, Crabo BG, Zaneveld LJ. Development of an assay to assess the functional integrity of the human sperm membrane and its relationship to other semen characteristics. J Reprod Fertil. 1984;70(1):219-28.
36. Nowicka-Bauer K, Szymczak-Cendlak M. Structure and function of ion channels regulating sperm motility—an overview. Int J Mol Sci. 2021;22(6):3259.
37. Calza N, Ciotti PM, Tranquillo ML, Notarangelo L, Zuffa S, Damiano G, et al. P–098 use of dimethylxanthine theophylline in surgical retrieved sperms that do not recover motility after thawing. Hum Reprod. 2021;36:deab130.097.
38. Oei SG, Helmerhorst FM, Keirse MJ. When is the post-coital test normal? A critical appraisal. Hum Reprod. 1995;10(7):1711-4.
39. Moghissi KS. Postcoital test: physiologic basis, technique, and interpretation. Fertil Steril. 1976;27:117-29.
40. Mortimer D, Mortimer ST, Shu MA, Swart R. A simplified approach to sperm-cervical mucus interaction testing using a hyaluronate migration test. Hum Reprod. 1990;5(7):835-41.
41. Turek PJ. Immunopathology and infertility. Infertility in the Male. Philadelphia: Mosby Year Book; 1997.
42. Sikka SC, Hellstrom WJG. Tests for antisperm antibodies. In: Lipshultz LI, Howards SS, Niederberger CS (Eds). Infertility in the Male, 4th edition. Cambridge: Cambridge University Press; 2009.
43. Visconti PE, Kopf GS. Regulation of protein phosphorylation during sperm capacitation. Biol Reprod. 1998;59(1):1-6.
44. Zaneveld LJ, De Jonge CJ, Anderson RA, Mack SR. Human sperm capacitation and the acrosome reaction. Hum Reprod. 1991;6:1265-74.
45. Zaneveld LJ, Anderson RA, Mack SR, De Jonge CJ. Mechanism and control of the human sperm acrosome reaction. Hum Reprod. 1993;8(12):2006-8.
46. De Jonge CJ, Barratt CL, Radwanska E, Cooke ID. The acrosome reaction-inducing effect of human follicular and oviductal fluid. J Androl. 1993;14(5):359-65.
47. Storey BT. Interactions between gametes leading to fertilization: the sperm's eye view. Reprod Fertil Dev. 1995;7(4):927-42.
48. Baldi E, Luconi M, Bonaccorsi L, Krausz C, Forti G. Human sperm activation during capacitation and acrosome reaction: role of calcium, protein phosphorylation and lipid remodelling pathways. Front Biosci. 1996;1:d189-205.
49. Goodson SG, White S, Stevans AM, Bhat S, Kao CY, Jaworski S, et al. Casanova: a multiclass support vector machine model for the classification of human sperm motility patterns. Biol Reprod. 2017;97(5):698-708.
50. Saling PM, Storey BT. Mouse gamete interactions during fertilization in vitro. Chlortetracycline as a fluorescent

probe for the mouse sperm acrosome reaction. J Cell Biol. 1979;83(3):544-55.
51. Yanagimachi R. Mammalian fertilization. In: Knobil E, Neill JD (Eds). The Physiology of Reproduction, 2nd edition. New York: Raven Press; 1994. pp. 189-317.
52. Cross NL, Meizel S. Methods for evaluating the acrosomal status of mammalian sperm. Biol Reprod. 1989;41(4):635-41.
53. De Jonge CJ, Barratt CL. Methods for the assessment of sperm capacitation and acrosome reaction excluding the sperm penetration assay. Methods Mol Biol. 2013;927:113-8.
54. Talbot P, Chacon RS. A triple-stain technique for evaluating normal acrosome reactions of human sperm. J Exp Zool. 1981;215(2):201-8
55. Freund M. Standards for the rating of human sperm morphology. A cooperative study. Int J Fertil. 1966; 11(1):97-180.
56. Macleod J. A possible factor in the etiology of human male infertility: preliminary report. Fertil Steril. 1962;13:29-33.
57. Allen JW, Dix DJ, Collins BW, Merrick BA, He C, Selkirk JK. Hsp70-2 is part of the synaptonemal complex in mouse and hamster spermatocytes. Chromosoma. 1996;104(6):414-21.
58. Dix DJ, Allen JW, Collins BW, Mori C, Nakamura N, Poorman-Allen P, et al. Targeted gene disruption of Hsp70-2 results in failed meiosis, germ cell apoptosis, and male infertility. Proc Natl Acad Sci U S A. 1996;93(8):3264-8.
59. Huszar G, Stone K, Dix D, Vigue L. Putative creatine kinase M-isoform in human sperm is identified as the 70-kilodalton heat shock protein HspA2. Biol Reprod. 2000;63(3):925-32.
60. Huszar G, Ozenci CC, Cayli S. Hyaluronic acid binding by human sperm indicates cellular maturity, viability, and unreacted acrosomal status. Fertil Steril. 2003;79(Suppl. 3): 1616-24.
61. Worrilow KC, Eid S, Matthews JM, Pelts EJ, Khoury C, Liebermann J. A multi-site clinical trial evaluating PICSI® versus intracytoplasmic sperm injection (ICSI): positive clinical outcomes observed in a prospective, randomized and double-blinded study. Fertil Steril. 2009;92:S36-7.
62. Worrilow KC, Eid S, Woodhouse D, Perloe M, Smith S, Witmyer J, et al. Use of hyaluronan in the selection of sperm for intracytoplasmic sperm injection (ICSI): significant improvement in clinical outcomes—multicenter, double-blinded and randomized controlled trial. Hum Reprod. 2013;28(2):306-14.
63. Oehninger S, Toner J, Muasher SJ, Coddington C, Acosta AA, Hodgen GD. Prediction of fertilization in vitro with human gametes: is there a litmus test? Am J Obstet Gynecol. 1992;167(6):1760-7.
64. Oehninger S, Franken D, Alexander N, Hodgen GD. Hemizona assay and its impact on the identification and treatment of human sperm dysfunctions. Andrologia. 1992;24(6):307-21.
65. Oehninger S. Clinical and laboratory management of male infertility: an opinion on its current status. J Androl. 2000;21(6):814-21.
66. Oehninger S. Molecular basis of human sperm-zona pellucida interaction. Cells Tissues Organs. 2001;168(1-2):58-64.
67. Liu DY, Baker HW. Tests of human sperm function and fertilization in vitro. Fertil Steril. 1992;58(3):465-83.
68. ESHRE Andrology Special Interest Group. Consensus workshop on advanced diagnostic andrology techniques. Hum Reprod. 1996;11(7):1463-79.
69. Liu DY, Garrett C, Baker HW. Clinical application of sperm-oocyte interaction tests in in vitro fertilization—embryo transfer and intracytoplasmic sperm injection programs. Fertil Steril. 2004;82(5):1251-63.
70. Burkman LJ, Coddington CC, Franken DR, Krugen TF, Rosenwaks Z, Hogen GD. The hemizona assay (HZA): development of a diagnostic test for the binding of human spermatozoa to the human hemizona pellucida to predict fertilization potential. Fertil Steril. 1988;49(4):688-97.
71. Oehninger S, Morshedi M, Franken D. The hemizona assay for assessment of sperm function. Methods Mol Biol. 2013;927:91-102.
72. Arslan M, Morshedi M, Arslan EO, Taylor S, Kanik A, Duran HE, et al. Predictive value of the hemizona assay for pregnancy outcome in patients undergoing controlled ovarian hyperstimulation with intrauterine insemination. Fertil Steril. 2006;85(6):1697-707.
73. Oehninger S, Coddington CC, Scott R, Franken DA, Burkman LJ, Acosta AA, et al. Hemizona assay: assessment of sperm dysfunction and prediction of in vitro fertilization outcome. Fertil Steril. 1989;51(4):665-70.
74. Franken DR, Kruger TF, Oehninger S, Coddington CC, Lombard C, Smith K, et al. The ability of the hemizona assay to predict human fertilization in vitro in different and consecutive IVF/GIFT cycles. Hum Reprod. 1993;8(8):1240-4.
75. Franken DR, Oehninger SC. The clinical significance of sperm-zona pellucida binding: 17 years later. Front Biosci. 2006;11:1227-33.
76. Oehninger S, Franken D, Kruger T. Approaching the next millennium: how should we manage andrology diagnosis in the intracytoplasmic sperm injection era? Fertil Steril. 1997;67(3):434-6.
77. Oehninger S, Mahony M, Ozgür K, Kolm P, Kruger T, Franken D. Clinical significance of human sperm-zona pellucida binding. Fertil Steril. 1997;67(6):1121-7.
78. Oehninger S, Franken DR, Sayed EM, Barroso G, Kolm P. Sperm function assays and their predictive value for fertilization outcome in IVF therapy: a meta-analysis. Hum Reprod Update. 2000;6(2):160-8.
79. Vogiatzi P, Chrelias C, Cahill DJ, Creatsa M, Vrachnis N, Iliodromiti Z, et al. Hemizona assay and sperm penetration assay in the prediction of IVF outcome: a systematic review. Biomed Res Int. 2013;2013:945825.
80. Mol BW, Meijer S, Yuppa S, Tan E, de Vries J, Bossuyt PM, et al. Sperm penetration assay in predicting successful in vitro fertilization. A meta-analysis. J Reprod Med. 1998;43:503-8.
81. Oehninger S. Clinical management of male infertility in assisted reproduction: ICSI and beyond. Int J Androl. 2011; 34:e319-29.
82. Franken DR, Oehninger S. Semen analysis and sperm function testing. Asian J Androl. 2012;14:6-13.
83. World Health Organization. WHO laboratory manual for the examination and processing of human semen, 6th edition. 2021.
84. Mendizabal-Ruiz G, Chavez-Badiola A, Aguilar Figueroa I, Martinez Nuño V, Flores-Saiffe Farias A, Valencia-Murilloa R, et al. Computer software (SiD) assisted real-time single sperm selection associated with fertilization and blastocyst formation. Reprod Biomed Online. 2022;45:703-11.

CHAPTER

99

# Selection of Sperm

Muthukumar K

## INTRODUCTION

Assisted reproductive technology (ART) includes intrauterine insemination (IUI), in vitro fertilization (IVF), and intracytoplasmic sperm injection (ICSI) techniques. Over the decades, various attempts have been made to optimize the sperm recovery by efficient processing methods for IUI and selection of individual sperm for ICSI. The glass wool filtration (GWF),[1] swim-up,[2] and density gradient centrifugation (DGC) methods[3] are most commonly used for the separation of morphologically normal, motile, and viable sperm. Advanced sperm selection methods for ICSI were approached based on the structural characteristics with very high magnification,[4] physiological properties of binding ability,[5] chromatin organization,[6] and removal of apoptotic sperm by processing,[7] and were reported by different authors. The validation of different selection methods by evidence-based study has drawn different conclusions in routine clinical application.

## SPERM SELECTION FOR INTRAUTERINE INSEMINATION

The processing of semen from normal to mild Oligo Asthenozoospermic sample while handling IUI. Two techniques were preferred to maximize the yield of spermatozoa with potential fertilizing ability. Swim-up methods were recommended for normozoospermic samples by the World Health Organization (WHO). In contrast, the gradient method was found better for mild oligoasthenozoospermic samples.

### Migration Method

#### *Swim-up Procedure*

The swim-up method of processing the sample is done by direct or indirect method.[8,9] In the direct swim-up method, the sample was overlaid with human tubal fluid (HTF) buffered with HEPES [4-(2-hydroxyethyl)-1-piperazine ethanesulfonic acid] for nearly 45 minutes at 37°C, and the sperm migrated over the fluid collected for insemination. The direct swim-up avoids the centrifugation process and potential damage caused by reactive oxygen species (ROS). But, the chances of seminal plasma contamination into the fluid cannot be avoided. The indirect swim-up method recommends to add equal amount of HTF–HEPES to the semen and aliquot of 1 mL per round, and bottom tubes were further made to centrifuge at 500 g for 10 minutes. The supernatant of centrifuged sample is removed carefully without disturbing the pellet, and the 1 mL of HEPES-HTF is overlaid and left incubated for 45 minutes at 37°C for sperms to migrate and to harvest the spermatozoa. While processing by swim-up method, hyperactivation may not occur immediately, and sufficient incubation in HTF assures capacitation.

The swim-up procedure yields high population of motile spermatozoa with less contamination of other cells, debris, and proteins.

#### *Migration Sedimentation*

This method is an extension of swim-up to evaluate the sperm function with additional sedimentation step using a special glass or plastic tube with inner cone.[10] The limitation of this method was of lower yield and not widely accepted in ART.[11]

#### *Transmembrane Migration*

The transmembrane migration method employs migration via membrane filter through the cylindrical pores at right angles to the plane of the membrane.[12] The yield of sperm is found to be less despite after modification of the method and not clinically applied in routine processing of semen sample.

### Density Gradient Method

The DGC method of sperm preparation utilizes conical bottom tube with 80% gradient overlaid with 40% gradient. The principle of DGC is based on the density-based separation and the mature morphologically normal sperm found to be higher than 80% gradient found to collect as a soft pellet at conical bottom on centrifugation at 300 g for 20 minutes and soft pellet transferred into a 9 mL of HTF-HEPES. Final spin was done for 5 minutes to remove the plasma and utilized for IUI.[13] DGC yields more morphologically normal,[14] hyperactivated spermatozoa with less DNA-fragmented spermatozoa and less of aneuploid sperm[15] compared to swim-up method. Historically, Percoll was a compound used for density gradient but later discontinued due to the presence of endotoxins and potential in vivo toxicity[16,17] and later replaced by silane-coated silica particles with equal potential of sperm isolation of morphologically normal and motile spermatozoa. DGC was shown to have less of caspase activation, disruption of mitochondrial membrane potential, and externalized phosphatidylserine.[18-21]

A combination of DGC and modified swim-up was recommended to remove human immunodeficiency virus (HIV)-1 RNA and proviral DNA.[22]

### Filtration Techniques

The filtration techniques of sperm separation were followed using the glass wool, glass bead, and Sephadex columns for sperm separation.

#### *Glass Wool Filtration*

The GWF method separates spermatozoa according to the motility and size of sperm head. This method efficiently separates the leukocytes and prevents ROS-induced sperm damage. The densely packed glass wool fibers using gravitational force separates motile spermatozoa with self-propelled motion of the cells. The efficacy of each filtration depends on the properties of glass wool used and the chemical nature of glass, surface structure, charge, and thickness of glass wool which influences the efficacy of the filtration.[23,24] Transmission of glass particles into the filtration and acrosome-damaged sperm found is the limitation of this technique. In terms of functional integrity, this technique is found superior over DGC and has optimized recovery than swim-up method.

#### *Glass Bead Filtration*

Spheres of glass bead arranged in a column are used to separate highly motile spermatozoa.[25] This technique was found to be better than swim-up and also found to have positive post-thaw outcome of cryopreserved sample. The limitation of this technique was found to be due to transfer of glass bead into the filtrate.[26]

#### *Sephadex Columns*

This technique is based on the chromatographic media[27] composed of microscopic beads synthetically derived from the polysaccharide dextran. In comparison to swim-up and DGC, a high yield and more motile spermatozoa separation were reported.[28] A higher pregnancy rate in IUI using Sephadex columns sperm preparation was reported than swim-up.[29] But chromatin condensation and morphologically normal spermatozoa were found better in DGC than in Sephadex columns.[30]

## SPERM SELECTION FOR INTRACYTOPLASMIC SPERM INJECTION

The sperm selection for ICSI can be broadly divided based on the motile and nonmotile spermatozoa. The selection approaches now in current practice are based on the following principles:

- Morphological analysis using ultrastructural evaluation and sperm birefringence pattern
- Physiological method of hyaluronic acid binding
- Selection based on sperm membrane surface charge
- Magnetic-activated cell sorting system (MACS)
- Microfluidics
- Selection of nonmotile but viable spermatozoa.

The different approaches are in detail below, with merits and demerits.

### Morphological Analysis—Ultrastructural Evaluation

Assessing the motile-sperm organelle morphology examination (MSOME) was introduced as an advanced sperm selection method.[4] The fine nuclear morphology of motile spermatozoa was examined in real time at very high magnification. The inverted light microscope is equipped with high-power differential interference contrast (DIC) optics, resulting in an optical magnification of ×1,500, and further enhancement by digital imaging allows achieving a total magnification of up to ×6,600. This magnification allows to identify a spermatozoon with a normal nucleus, defined by an oval shape with a smooth configuration and a normal nuclear content (with <4% of the nucleus occupied by vacuoles). MSOME assessment over six sperm organelles (acrosome, postacrosomal lamina, nucleus, neck, tail, and mitochondria) found the sperm nucleus appeared to have an association with ICSI outcome[31] and a positive correlation between MSOME selected with successful ICSI outcome with previous failures.[32-34]

The vacuoles in the sperm nucleus found to have an association with apoptosis of spermatozoa and negative correlation with ICSI outcome. MSOME criteria grade vacuoles in the nucleus with large size have the most DNA-fragmented spermatozoa. The larger size vacuoles vary by definition ranging from space occupied by 4 to 50%. The number of vacuoles was considered to be significant while selecting spermatozoa.

Injection of morphologically selected spermatozoa (IMSI) with MSOME criteria does not found to improve the fertilization and cleavage rate in consensus between different groups, and contradictory report on embryo quality, blastocyst formation.[34-37] The application of IMSI has supported improvement in ongoing pregnancy rates with low abortion rates over repeated implantation failures.[38] Sperm selection by conventional ICSI seems sufficient for an unselected population,[39] as evidenced by similar pregnancy and delivery rates for ICSI and IMSI in the very first ART cycle of a couple. The technique advocated only in highly DNA-fragmented sperms as a prospective randomized control trial on frozen spermatozoa.

The practical limitation of the IMSI would be the cost and time consumption of procedure. The technique involves sperm selection at room temperature with glass Petri dish and subsequent change to another dish for ICSI.

## Morphological Analysis—Sperm Birefringence

The acrosome-reacted spermatozoa with proper chromatin organization and protoplasmic nature exhibit specific birefringence when analyzed through polarized microscopy. The basis of the selection considers that human spermatozoa have characteristics of birefringence that reflect the state of inner protoplasmic structures. This noninvasive technique utilized polarized microscopy with added feature to detect type and intensity of birefringence with additional optical system.[6] Acrosome-reacted spermatozoa selected by this method, in comparison to nonreacted spermatozoa, were found to improve fertilization rate.

## Physiological Method of Hyaluronic Acid Binding

The hyaluronic acid binding-based sperm selection is considered to be a physiological method. In this method, the mature normal spermatozoa considered to be only having binding ability to hyaluronic acid was claimed to get selected for ICSI.[5] In routine practice, either a commercially available Petri dish intracytoplasmic sperm injection (PICSI) dish with hyaluron gel coated as a dot or a solution form of hyaluronic acid can be utilized while selecting the population of normal spermatozoa for ICSI. The sperm preparation has to be adequate and clean to add in the coated area to assess the binding, and the room temperature is recommended for 15 minutes of incubation in hyaluronic acid to ensure the binding. The sperm selected by this method was found to show less DNA fragmented and found normal as per MSOME criteria. A combination of hyaluron-bound sperm and subsequent IMSI also has been advocated. The hyaluronic acid binding has reports on improved fertilization rates but no impact on pregnancy rates,[40] while other reports have shown improvement in embryo development rate without influencing fertilization and pregnancy rate,[41] and the discrepancy was attributed to study design. One multicenter study supports higher clinical pregnancy rates than conventional ICSI.[42]

## Sperm Selection Based on Surface Charge

### *Electrophoretic Method*

The electrophoresis-based technology (Microflow CS-10, Nusep Ltd., Frenchs Forest, Australia) separates spermatozoa based on size and electronegative charge. The sperm sample solution is loaded into the apparatus reservoirs and allowed to equilibrate with special buffer for only 5 minutes prior to application of an electric field in the form of constant applied current of 75 mA and a variable voltage of 18–21 V. Sorted sperm is retrieved from the collection chamber.[43] This method was considered relatively quick without centrifugation and found superior than density gradient separation. But this method found decreased motility and equal kinetics as compared to density gradient method. The complexity of the apparatus used limits the use of the technology.

### *Zeta Potential Method*

This method is based on the electrokinetic potential of the sperm, an electric potential between the sperm membrane and its surrounding measuring –16 to –20 mV in mature sperm.[44] In this method, washed sperm placed into a positively charged centrifuge tubes prepared by simply rotating a tube two or three times in a latex glove. After 1 minute, the tube is centrifuged and inverted to remove all the nonadhering sperm and other contaminants. Thereafter, adhering (negatively charged, mature) sperm can be retrieved by rinsing the tube with serum-supplemented media. The zeta potential method is found simple and inexpensive, but the limitation includes low recovery over oligoasthenozoospermic sample and is not applicable over surgically retrieved sperm and charges may get neutralized if humid environment. The zeta potential selection method provided higher morphology, hyperactivation, DNA integrity, and mature sperms, but not motility, in comparison with density gradient method.[44-46]

## Magnetic-activated Cell Sorting of Nonapoptotic Spermatozoa

The externalization of phosphatidylserine by apoptotic sperm forms the basis of this method. It allows for its binding with annexin-V-conjugated paramagnetic microbeads, which could be used to label and separate apoptotic spermatozoa using MACS (Miltenyi Biotec GmbH, Bergisch Gladbach, Germany).[47] The bead/sperm mixture is allowed to run through the MACS column, which is placed inside a magnet. The magnetic force will cause the retention of the cells labeled with microbeads inside the column, while the nonlabeled cells will freely flow. This method needs to be combined with density gradient to remove leukocytes and other plasma contaminants.[48] Although this method is fast and inexpensive, the low recovery rate limits its application. Additionally, the retention of microbeads in processed samples advocates modifying by combining annexin to glass wool to improve the efficacy of the system. MACS combined with density gradient yields spermatozoa with higher membrane potential, lower active caspase-3, and phosphatidylserine externalization[49-51] compared to only density gradient separation with proven benefit with fresh and cryopreserved samples. A higher embryo development rate and clinical pregnancy rate using MACS in comparison to density gradient with abnormal semen parameters were reported with live birth in previous failed ICSI cycles due to poor fertilization and embryo development.[52]

## Microfluidics-based Sperm Selection

The application of microfluidics on sperm selection was found to be of greater advantage compared to swim-up and density gradient methods. It was demonstrated in a pump-less hydrostatic pressure microfluidic device in which the sperm swim through laminar flows to reach a collecting area for motile sperm. This device differentiates motile sperm from immotile sperm, dead sperm or dead cells, and debris in raw semen, and thus opened a new era of microfluidic applications in ART. Briefly, microfluidics involves constructing the channel structures, which were fabricated from polydimethylsiloxane (PDMS) using standard photolithography and micromolding techniques. These structures were then plasma bonded to a glass microscope slide, which constituted the base of the device and the bottom surface of the microchannels. The device consisted of a 250 mm diameter microchannel with an inlet to insert media and sperm and an outlet to let air out as these elements are inserted. The length of microfluidic channels was about 3 cm. A study comparing the sperm separated by above microfluidic device in comparison to swim-up and density gradient had higher rates of average ratio of sperm, fast swimming forward average sperm activity ratio, value derivation for the curvilinear, value derivation for straight-line velocities, value derivation for average path, amplitude of lateral head displacement, amplitude of cross-frequency, progression ratios of linearity, progression ratios of wobble, progression ratios of straightness, and lower rates of deformity. In addition, the DNA integrity of sperm selection was better maintained than that selected by traditional methods.[53]

Recent advances attempted to integrate optics with microfluidics-based sperm separation.[54]

Raman spectroscopy principle plays a vital role in integrating microfluidics and optics that allows to distinguish sperm with improved nuclear integrity.[55,56] Microfluidics, along with dynamic, high-speed imaging, improved more accurate observation and quantification of the dynamics of sperm movement in a setting that mimics their natural environment by simultaneously visualizing the processes at small length and fast time scales. On-chip digital imaging approaches, within microfluidic systems, label-free 3D imaging of sperm is possible.[57] These methods employ a digital optoelectronic sensor, such as a complementary metal-oxide semiconductor chip, to digitally reconstruct the volume of the cell in 3D space by recording the interference pattern difference between a reference light wave and a light wave scattered by the specimen.[57]

## Selection of Viable Nonmotile Spermatozoa

One of the challenges while encountering either ejaculate or surgically retrieved sperms while doing ICSI is the presence of only immotile sperm available and selection of viable sperm that have fertilizing ability and achieving further ongoing clinical pregnancy and live birth. Various approaches were documented in the literature to select the viable spermatozoa as discussed here.

### *Modified Hypoosmotic Swelling Test*

The conventional hypoosmotic swelling (HOS) test described was found to induce some detrimental changes in sperm structure, found not preferred over ICSI was modified as to have a solution containing 50% culture medium and 50% deionized water. Spermatozoa are left for 10 seconds, and viable sperms chosen based on curved or swollen tail. Reactive sperms are transferred into a fresh drop and washed thrice for osmotic re-equilibration. Washed sperms are then transferred to PVP drop for ICSI. A randomized trial using the modified hypoosmotic-based sperm selection has shown higher clinical pregnancy rate of immotile testicular sperms of fresh and cryopreserved samples in comparison to no treatment.[58]

### *Sperm Tail—Mechanical Touch*

This method is based on the mechanical stimuli and reflex observation to select viable and nonviable spermatozoa by injection pipette of ICSI. In detail, laterally pressing the sperm in the upper one third of immotile spermatozoa tail with ICSI dish forcing the tail to one side, and the response is observed. The viable spermatozoa recover and reposition the tail with flexibility. Rigid sperms are not capable to recover signs as not viable. Also, the movement of head along with the direction of tail movements is considered not viable, and the movement of head on opposite direction is found to be viable. Acceptable pregnancy rate is achieved using fresh and frozen immotile spermatozoa by the mechanical touch method.[59]

### Laser-assisted Sperm Selection

The use of lasers for sperm selection was the development of a technique for the identification of viable but immotile spermatozoa.[60] A single laser shot of 129 μJ for approximately 1.2 ms being directed to the tip of the flagellum. The live but immotile spermatozoa cause a curling or coiling of the tail. If no such change is observed, then the spermatozoon is considered as nonviable. The successful application of this laser selection was the identification of viable spermatozoa in a patient with primary ciliary dyskinesia that resulted in a pregnancy.[61] The use of the technique on ejaculated asthenozoospermic samples and immotile spermatozoa from testicular biopsies demonstrated its ability to identify numbers of viable spermatozoa in a sample was comparable to that of the HOS test (22.0 vs. 21.5%). Fertilization rate increased significantly from 20.4% in the randomly selected testicular sperm extraction (TESE) spermatozoa group to 45.4% in the laser selection group; accordingly, the take-home baby rate increased from 5.9% to 19.0%. Furthermore, if laser-selected spermatozoa from asthenozoospermic samples were used for ICSI, significantly higher fertilization and embryo cleavage rates were achieved in comparison to those resulting from randomly selected spermatozoa. Laser-tested TESE spermatozoa selection over immotile situation was found to be quick, easy, repeatable, and a safe means of viability testing.[62]

### Chemical Stimulators-mediated Sperm Selection

The use of pentoxifylline and theophylline to induce sperm motility by inhibiting the phosphodiesterase activity, and thus increasing intracellular cAMP levels was found to ensure motile sperm selection from a population of immotile sperms that have viability and can become motile on stimulation.[63]

In conditions of oligozoospermia or asthenozoospermia where fertilization failure in previous IVF cycles was overcome by incubation with pentoxifylline[63] with no influence on acrosome reaction[64] under different concentrations. In testicular samples,[65] the addition of 3.6 mM pentoxifylline was found to induce significant motility after only 30 minutes incubation. It is recommended to wash the exposed sperm thoroughly before using ICSI. An improved fertilization rate and embryo development were reported in comparison to no artificial activation without improvement in clinical pregnancy rate.[66] The use of pentoxifylline significantly reduces the time spent finding and selecting motile spermatozoa.[67] In a study where pentoxifylline treated against HOS-identified spermatozoa,[68] the addition of pentoxifylline proved to significantly increase the fertilization (62.05 vs. 41.07%) and clinical pregnancy rates (32 vs. 16%).

The compound pentoxifylline is efficient in the selection of spermatozoa with structural defects such as axonemal, enzymatic, or functional tail defects[69] and is able to activate ejaculated spermatozoa from a patient with Kartagener's syndrome that resulted in a viable pregnancy.[70]

Theophylline, another member of xanthine family, has been used in a prospective clinical sibling oocyte trial where it was found to have an immediate but short-term effect on sperm motility and showed to have the additional benefits of shorter searching time, significantly higher fertilization rates increasing from 63.3 to 79.9% in the treatment group. The concerns with respect to the safety of these chemical compounds recommend the benefit on shorter exposure.

### Birefringence

The sperm birefringence property was explored while choosing immotile but viable for ICSI. In one study, it has proved patients with complete asthenozoospermia superior quality zygotes, embryos and pregnancy rates can be produced than the HOS test.[71] In immotile testicular sperm selection for ICSI, the birefringence property can be applied to optimize the outcome. The cost of the polarizing microscopy arrangement has limitations to apply universally in all clinics.

## CONCLUSION

Sperm selection for ICSI found to be approached by various methods but still not found one approach as highly superior than other methods. It is suggestive to individualize the technique according to each type of sample. The available evidence remains preliminary to draw strong conclusion on various methods.

## KEY POINTS

- The sperm preparation for ART found to be approached with different modalities and the single sperm selection was also found to be with various advanced techniques.
- Systematic review published early concluded application of advanced sperm selection techniques are encouraging in terms of fertilization and pregnancy rates but most of the studies are underpowered to conclude the benefit over pregnancy and live birth rate.[74]
- The advanced technique like IMSI involves cost and time factor as well as reports of certain detrimental effects.[75]
- Most of the techniques also involves approaches with combination of techniques with prolonged exposure in vitro during sperm selections that may cause iatrogenic damage to the sperm and long-term effects on the offspring but remains inconclusive due to lacking evidence and further to conclude, considering all the present constraints over sperm selection the future research can evolve a safer and rapid alternative to sperm selection.
- In an retrospective study of data[76] comparing neonatal outcomes between IMSI and ICSI found no significant

difference. The mean pregnancy duration and mean birth weight were almost identical in both groups. There was no significant difference in major congenital malformations between the two groups.

- Recent evidence from Cochrane study[77] after careful meta-analysis of available evidence found sperm selected by hyaluronic acid binding may have little or no effect on live birth or clinical pregnancy but may reduce the miscarriage rate and uncertain about zeta sperm selection on live birth, clinical pregnancy and miscarriage rate as available evidence of very low quality. Further MACS-based selection in comparison to conventional ICSI also found to be very low quality evidence uncertain to provide reducing miscarriage and improving clinical pregnancy rate.
- With regard to IMSI over ICSI and birth defects a recent meta-analysis study reported[78] as children conceived after IMSI have decreased structural chromosomal defect compared to ICSI. The other chromosomal abnormalities like trisomy 13, 18, 21 and triple X similar between children conceived after IMSI and ICSI.

## REFERENCES


1. Paulson JD, Polakoski KL. A glass wool column procedure for removing extraneous material from the human ejaculate. Fertil Steril. 1977;28:178-81.
2. Mahadevan M, Baker G. Assessment and preparation of semen for in vitro fertilization. In: Wood C, Trounson A (Eds). Clinical In Vitro Fertilization. Berlin: Springer-Verlag; 1984. pp. 83-97.
3. Arcidiacono A, Walt H, Campana A, Balerna M. The use of Percoll gradients for the preparation of subpopulations of human spermatozoa. Int J Androl. 1983;6:433-45.
4. Bartoov B, Berkovitz A, Eltes F, Kogosovsky A, Yagoda A, Lederman H, et al. Pregnancy rates are higher with intracytoplasmic morphologically selected sperm injection than with conventional intracytoplasmic injection. Fertil Steril. 2003;80:1413-9.
5. Huszar G, Jakab A, Sakkas D, Ozenci CC, Cayli S, Delpiano E, et al. Fertility testing and ICSI sperm selection by hyaluronic acid binding: clinical and genetic aspects. Reprod Biomed Online. 2007;14:650-66.
6. Gianaroli L, Magli MC, Ferraretti AP, Crippa A, Lappi M, Capitani S, et al. Birefringence characteristics in sperm heads allow for the selection of reacted spermatozoa for intracytoplasmic sperm injection. Fertil Steril. 2010;93:807-13.
7. Alvarez Sedo C, Uriondo H, Lavolpe M, Noblia F, Papier S, Nodar F. Clinical outcome using non-apoptotic sperm selection for ICSI procedures: report of 1 year experience. Fertil Steril. 2010;94:S23.
8. Canale D, Giorgi PM, Gasperini M, Pucci E, Barletta D, Gasperi M, et al. Inter- and intra-individual variability of sperm morphology after selection with three different techniques: layering, swimup from pellet and Percoll. J Endocrinol Invest. 1994;17:729-73.
9. Cooper TG, Aitken J, Auger J, Baker GHW, Barratt CLR, Behre HM, et al. Sperm preparation techniques. WHO Laboratory Manual for the Examination and Processing of Human Semen, 5th edition. Switzerland: WHO Press; 2010.
10. Harrison RF, Bonnar J, Thompson W (Eds). Fertility and Sterility: The Proceedings of the XIth World Congress on Fertility and Sterility, Dublin, June 1983, held under the Auspices of the International Federation of Fertility Societies. Springer Netherlands; 2012.
11. Yener C, Mathur S, Parent B. Comparison of two sperm preparation techniques using automated sperm motion analysis: migration sedimentation versus swim-up. Arch Androl. 1990;25:17-20.
12. Chijioke PC, Crocker PR, Gilliam M, Owens MD, Pearson RM. Importance of filter structure for the trans-membrane migration studies of sperm motility. Hum Reprod. 1988;3:241-4.
13. Mortimer D, Mortimer ST. Methods of sperm preparation for assisted reproduction. Ann Acad Med Singap. 1992;21:517-24.
14. Glander HJ. Effektivität der Methoden für die Spermienkollektion, -separation und konzentrierung. Hautnah Derm. 1993;9:52-60.
15. Jakab A, Kovacs T, Zavaczki Z, Borsos A, Bray-Ward P, Ward D, et al. Efficacy of the swim-up method in eliminating sperm with diminished maturity and aneuploidy. Hum Reprod. 2003;18:1481-8.
16. Pickering SJ, Fleming TP, Braude PR, Bolton VN, Gresham GA. Are human spermatozoa separated on a Percoll density gradient safe for therapeutic use? Fertil Steril. 1989;51: 1024-9.
17. Pharmacia Biotech. Important Notice: Percoll® NOT to be used in Assisted Reproduction Technologies in Humans. Uppsala, Sweden: Pharmacia Biotech; 1996.
18. Larson KL, Brannian JD, Timm BK, Jost LK, Evenson DP. Density gradient centrifugation and glass wool filtration of semen remove spermatozoa with damaged chromatin structure. Hum Reprod. 1999;14:2015-9.
19. Ollero M, Gil-Guzman E, Lopez MC, Sharma RK, Agarwal A, Larson K, et al. Characterization of subsets of human spermatozoa at different stages of maturation: implications in the diagnosis and treatment of male infertility. Hum Reprod. 2001;16:1912-21.
20. Barroso G, Taylor S, Morshedi M, Manzur F, Gavino F. Oehninger S. Mitochondrial membrane potential integrity and plasma membrane translocation of phosphatidylserine as early apoptotic markers: a comparison of two different sperm subpopulations. Fertil Steril. 2006;85:149-54.
21. Paasch U, Agarwal A, Gupta AK, Sharma RK, Grunewald S, Thomas Jr AJ, et al. Apoptosis signal transduction and the maturity status of human spermatozoa. Ann N Y Acad Sci. 2003;1010:486-9.
22. Kato S, Hanabusa H, Kaneko S, Takakuwa K, Suzuki M, Kuji N, et al. Complete removal of HIV-1 RNA and proviral DNA from semen by the swim-up method: assisted reproduction technique using spermatozoa free from HIV-1. AIDS. 2006;20:967-73.
23. Sanchez R, Concha M, Ichikawa T, Henkel R, Schill WB. Glass wool filtration reduces reactive oxygen species by elimination of leukocytes in oligozoospermic patients with leukocytospermia. J Assist Reprod Genet. 1996;13:489-94.
24. Ford WCL, McLaughlin EA, Prior SM, Rees JM, Wardle PG, Hull PG. The yield, motility and performance in the

hamster egg test of human spermatozoa prepared from cryopreserved semen by four different methods. Hum Reprod. 1992;7:654-9.
25. Daya S, Gwatkin RB, Bissessar H. Separation of motile human spermatozoa by means of a glass bead column. Gamete Res. 1987;17:375-80.
26. Lechtzin N, Garside W, Heyner S, Hillman N. Glass-bead column separation of motile and nonmotile human spermatozoa. J In Vitro Fert Embryo Transf. 1991;8:96-100.
27. Drobnis EZ, Zhong CQ, Overstreet JW. Separation of cryopreserved human semen using Sephadex columns, washing, or Percoll gradients. J Androl. 1991;12:201-8.
28. Gabriel LK, Vawda AI. Preparation of human sperm for assisted conception: a comparative study. Arch Androl. 1993;30:1-6.
29. Zavos PM, Centola GM. Methods of semen preparation for intrauterine insemination and subsequent pregnancy rates. Tohoku J Exp Med. 1992;168:583-90.
30. Hammadeh ME, Zavos PM, Rosenbaum P, Schmidt W. Comparison between the quality and function of sperm after semen processing with two different methods. Asian J Androl. 2001;3:125-30.
31. Bartoov B, Berkovitz A, Eltes F, Kogosowski A, Menezo Y, Barak Y. Real-time fine morphology of motile human sperm cells is associated with IVF-ICSI outcome. J Androl. 2002;23(1):1-8.
32. Berkovitz A, Eltes F, Yaari S, Katz N, Barr I, Fishman A, et al. The morphological normalcy of the sperm nucleus and pregnancy rate of intracytoplasmic injection with morphologically selected sperm. Hum Reprod. 2005;20:185-90.
33. Berkovitz A, Eltes F, Lederman H, Peer S, Ellenbogen A, Feldberg B, et al. How to improve IVF-ICSI outcome by sperm selection. Reprod Biomed Online. 2006;12:634-8.
34. Hazout A, Dumont-Hassan M, Junca A, Cohen Bacrie P, Tesarik J. High-magnification ICSI overcomes paternal effect resistant to conventional ICSI. Reprod Biomed Online. 2006;12:19-25.
35. Antinori M, Licata E, Dani G, Cerusico F, Versaci C, d'Angelo D, et al. Intracytoplasmic morphologically selected sperm injection: a prospective randomized trial. Reprod Biomed Online. 2008;16:835-41.
36. Mauri AL, Petersen CG, Oliveira JB, Massaro FC, Baruffi RL, Franco Jr JG. Comparison of day 2 embryo quality after conventional ICSI versus intracytoplasmic morphologically selected sperm injection (IMSI) using sibling oocytes. Eur J Obstet Gynecol Reprod Biol. 2010;150:42.
37. De Vos A, Van de Velde H, Bocken G, Eylenbosch G, Franceus N, Meersdom G, et al. Does intracytoplasmic morphologically selected sperm injection improve embryo development? A randomized sibling-oocyte study. Hum Reprod. 2013;28:617-26.
38. Oliveira JB, Cavagna M, Petersen CG, Mauri AL, Massaro FC, Silva LFI, et al. Pregnancy outcomes in women with repeated implantation failures after intracytoplasmic morphologically selected sperm injection (IMSI). Reprod Biol Endocrinol. 2011;9:99-105.
39. Klement AH, Koren-Morag N, Itsykson P, Berkovitz A. Intracytoplasmic morphologically selected sperm injection versus intracytoplasmic sperm injection: a step toward a clinical algorithm. Fertil Steril. 2013;99:1290-3.
40. Nasr-Esfahani MH, Razavi S, Vahdati AA, Fathi F, Tavalaee M. Evaluation of sperm selection procedure based on hyaluronic acid binding ability on ICSI outcome. J Assist Reprod Genet. 2008;25:197-203.
41. Parmegiani L, Cognigni GE, Bernardi S, Troilo E, Ciampaglia W, Filicori M, et al. 'Physiologic ICSI': hyaluronic acid (HA) favors selection of spermatozoa without DNA fragmentation and with normal nucleus, resulting in improvement of embryo quality. Fertil Steril. 2010;93:598-604.
42. Worrilow KC, Eid S, Mathews JM, Pelts EJ, Khoury C, Liebermann J. A multi-site clinical trial evaluating PICSI versus intracytoplasmic sperm injection (ICSI): positive clinical outcomes observed in a prospective, randomized and double-blinded study. Fertil Steril. 2009;92:S36.
43. Ainsworth C, Nixon B, Jansen RP, Aitken RJ. First recorded pregnancy and normal birth after ICSI using electrophoretically isolated spermatozoa. Hum Reprod. 2007;22:197-200.
44. Chan PJ, Jacobson JD, Corselli JU, Patton WC. A simple zeta method for sperm selection based on membrane charge. Fertil Steril. 2006;85:481-6.
45. Kam TL, Jacobson JD, Patton WC, Corselli JU, Chan PJ. Retention of membrane charge attributes by cryopreserved-thawed sperm and zeta selection. J Assist Reprod Genet. 2007;24:429-34.
46. Razavi SH, Nasr-Esfahani MH, Deemeh MR, Shayesteh M, Tavalaee M. Evaluation of zeta and HA-binding methods for selection of spermatozoa with normal morphology, protamine content and DNA integrity. Andrologia. 2010;42:13-9.
47. Grunewald S, Paasch U, Glander HJ. Enrichment of non-apoptotic human spermatozoa after cryopreservation by immunomagnetic cell sorting. Cell Tissue Bank. 2001;2:127-33.
48. Said TM, Grunewald S, Paasch U, Glander HJ, Baumann T, Kriegel C, et al. Advantage of combining magnetic cell separation with sperm preparation techniques. Reprod BioMed Online. 2005;10:740-6.
49. Said TM, Agarwal A, Zborowski M, Grunewald S, Glander HJ, Paasch U. Utility of magnetic cell separation as a molecular sperm preparation technique. J Androl. 2008;29:134-42.
50. Grunewald S, Paasch U, Said TM, Rasch M, Agarwal A, Glander HJ. Magnetic-activated cell sorting before cryopreservation preserves mitochondrial integrity in human spermatozoa. Cell Tissue Bank. 2006;7:99-104.
51. Grunewald S, Said TM, Paasch U, Glander HJ, Agarwal A. Relationship between sperm apoptosis signalling and oocyte penetration capacity. Int J Androl. 2008;31:325-30.
52. Rawe VY, Boudri HU, Sedo CA, Carro M, Papier S, Nodar F. Healthy baby born after reduction of sperm DNA fragmentation using cell sorting before ICSI. Reprod Biomed Online. 2010;20:320-3.
53. Zhang B, Yin TL, Yang J. A novel microfluidic device for selecting human sperm to increase the proportion of morphologically normal, motile sperm with uncompromised DNA integrity. Anal Methods. 2015;598:1-5988.
54. Eravuchira PJ, Mirsky SK, Barnea I, Levi M, Balberg M, Shaked NT. Individual sperm selection by microfluidics integrated with interferometric phase microscopy. Methods. 2018;136:152-9.
55. Stiavnicka M, Abril-Parreno L, Nevoral J, Kralickova M, Garcia-Alvarez O. Non-invasive approaches to epigenetic-based sperm selection. Med Sci Monit. 2017;23:4677-83.

56. Amaral S, Da Costa R, Wubbeling F, Redmann K, Schlatt S. Raman microspectroscopy analysis of different sperm regions: a species comparison. Mol Hum Reprod. 2018;24:185-202.
57. Di Caprio G, Ferrara MA, Miccio L, Merola F, Memmolo P, Ferraro P, et al. Holographic imaging of unlabelled sperm cells for semen analysis: a review. J Biophotonics. 2015;8:779-89.
58. Sallam HN, Farrag A, Agameya AF, El-Garem Y, Ezzeldin F. The use of the modified hypo-osmotic swelling test for the selection of immotile testicular spermatozoa in patients treated with ICSI: a randomized controlled study. Hum Reprod. 2005;20:3435-40.
59. De Oliveira NM, Vaca Sanchez R, Rodriguez Fiesta S, Lopez Salgado T, Rodriguez R, Bethencourt JC, et al. Pregnancy with frozen-thawed and fresh testicular biopsy after motile and immotile sperm microinjection, using the mechanical touch technique to assess viability. Hum Reprod. 2004;19:262-5.
60. Aktan TM, Montag M, Duman S, Gorkemli H, Rink K, Yurdakul T. Use of a laser to detect viable but immotile spermatozoa. Andrologia. 2004;36:366-9.
61. Geber S, Lemgruber M, Taitson PF, Valle M, Sampaio M. Birth of healthy twins after intracytoplasmic sperm injection using ejaculated immotile spermatozoa from a patient with Kartagener's syndrome. Andrologia. 2012;44(Suppl. 1):842-4.
62. Nordhoff V, Schuring AN, Krallmann C, Zitzmann M, Schlatt S, Kiesel L, et al. Optimising TESE-ICSI by laser-assisted selection of immotile spermatozoa and polarisation microscopy for selection of oocytes. Andrology. 2013;1:67-74.
63. De Turner E, Aparicio NJ, Turner D, Schwarzstein L. Effect of two phosphodiesterase inhibitors, cyclic adenosine 3':5'-monophosphate, and a beta-blocking agent on human sperm motility. Fertil Steril. 1978;29:328-31.
64. Yovich JM, Edirisinghe WR, Cummins JM, Yovich JL. Preliminary results using pentoxifylline in a pronuclear stage tubal transfer (PROST) program for severe male factor infertility. Fertil Steril. 1988;50:179-81.
65. Mladenovic I, Micic S, Pearson RM, Genbacev O, Papic N. Effects of pentoxifylline on human sperm parameters in vitro. J Assist Reprod Genet. 1994;11:495-9.
66. Tasdemir I, Tasdemir M, Tavukcuoglu S. Effect of pentoxifylline on immotile testicular spermatozoa. J Assist Reprod Genet. 1998;15:90-2.
67. Kovacic B, Vlaisavljevic V, Reljic M. Clinical use of pentoxifylline for activation of immotile testicular sperm before ICSI in patients with azoospermia. J Androl. 2006;27:45-52.
68. Griveau JF, Lobel B, Laurent MC, Michardiere L, Le Lannou D. Interest of pentoxifylline in ICSI with frozen-thawed testicular spermatozoa from patients with non-obstructive azoospermia. Reprod Biomed Online. 2006;12:14-8.
69. Mangoli V, Mangoli R, Dandekar S, Suri K, Desai S. Selection of viable spermatozoa from testicular biopsies: a comparative study between pentoxifylline and hypoosmotic swelling test. Fert Steril. 2010;95:631-4.
70. Yildirim G, Ficicioglu C, Akcin O, Attar R, Tecellioglu N, Yencilek F. Can pentoxifylline improve the sperm motion and ICSI success in the primary ciliary dyskinesia? Arch Gynecol Obstet. 2009;279:213-5.
71. Ghosh S, Chattopadhyay R, Bose G, Ganesh A, Das S, Chakravarty BN. Selection of birefringent spermatozoa under Polscope: effect on intracytoplasmic sperm injection outcome. Andrologia. 2012;44:734-8.
72. Said TM, Land JA. Effects of advanced selection methods on sperm quality and ART outcome: a systematic review. Hum Reprod Update. 2011;17(6):719-33.
73. Junca AM, Dumont M, Cornet D, Douard S, De Mouzon J, Prisant N. Is intracytoplasmic morphologically sperm injection (IMSI) detrimental for pregnancy control? Fertil Steril. 2010;94:S31.
74. Gaspard O, Vanderzwalmen P, Wirleitner B, Ravet S, Wenders F, Eichel V, et al. Impact of high magnification sperm selection on neonatal outcomes: a retrospective study. J Assist Reprod Genet. 2018;35:1-9.
75. Lepine S, McDowell S, Searle LM, Kroon B, Glujovsky D, Yazdani A. Advanced sperm selection techniques for assisted reproduction. Cochrane Database Syst Rev. 2019;7(7):CD010461.
76. Dieamant F, Petersen CG, Vagnini LD, Renzi A, Petersen B, Massaro F, et al. Impact of intracytoplasmic morphologically selected sperm injection (IMSI) on birth defects: a systematic review and meta-analysis. J Assist Reprod Genet. 2021;25(3):466-72.

CHAPTER

# 100 Sperm Chromatin Assessment

*Priya Kannan*

## INTRODUCTION

Male fertility assessment has been traditionally assessed by measuring the concentration, motility, and morphology of the sperms in the ejaculate.

The primary function of the sperm is to deliver the paternal genome to the oocyte. The head of a mature spermatozoon has deoxyribonucleic acid (DNA) in a condensed and compact structure in insoluble form. Up to 85% of the sperm DNA is bound by protamine and exists as DNA-protamine complexes. The DNA-protamine complexes are more compact than DNA-histamine complexes.[1,2]

During spermiogenesis, protamines, which are half the size of histones, replace the majority of histones, and the sperm chromatin is wound into a supercoiled structure named toroids.[3] As the sperm passes through the epididymis, the protamines are cross-linked by sulfide bonds reducing the chromatin to one-sixth of volume taken up in somatic cells.[4] The sperm DNA is thus protected while the sperm is transported through the male and female genital tract. Postfertilization, the chromatin in the sperm must decondense correctly. Any abnormality in the sperm DNA, such as protamine deficiency,[5] oxidative stress[6] or failure to repair DNA strand breaks,[7] has the capacity to reduce the ability of the sperm to produce viable embryo. Damage can also occur due to iatrogenic factors, such as storage temperatures, handling conditions, lapse of time after ejaculation, infections, and reactions to medicines or post-testicular oxidative stress.[8]

Sperm DNA damage can be defined as any chemically induced change in the structure of the DNA. Sperm DNA fragmentation (sDF) is one of the most common disturbances that affects the genetic material. It can occur as single or double strand breaks. sDF may be triggered by different processes, including the defective packaging of the DNA during spermatogenesis, and processes of cell death and oxidative stress, which may be associated with several pathological and environmental conditions.

## CLINICAL SIGNIFICANCE

The clinical relevance of sperm DNA integrity to human reproduction and its influence on both natural and assisted reproductive technology (ART), conceptions have been researched over the past decade. During intracytoplasmic sperm injection (ICSI), only morphologically normal and motile spermatozoa are used to fertilize an oocyte. It has been reported that spermatozoa with apparently normal morphology may have DNA fragmentation. With this, it is but a natural conclusion that spermatozoa with normal-shaped appearance, but with DNA fragmentation could be mistakenly selected to fertilize oocytes during ICSI. This concern became more clinically significant following a study that suggested a highly statistically significant negative correlation between the percentage of sperm DNA fragmentation and embryo quality.[9] Accumulating evidence indicates that a negative correlation exists between disturbances in the organization of the genomic material in sperm nuclei and the fertility potential of spermatozoa, whether in vivo or in vitro.

There have been certain areas in reproduction where the integrity of sperm nucleus seems to be important.

- *Reduced fertility:*
  - Increased DNA fragmentation has been associated with reduced fertility.[10-12]
  - There have been studies that found correlation between sperms with abnormal DNA integrity and impaired sperm concentration and motility.[13]
- *Time to pregnancy:*
  - In some studies, it was found that sperm DNA integrity correlated with time to pregnancy using procedures such as intrauterine insemination (IUI), in vitro fertilization (IVF), and ICSI.[1,14-16]
  - But there is insufficient evidence to use sperm DNA fragmentation as predictor of fertility.[15]
- *Predictor of outcome in IVF/ICSI:*
  - There are varying results regarding the correlation between sperm DNA fragmentation with pregnancy

in IVF/ICSI cycles. Some studies have shown a highly statistically significant negative correlation between the percentage of sperm DNA fragmentation and embryo quality.[9,17] There are some meta-analyses that suggested small but statistically significant correlation between sperm DNA integrity tests and pregnancy in IVF/ICSI cycles.[18] As the evidence is inconclusive, routine testing for DNA integrity for patients undergoing IVF/ICSI is not recommended.[19]

- *Spontaneous abortion rates:* There has been evidence, including a recent systematic review and meta-analysis, suggesting that a higher rate of DNA fragmentation in sperms may be significantly associated with pregnancy loss after IVF or ICSI.[20-22]

## CAUSES OF SPERM DNA DAMAGE

The DNA repair systems in sperms are thought to be less active in the later stages of spermatogenesis and so sperms with breaks in DNA are found in the ejaculate.[6]

There are many causes that can cause sperm DNA damage. But the mechanism is not well elucidated. Some of the accepted causes are protamine deficiency or mutation, genetic disorders,[14] and oxidative stress such as varicocele.[12]

Factors, such as irradiation, leukocytospermia, chemotherapy, and high speed centrifugation, also contribute to damages to the sperm chromatin.

## ASSAYS FOR DETECTION OF SPERM DNA INTEGRITY

There are many tests that measure sperm DNA integrity and report the percentage of sperms with DNA fragmentation. At the present time, it has been suggested that a sperm chromatin structure of poor quality may be indicative of male subfertility. Sperm chromatin structure evaluation has been evolving as an independent measure of sperm quality.

Two different methods have been used to assess DNA fragmentation. The first one includes those methodologies that are used to detect DNA breaks. This group would include tests such as the terminal deoxyuridine triphosphate (dUTP) nick-end labeling (TUNEL), or *in situ* nick translation (ISNT). The second type of technique measures the susceptibility of chromatin to denaturation under certain treatments. This group would include the sperm chromatin structure assay (SCSA), the DNA breakage detection-fluorescence in situ hybridization (DBD-FISH), a methodology that uses in situ acid nucleic hybridization, the comet assay, and sperm chromatin dispersion (SCD). The standardized methodology for the methods has been published in the 6th edition of WHO laboratory manual for the examination and processing of human semen.[40]

The tests that are used to assess sperm chromatin assessments are:

- SCSA
- TUNEL
- Comet
- SCD
- Acridine orange test
- Acidic aniline blue
- Toluidine blue stain
- DBD-FISH
- ISNT
- Chromomycin A3
- 8-hydroxy-2′-deoxyguanosine (8-OHdG) measurement.

### Sperm Chromatin Structure Assay

Sperm chromatin structure assay technique, developed by Evenson et al.[23] almost 25 years ago, is considered a reference in the analysis of spermatic DNA fragmentation. This test is based on the principle that abnormal sperm chromatin has a greater susceptibility to the physical induction of partial DNA denaturation *in situ*. It measures the stability of the sperm DNA in hot or acid media. The assay utilizes acridine orange, a DNA probe and flow cytometry. This protocol has been classified as SCSA acid and SCSA heat to distinguish the means of inducing DNA denaturation.

The proportion of the sperm with fragmented DNA is measured and expressed as DNA fragmentation index (DFI). This is the most commonly used assay. Sperm chromatin structure assay data are not well correlated with classical sperm quality parameters and have been solidly shown to predict sub/infertility. This assay is ideally suited to human and animal fertility clinics to assess male sperm DNA integrity as related to fertility potential and embryo development as well as effects of reproductive toxicants.[24] A DFI threshold was established that identifies samples compatible with pregnancy (<30%).[25] SCSA is the most successful assay in predicting the various outcomes of ART including the fertilization and implantation rates.[26]

The SCSA requires the presence of expensive instrumentation and highly skilled technicians, but has a cutoff point (30% DFI) to differentiate between fertile and infertile samples.

### Terminal dUTP Nick End Labeling (TUNEL) Assay

In this assay, in a reaction catalyzed by the terminal transferase, the ends of the fragmented DNA are tagged with labeled nucleotides. Later, the modified nucleotides are detected by a fluorochrome antibody.[27] The TUNEL assay quantifies the incorporated dUTP at single-strand and double-strand DNA breaks. Sperms with normal DNA show only background staining or fluorescence, while the sperms with fragmented DNA are seen with bright stain or fluoresce. This assay is also popularly used.

Presently, many commercial kits have been made available. The kits provide tagged probes and the enzyme necessary to bind the probe to the DNA breaks. After labelling, the percentage of fluorescent spermatozoa can be determined by fluorescent microscopy or a flow cytometer. For assessment of clinical semen samples, TUNEL is best coupled with flow-cytometry. When using fluorescent microscope, at least 200 spermatozoa should be scored.

## Comet

The comet assay is a method to evaluate sperm DNA fragmentation and the principle is alkaline denaturation of DNA. It is based on the differential migration of broken DNA strands in an electric field depending on the charge. The name of the test is so because of the "comet" like appearance of the stained unwound DNA fragments under fluorescence microscope. It is a single cell electrophoresis assay that quantifies single and double-stranded breaks in fluorochrome-labeled sperms. It was first introduced by Ostling and Johanson in 1984.[28] This test is based on the principle that abnormal chromatin structure with DNA breaks, will mobilize and more freely toward the positive pole in an electric field neutral.[29] The test was originally set in neutral buffer. This was modified by Singh et al. in 1988 by using alkaline electrophoresis buffer that increased the sensitivity of this test.[30]

During electrophoresis, strands of DNA move in the gel sideways to form a tail of the comet. DNA without breaks remains in the head of the comet. This migration of the genetic material resulted in the "Comet Head and Tail". The extent of migration was proportional to the extent of damage inflicted on the cell.[28] Hence, the length of the tail is indicative of the extent of damage. The comet is a well-standardized assay that correlates significantly with TUNEL and SCSA assays. It is recommended that least 50 comets per duplicate slide should be scored. Commercial kits and detection software are also available.

## Sperm Chromatin Dispersion

Calvin and Bedford in 1971,[31] reported the role of disulfide bridges in the compaction and stabilization of the sperm nucleus. If disulfide cross-links break and a specific lysis solution is used to extract proteins, DNA's loops relax constituting haloes around the residual nuclear central structure. This method involves light microscopy method to evaluate the susceptibility of sperm DNA to acid denaturation. This method is based on the principle that intact DNA loops expand following denaturation, however when DNA is fragmented, expansion does not happen or is minimal. The SCD test is based on the principle that sperm with fragmented DNA fail to produce a characteristic halo when mixed with an aqueous agarose following acid denaturation and removal of nuclear proteins.[32,33] In this test, after dissolution of the nuclear protein using acid/salt treatment, the sperms are mixed with agarose. The sperms which fail to produce the "halo" are identified as sperms with fragmented DNA.

This valuation can be automated, using computer programs associated with systems type computer-assisted sperm analyzer (CASA). The technique needs the inclusion of sperms in agarose gels, but without electrophoresis. The principal advantage of this technique is that result interpretation does not need color determination or fluorescence intensity. Neither does it require complex equipment, nor specialized personnel.[34] Due to the simplicity of this methodology, it has been proposed that SCD can be potentially used as a routine test in the study of spermatic DNA fragmentation in basic andrology laboratories. The SCD test is available as commercial kits. The kits which provide all the reagents of the assay to ensure its easy application and technical operation and to provide repeatable and consistent results in different clinical laboratories.

## Acridine Orange Test

The test uses the metachromatic properties of acridine orange. This test is based on the unique property of acridine orange to emit green fluorescence when intercalated between double-stranded DNA, and red fluorescence when associated with single-stranded DNA. This test is also based on fluorescence, similar to SCSA but lacks the precision in measurement. The fluorochrome acridine orange intercalates into double-stranded DNA and binds to single-stranded DNA as an aggregate. The acridine orange bound to native DNA fluoresces green, whereas the aggregated acridine orange on denatured DNA fluoresces red.[35]

## DNA Breakage Detection-Fluorescence In Situ Hybridization

It is a relatively recent methodology. Discrimination of sperm cells containing fragmented DNA relies on high pH induced DNA denaturation originated in simple or double-strand breaks. After denaturation and extraction of proteins using a lysis solution, the simple strand generated DNA is hybridized with a DNA probe.

This test allows a direct estimation of DFI in a sperm sample.[36,37] From the research point of view, this methodology has a lot of interest, since it is the only available technique that allows evaluation of damage cell to cell, *in situ*, in specific DNA sequences.

## *In Situ* Nick Translation Test

*In situ* nick translation test, similar to TUNEL, quantifies the degree of DNA damage. This assay quantifies the incorporation of biotinylated dUTP at single-strand DNA breaks in a reaction that is catalyzed by the template-dependent enzyme DNA polymerase I.

The results of ISNT analysis have been used for the study of the anomalies originated during the remodeling of the spermatic chromatin. From a practical point of view, this technique would have the same provisions and disadvantages as the TUNEL, but there is no commercial kit available for its direct application on sperms.

### Toluidine Blue

Toluidine is a sensitive structural probe for DNA structure and packaging. When this stain joins chromatin rich in histones, it presents a violet-bluish coloration. But when it joins with chromatin rich in protamines, it gives a pale blue coloration.[38]

This technique is simple, low cost and has the advantage of providing permanent preparations for its use in an ordinary microscope, though the intermediate tints are of difficult valuation. Unfortunately, the results have a poor reproducibility.

### Chromomycin A3

The chromomycin A3 (CMA3) anchors specifically to rich guanine-cytosine regions and competes with protamines. Therefore, when sperms present an intense CMA3 staining, it is interpreted that this cellular population shows protamine deficiency. Therefore, high CMA3 fluorescence is a strong indicator of the low protamination state of spermatozoa.[39] One of the most important limitations of this technique is the interobserver subjectivity.

## DRAWBACK OF SPERM DNA TESTING

The tests used for measuring DNA fragmentation have been under the scanner as the results are not always consistent. This is due to a variety of factors such as lack of RCTs, different testing assays with varying cut-off values, inconsistent cut-off values defining the normal and abnormal ranges and non-standardized protocols.

## CLINICAL GUIDELINE FOR USE OF SPERM DNA FRAGMENTATION

As per the ASRM-AUA Guidelines, published in 2020:[41]

1. Sperm DNA fragmentation analysis is not recommended in the initial evaluation of the infertile couple (moderate recommendation-evidence level grade: (c) as there were no prospective studies that had directly evaluated the impact of DNA fragmentation testing on the clinical management of infertile couples.
2. Further, the committee concluded that the presently available data were inadequate to recommend SDF assay to be routinely performed in the initial evaluation of the infertile male.
3. Although in presently available studies, high sperm DNA fragmentation was negatively associated with pregnancy rates and positively associated with miscarriages, the association was unclear due to the variability in the normal range in different studies and the use of different tests. Hence it was recommended that for male partners with high sperm DNA fragmentation, a clinician may choose to counsel the possible association with infertility and compromised outcome after ART.
4. In a patient with high sperm DNA fragmentation, a clinician may consider using surgically obtained sperm for ICSI. Hence it was recommended that, DNA fragmentation testing may be advantageous for men in couples undergoing IVF especially in a clinical situation of repeated IVF failure. This was based on a prospective cohort study of over 100 couples with high DNA fragmentation, testicular sperm yielded substantially higher live birth rates than ejaculated sperm.

## CONCLUSION

The sperm chromatin quality is being considered a new parameter of seminal quality, possibly related to the fertility of the individual and will continue to evolve. The threshold for DNA fragmentation value proposed by Evenson, establishes that the probability of fertilization *in vivo* is near to zero if the proportion of damaged sperms exceeds 30%. Though DNA fragmentation does not have correlation with the classic parameters of seminal quality, it may be used as a predictor of the fertilizing capacity of an individual. Therefore, its study is advised in order to have a more complete vision of the seminal quality.

In view of the current level of knowledge and with easy-to-use commercial kits, which does not require expensive equipment being rolled out for use in clinical laboratories, the most appropriate thing is to diagnose and treat DNA fragmentation, when necessary. Sperm chromatin assessment, as an additional parameter, would complement the study of the semen, in order to obtain a much more complete vision of each particular situation. However, regular use of this test is not warranted and scientifically not supported at this point in time.

## REFERENCES


1. Lin MH, Kuo-Kuang Lee R, Li SH, Lu CH, Sun FJ, Hwu YM. Sperm chromatin structure assay parameters are not related to fertilization rates in in vitro fertilization and intracytoplasmic sperm injection, but might be related to spontaneous abortion rates. Fertil Steril. 2008;90(2):352-9.
2. Erenpreiss J, Spano M, Erenpresia J, Bungum M, Giwercman A. Sperm chromatin structure and male fertility: biological and clinical aspects. Asian J Androl. 2006;8:11-29.
3. Conwell CC, Vilfan ID, Hud NV. Controlling the size of nanoscale toroidal DNA condensates with static curvature and ionic strength. Proc Natl Acad Sci USA. 2003;100(16):9296-301.
4. Barratt CL, Aitken RJ, Björndahl L, Carrell DT, de Boer P, Kvist U, et al. Sperm DNA: organization, protection and

vulnerability: from basic science to clinical applications—A position report. Hum Reprod. 2010;25(4):824-38.

5. Carrell DT, Liu L. Altered protamine 2 expression is uncommon in donors of known fertility, but common among men with poor fertilizing capacity and may reflect other abnormalities in spermiogenesis. J Androl. 2001;22(4):604-10.
6. Saleh RA, Agarwal A, Sharma RK, Said TM, Sikka SC, Thomas AJ Jr. Evaluation of nuclear DNA damage in spermatozoa from infertile men with varicocoele. Fertil Steril. 2003;80(6):1431-6.
7. Lewis SE, Aitken RJ. DNA damage to spermatozoa has impact on fertilization and pregnancy. Cell Tissue Res. 2005;322(1):33-41.
8. Gonazalez-Marin C, Gosalvez J, Roy R. Types, causes, detection and repair of DNA fragmentation in Animal and Human Sperm Cells. Int J Mol Sci. 2012;13(11):14026-52.
9. Avendaño C, Franchi A, Duran H, Oehninger S. DNA fragmentation of normal spermatozoa negatively impacts embryo quality and intracytoplasmic sperm injection outcome. Fertil Steril. 2010;94(2):549-57.
10. Evenson DP, Jost LK, Marshall D, Zinaman MJ, Clegg E, Purvis K, et al. Utility of sperm DNA chromatin assay as a diagnostic and prognostic tool in the human fertility clinic. Hum Reprod. 1999;14(4):1039-49.
11. Evenson DP, Wixon R. Meta-analysis of sperm DNA fragmentation using the sperm chromatin assay. Reprod Biomed Online. 2006;12(4):466-72.
12. Simon L, Lewis SE. Sperm DNA damage or progressive motility: which one is the better predictor of fertilization in vitro? Syst Biol Reprod Med. 2011;57(3):133-8.
13. Sharma RK, Said T, Agarwal A. Sperm DNA damage and its clinical relevance in assessing reproductive outcomes. Asian J Androl. 2004;6(2):139-48.
14. O'Brien J, Zini A. Sperm DNA integrity and male infertility. Urology. 2005;65(1):16-22.
15. Bungum M, Humaiden P, Spano M, Spano M, Bungum L, Erenpreiss J, et al. Sperm DNA assessment in prediction of assisted reproductive technology outcome. Hum Reprod. 2007;22(1):174-9.
16. Bungum M, Humaiden P, Spano M, Jepson K, Bungum L, Giwercman A, et al. The predictive value of sperm chromatin structure assay parameters for the outcome of intrauterine insemination, IVF and ICSI. Hum Reprod. 2004;19(6):1401-8.
17. Zini A. Are sperm chromatin and DNA defects relevant in the clinic? Syst Biol Reprod Med. 2011;57(1-2):78-85.
18. Bronet F, Martínez E, Gaytán M, Liñán A, Cernuda D, Ariza M, et al. Sperm DNA fragmentation index does not correlate with the sperm or embryo aneuploidy rate in recurrent miscarriage or implantation failure patients. Hum Reprod. 2012;27(7):1922-9.
19. Simon L, Lutton D, Mcmanus J, Lewis SE. Sperm DNA measured by the alkaline Comet assay as an independent predictor of male infertility and in vitro fertilization success. Fertil Steril. 2011;95(2):652-7.
20. Zini A, Boman JM, Belzile E, Ciampi A. Sperm damage is associated with an increased risk of pregnancy loss after IVF and ICSI: Systematic review and meta-analysis. Hum Reprod. 2008;23(12):2663-8.
21. Robinson L, Gallos ID, Conner SJ, Rajkhowa M, Miller D, Lewis S, et al. The effect of sperm DNA fragmentation on miscarriage rates: a systematic review and meta-analysis. Hum Reprod. 2012;27(10):2908-17.
22. Dar S, Grover SA, Moskovtsev SI, Swanson S, Baratz A, Librach CL. In vitro fertilization-intracytoplasmic sperm injection outcome in patients with a markedly high DNA fragmentation index (>50%). Fertil Steril. 2013;pii:S0015-0282(13)00412-3.
23. Evenson DP, Darzynkiewicz Z, Melamed MR. Relation of mammalian sperm chromatin heterogeneity to fertility. Science. 1980;210(4474):1131-3.
24. Evenson D, Jost L. Sperm chromatin structure assay is useful for fertility assessment. Methods Cell Sci. 2000;22(2-3):169-89.
25. Evenson DP, Larson KL, Jost LK. Sperm chromatin structure assay: its clinical use for detecting sperm DNA fragmentation in male infertility and comparisons with other techniques. J Androl. 2002;23(1):25-43.
26. Larson K, DeJonge C, Barnes A, Jost LK, Evenson DP. Sperm chromatin structure assay parameters as predictors of failed pregnancy following assisted reproductive techniques. Hum Reprod. 2000;15(8):1717-22.
27. Barroso G, Morshedi M, Oehninger S. Analysis of DNA fragmentation, plasma membrane translocation of phosphatidylserine and oxidative stress in human spermatozoa. Hum Reprod. 2000;15(6):1338-44.
28. Ostling O, Johanson K. Microelectrophoretic study of radiation-induced DNA damages on individual cells. Biochem Biophys Res Commun. 1984;123(1):291-8.
29. Aravindan GR, Bjordahl J, Jost LK, Evenson DP. Susceptibility of human sperm to in situ DNA denaturation is strongly correlated with DNA strand breaks identified by single-cell electrophoresis. Exp Cell Res. 1997;236(1):231-7.
30. Singh NP, McCoy MT, Tice RR, Schneider EL. A simple technique for quantitation of low levels of DNA damage in individual cells. Exp Cell Res. 1988;175(1):184-91.
31. Calvin HI, Bedford JM. Formation of disulfide bonds in the nucleus and accessory structures of mammalian spermatozoa during maturation in the epididymis. J Reprod Fertil Suppl. 1971;13(Suppl 13):65-75.
32. Fernández JL, Muriel L, Goyanes V, Segrelles E, Gosálvez J, Enciso M, et al. Simple determination of human sperm DNA fragmentation with an improved sperm chromatin dispersion test. Fertil Steril. 2005;84(4):833-42.
33. Zhang LH, Qiu Y, Wang KH, Wang Q, Tao G, Wang LG. Measurement of sperm DNA fragmentation using bright-field microscopy: comparison between sperm chromatin dispersion test and terminal uridine nick-end labeling assay. Fertil Steril. 2010;94(3):1027-32.
34. Cortés-Gutiérrez EI, Dávila-Rodríguez MI, López-Fernández C, Fernández JL, Gosálvez J. Assessing sperm DNA damage. Actas Urol Esp. 2007;31(2):120-31.
35. Gopalkrishnan K, Hurkadli K, Padwal V, Balaiah D. Use of acridine orange to evaluate chromatin integrity of human spermatozoa in different groups of infertile men. Andrologia. 1999;31(5):277-82.
36. Fernández J, Goyanes V, Ramiro-Díaz J, Gosálvez J. Application of FISH for in situ detection and quantification of DNA breakage. Cytogenet Cell Genet. 1998;82(3-4):251-6.
37. Fernández JL, Vazquez-Gundin F, Delgado A, Goyanes VJ, Ramiro-Díaz J, de la Torre J, et al. DNA breakage detection-FISH (DBD-FISH) in human spermatozoa: technical

variants evidence different structural features. Mutat Res. 2000;453(1):77-82.

38. Andreetta AM, Stockert JC, Barrera C. A simple method to detect sperm chromatin abnormalities: cytochemical mechanism and possible value in predicting semen quality in assisted reproductive procedures. Int J Androl. 1995; 18(Suppl 1):23-8.
39. Manicardi GC, Bianchi PG, Pantano S, Azzoni P, Bizzaro D, Bianchi U, et al. Presence of endogenous nicks in DNA of ejaculated human spermatozoa and its relationship to chromomycin A3 accessibility. Biol Reprod. 1995;52(4):864-7.
40. World Health Organization. (2021). WHO laboratory manual for the examination and processing of human semen, 2021. Accessed at: https://www.who.int/publications/i/item/9789240030787.
41. Schlegel PN, Sigman M, Collura B, De Jonge CJ, Eisenberg ML, Lamb DJ, et al. 2020 Diagnosis and Treatment of Infertility in Men: AUA/ASRM Guideline. Fertil Steril. 2021;115(1):62-9.

CHAPTER 101

# Advanced Sperm Preparation Techniques in Assisted Reproductive Technology

*Natchandra Chimote, Bindu Chimote*

## INTRODUCTION

About 12–15% couples all over the world face the problem of infertility for various reasons. Out of which almost 50% of the infertility cases are due to male factor. For last five decades, assisted reproductive technology (ART) has been trying to become a viable solution to overcome the inability of male patients' spermatozoa to fertilize the oocyte and obtain a viable pregnancy and subsequently a healthy child, yet the efficiency of the different techniques has still the scope to improve on the results of ART. According to the latest reports of the European Society of Human Reproduction and Embryology (ESHRE) and the Centers for Disease Control and Prevention (CDC) of the United States, the percentages of deliveries per ART cycle in 2014 and 2016 were 21 and 22%, respectively. Among many reasons for this relatively low efficiency, the quality of the spermatozoa has been turned out to be critical factor. Mainly the occurrence of high percentages of fragmented deoxyribonucleic acid (DNA) of spermatozoa in ejaculates is possibly one of the major factors causing limited outcomes in ART. Thus, to ensure separation or selection of highest quality of spermatozoa has become one of the main challenges in reproductive medicine, particularly their genetic integrity. The most modern techniques for separation and selection of human spermatozoa are discussed in this chapter with a main focus on sperm DNA integrity, the fertilizing potential, top quality embryo development in vitro, implantation potential, viable pregnancy and live birth following in vitro fertilization (IVF) and intracytoplasmic sperm injection (ICSI).

At ejaculation, tens of millions of spermatozoa are deposited by the human male into the upper part of the vagina near the cervical orifice. Their journey starts from here through the genital tract like a competitive race to reach the oocyte first and fertilize it in ampulla part of fallopian tube.[1,2] In the human, out of the total number of ejaculated spermatozoa, only about 10% will enter the cervix, 1% the uterus, and 0.1% the fallopian tube. Eventually, out of the $10^2$–$10^3$ spermatozoa that will reach the cumulus-oocyte complex, usually only one spermatozoon will fertilize the egg.[1] Hence, it follows that an extremely stringent selection process of spermatozoa, which is essential for fertilization to produce healthy offspring, is occurring, in which the female genital tract is involved. With the advent of ART, sperm separation strategies from seminal plasma were developed, which are mainly based on motility, and adhesion and filtration processes.[3,4] While in the early years of ART, the focus was rather on obtaining motile spermatozoa, in later years, the focus shifted to the isolation of functional spermatozoa, a requirement dictated by the observations that functional sperm parameters are correlated with the results of fertilization in vitro.[5] The spermatozoa of all placental (eutherian) mammals, including humans, are in a protective, nonlabile state at ejaculation and are incapable of fertilization even if they are placed in direct contact with an oocyte. Consequently, they must undergo a subsequent period of final maturation during which they acquire the capacity to interact with the oocyte-cumulus complex and achieve fertilization. This process, which was discovered independently by Austin and Chang in 1951, was termed capacitation, and spermatozoa in the ejaculate are prevented from undergoing capacitation by one or more decapacitation factors that are present in the seminal plasma.[6] Capacitation of eutherian spermatozoa is essential for fertilization not only in vivo but also in vitro, and underlies the manipulation of spermatozoa for clinical IVF.

Seminal plasma not only contain one or more decapacitation factors that prevent natural capacitation of spermatozoa after ejaculation, but also contains one or more factors that have adverse effects on sperm functions such as its ability to penetrate though viscous cervical mucus[7], to undergo acrosome reaction in vitro, and overall fertilization process.[8-10] Therefore, to avoid these factors and to retain capacity to fertilize oocyte, separation of spermatozoa from seminal plasma is the essential prerequisite step to maintain ability for capacitation and express their intrinsic fertilizing ability. In ART laboratories, this requirement is manifested in the process commonly referred to as *sperm washing*, in which spermatozoa are removed from the seminal plasma and resuspended in culture medium.

It must be noted that, prolonged exposure to seminal plasma (>30 minutes) can permanently diminish the fertilizing potential of spermatozoa after ejaculation in vitro.[8] Even contamination caused by small traces of seminal plasma in the prepared sperm sample can diminish or totally inhibit their fertilizing potential.[11] Therefore, spermatozoa for clinical procedures such as intrauterine insemination (IUI) or IVF (and also for laboratory tests of sperm fertilizing ability) must be separated from the seminal plasma environment not only as soon as possible after ejaculation (allowing for the required waiting time for liquefaction) but also as efficiently as possible.

Approximately 2–4% of births in developed countries involve the use of ART.[12] With ART, semen samples must first be processed before they can be used for insemination. In fact, sperm preparation methods in vitro imitate the natural process in which viable sperm are separated from other constituents of the ejaculate as they actively migrate through the cervical mucus.[13]

If spermatozoa are not separated from seminal plasma within 30 minutes of ejaculation, the fertilizing capacity permanently diminishes[14], hence the World Health Organization (WHO)[15] recommends separating sperm cells from the seminal plasma within 1 hour after ejaculation to limit damage from leukocytes and other cells present in the seminal plasma.

Various sperm separation or isolation methods exist to select sperm cells. These include swim-up methods, two-layer discontinuous gradient centrifugation, pentoxifylline wash, test-yolk buffer, sedimentation methods and polyvinylpyrrolidone (PVP) droplet swim-out, electrophoresis, and fluorescence cell sorting methods.[16] A number of these have been developed to separate viable sperm from the seminal ejaculate for use in ART such as swim-down, swim-up, migration-sedimentation, density gradient centrifugation, magnetic activated cell sorting (MACS), and glass wool filtration. This chapter will discuss these techniques—the more commonly used procedures are explained in detail. It will also explain the procedures used to prepare viscous semen samples as well as when to obtain and prepare semen samples using epididymal and testicular spermatozoa, assisted ejaculation, and retrograde ejaculation. The ideal sperm separation technique should:

- Be quick, easy, and cost-effective,
- Isolate as much motile spermatozoa as possible,
- Not cause sperm damage or nonphysiological alterations of the separated sperm cells,
- Eliminate dead spermatozoa and other cells, including leukocytes and bacteria,
- Eliminate toxic or bioactive substances like decapacitation factors or reactive oxygen species (ROS), and
- Allow processing of larger volumes of ejaculates.

Since none of the methods available meets all these requirements, a variety of sperm separation techniques are mandatory in clinical practice to obtain an optimal yield of functionally competent spermatozoa for insemination purposes. Depending on the ejaculate quality, these methods have different efficiency and areas of use. In the conventional swim-up technique, functional spermatozoa can come into close cell-to-cell contact with defective sperm or leukocytes by centrifugation, thus causing massive oxidative damages of the sperm plasma membrane by ROS and consequently of sperm functions.[17] Therefore, the quality of the ejaculates has direct consequences on the choice of a sperm separation method.

## SIMPLE WASH METHOD

In the simple wash method, following complete liquefaction, culture medium is added to the ejaculate (2:1 parts ratio) and centrifuged twice to remove the seminal plasma. It is essential to use lower centrifugal forces (<500 g) and fewer centrifugation steps to minimize the damage caused by formation of ROS by nonviable spermatozoa and leukocytes.[14] Increased levels of ROS result in DNA damage in spermatozoa, decreased sperm motility, increased numbers of apoptotic spermatozoa, and decreased sperm plasma membrane integrity.[18] Additionally, the presence of large numbers of nonviable spermatozoa in the prepared sample can inhibit capacitation a physiological process that confers spermatozoa with the ability to fertilize an oocyte.[18] The simple wash technique is usually used when the semen sample has optimal parameters. This technique is often used to prepare sperm cells for IUI because it produces very high-yields of spermatozoa.

## MIGRATION-BASED TECHNIQUES

### Swim-up

Swim-up is one of the most commonly used techniques for sperm preparation. Swim-up can be performed using a cell pellet or a liquefied semen sample. In conventional swim-up, a prewashed sperm pellet obtained by a soft spin is placed in an overlaying culture medium in a conical tube **(Fig. 1)**. The common steps of this method (using a cell pellet) are as follows:

- Allow specimen to liquefy completely for 15–30 minutes in a 37°C incubator before processing.
- Measure volume using a sterile 2 mL pipette.
- Transfer specimen from a plastic cup to a sterile 15 mL-conical centrifuge tube. If specimen is >3 mL, split the specimen into two aliquots.

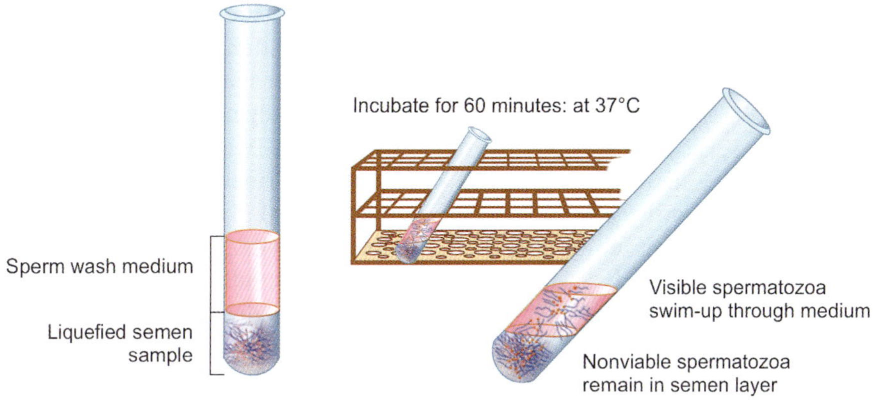


**Fig. 1:** A prewashed sperm pellet obtained by a soft spin.

- Gently mix the specimen with Quinn's Sperm Wash Media [human tubal fluid (HTF)] in a ratio of 1:4 using a sterile Pasteur Pipette.
- Centrifuge the tubes at 1,600 rpm for 10 minutes.
- Examine for sperm count and motility. Carefully aspirate the supernatant without disturbing the pellet and resuspend the pellet in 3 mL of fresh HTF. Transfer the resuspended sample into two 15 mL sterile round bottom tubes using a sterile serological pipette (1.5 mL in each).
- Centrifuge the tubes at 500 rpm for 5 minutes.
- Incubate the tubes at a 45° angle for 1 hour for swim-up in vertical rack in a 37°C incubator.
- After the incubation period, aspirate the entire supernatant from the round bottom tube. Use a Pasteur Pipette, with the tip placed just about the pellet surface.
- Pool supernatant from the two round bottom tubes into a single 15 mL conical centrifuge tube. Centrifuge the tube at 1,600 rpm for 7 minutes.
- Aspirate the supernatant from the top of the meniscus using a Pasteur Pipette.
- Resuspend the pellet in a volume of 0.5 mL HTF using a 1 mL sterile pipette. Record the final volume.

*Note:* Sterile techniques should be used throughout specimen processing. When examining the specimen, it is important to pay particular attention to extraneous round cells, debris, and bacteria that may be present. The medium used in this technique provides the sperm with a nourishing environment and attracts the sperm cells. The spermatozoa leave the pellet and swim into the medium. The sperm cells furthest away from the pellet are retrieved since they have the greatest probability of being motile and morphologically normal.

The swim-up method has been modified for oligozoospermic men.[19] This modified method is called direct swim-up and involves swim-up from semen rather than swim-up from the cell pellet. Direct swim-up is the simplest and fastest method for separating sperm by migration. Round-bottom tubes are used for direct swim-up to maximize the surface area between the semen and medium.[14] Multiple tubes with small volumes can be used to further increase this interface area and increase the number of motile sperm retrieved.[19] With this particular procedure, incubation is performed at 34.5°C, which has been reported to result in higher motility than incubation at 37°C.[20]

The swim-up method is simple and relatively inexpensive.[3] Yet, it has some disadvantages:

- Centrifugation, which is performed to create a cell pellet before conventional swim-up, has been shown to generate ROS.[21]
- The amount of motile spermatozoa retrieved is relatively low.
- Only 5–10% of the sperm cells subjected to swim-up are retrieved.
- When a concentrated cell pellet is used, some motile spermatozoa may be trapped in the middle of the pellet and thus may not travel as far as the sperm cells at the edges of the pellet.

Considering that the efficiency of the technique is based on the surface of the cell pellet and the initial sperm motility in the ejaculate, the yield of motile spermatozoa is limited. Many layers of cells in the pellet may cause potentially motile spermatozoa in the lower levels of the pellet never to reach the interface with the culture medium layer. In addition, a significant decrease in the percentage of normally chromatin-condensed spermatozoa has been reported after the swim-up procedure.[22] Another major disadvantage of this technique is the fact that for its use spermatozoa are pelleted, thus coming into close cell-to-cell contact with each other, cell debris and leukocytes, which are known to produce very high levels of ROS.[23] Due to the extraordinary high amount of polyunsaturated fatty acids in the sperm's plasma membranes,[24] these ROS cause lipid peroxidation and therefore a dramatic decrease in sperm functions, including motility.[25] Overall, although many men's spermatozoa may not be impaired to the extent of inhibiting fertilization, some couples' chances of successful IVF will certainly be

**TABLE 1:** Advantages and disadvantages of the original migration-sedimentation method according to Tea, et al., (1984).

| *Advantages* | *Disadvantages* |
|---|---|
| Usually very clean fraction of highly motile spermatozoa | The original method is restricted to ejaculates of high sperm count and good motility. The original method has a very low recovery rate |
| Reactive oxygen species are reduced | • Special glass or plastic tubes are required<br>• Tubes are more expensive and relatively sensitive |
| Very gentle separation method | For repeated use in in vitro fertilization, glass and plastic tubes must be sterilized |

compromised. It is therefore not reasonable to continue and to use a technique, such as swim-up from pelleted semen with the inherent potential to cause irrevocable damage to spermatozoa prejudicial to a desired functional endpoint. Eventually, this knowledge led to the development of other more gentle sperm separation methods that also allow a higher recovery of motile and functional spermatozoa. The advantages and disadvantages of the conventional swim-up are summarized in **Table 1**.

## Migration-sedimentation

Direct swim-up from semen is used for sperm samples with average or good motility. On the other hand, migration-sedimentation is usually used for samples with low motility.[26] Migration-sedimentation uses the swim-up technique but also relies on the natural settling of spermatozoa due to gravity. Sperm cells migrate from a ring-shaped well into a culture medium above and then settle through the central hole of the ring. Special tubes called Tea-Jondet tubes are used for migration-sedimentation.[26]

The advantage of this technique is that it is a gentle method, and thus the amount of ROS produced is not very significant. On the other hand, the special tubes that are needed are relatively expensive.[24]

## Swim-down

This technique relies on the natural movement of spermatozoa. A discontinuous bovine serum albumin medium is prepared. This medium becomes progressively less concentrated moving from top to bottom. The semen sample is placed onto the top of the medium, and the tube is incubated at 37°C for 1 hour.[26] During migration, the most motile sperm move downward into the gradient.

## Density Gradient Centrifugation

Density gradient centrifugation separates sperm cells based on their density. Thus, at the end of centrifugation, each spermatozoon is located at the gradient level that matches its density.[14] Morphologically, normal and abnormal spermatozoa have different densities. A mature morphologically normal spermatozoon has a density of at least 1.10 g/mL whereas an immature and morphologically abnormal spermatozoon has a density between 1.06 g/mL and 1.09 g/mL.[27] As a result, the resulting interphases between seminal plasma and 40% density gradient, 40 and 80% density gradients containing leukocytes, cell debris and morphologically abnormal sperm with poor motility, are discarded. The highly motile, morphologically normal, viable spermatozoa form a pellet at the bottom of the tube. Centrifugal force and time should be kept at the lowest possible values (<300 g) in order to minimize the production of ROS by leukocytes and nonviable sperm cells.[28] Also, nonviable sperm cells and debris should be separated from viable sperm cells as soon as possible to minimize oxidative damage.[29]

Density gradients can either be continuous or discontinuous. Density gradually increases from the top of a continuous gradient to its bottom. There are clear boundaries between layers of discontinuous gradients.[3] The latter gradient is formed when a number of layers of decreasing density are placed on top of each other.[14] Double density gradients comprise the commonly used sperm preparation protocol for ART.[14] Components of the density gradient sperm separation procedure include a colloidal suspension of silica particles stabilized with covalently bonded hydrophilic silane supplied in {[4-(2-hydroxyethyl)-1-piperazine ethane sulfonic acid] HEPES}. There are two gradients: (1) a lower phase (90%) and (2) an upper phase (45%). Sperm washing medium (modified HTF with 5.0 mg/mL human albumin) is used to wash and resuspend the final pellet **(Fig. 2)**.

Below are some of the main steps of the process:

- Place all components of the upper and lower phase and semen samples in an incubator at 37°C for 20 minutes.
- Transfer 2 mL of the lower phase into a sterile conical-bottom, disposable centrifuge tube.
- Layer 2 mL of the upper phase on top of the lower phase using a transfer pipette. Slowly dispense the upper phase lifting the pipette up the side of the tube as the level of the upper phase rises. A distinct line separating the two layers will be observed. This two-layer gradient is stable for up to 2 hours.
- Measure semen volume to be loaded using a sterile 2 mL pipette. Remove a drop of semen using sterile technique for count, percent motility, and presence of round cells.
- Gently place up to 3 mL of liquefied semen onto the upper phase (leaving approximately 0.1 mL in original container for a prewash analysis). If volume is >3 mL, it may be necessary to split the specimen into two tubes before processing.
- Centrifuge for 20 minutes at 1,600 rpm.

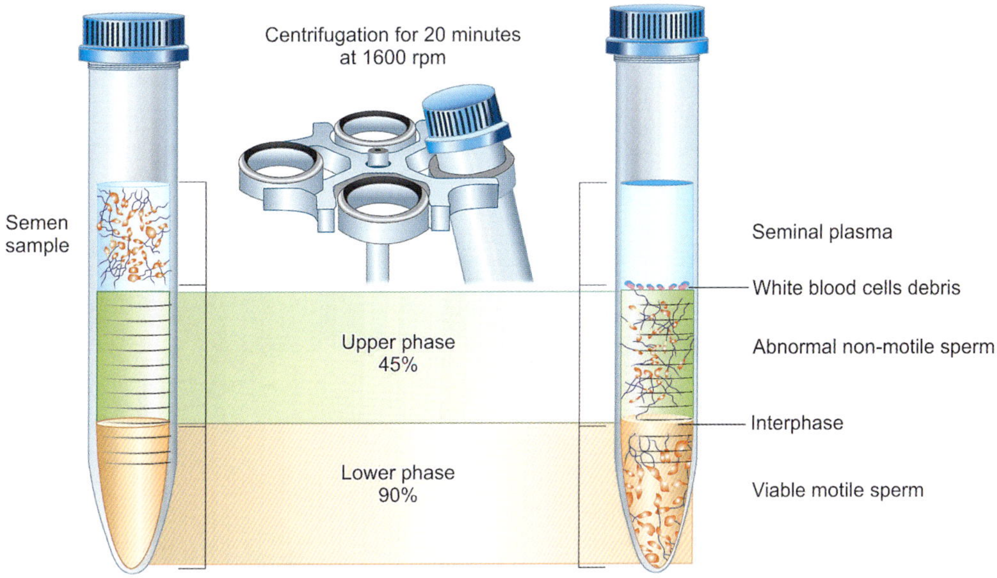


**Fig. 2:** Density gradient centrifugation. The lower and upper gradients are carefully layered and the seminal ejaculate layered on the top. The sample is centrifuged at 1,600 rpm for 20 minutes. Clear seminal plasma is retained on the uppermost part of the gradient followed by a clear separation of white blood cells, debris, and other cells. The immature, abnormal sperm are seen along the gradient based on their density and motility. Highly motile normal sperm move actively to the bottom of the gradient and collected as a pellet.

*Note:* Occasionally, samples that do not liquefy properly and remain too viscous to pass through the gradient will be encountered. Increasing the centrifugal force up to but no >600 × g will aid in separating the sperm in these cases.

- Using a transfer pipette, add 2 mL of HTF and resuspend pellet. Mix gently with pipette until sperm pellet is in suspension.
- Centrifuge for 7 minutes at 1,600 rpm.
- Again, remove supernatant from the centrifuge tube using a transfer pipette down to the pellet.
- Resuspend the final pellet in a volume of 0.5 mL using a 1 mL sterile pipette with HTF. Record the final volume.
- The advantages and disadvantages of density gradient centrifugation are listed in **Table 2**.

**TABLE 2:** The advantages and disadvantages of density gradient centrifugation.

| *Advantages of density gradient centrifugation* | *Disadvantages of density gradient centrifugation* |
|---|---|
| Density gradient centrifugation requires maximally a 30 minutes centrifugation. It takes less time than the swim-up technique which requires 1 hour incubation | Production of good interphases between layers can take some time |
| Density gradient centrifugation is relatively easy to perform under sterile conditions | There is a risk of contamination with endotoxins |
| Spermatozoa from oligozoospermic semen can be effectively separated with density gradient centrifugation[3] | Some scientists have claimed that density gradient centrifugation negatively affects sperm DNA integrity. For instance, spermatozoa recovered after density gradient centrifugation possess lower DNA integrity than spermatozoa recovered after swim-up[23] |
| Density gradient centrifugation eliminates the majority of leukocytes in the ejaculate | |

## TIPS TO MAXIMIZE THE SPERM YIELD

- It is important to make sure that all components of the gradient and sperm wash medium are at room to body temperature before use. This will protect spermatozoa from *cold shock*. In addition, any condensation on the media bottles will disappear, which aids in the visual detection of contamination. Any bottle whose contents appear in any way cloudy or hazy should not be used.
- Do not use the same pipette in more than one bottle of media.
- Prolonged exposure to a 5% $CO_2$ environment will alter the pH of these products, which may in turn affect their nature and performance.
- Highly viscous semen usually should be treated with 5 mg of trypsin, dissolved in 1.0 mL of sperm washing media and added to the ejaculate 5 minutes before loading on the upper gradient. This will increase the motile sperm yield without causing any measurable damage to the motile sperm.
- Avoid overloading the gradient as it causes a phenomenon called *rafting*. Rafting is the aggregation of desirable as

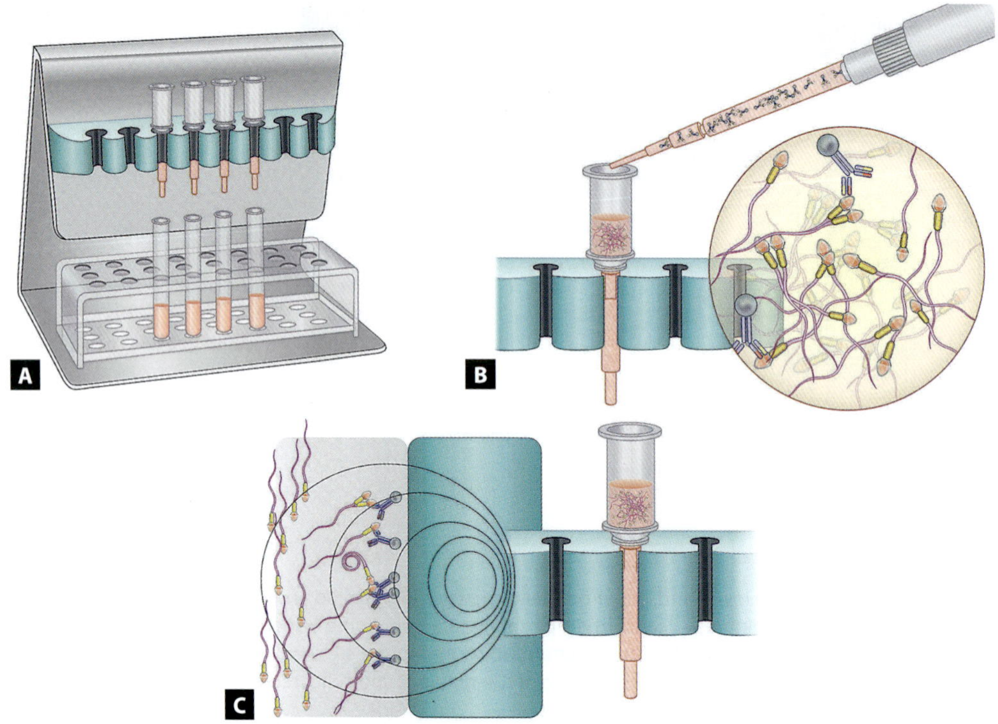


**Figs. 3A to C:** Magnetic activated cell sorting: (A) The Octet magnetic collection device can be used for loading up to a maximum of 8 samples. The tubes are placed between each open slot surrounded by the magnetic field; (B) The apoptotic and the nonapoptotic cells are labeled with the annexin V antibody beads (magnetic). These attach to the outer surface of the sperm that are apoptotic. Annexin V beads (magnetic) do not bind to the sperm that are nonapoptotic and have intact membranes; (C) Apoptotic sperm with annexin V beads (magnetic) are retained in the column while the nonapoptotic sperm are eluted out and collected in a tube below the collection device.

well as undesirable components of the semen that will be present in the postcentrifugation pellet. Use the gradient within 1 hour after creating it—eventually the two phases over time blend into each other and a sharp interface will not exist.

- Percoll™, a colloidal suspension of silica particles coated with polyvinylpyrrolidone, was widely used by ART laboratories until it was withdrawn from the market for clinical use. Nowadays, media containing silane-coated silica particles are commonly used. Isolate™ (Irvine Scientific, Santa Ana, CA), Ixa Prep™, Sperm preparation medium™ and Supra Sperm™ (ORIGIO, MediCult, Copenhagen, Denmark), SpermGrad™ (Vitrolife, San Diego, CA), SilSelect™ (Ferti Pro NV, Beernem, Belgium), and PureSperm™ (Nidacon Laboratories AB, Gothenburg, Sweden) are commonly used.[3]

## MAGNETIC-ACTIVATED CELL SORTING

Magnetic-activated cell sorting separates apoptotic spermatozoa from nonapoptotic spermatozoa. During apoptosis (programmed cell death), phosphatidyl serine residues are translocated from the inner membrane of the spermatozoa to the outside. Annexin V has a strong affinity for phosphatidyl serine but cannot pass through the intact sperm membrane. Colloidal superparamagnetic beads (~50 nm in diameter) are conjugated to highly specific antibodies to annexin V and used to separate dead and apoptotic spermatozoa by MACS. Annexin V binding to spermatozoa indicates compromised sperm membrane integrity.

A 100 μL sperm sample is mixed with 100 μL of MACS microbeads and incubated at room temperature for 15 minutes. The mixture is loaded on top of the separation column which is placed in the magnetic field [0.5 Tesla (T) between the poles of the magnet and 1.5 T within the iron globes of the column]; 1 Tesla = 10,000 gauss **(Figs. 3A and B)**. The column is rinsed with buffer. All the unlabeled (annexin V-negative) nonapoptotic spermatozoa pass through the column **(Fig. 3C)**. The annexin V-positive (apoptotic) fraction is retained in the column. The column is removed from the magnetic field, and annexin V-positive fraction is eluted using the annexin V-binding buffer.[16] The procedure is explained in **Figures 3A to C**.

Spermatozoa prepared by density gradient centrifugation followed by MACS have a higher percentage of motility, higher percentage viability, and a lower expression of apoptotic markers than spermatozoa prepared by density gradient centrifugation alone.[30] Annexin V-negative spermatozoa have a higher motility, lower caspase activation, lower membrane mitochondrial potential disruption, lowers amount of DNA damage, and

**TABLE 3:** The advantages and disadvantages of magnetic activated cell sorting (MACS).

| *Advantages of MACS* | *Disadvantages of MACS* |
|---|---|
| • MACS acts at the molecular level as opposed to routine sperm preparation techniques that rely on sperm density and motility<br>• MACS is the only known technique which separates apoptotic spermatozoa from nonapoptotic spermatozoa<br>• MACS is rapid, convenient, and noninvasive<br>• Bead detachment after MACS is not necessary<br>• MACS provides optimal purity and recovery with reliable and consistent results<br>• MACS can used to optimize the cryopreservation-thawing outcome and enhance cryosurvival rates following cryopreservation | Viable spermatozoa ought to be separated from all substances in the ejaculate such as apoptotic spermatozoa, leukocytes, and seminal plasma. MACS, which removes apoptotic spermatozoa, needs to be used in conjunction with other techniques such as density gradient centrifugation to remove the other substances |

higher oocyte penetration capacity than annexin V-positive spermatozoa.[29] MACS improves the acrosome reaction in couples with unexplained fertility.[27,31] Annexin V-negative sperm cells show significantly higher motility and survival rates following cryopreservation than annexin V-positive sperm cells.[32] Dirican, et al.,[33] reported that spermatozoa selected by MACS were associated with higher cleavage and pregnancy rates than spermatozoa selected by density gradient centrifugation in oligoasthenozoospermia cases.

The advantages and disadvantages of MACS are outlined in **Table 3**.

## GLASS WOOL FILTRATION

During glass wool filtration, which has already been described by Paulson and Polakoski in 1977,[34] motile spermatozoa are separated from immotile sperm cells by means of densely packed glass wool fibers. The principle of this sperm separation technique lies in both the self-propelled movement of the spermatozoa and the filtration effect of the glass wool. The success of this method is directly linked to the kind of glass wool used.[35] Thus, factors like the chemical nature of the glass (i.e., borate glass, silicate glass, or quartz glass), the surface structure and charge of the glass wool, thickness of the glass wool fibers or the pore size of the filter have to be taken into consideration. Potential risks of the technique such as damages of the spermatozoa or the occurrence of glass wool fragments in the filtrate essentially depend on the kind of glass wool used and on the intensity of the washing prior to the filtration.

Compared with the swim-up or migration-sedimentation, glass wool filtration, just as density gradient centrifugation, is a technique that uses the whole volume of the ejaculate and therefore yields a significantly higher total number of motile spermatozoa.[22,36] Thus, it can also be used for patients with oligo- and/or asthenozoospermia.[36] Like density gradient centrifugation, glass wool filtration also provides the advantage that the sperm separation can directly be performed from the ejaculate. Only after the separation of the functional spermatozoa from the immotile ones, leukocytes and debris, a centrifugation step will be necessary to remove the seminal plasma. This is an important aspect as this procedure reduces cellular damage by ROS.

By means of glass wool filtration, it is even possible to prepare motile spermatozoa from patients with retrograde ejaculation.[4] In these cases, the procedure includes adjustment of the osmolarity of the patient's urine to values of about 350 mOsmol/kg by drinking water. Prior to the ejaculation, the patients are requested to urinate most of the urine in the bladder. The small amount of antegrade-produced ejaculate is collected in a plastic beaker, while the retrograde fraction of the ejaculate needs to be urinated immediately into a jar with 50 mL culture medium containing human serum albumin to dilute the urine. Finally, the urine/medium mixture has to be centrifuged, resuspended in 3–4 mL of fresh medium and filtrated on the glass wool column. As constituents of the urine can damage the spermatozoa, a speedy work-up of such ejaculates is mandatory. In addition to the separation of spermatozoa, glass wool filtration has been shown to eliminate leukocytes to an extent of up to 90%.[37] Since leukocytes are frequent even in normal ejaculates[38] and produce 100-times more ROS than spermatozoa,[23] this effect significantly contributes to a reduction of free radicals in the ejaculate.[35,37] This is of paramount importance for the functionality of spermatozoa because the male germ cells are particularly susceptible to oxidation by ROS because of their extraordinary high content of polyunsaturated fatty acids in their plasma membrane.[24,39,40]

Another clinically interesting aspect related to glass wool filtration is chromatin condensation, which has repeatedly been shown to be predictive of fertilization in vitro.[40-43] Glass wool filtration[22] like the density gradient centrifugation with Pure Sperm®[44] or the migration-sedimentation technique[45] significantly selects normally chromatin-condensed spermatozoa, while conventional swim-up or Percoll® centrifugation decrease this sperm parameter. As human sperm chromatin condensation follows a seasonal rhythm, which even shows a shift of about half a year on the southern hemisphere,[46] this might have a clinical impact on the results in IVF. Should a patient be examined in winter when the quality of sperm chromatin condensation is high[46] and referred to IVF in summer when the percentage of normally chromatin-condensed spermatozoa is significantly lower,

**TABLE 4:** The advantages and disadvantages of glass wool filtration.

| Advantages | Disadvantages |
|---|---|
| • Simple to perform<br>• Normally, recovery of spermatozoa with good motility<br>• Spermatozoa from ejaculates with a very low sperm density can be separated<br>• Good yield<br>• Leukocytes are eliminated to a large extent<br>• Reactive oxygen species are significantly reduced | • Bit more expensive<br>• The filtrate is not as clean as it is with other sperm separation methods<br>• Remnants of debris are still present |

IVF for this patient might fail. Thus, for these patients a sperm separation by means of glass wool filtration, Pure Sperm® or migration-sedimentation might be beneficial.

The advantages and disadvantages of this method are summarized in **Table 4**.

## GLASS BEADS

This method has been used for the preparation of hamster spermatozoa for in vitro capacitation[47] and resulted in an efficient, high-yield selection of motile human spermatozoa from semen.[48] However, there were concerns regarding the possible spillover of beads into the insemination medium. As a result, the use of glass beads for effective sperm preparation for assisted reproduction has not widely been accepted.

## SEPHADEX COLUMNS

In the early nineties sperm separation by means of Sephadex beads emerged[49] and a commercial sperm separation kit based on this principle (Sperm Prep®) has become available. Compared to migration-sedimentation and swim-up from pelleted semen it produced significantly higher yields.[50] Moreover, morphologically normal sperm cells could be enriched in the filtrate after Sperm Prep® separation as well as significantly higher pregnancy rates for IUI as compared with the conventional swim-up method.[51] Sperm Prep® method when compared to and Percoll® centrifugation, Percoll® separated spermatozoa showed a significantly higher percentage of normally chromatin-condensed and morphologically normal spermatozoa.[52] However, the fertilization rates reported by these authors were similar. López, et al.,[53] used a prepacked PD-10 column containing Sephadex G-25 particles (Pharmacia Biotechnology, Uppsala, Sweden), which is normally used to desalt proteins in solutions, to separate human spermatozoa and compared the results with the Sperm Prep® method and Percoll® centrifugation. The PD-10 column and density gradient centrifugation in Percoll® yielded a comparable number of spermatozoa and showed similar percentages of morphologically normal spermatozoa after sperm separation. On the contrary, the Sperm Prep® method resulted in significantly lower values of sperm count and morphology.

## TRANSMEMBRANE MIGRATION

Another alternative sperm separation technique that was also developed in the late eighties is migration/filtration of motile spermatozoa through a Nuclepore membrane filter. These filters are unusual because their pores are cylindrical and at right angles to the plane of the membrane.[54] The spermatozoa, therefore, have straight channels to swim through the membrane. Unfortunately, these membranes had a very low ratio of the total cross-sectional area of the pores to the overall membrane area. Consequently, the yield is extremely low. Primarily, this method was used for testing the motility of sperm populations treated with various pharmacological agents, but not as a preparation method for assisted reproduction.[55]

Another approach of separating viable human spermatozoa by means of membranes was undertaken by Agarwal, et al.,[56] using a membrane which has been developed for selective removal of leukocytes (L4 membrane). Besides, a significant increase of motility, ejaculates filtered through this membrane have been shown to contain fewer leukocytes. This fact is, of course, of importance in those cases that have increased numbers of leukocytes in the ejaculate as a result of infections. Moreover, this membrane seems to be selective for spermatozoa with normal membrane integrity [57, 58] and sperm producing low amounts of ROS.[59] However, despite these advantages of the membrane it has never come into practical clinical use for human assisted reproduction.

## REDUCTION OF SEMEN VISCOSITY

Human semen normally liquefies within 5–20 minutes after ejaculation.[9] However, some ejaculates fail to liquefy and some are viscous by nature. Semen viscosity is a problem since it can reduce sperm motility. To reduce viscosity, the semen can be mixed with a medium. Liquefaction achieved by this method might not be adequate for highly viscous samples. Forcing the viscous semen through a needle with a narrow gauge is another option. However, this technique damages the sperm cells.[9] A commonly used viscosity treatment system involves enzymatic liquefaction using trypsin (5 mg). These can also be obtained prepackaged in 5 mg vials (VTS; Vitrolife, San Diego, CA). If the sample fails to completely liquefy following 20 minutes of incubation at 37°C, trypsin is added directly to the semen specimen. The specimen is then swirled and incubated for an additional 10 minutes. This results in complete liquefaction of the sample.

## WHEN TO USE A PARTICULAR SPERM PREPARATION TECHNIQUE

The choice of sperm preparation method depends on the characteristics of the semen sample. When sperm parameters such as concentration and motility are within the normal ranges, the direct swim-up technique is preferred.[15] For significantly oligozoospermic, teratozoospermic, and asthenozoospermic samples, density gradient centrifugation is preferred since density gradient centrifugation leads to a higher recovery of motile sperm cells than the swim-up technique. Also, density gradient centrifugation can be modified to address the issues of each individual specimen, and it is the method of choice for sperm preparation in the majority of ART and andrology laboratories.[4] Glass wool filtration is also effective for the separation of sperm cells from semen with suboptimal parameters.[15]

### Sperm Preparation for Assisted Reproductive Techniques

Density gradient centrifugation is usually used to prepare sperm cells for standard IVF. If the semen sample is poor in terms of motility and concentration, ICSI should be considered.[29]

The sperm sample can be prepared for ICSI with density gradient centrifugation or swim-up. Oligozoospermic samples can be prepared using the swim-up technique if there are some viable spermatozoa with forward motility.[29] If needed, sperm cells in oligozoospermic samples can be concentrated with a wash and resuspension. These concentrated samples can be used directly or be subjected to density gradient centrifugation or swim-up before being used. Density gradient centrifugation is a better option than swim-up for significantly oligozoospermic and significantly asthenozoospermic samples as well as for samples with high quantities of debris.[29] The hyposmotic swelling test is also an efficient method for selecting sperm for ICSI.[60]

### Preparation of Epididymal and Testicular Spermatozoa

In case of epididymal obstruction or complete azoospermia, spermatozoa can be obtained from the epididymis or the testicular tissue, both require special preparation. Usually, large numbers of sperm cells can be collected from the epididymis. Sperm samples obtained from the epididymis do not contain a significant amount of nongerm cells such as red blood cells. If sufficient numbers of epididymal sperm cells are collected, density gradient centrifugation can be used to prepare the spermatozoa for ART. On the other hand, the simple wash technique will be used if the number of spermatozoa aspirated is low.[15]

Spermatozoa can be retrieved from the testes by open biopsy or by percutaneous needle biopsy.[15] Testicular samples contain large numbers of nongerm cells such as red blood cells. Spermatozoa need to be separated from these nongerm cells. Also, the elongated spermatids, which are bound to the seminiferous tubules, must be freed. Sperm cells collected from the testes are used in ICSI because low numbers of spermatozoa with poor motility are generally aspirated. Pentoxifylline is occasionally used to increase the motility of epididymal and testicular spermatozoa before ICSI.

### Preparation of Assisted Ejaculation Samples

Direct penile vibratory stimulation or indirect rectal stimulation is used to retrieve semen from men who have disturbed ejaculation or who cannot ejaculate due to health issues such as spinal cord injury. Patients with spinal cord injury often have ejaculates with a high sperm concentration and low sperm motility. These ejaculates are also contaminated with red blood cells and white blood cells.[15] Ejaculates obtained by electroejaculation are most effectively prepared with density gradient centrifugation.[4] It has been reported that semen obtained by vibratory stimulation is of better quality than semen obtained by electroejaculation for men with spinal cord injuries.[61]

### Preparation of Retrograde Ejaculation Samples

Retrograde ejaculation occurs when semen is directed into the urinary bladder during ejaculation. If there is an inadequate number of spermatozoa in the ejaculate, sperm cells in the urine need to be retrieved. At the laboratory, the patient is first asked to urinate without entirely emptying his bladder. Then, he is asked to ejaculate and urinate again into another specimen cup containing 5–6 mL of culture medium, which alkalinizes the urine. The urine sample volume is noted and analyzed after centrifugation.[62] The concentrated retrograde specimen and the antegrade specimen are usually prepared with density gradient centrifugation.[15] The Liverpool solution containing sodium bicarbonate given orally to alkalinize urine have been recently described and was demonstrated to be associated with improved sperm motility.[63]

## LIMITATIONS OF CONVENTIONAL SPERM PREPARATION TECHNIQUES

By employing conventional sperm preparation strategies for ART, natural sperm selection processes taking place at various levels of the female genital tract are bypassed to varying extents. In the case of ICSI, where a single spermatozoon is injected into the oocyte, all natural barriers for fertilization are bypassed and even sperm components that normally do not enter the female gamete are introduced. Thereby, oocyte activation and embryo development could possibly be impaired.[63] Since spermatozoa with nuclear DNA damage are capable of fertilizing oocytes,[64,65] this, depending on the severity of the damage, may cause recurrent pregnancy loss.[66] Additionally, serious concerns regarding the health of the offspring were raised.[67-69] On the other hand, embryos deriving from such germ cells can develop to full term.[70,71] Thus, conventional sperm separation techniques show distinct limitations in that they do not necessarily select spermatozoa according to their functional competence or genetic quality as it is achieved in the female genital tract.

## ADVANCED STRATEGIES OF SPERM SELECTION

Advanced strategies of sperm selection are defined as being based on sophisticated principles that employ physiological selection procedures. These principles are founded either on a more stringent assessment of sperm morphology, which is a sperm characteristic selected for at three different sites in the female **(Fig. 4)**, or on molecular characteristics of mature spermatozoa, which are associated with proper cellular function and genomic integrity.

Currently, advanced selection procedures can be divided into three groups, on the basis of:

1. Sophisticated morphological assessment
2. Electrical charge
3. Molecular binding.

The latter two principles in part mimic female selection mechanisms.

### Selection Based on Morphology

Normal sperm morphology evaluated after fixation on the basis of strict criteria[72] at ×1,000 magnification is regarded as a good predictor of fertilization success in vitro.[73] For ICSI, however, the embryologist selects the most normal (least abnormal)-looking spermatozoon on the basis of light microscopy at magnifications of ×400 in unfixed, unstained, and wet sperm preparations. Success of assisted reproduction is also dependent on the ultramorphology of the spermatozoon that is taken for injection. Therefore, morphological discrimination by means of light microscopy is not good enough as subtle malformations, particularly DNA damage and chromosomal aberrations,[74,75] cannot be detected and defective spermatozoa might be accepted for normal ICSI procedure.[76,77] Ryu, et al.,[78] highlighted the relationship between sperm morphology and genetic abnormalities by showing significantly higher frequencies of aneuploidy in infertile patients.

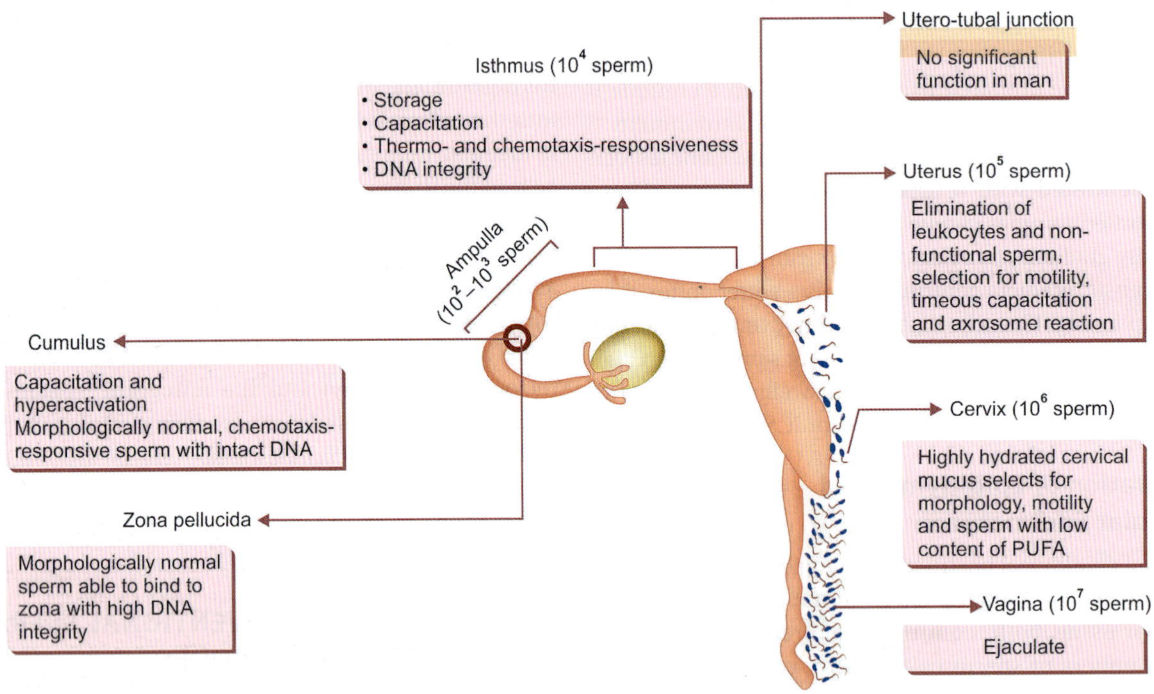


**Fig. 4:** Sites of sperm selection in the human female. Estimated numbers of spermatozoa in the respective sections of the female genital tract are given in brackets. Soon after deposition in the vagina, spermatozoa move out of the seminal plasma and enter the highly hydrated cervical mucus where sperm selection for morphology and motility takes place. Spermatozoa that are selected here are characterized by a low plasma membrane content of polyunsaturated fatty acids (PUFA). Subsequently, spermatozoa are transported through the uterus where male germ cells are selected for motility and timely capacitation. Dysfunctional spermatozoa are eliminated. After passing the uterotubal junction, which has, in contrast to numerous animal species, no significant functions in man, spermatozoa enter the isthmus of the fallopian tube. In the isthmus, spermatozoa can be stored for up to 5 days. In the isthmus and the cumulus, spermatozoa are selected for capacitation, thermo- and chemotaxis-responsiveness and DNA integrity. Finally, after passing through the cumulus, spermatozoa bind to the zona pellucida where another morphological selection takes place. Moreover, male germ cells are further selected for zona-binding ability and DNA integrity PUFA.

## Motile Sperm Organelle Morphological Examination

Since light microscopically invisible damage may be the reason that chromosomal or DNA damage in spermatozoa can be transferred to the progeny,[79] a method that evaluates sperm morphology at higher, digital magnification (×6,300) using Nomarski interference contrast has been developed.[80] With motile sperm organelle morphological examination (MSOME), the morphological status of the acrosome, postacrosomal lamina, neck, mitochondria, flagellum, and the sperm nucleus is examined. For the latter, the shape, as well as the presence and size of vacuoles, is observed. MSOME is now included into ICSI protocols in an increasing number of centers for ART. The combination of MSOME and ICSI has been named intracytoplasmic morphologically selected sperm injection (IMSI) **(Fig. 5)**.[81] Compared with standard ICSI procedures, IMSI has been shown not only to increase fertilization rates,[81] but also implantation and pregnancy rates.[81,82] Concerns have been raised about IMSI because it is expensive and takes with 1.5–5 hours[83] longer than ICSI. Since the normal ICSI procedure is performed at 37°C, the extended exposure of spermatozoa to this temperature might pose a risk to the male germ cell. Peer et al.,[84] exposed human spermatozoa to different temperatures for extended times and found that sperm morphology deteriorated significantly after incubation for 2 hours at 37°C, which was not the case after incubation at 21°C. Therefore, the authors recommended the performance of IMSI at 21°C.

### *Indications for Intracytoplasmic Morphologically Sperm Injection*

The only confirmed indication of IMSI is recurrent implantation failure following ICSI. The literature review results suggest that IMSI is only of value (in terms of higher clinical pregnancy and live birth rates) for patients with one or more previous ICSI failure and not for unselected patients or those undergoing their first treatment attempt.

i. Vacuoles were shown to be linked to chromatin condensation failure[85-88]
ii. Chromatin condensation failure is associated with recurrent abortions[89,90], and
iii. A growing body of evidence suggests that the degree of sperm chromatin condensation at the time of fertilization can influence early and late embryo development.[91]

Current work postulates that the higher pregnancy and delivery rates and lower miscarriage rates observed for IMSI after ICSI failure can be explained (at least in part) by the exclusion of spermatozoa containing sperm head vacuoles of nuclear origin.

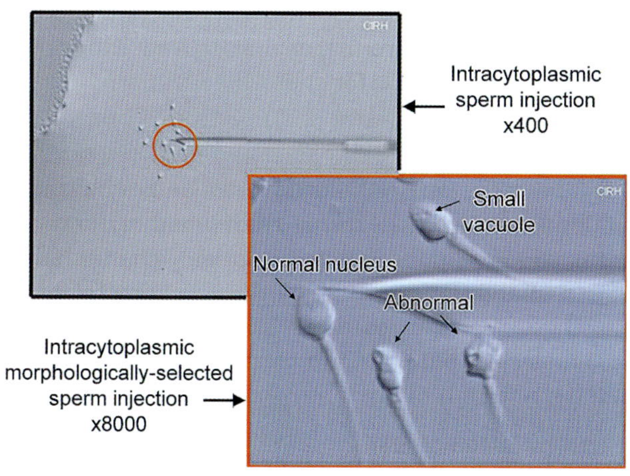


**Fig. 5:** Magnetic sperm organelle morphological examination–intracytoplasmic sperm injection (ICSI): intracytoplasmic morphologically sperm injection (IMSI).

### *Potential Indications of Intracytoplasmic Morphologically Sperm Injection*

*Teratozoospermia:* It has already been shown that individual spermatozoa differ in their ability to produce an embryo capable of implanting. Indeed, the use of morphometrically normal spermatozoa with no vacuoles or less than two small vacuoles has been associated with significantly higher blastocyst rates than all other types of spermatozoa (i.e., those with more than two small vacuoles, those with one large vacuole and those with morphometric abnormalities).[92,93] In contrast, one study has reported lower blastocyst rates when vacuole-free spermatozoa were used for injection (relative to spermatozoa with vacuoles).

In summary, IMSI might be indicated in some cases of teratozoospermia. However, given that only one randomized study observed higher clinical pregnancy rates for IMSI than for ICSI in patients with teratozoospermia and the threshold for the number of morphometrically normal spermatozoa (as assessed by MSOME) below which IMSI might produce higher clinical pregnancy and delivery rates than ICSI remains to be determined, further studies of the potential value of IMSI in patients with teratozoospermia are required.

### *Intracytoplasmic Morphologically Sperm Injection and Spermatozoa with Nuclear Abnormalities*

The use of IMSI might help to avoid the selection of spermatozoa with nuclear abnormalities such as chromatin condensation failure, DNA fragmentation, and an abnormal chromosomal content. First, given that the nuclear origin of sperm head vacuoles has been linked to chromatin condensation failure, a high proportion of noncondensed chromatin could be considered as an indication for IMSI. No data are available but this question deserves to be evaluated in large-scale, randomized trials.

A second potential indication of interest is sperm DNA fragmentation. Indeed, it has been shown that spermatozoa judged to be normal at ICSI-like magnifications can present DNA fragmentation and that normal vacuole-free spermatozoa selected at an IMSI-like magnification are less DNA fragmented than normal spermatozoa selected at an ICSI-like magnification.[94]

Thirdly, sperm aneuploidy may be considered. Although two studies have reported that spermatozoa with large vacuoles are more likely to be aneuploid than normal, vacuole-free spermatozoa[74] or spermatozoa from whole semen,[88] IMSI was found to be no more efficient than ICSI for selecting euploid spermatozoa in patients with a high proportion of aneuploid spermatozoa (e.g., patients with a high proportion of spermatozoa with enlarged heads[95] or translocations.[96,97] Hence, it has not been proved that IMSI can be used to efficiently select euploid spermatozoa. Indeed, one can even consider that the opposite is true (i.e., a demonstrated lack of efficiency).

### *Intracytoplasmic Morphologically Sperm Injection for Older Women*

Interestingly, only one research group has evaluated IMSI in older women. In a randomized study of patients with a mean age of 37 years, preimplantation genetic diagnosis showed that ICSI (n = 60) was associated with significantly higher sex chromosome aneuploidy in the embryo and a significantly greater proportion of chaotic embryos (i.e., with two or more chromosomal number abnormalities) relative to IMSI (n = 60). The researchers postulated that, in older women, oocytes were less able to repair the injected spermatozoon's DNA and hence that use of IMSI to select spermatozoa with fewer nuclear abnormalities could be of value for aged oocytes and older women.[98] This indication also deserves to be evaluated in large-scale, randomized trials.

## CONCLUSION

Almost two decade after the introduction of IMSI, this technique continues to divide assisted reproduction professionals. There are few confirmed indications of IMSI, partly because few randomized, head-to-head studies have been performed. According to this systematic literature review, the only currently and consistently acknowledged indication of IMSI is recurrent implantation failure following ICSI. All other potential indications of IMSI must be further assessed.

## ZETA POTENTIAL

The electrical charge (216 mV–220 mV) of the sperm plasma membrane is called electrokinetic potential or *zeta potential*[16] **(Fig. 6)**. Sperm membrane is negatively charged.[16,99] On this basis, methods for separating X- and Y-bearing spermatozoa[99] and for the separation of pure sperm heads from disintegrated mammalian spermatozoa[100] were developed decades ago. Later, the methods developed by Ainsworth, et al., (2005)[101] allowed to collect the

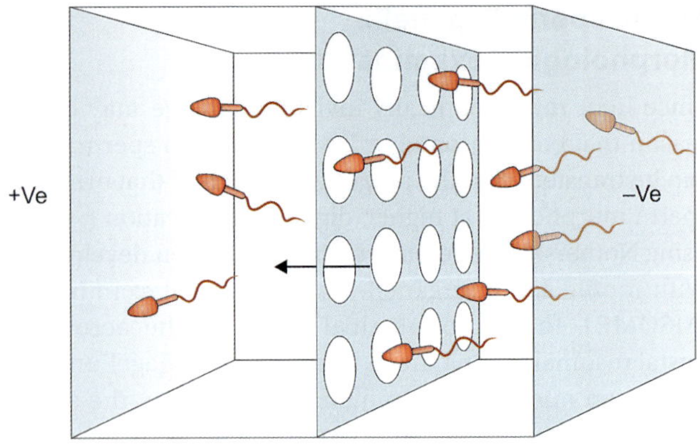


**Fig. 6:** Example of sperm selection by the Z-method developed by Ainsworth, et al., (2005): Spermatozoa are placed in a well-isolated from another adjacent well by a porous membrane and filled with a medium free of cells. An electric field is then applied with the anode in the well free of cells and the cathode in the well containing the sperm suspension. Due to the negative charge of the sperm membrane, spermatozoa migrate toward the compartment free of cells passing through the porous membrane. Spermatozoa can be then collected for downstream applications.

charged spermatozoa adhered to the wall of a centrifuge tube or migrating within an electric field, respectively. With both methodologies, downstream analysis of the selected spermatozoa revealed an increased percentage of spermatozoa with higher quality and porting high integrity DNA.[102-104]

This procedure, known as Zeta method, has allowed the selection of spermatozoa with reduced DNA fragmentation compared to the HA-coated dish selection.[105] Also, sperm DNA fragmentation has been proven to be lower using DGC-Zeta than DGC by itself[103] or MACS-DGZ.[104] However, despite these promising results, only one randomized study has been published using spermatozoa selected by Zeta method in patients undergoing ICSI.[105] In this research, significant increases in top quality embryos [45.83 ± 3.11% versus 35.38 ± 4.64% (P = 0.04)] and pregnancy rates [39.2 versus 21.8% (P = 0.009)] were obtained with DGC/Zeta compared to DGC, respectively. However, further analysis is needed to know the potential of Zeta method for improving ARTs.

## MOLECULAR BINDING

Now it has been very well-documented and established by numerous studies that during epididymal maturation of sperm, certain surface molecules not only change but also get associated with normal sperm function. To identify capability of spermatozoa to fertilize human oocyte, based on these molecular bindings, two methods are being currently used: (1) sperm binding to Annexin V and (2) hyaluronic acid (HA).

The plasma membrane of the spermatozoa takes part in number of cell metabolism, capacitation, zona binding, and acrosome reaction which are very crucial for their functionality. Its accessibility and relation with sperm vitality and quality make this organelle, its integrity, and variable characteristics, a logical target for the development of selection methods of high quality spermatozoa for their use in ART.

## Annexin V Magnetic Activated Cell Sorting

Magnetic activated cell sorting is a method that allows the separation of cell populations based on their surface antigens.[106] These antigens are coated with a molecule with magnetic nanoparticles that have affinity for these antigens. This coating allows the trapping of the desired cell subpopulation and its separation within a column subject to a strong magnetic field as described earlier. Thus, trapped cell expressing the antigen remain in the column while other undesired cells flow through for downstream applications. If membrane integrity is lost in an early event of the apoptotic response, it leads to the extrusion of phosphatidylserine.[107] On this basis, Annexin V, a molecule showing high affinity for phosphatidylserine,[108] is coated on nanoparticles which bind to apoptotic spermatozoa so that they are retained in the MACS column, allowing the recovery of nonapoptotic spermatozoa for their use in ARTs[109] **(Fig. 7)**.

This technique was first used by Grunewald, et al.,[110] in 2001 for selection of sperm enriched in nonapoptotic spermatozoa which retained membrane integrity using Annexin V MACS (AV-MACS) in the human clinical practice, demonstrating the utility of this technique. In a study of selection of sperm from semen samples of 35 healthy donors by Said, et al., (2006)[30], AV-MACS method reported spermatozoa enriched with lower DNA fragmentation and higher oocyte penetration capacity. Similarly, using this method, Zahedi, et al., (2013)[103] also reported in both fertile and nonfertile (terato- and asthenozoospermia) males, an enrichment of spermatozoa with lower DNA fragmentation. Interestingly, spermatozoa from idiopathic infertile males and patients affected by varicocele, in the studies carried out by Lee, et al., (2010)[31] and Degheidy, et al., (2015)[111], when subjected to AV-MACS technique of sperm selection showed significantly low DNA fragmentation and intact motility compared to original semen sample. However, a number of studies comparing AV-MACS with SU and DGC questioned the actual efficiency of this technique for the enhancement of spermatozoa with higher quality. So, semen form infertile patients with variable etiologies were treated with AV-MACS followed by DGC by Tavalaee, et al., (2012).[112] The combination of these two techniques proved to be more efficient at enriching permatozoa with lower DNA fragmentation than both procedures individually or DGC followed by AV-MACS. Nadalini, et al., (2014)[113] obtained better results with DGC followed by SU than with DGC followed by AV-MACS in terms of sperm quality. However, no significant differences were found in overall sperm quality and DNA fragmentation by using AV-MACS, SU, DG, SU/AV-MACS, and DG/AV-MACS[114] perhaps due to the low sample size of the study.

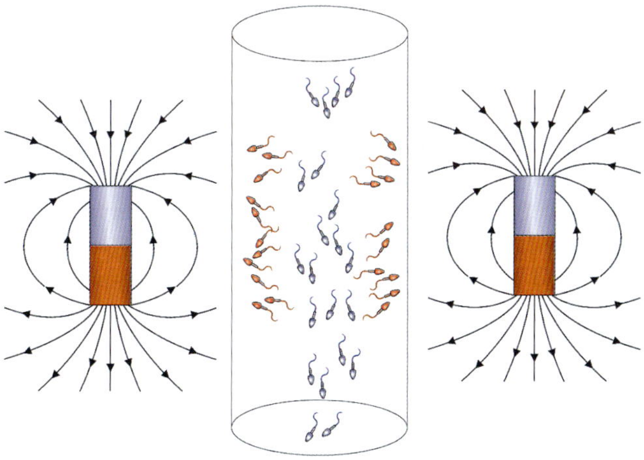

**Fig. 7:** Example of Annexin V magnetic activated cell sorting: Apoptotic spermatozoa (red in the figure) are bound to magnetic nanoparticles coated with Annexin V and affinity to the externalized phosphatidylserine in this sperm population. Semen is then passed through a column with magnetos on the side, thus apoptotic spermatozoa are retained and nonapoptotic are washed out for downstream applications.

On the contrary, a better quality of motility and DNA fragmentation in spermatozoa selected by AV-MACS followed by DCG was obtained by Berteli, et al., (2017)[115] compared to the other combinations tested: DCG and AV-MACS alone or DCG followed by AV-MACS. Recently, Zhang et al. (2018)[116] reported similar results with the combination of DCG followed by AV-MACS in immotile sperm samples resulting in the recovery of a sperm population with lower DNA fragmentation compared to DGC alone. This result is in agreement with Esbert, et al., (2017)[117] who reported that DGC followed by AV-MACS reduced the number of spermatozoa having chromosomal abnormalities.

Earlier, the results were scarce and unclear in using sperm selection technique of AV-MACS for ART. In comparison with DGC, sperm selected by AV-MACS prior to ICSI in 196 oligoasthenozoospemic patients showed higher cleavage and pregnancy rates in an early study by Dirican, et al., (2008).[33] Sperm selected from cryopreserved semen samples in 237 infertile couples by SU preparation method or SU followed by AV-MACS method before ICSI in donor oocyte cycles resulted in no difference in fertilization rates, embryo quality, implantation and live birth rates.[118] García-Ferreyra et al. (2014)[119] reported higher, but not statically significant pregnancy and implantation rates when semen showing basal high DNA fragmentation was selected by AV-MACS followed by DGC, compared to DGC alone in ICSI treatments. These results are supported by those reported by Stimpfel et al. (2018)[120] in couples of teratozoospermic patients and women over 30 years old undergoing ICSI, showing higher quality blastocysts when spermatozoa were selected by DGC/SU followed by AV-MACS, compared to

DGC/SU. Recently, a significantly higher top quality embryos and clinical pregnancies were reported by Ziarati, et al., (2019)[121] reported a significant increase in the percentage of high-quality embryos and clinical pregnancies in 80 infertile couples undergoing ICSI with mainly moderate or severe male factor employing DGC followed by when compared to DGC alone.

Collectively these studies indicate that the combination of DGC and MACS can provide slight benefits in patients with male factor undergoing ICSI in terms of clinical pregnancy. However, it is not clear to which extent live birth rate is actually improved. Thus, the combination of AV-MACS with other sperm preparation methods could be determinant for improving ART. More experiments, comprising larger number of patients, and exploring the different variables involved, are needed in order to confirm the utility of AV-MACS for the human clinical practice.

## HYALURONIC ACID BINDING

One of the main components of the extracellular matrix surrounding the cumulus-oocyte complex (COC) is the hyaluronic acid (HA).[122] During completion of spermatogenesis followed by adequate maturation in spermiogenesis, mature human sperm membrane develop and exhibit binding sites to it.[123,124] Based on sperm–HA interaction or binding, two techniques of sperm selection have been developed:

i. Recovering spermatozoa that are trapped and stuck on the surface of HA coated dish.[124]
ii. Picking up spermatozoa those move very slowly while swimming in a medium containing HA in solution[125] **(Fig. 8)**.

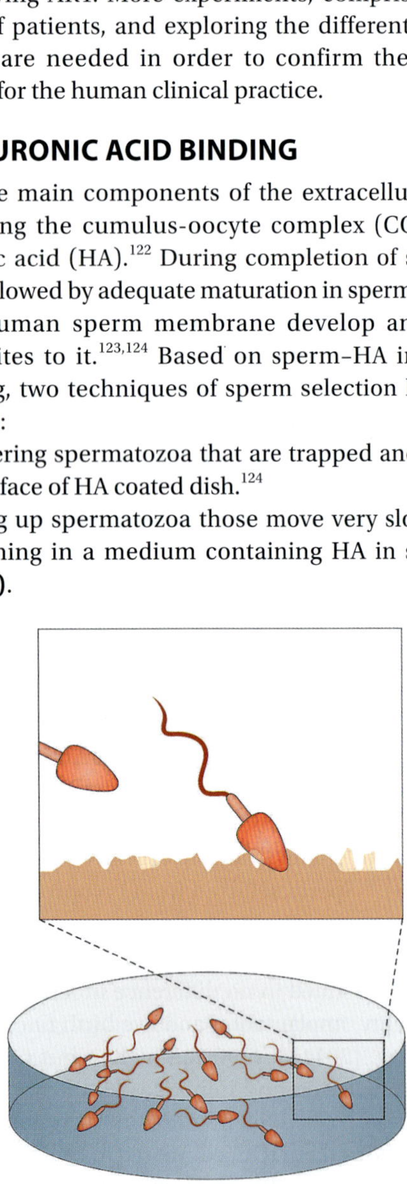

**Fig. 8:** Example of method for sperm selection based on hyaluronic acid-binding. Spermatozoa are placed on a dish coated with hyaluronic acid (HA, orange in the figure). Matured spermatozoa bind to the surface due to their interaction with the HA. These spermatozoa can be then recovered for ICSI using a micromanipulation system.

To date, two methods for HA binding are in use, namely, the picked spermatozoa for ICSI (PICSI) dish (hyaluronan-coated chamber) and a hyaluronan-containing medium. Both methods are ready to use systems that are commercially available and have received official recognition for conformity with health and safety requirements in the EU and the United States.

## PICSI DISH

Principally, the PICSI dish is a Petri dish that has spots of immobilized HA on it as shown in **Figures 9A to C**. Washed or density gradient-prepared spermatozoa suspensions are placed on top of these spots of HA and incubated for 15 minutes at 37°C. Subsequently, the freely moving spermatozoa are removed by gently rinsing the HA droplet and removing the nonbound sperm. Finally, the bound spermatozoa can be picked (P) with an ICSI pipette (hence, PICSI)[126] as shown in **Figures 9A to C**.

## HYALURONAN-CONTAINING MEDIUM

The alternative to the PICSI dish is a viscous medium containing HA. Here, a 5 mL droplet of density gradient-prepared spermatozoa is connected with a pipette tip to a 5 mL droplet of sperm slow medium by dragging the suspension into contact and incubated for 15 minutes at 37°C under oil. Afterward, spermatozoa bound to HA at the interface of the two droplets are selected with an ICSI pipette[127] as shown in **Figure 10**.

Both these methods have capacity to select spermatozoa which have reduced DNA fragmentation. While using HA-coated dish for sperm selection, an inverse correlation was established, among HA bound spermatozoa and protamine deficiency, DNA fragmentation, and abnormal sperm morphology in original sample.[128] In contrast, Razavi, et al., (2010)[104] reported same DNA fragmentation in spermatozoa isolated using HA coated dish and the ones in which dish was not used. But very soon, many others reported higher DNA integrity in spermatozoa selected by HA-binding technique.[126,129,130] Furthermore, Parmegiani, et al., (2010)[128] and Huang, et al., (2015)[131] observed lower DNA fragmentation in spermatozoa selected in HA solution compared to SU, and by HA coated dishes compared to DGC, respectively. However, both HA and HA coated dish studies reported similar levels of DNA fragmentation when compared to spermatozoa selected under the microscope regarding motility and morphological features. Similarly, Mongkolchaipak and Vutyavanich (2013)[129,130] did not find any difference between DGC/HA coated dishes and DGC/intracytoplasmic IMSI respect to sperm DNA fragmentation. These results question the utility of sperm selection based on HA-binding.

Parmegiani, et al., (2010)[132] compared reproductive outcome in 331 patients undergoing ICSI using HA solution

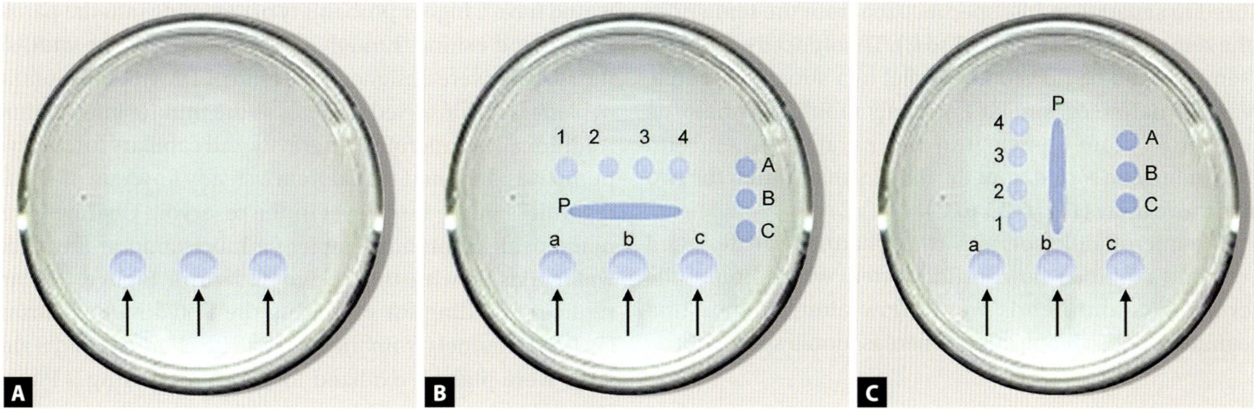


**Figs. 9A to C:** PICSI dish.

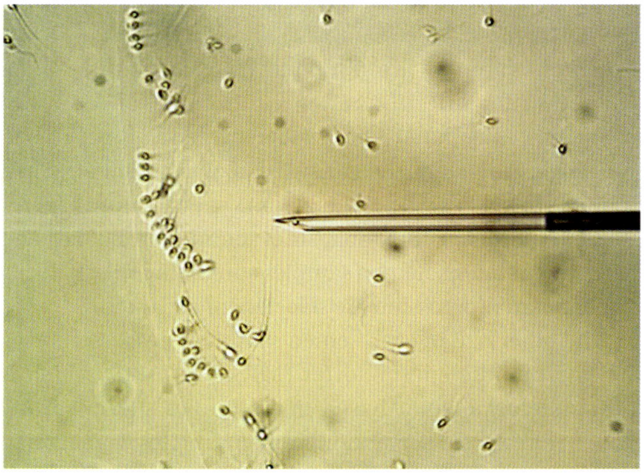

**Fig. 10:** Hyaluronan containing medium.

(293 patients) and conventional ICSI (86 patients) with no differences in clinical pregnancies or live birth ratios though an improved in embryo quality and implantation rate was observed. In another study, the same authors reported comparable results employing 206 oligozoospermic patients (Parmegiani, et al., 2010).[126] Subsequent studies reported similar results using either HA-coated dishes or HA solution.[133-136] Interestingly however, Worrilow, et al., (2013)[137] found that HA-coated dishes in sperm selection significantly increased pregnancy [136,137] and live birth rate (Mokánszki, et al., 2014)[136] in patients undergoing ICSI when selected sperm had HA-binding capacity ≤65%, as measured by the Hyaluronan binding assay. As a result of which a conclusion can be derived that the HA-binding selection method could be useful only in specific cases and indicates the need of a basic semen analysis for determining the suitability of the technique. Erberelli, et al., (2017)[138] therefore reported a significant improvement of ICSI using HA-coated dishes in patients with various categories of male factor. The results suggested that the benefit of this method could be higher for teratozoospermic patients. In a randomized study employing a large number of patients (2772 couples), Miller et al. (2019)[139] did not find any significant benefit of HA-coated dishes compared to conventional ICSI and either detected an association between results of Hyaluronan binding assay and ICSI outcomes, contradicting previous works above described. These results collectively show a poor capacity of HA binding methods for improving ICSI; however, more studies are needed to identify the types of patients that could benefit from this procedure.

## MICROFLUIDIC ISOLATION OF MOTILE SPERMATOZOA

With the advent of (ICSI), men with severe oligozoospermia are now offered the opportunity to reproduce their own child. In addition to low sperm counts, semen samples from these patients often have large amounts of cellular debris. Consequently, swim-up from a pellet is not a viable option to prepare these sperm samples. Additionally, due to the extremely low yield of motile spermatozoa with the other isolation methods discussed, the number of viable spermatozoa available after processing for use in ICSI is limited and occasionally prohibitive for this group of men. Because of this, new sperm isolation methods are required for this patient population.

The field of microfluidics is a new area of biomedical engineering concerned with the microscopic flow of fluids. At the microscopic level, streams of fluid will maintain laminar rather than turbulent flow. Because viscous forces dominate over inertial forces in these small flows, two separate streams of fluid with laminar flow can be placed parallel to each other with the two streams mixing only by diffusion despite there being no physical barrier between them. Multiple laminar flow systems have previously been utilized to perform diffusion based separation,[140] to detect molecules,[141] to fabricate microstructures in capillaries,[142] and to pattern cells and their environments.[143] It was thought that this unique feature of microscopic fluid flow could be utilized to separate motile spermatozoa from the remainder of the semen sample **(Figs. 11A to C)**. Theoretically, a stream of semen could be flowed in parallel to a stream of media. Given the nature of laminar flow, only motile spermatozoa could cross from semen into the parallel stream and subsequently be sorted from the initial stream when the two fluids move away **(Figs. 12A to C)**.

The microfluidic sperm sorting channel was designed to provide a laminar flow sorting system where nonmotile spermatozoa and debris would flow along their initial streamlines and exit one outlet whereas motile spermatozoa would have a higher probability of deviating into the parallel stream and exiting through a different outlet. The widths of the streams were designed for a ratio of 1:3 with the intention of placing the unsorted samples in the thinner inlet channel. Additionally, a microfluidic gravity and capillary force driven pump was designed to maintain a steady flow rate of ~8 nL/s regardless of the fluid level in the reservoir. Channels were made using photolithography for fabrication of the silicon wafer master with the design shown in **Figure 11B** and replica moulding for preparing the polydimethylsiloxane (PDMS) channels from the master. The channels and a glass slide were plasma oxidized for 5 minutes using a Plasma Prep IITM Chamber. This allowed the channels to seal onto the slide and to make the inner surface of the channels hydrophilic, which improved liquid flow inside the channels enough that no additional bovine serum albumin (BSA) was needed for most semen samples.

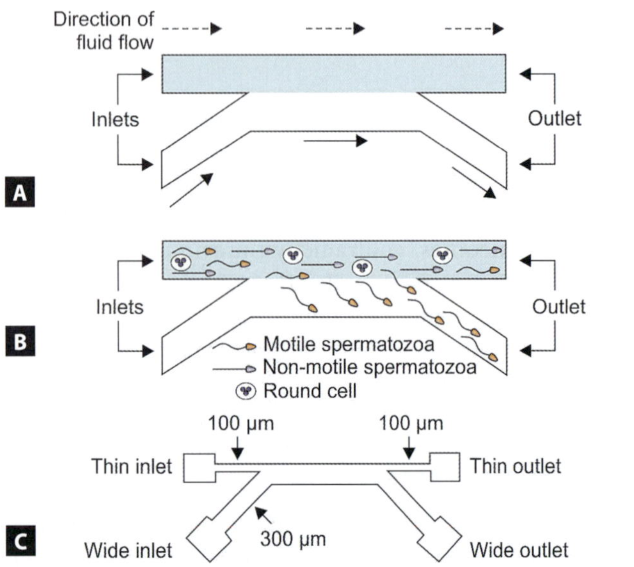


**Figs. 11A to C:** Passively driven microfluidic device for sperm sorting based on motility. (A) Represents the flow direction; (B) Illustrates the sperm cells crossing streams; (C) Dimensions of the channels are at the micrometer scale.

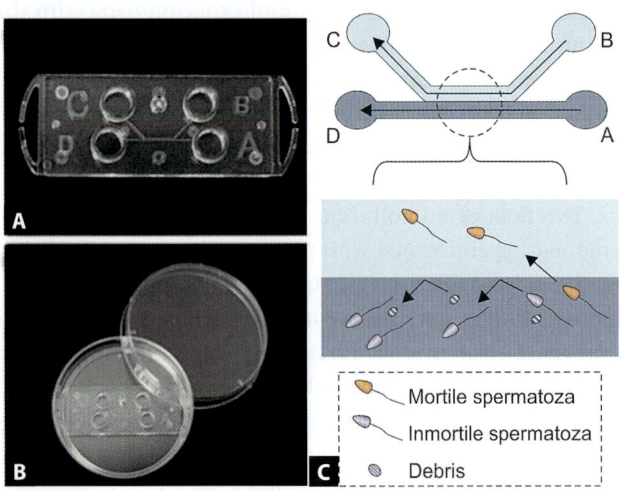


**Figs. 12A to C:** (A) A microfluidic sperm sorter (MFSS) device; (B) The MFSS fixed in a 60-mm dish for easy handling; (C) Schematic representation of the microfluidic sperm sorting principle: an illustration of two laminar flows (A→D and B→C) in the MFSS channel.

Semen samples are obtained from men undergoing evaluation for infertility after a minimum of 3 days of abstinence. After liquefaction, a semen analysis is performed by a single individual and consisted of assessment of semen volume, pH, viscosity, liquefaction, sperm count, sperm motility, sperm agglutination, strict sperm morphology, and cell contamination. Semen samples containing spermatozoa with forward progression are selected for separation.

The other half of each semen sample is processed using the microfluidic sperm sorter (MFSS) QUALIS, which is a cycloolefin polymer-based microfluidics sperm sorting chip. Before sperm separation, semen samples were filtered using a 20 mm pore size filter to remove foreign bodies. Each ejaculated sample was carefully diluted 1:1 with sperm sorting medium [HTF medium with 10% serum substitute supplement (SSS)] and maintained at approximately 37°C before using the MFSS.

After fixing the MFSS in a 60 mm dish, 100 mL of the sperm-sorting medium was loaded in chambers A, B, C, and D to create streamlines in the microfluidics channels as shown in lower half of **Figure 12B**. After the medium was removed from all chambers, 20 µL of the medium is loaded in chambers C and D, 100 µL of the medium is loaded in chamber B, and 65 µL of sperm suspension is loaded in chamber A. The average number of spermatozoa in 65 µL of sperm suspension is 300 x $10^3$ sperm. The amount of medium in chamber B is adjusted such that the width of the laminar flow from chamber A is approximately 40% of the overall width of the central microchannel under the microscope. After 30 minutes, completely isolated spermatozoa (25–30 mL) were extracted from chamber C. The contents of chamber C are collected and stored together before IUI, IVF, or ICSI depending quality of semen.

In a study,[144] the MFSS method was significantly more effective than the centrifugation and swim-up procedure in regards to higher motility and lower DNA fragmentation index (DFI) of sperm but not for number of sperm isolated. The MFSS method allows selection of sperm with high DNA integrity.[145] The study reported the possibility of decreasing sperm DFI to 1% by using an MFSS device. In a previous study,[146] DNA fragmentation after the centrifugation and swim-up processing was 12 and 6%, respectively, and motility after only centrifugation and combination with centrifugation and swim-up processing was 67 and 84%, respectively.

Thus, the MFSS method is considerably more efficient than the centrifugation and swim-up procedure. The risk of selecting sperm with DNA fragmentation decreases to 1 in 10 by using the MFSS method compared with the centrifugation and swim-up procedure.

A very small quantity of sperm can be collected from compromised semen quality samples using the MFSS. However, even a small number of normal sperm are sufficient for ICSI. The MFSS is adequate for clinical use in ICSI. Semen processing using the centrifugation and swim-up procedure may take up to 2 hours. However, with the MFSS, a one-step sorting protocol without centrifugation is possible and it can complete processing within 30–45 minutes.[147] Reducing the treatment time and eliminating the centrifugation step may minimize sperm exposure to concentrated ROS and prevent DNA fragmentation.[25]

## SPERM SELECTION BASED ON GUIDANCE MECHANISMS

A physiological mechanism for guidance of sperm within the female genital tract has been suggested for selection of spermatozoa which are capable of fertilizing an oocyte, development of a viable embryo to ensure implantation that is carried forward to full term. Hence, a strategy should be employed to develop new sperm selection technique in vitro that is based on the same principle of guidance of spermatozoa in the female genital tract. As a result of which, three known mechanisms have been proposed to guide the spermatozoa within the oviduct and they are being tested accordingly for their capacity to select spermatozoa with the aim of improving ART results.

### Rheotaxis

It is proved that human and mice spermatozoa swim against the direction of fluid flow.[148,149] This natural feature of sperm is known as "rheotaxis." The first study conducted by De Martin, et al.,[150] (2017) to select sperm from donors with normozoospermia employing rheotaxis process. It reported that sperm selected in this manner were enriched with higher chromatin compaction (99%) as compared to (71%) in original sample before selection. It was higher than even sperm selected using DGC (83%) **(Fig. 13)**.

Thus, the results in animal studies reported to date are promising, but the passive nature of rheotaxis, which is

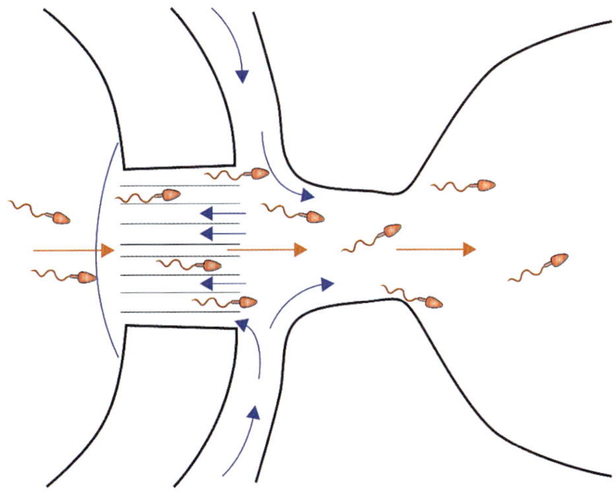

**Fig. 13:** Method of sperm selection by rheotaxis developed by Nagata, et al., (2018). A flow (blue arrows) is created through a serial of microchannels toward a well were sperm sample is placed. In response to the flow the spermatozoa swim toward it passing through the microchannels and accumulating in a receptive well where they can be collected for downstream applications (red arrows indicate migration of the sperm).

based on the hydrodynamics of the motile spermatozoa,[151] indicates that this mechanism has poor selective potential beyond the separation of those spermatozoa with a correct swimming behavior. Although this is the in vitro situation, the in vivo picture could be drastically different.

So, rheotaxis would be part of a selection system of capacitated spermatozoa allowing only this subpopulation of spermatozoa to migrate toward the in vivo fertilization site. In vitro developed procedures could test this hypothesis for sperm selection by rheotaxis. That would be an effective way of selecting capacitated spermatozoa for improving ART results.

### Chemotaxis

Chemotaxis, a mechanism of navigation used by spermatozoa when they come in the proximity of oocyte where chemical components released by combined estrogen and progestin oral contraceptive pill (COC) such as progesterone (P4) attracts them (P4 acts as chemoattractant) to orient their swimming pattern toward zona of an oocyte.[152] It is important to note that only capacitated spermatozoa are attracted by chemotaxis. That is how the property of capacitated sperm allows the selection of this specific subpopulation[152] **(Fig. 14)**.

Gatica, et al.,[153] (2013) selected spermatozoa from both normozoospermic donors and subfertile patients by employing P4 gradient in a simple device named "Sperm Selection Assay" (SSA). It was found that the selected spermatozoa had three fold capacitated sperm with much lesser DNA fragmentation and less oxidative stress than the original semen sample, in both the cases. Li, et al.,[154]

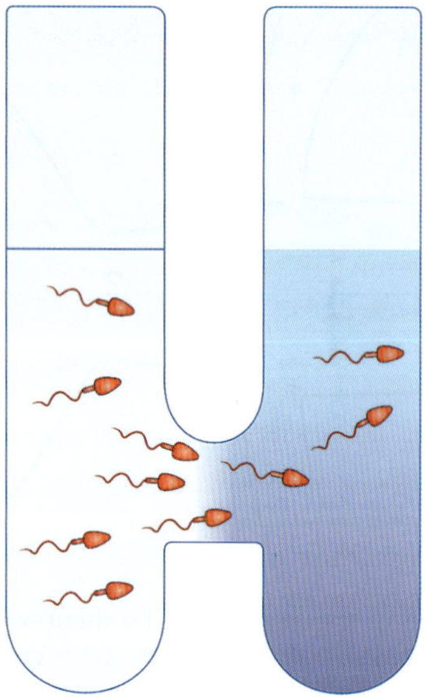

**Fig. 14:** Method of sperm selection by chemotaxis developed by Gatica, et al., (2013): Two wells are connected by a 2 mm length per 2.5 mm diameter tube. One of the wells is filled with a medium containing the chemoattractant molecule in solution (colored in blue) and the other well is filled with the spermatozoa suspension. The chemoattractant diffuses through the connecting tube generating a gradient and the spermatozoa respond by migrating toward the higher concentration and accumulating in the initial well free of cells where they can be collected for downstream applications.

(2018) also reported an improvement in the sperm quality from normozoospermic donors in terms of normal morphology, lower DNA fragmentation, and lower percentage of apoptotic spermatozoa when using another device composed of a system of microfluidic channels. However, the effectiveness of sperm selection by chemotaxis in the improvement of ART in clinical practice has not been studied to date.

### Thermotaxis

Thermotaxis is a process in which sperm is oriented to swim in the direction of higher temperature in a gradient.[155] Evidence indicates that this mechanism allows sperm to orient itself in the fallopian tubes to ascend to the ampulla.[148] As in chemotaxis, only capacitated spermatozoa respond to thermotactic stimuli, so based on it, this subpopulation could be selected[155] **(Fig. 15)**.

The use of these selected spermatozoa for ICSI in mice increased cleavage rates and blastocyst production, as well as implantation and live birth rate as opposed to the use of spermatozoa selected by SU. Although this is the only work in thermotaxis in ART, a recent study carried out in bulls has shown that seminal samples delivering high pregnancy rates after artificial insemination show a greater response to thermotaxis.[156] However, as in the case of rheotaxis and chemotaxis, there are still no available publications showing the capability of sperm selection by thermotaxis to improve the ART efficiency in the human clinic.

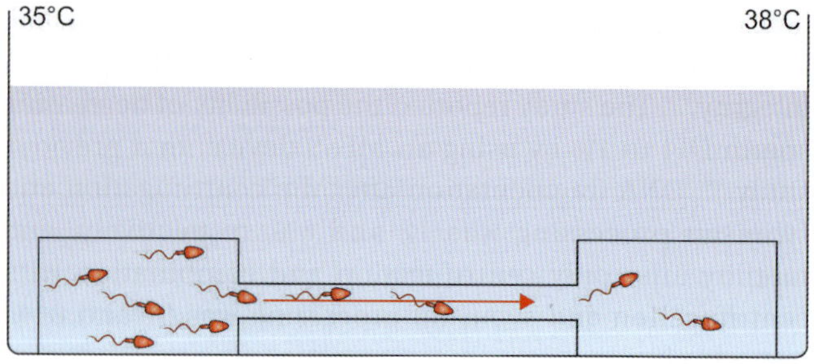


**Fig. 15:** Method of sperm selection by thermotaxis developed by Pérez-Cerezales, et al., (2018). Spermatozoa are placed on a drop of a medium connected by a capillary to a second drop free of cells. A temperature gradient is generated between both drops being the highest temperature at the place of the drop free of cells. Spermatozoa respond by thermotaxis migrating toward the warmer temperature and accumulating in the second drop where they can be collected for downstream applications (2003).

## CONCLUSION

The efficiency of ART has tremendous scope for improvement in terms of laboratory techniques, developmental embryology and pregnancy outcome. Sperm selection is an important factor for achieving higher live birth rates in ART, especially in compromised male factor. However, the techniques developed to date have failed partially to be useful for their routine application in the clinical practice and seemed to have limited scope only in specific cases of malefactor. Some novel methods described in this chapter based on the principles of physiological selection operating in vivo and on microfluidic environments have delivered promising results yet to be confirmed in large studies in the context of clinical practice. These studies should be randomized and strict in the confrontation of results with several compromised semen samples minimizing the female factor. The key factor is to combine various sperm selection techniques to increase the efficiency of the ART.

## FUTURE DEVELOPMENT OF SPERM PREPARATION TECHNIQUES

As sperm selection by a fertile female usually permits only those male germ cells that exhibit normal nuclear DNA integrity access to the oocyte, any artificial selection method mimicking the biological situation should monitor this essential parameter. However, all currently employed methods to determine DNA damage (TUNEL assay, SCSA, COMET assay, Halosperm assay, etc.) are invasive and therefore consumptive.

Clinical application of novel, more physiological sperm selection techniques demands that such techniques are noninvasive, safe, highly discriminative, and relatively easy to perform. Moreover, it is imperative for any new method that sperm functions are maintained as much as possible and not compromised. These requirements might come at the cost of relatively expensive equipment or procedures.

Recently developed techniques that are noninvasive and therefore have the potential to be used for isolation of potentially fertilizing spermatozoa are more sophisticated and more expensive than those that are currently used in ART and include Raman microspectrometry, confocal light absorption, and scattering spectroscopic microscopy and polarization microscopy. At present, all of these are only in experimental stages and specific recommendations for routine application cannot be made.

## KEY POINTS

Despite significant improvements in human sperm preparation methods during recent years, our knowledge about the physiological sperm selection processes in the female reproductive tract is still fragmentary, as can be noticed from contradictory reports of the effect of certain selection methods on sperm function and IVF/ICSI results. If the physiological processes could be mimicked, the number of spermatozoa used for insemination in IUI or IVF would not only be drastically reduced, but the quality of spermatozoa that would be used for ICSI would increase. Additionally, success rates of assisted reproduction would improve, as good quality spermatozoa bearing a genome of highest integrity would be selected.

Nevertheless, no simple solution to this dilemma is available, and certainly, the efforts in minimizing mutagenic or lethal effects of DNA damage will not come cheap, which might also be a problem, particularly in developing countries. Human reproductive scientists and clinicians are not only doing their utmost to assist infertile couples to fulfil their wish for a child, as the WHO recognizes infertility as disease, but have also the duty to minimize the risks of ART for both the parents and progeny. Consequently, scientists have to understand the fertilization process better and search for the most physiological methods for human sperm selection. Nevertheless, despite progress that has been made to select and identify the most suitable spermatozoa for human-assisted reproduction, most of the new techniques are large-scaled and therefore expensive. With respect to future developments, more confirming and expanded data remain to be seen as individual groups have presented only preliminary results.

## REFERENCES


1. Williams M, Hill CJ, Scudamore I, Dunphy B. Sperm numbers and distribution within the human fallopian tube around ovulation. Hum Reprod. 1993;8(12):2019-26.
2. Eisenbach M, Giojalas LC. Sperm guidance in mammals—an unpaved road to the egg. Nat Rev Mol Cell Biol. 2006;7(4): 276-85.
3. Henkel RR, Schill WB. Sperm preparation for ART. Reprod Biol Endocrinol. 2003;14(1):108.
4. Henkel R. Sperm processing for IVF. In: Nagy ZP, Varghese A, Agarwal A, (Eds). Practical Manual of In Vitro Fertilization: Advanced Methods and Novel Devices: New York: Springer; 2012.
5. Franken DR, Henkel R. Sperm functional assays. In: Tandulwadkar S, Mittal B, (Eds). Optimizing IUI Results—A Guide to Gynecologists. New Delhi: Jaypee Brothers Medical Publishers (P) Ltd; 2010. pp. 155-67.
6. Yanagimachi R. Mammalian fertilization. In: Knobil E, Neill JD, (Eds). The Physiology of Reproduction, 2nd edition. New York: Raven Press; 1994.
7. Kremer J. The in vitro spermatozoal penetration test in fertility investigations. PhD dissertation. The Netherlands: University of Groningen; 1968.
8. Rogers BJ, Perreault SD, Bentwood BJ, McCarville C, Hale RW, Soderdahl DW. Variability in the human-hamster in vitro assay for fertility evaluation. Fertil Steril. 1983;39(2):204-11.
9. Mortimer D, Mortimer ST. Methods of sperm preparation for assisted reproduction. Ann Acad Med Singapore. 1992;21(4):517-24.
10. Mortimer ST, Swan MA, Mortimer D. Effect of seminal plasma on capacitation and hyperactivation in human spermatozoa. Hum Reprod. 1998;13(8):2139-46.
11. Kanwar KC, Yanagimachi R, Lopata A. Effects of human seminal plasma on fertilizing capacity of human spermatozoa. Fertil Steril. 1979;31(3):321-7.
12. Poenicke K, Grunewald S, Glander H. Sperm Selection in Assisted Reproductive Techniques. In: Rao KA, Agarwal A, Srinivas MS, (Eds). Andrology Laboratory Manual, 1st edition. New Delhi: Jaypee Brothers Pvt. Ltd; 2010. pp. 173-87.
13. Franken DR, Claasens OE, Henkel RR. Sperm Preparation Techniques, X/Y Chromosome Separation. In: Acosta AA, Kruger TF (Eds). Human Spermatozoa in Assisted Reproduction, 2nd edition. USA: Informa Healthcare; 1996. pp. 277-94.
14. Bjorndahl L, Mortimer D, Barratt CLR, Alvarez JG, Bjoerndahl L, Menkveld R, et al. Sperm Preparation. A Practical Guide to Basic Laboratory Andrology, 1st edition. USA: Cambridge University Press; 2010. pp. 167-87.
15. WHO. Sperm Preparation Techniques. In: Cooper TG, Aitken J, Auger J, Baker GHW, Barratt CLR, Behre HM, et al (Eds). World Health Organization Laboratory Manual for the Examination and Processing of Human Semen, 5th edition. Switzerland: WHO Press; 2010. pp. 161-8.
16. Chan PJ, Jacobson JD, Corselli JU, Patton WC. A simple zeta method for sperm selection based on membrane charge. Fertil Steril. 2006;85(2):481-6.
17. Aitken RJ, Clarkson JS. Significance of reactive oxygen species and antioxidants in defining the efficacy of sperm preparation techniques. J Androl. 1988;9(6):367-76.
18. Makker K, Agarwal A, Sharma R. Oxidative stress and male infertility. Indian J Med Res. 2009;129(4):357-67.
19. Jameel T. Sperm swim-up: a simple and effective technique of semen processing for intrauterine insemination. J Pak Med Assoc. 2008;58(2):71-4.
20. Otsuki J, Chuko M, Momma Y, Takahashi K. A comparison of the swim-up procedure at body and testis temperatures. J Assist Reprod Genet. 2008;25(8):413-5.

21. Ren SS, Sun GH, Ku CH, Chen D-C, Wu G-J. Comparison of four methods for sperm preparation for IUI. Arch Androl. 2004;50(3):139-43.
22. Henkel R, Franken DR, Lombard CJ, Schill WB. The selective capacity of glass wool filtration for normal chromatin condensed human spermatozoa: A possible therapeutic modality for male factor cases? J Assist Reprod Genet. 1994;11(8):395-400.
23. Ford WCL. The role of oxygen free radicals in the pathology of human spermatozoa: Implications of IVF. In: Matson PL, Lieberman BA. Clinical IVF Forum: Current Views in Assisted Reproduction. United Kingdom: Manchester University Press; 1990. pp. 123-39.
24. Aitken RJ, Clarkson JS. Cellular basis of defective sperm function and its association with the genesis of reactive oxygen species by human spermatozoa. J Reprod Fertil. 1987;81(2):459-69.
25. Mortimer D. Sperm preparation techniques and iatrogenic failures of in vitro fertilization. Hum Reprod. 1991;6(2):173-6.
26. Mortimer D. Sperm Washing. In: Mortimer D (Ed). Practical Laboratory Andrology, 1st edition. USA: Oxford University Press; 1994. pp. 267-86.
27. Oshio S, Kaneko S, Iizuka R, Mohri H. Effects of gradient centrifugation on human sperm. Arch Androl. 1987;19(1):85-93.
28. Bourne H, Edgar DH, Baker HWG. Sperm Preparation Techniques. In: Gardner DK, Weissman A, Howles CM, Shoham Z (Eds). Textbook of Assisted Reproductive Techniques: Laboratory and Clinical Perspectives, 2nd edition. USA: Informa Healthcare; 2004. pp. 79-91.
29. Said TM, Agarwal A, Grunewald S, Rasch M, Glander HJ, Paasch U. Evaluation of sperm recovery following annexin V magnetic activated cell sorting separation. Reprod Biomed Online. 2006;13(3): 336-9.
30. Said T, Agarwal A, Grunewald S, Rasch M, Baumann T, Kriegel C, et al. Selection of nonapoptotic spermatozoa as a new tool for enhancing assisted reproduction outcomes: an in vitro model. Biol Reprod. 2006;74(3):530-7.
31. Lee TH, Liu CH, Shih YT, Tsao HM, Huang CC, Chen HH, et al. Magnetic-activated cell sorting for sperm preparation reduces spermatozoa with apoptotic markers and improves the acrosome reaction in couples with unexplained infertility. Hum Reprod. 2010;25(4):839-46.
32. Said TM, Grunewald S, Paasch U, Rasch M, Agarwal A, Glander HJ. Effects of magnetic- activated cell sorting on sperm motility and cryosurvival rates. Fertil Steril. 2005;83(5):1442-6.
33. Dirican EK, Ozgun OD, Akarsu S, Akin KO, Ercan O, Uğurlu M, et al. Clinical outcome of magnetic activated cell sorting of nonapoptotic spermatozoa before density gradient centrifugation for assisted reproduction. J Assist Reprod Genet. 2008;25(8):375-81.
34. Van der Ven HH, Jeyendran RS, Tünnerhoff A, Hoebbel K, Diedrich K, et al. Glass wool column filtration of human semen: relation to swim-up procedure and outcome of IVF. Hum Reprod. 1988;3(1):85-8.
35. Sánchez R, Concha M, Ichikawa T, Henkel R, Schill WB. Glass wool filtration reduces reactive oxygen species by elimination of leukocytes in oligozoospermic patients with leukocytospermia. J Assisted Reprod Genet. 1996;13(6): 489-94.
36. Berger T, Marrs RP, Moyer DL. Comparison of techniques for selection of motile spermatozoa. Fertil Steril. 1985;43(2):268-73.
37. Henkel R, Ichikawa T, Sánchez R, Miska W, Ohmori H, Schill WB. Differentiation of ejaculates in which reactive oxygen species are generated by spermatozoa or leukocytes. Andrologia. 1997;29(6):295-301.
38. Wolff H. The biologic significance of white blood cells in semen. Fertil Steril. 1995;63(6):1143-57.
39. Aitken RJ, Clarkson JS, Fishel S. Generation of reactive oxygen species, lipid peroxidation, and human sperm function. Biol Reprod. 1989;41(10):183-97.
40. Iwasaki A, Gagnon C. Formation of reactive oxygen species in spermatozoa of infertile patients. Fertil Steril. 1992;57:409-16.
41. Terquem A, Dadoune JP. Aniline blue staining of human spermatozoon chromatin. Evaluation of nuclear maturation. In: André J (Ed). The Sperm Cell. The Hague: Martinus Nijhoff Publishers; 1983. pp. 249-52.
42. Auger J, Mesbah M, Huber C, Dadoune JP. Aniline blue staining as a marker of sperm chromatin defects associated with different semen characteristics between proven fertile and suspected infertile men. Int J Androl. 1990;13(6): 452-62.
43. Hammadeh ME, Stieber M, Haidl G, Schmidt W. Association between sperm cell chromatin condensation, morphology based on strict criteria, and fertilization, cleavage and pregnancy rates in an IVF program. Andrologia. 1998;30:29-35.
44. Hammadeh ME, Kuhnen A, Amer AS, Rosenbaum P, Schmidt W. Comparison of sperm preparation methods: effect on chromatin and morphology recovery rates and their consequences on the clinical outcome after in vitro fertilization embryo transfer. Int J Androl. 2001;24(6):360-8.
45. Hinting A, Lunardhi H. Better sperm selection for intracytoplasmic sperm injection with the side migration technique. Andrologia. 2001;33(6):343-6.
46. Henkel R, Menkveld R, Kleinhappl M, Schill WB. Seasonal changes of human sperm chromatin condensation. J Assisted Reprod Genet. 2001;18(7):371-7.
47. Lui CW, Mrsny RJ, Meizel S. Procedures for obtaining high percentages of viable in vitro capacitated hamster sperm. Gamete Res. 1979;2:207.
48. Daya S, Gwatkin RBL, Bissessar H. Separation of motile human spermatozoa by means of a glass bead column. Gamete Res. 1987;17(4):375-80.
49. Drobnis EZ, Zhong CQ, Overstreet JW. Separation of cryopreserved human semen using Sephadex columns, washing or Percoll gradients. J Androl. 1991;12:201-8.
50. Zavos PM, Centola GM. Methods of semen preparation for intrauterine insemination and subsequent pregnancy rates. Tohoku J Exp Med. 1992;168(4):583-90.
51. Pharmacia Biotech. Important notice: Percoll® NOT to be used in Assisted Reproduction Technologies in Humans. USA: Pharmacia Biotech Inc; 1996.
52. Hammadeh ME, Zavos PM, Rosenbaum P, Schmidt W. Comparison between the quality and function of sperm after semen processing with two different methods. Asian J Androl. 2001;3(2):125-30.
53. López O, Mata A, Antich M, Bassas L. Sperm selection by PD-10 sephadex columns: comparison with SpermPrep filtration and Percoll centrifugation. Hum Reprod. 1993;8(5):732-6.

54. Chijioke PC, Crocker PR, Gilliam M, Owens MD, Pearson RM. Importance of filter structure for the trans-membrane migration studies of sperm motility. Hum Reprod. 1988;3(2):241-4.
55. Raoof NT, Pearson RM, Turner P. A modified trans-membrane migration method for measuring the effect of drugs on sperm motility. Br J Clin Pharmacol. 1987;24(3):319-21
56. Agarwal A, Manglona A, Loughlin KR. Filtration of spermatozoa through L4 membrane: a new method. Fertil Steril. 1991;56(6):1162-5.
57. Agarwal A, Manglona A, Loughlin KR. Improvement in semen quality and sperm fertilizing ability after filtration through the L4 membrane: comparison of results with swim up technique. J Urol. 1992;147(6):1539-41.
58. Ikemoto I, Agarwal A, Fanning L, Loughlin KR. Improvement in membrane integrity and acrosin levels of human sperm by use of L4 membrane. Arch Androl. 1994;32(2):89-93.
59. Agarwal A, Ikemoto I, Loughlin KR. Levels of reactive oxygen species before and after sperm preparation: comparison of swim-up and L4 filtration. Arch Androl. 1994;32(3):169-74.
60. Liu J, Tsai YL, Katz E, Compton G, Garcia JE, Baramki TA. High fertilization rate obtained after intracytoplasmic sperm injection with 100% non-motile spermatozoa selected by using a simple modified hypo-osmotic swelling test. Fertil Steril. 1997;68(2):373-5.
61. Brackett NL, Padron OF, Lynne CM. Semen quality of spinal cord injured men is better when obtained by vibratory stimulation versus electroejaculation. J Urol. 1997;157(1):151-7.
62. Aust TR, Brookes S, Troup SA, Fraser WD, Lewis-Jones DI. Development and in vitro testing of a new method of urine preparation for retrograde ejaculation; the Liverpool solution. Fertil Steril. 2008;89(4):885-91.
63. Morozumi K, Shikano T, Miyazaki S, Yanagimachi R. Simultaneous removal of sperm plasma membrane and acrosome before intracytoplasmic sperm injection improves oocyte activation/embryonic development. Proc Natl Acad Sci U S A. 2006;103(47):17661-6.
64. Henkel R, Hajimohammad M, Stalf T, Hoogendijk C, Mehnert C, Menkveld R, et al. Influence of deoxyribonucleic acid damage on fertilization and pregnancy. Fertil Steril. 2004;81(4):965-72.
65. Twigg JP, Irvine DS, Aitken RJ. Oxidative damage to DNA in human spermatozoa does not preclude pronucleus formation at intracytoplasmic sperm injection. Hum Reprod. 1998;13:1864-71.
66. Carrell DT, Liu L, Peterson CM, Jones KP, Hatasaka HH, Erickson L, et al. Sperm DNA fragmentation is increased in couples with unexplained recurrent pregnancy loss. Arch Androl. 2003;49(1):49-55.
67. Aitken RJ, Krausz C. Oxidative stress, DNA damage and the Y chromosome. Reproduction. 2001;122(4):497-506.
68. Hansen M, Kurinczuk JJ, Bower C, Webb S. The risk of major birth defects after intracytoplasmic sperm injection and in vitro fertilization. N Engl J Med. 2002;346(10):725-30.
69. Wen SW, Leader A, White RR, Léveillé MC, Wilkie V, Zhou J, et al. A comprehensive assessment of outcomes in pregnancies conceived by in vitro fertilization/intracytoplasmic sperm injection. Eur J Obstet Gynecol Reprod Biol. 2010; 150(2):160-5.
70. Gandini L, Lombardo F, Paoli D, Caruso F, Eleuteri P, Leter G, et al. Full-term pregnancies achieved with ICSI despite high levels of sperm chromatin damage. Hum Reprod. 2004;19(6):1409-17.
71. Morrell JM, Rodriguez-Martinez H. Biomimetic techniques for improving sperm quality in animal breeding: a review. Open Androl J. 2009;1:1-9.
72. Menkveld R, Stander FS, Kotze TJ, Kruger TF, van Zyl JA. The evaluation of morphological characteristics of human spermatozoa according to stricter criteria. Hum Reprod. 1990;5(5):586-92.
73. Oehninger S, Kruger T. The diagnosis of male infertility by semen quality. Clinical significance of sperm morphology assessment. Hum Reprod. 1995;10(5):1037-8.
74. Garolla A, Fortini D, Menegazzo M, De Toni L, Nicoletti V, Moretti A, et al. High-power microscopy for selecting spermatozoa for ICSI by physiological status. Reprod Biomed Online. 2008;17(5):610-6.
75. Avendano C, Franchi A, Taylor S, Morshedi M, Bocca S, Oehninger S. Fragmentation of DNA in morphologically normal human spermatozoa. Fertil Steril. 2009;91(4): 1077-84.
76. Berkovitz A, Eltes F, Soffer Y, Zabludovsky N, Beyth Y, Farhi J, et al. ART success and in vivo sperm cell selection depend on the ultramorphological status of spermatozoa. Andrologia. 1999;31(1):1-8.
77. Wilding M, Coppola G, di Matteo L, Palagiano A, Fusco E, Dale B. Intracytoplasmic injection of morphologically selected spermatozoa (IMSI) improves outcome after assisted reproduction by deselecting physiologically poor quality spermatozoa. J Assist Reprod Genet. 2011;28(3):253-62.
78. Ryu HM, Lin WW, Lamb DJ, Chuang W, Lipshultz LI, Bischoff FZ. Increased chromosome X, Y, and 18 nondisjunction in sperm from infertile patients that were identified as normal by strict morphology: implication for intracytoplasmic sperm injection. Fertil Steril. 2001;76(5):879-83.
79. Aitken RJ, de Iuliis GN. Origins and consequences of DNA damage in male germ cells. Reprod Biomed Online. 2007;14(6):727-33.
80. Bartoov B, Berkovitz A, Eltes F, Kogosowski A, Menezo Y, Barak Y. Real-time fine morphology of motile human sperm cells is associated with IVF–ICSI outcome. J Androl. 2002;23(1):1-8.
81. Bartoov B, Berkovitz A, Eltes F, Kogosovsky A, Yagoda A, Lederman H, et al. Pregnancy rates are higher with intracytoplasmic morphologically selected sperm injection than with conventional intracytoplasmic injection. Fertil Steril. 2003;80(6):1413-9.
82. Hazout A, Dumont-Hassan M, Junca AM, Cohen Bacrie P, Tesarik J. High magnification ICSI overcomes paternal effect resistant to conventional ICSI. Reprod Biomed Online. 2006;12(1):19-25.
83. Berkovitz A, Eltes F, Yaari S, Katz N, Barr I, Fishman A, et al. The morphological normalcy of the sperm nucleus and pregnancy rate of intracytoplasmic injection with morphologically selected sperm. Hum Reprod. 2005;20(1):185-90.
84. Peer S, Eltes F, Berkovitz A, Yehuda R, Itsykson P, Bartoov B. Is fine morphology of the human sperm nuclei affected by in vitro incubation at 37 degrees C? Fertil Steril. 2007;88(6): 1589-94.

85. Boitrelle F, Ferfouri F, Petit JM, Segretain D, Tourain C, Bergere M, et al. Large human sperm vacuoles observed in motile spermatozoa under high magnification: nuclear thumbprints linked to failure of chromatin condensation. Hum Reprod. 2011;26:1650-8.
86. Boitrelle F, Albert M, Petit JM, Ferfouri F, Wainer R, Bergere M, et al. Small human sperm vacuoles observed under high-magnification are pocket-like nuclear concavities linked to chromatin condensation failure. Reprod Biomed Online. 2013;27:201-11.
87. Franco Jr JG, Mauri AL, Petersen CG, Massaro FC, Silva LF, Felipe V, et al. Large nuclear vacuoles are indicative of abnormal chromatin packaging in human spermatozoa. Int J Androl. 2012;35:46-51.
88. Perdrix A, Travers A, Chelli MH, Escalier D, Do Rego JL, Milazzo JP, et al. Assessment of acrosome and nuclear abnormalities in human spermatozoa with large vacuoles. Hum Reprod. 2011;26:47-58.
89. Kazerooni T, Asadi N, Jadid L, Kazerooni M, Ghanadi A, Ghaffarpasand F, et al. Evaluation of sperm's chromatin quality with acridine orange test, chromomycin A3 and aniline blue staining in couples with unexplained recurrent abortion. J Assist Reprod Genet. 2009;26:591-6.
90. Talebi AR, Vahidi S, Aflatoonian A, Ghasemi N, Ghasemzadeh J, Firoozabadi RD, et al. Cytochemical evaluation of sperm chromatin and DNA integrity in couples with unexplained recurrent spontaneous abortions. Andrologia. 2012;44 (Suppl. 1):462-70.
91. Hammoud SS, Nix DA, Hammoud AO, Gibson M, Cairns BR, Carrell DT. Genome-wide analysis identifies changes in histone retention and epigenetic modifications at developmental and imprinted gene loci in the sperm of infertile men. Hum Reprod. 2011;26:2558-69.
92. Knez K, Tomazevic T, Zorn B, Vrtacnik-Bokal E, Virant-Klun I. Intracytoplasmic morphologically selected sperm injection improves development and quality of preimplantation embryos in teratozoospermia patients. Reprod. Biomed Online. 2012;25:168-79.
93. Vanderzwalmen P, Hiemer A, Rubner P, Bach M, Neyer A, Stecher A, et al. Blastocyst development after sperm selection at high magnification is associated with size and number of nuclear vacuoles. Reprod Biomed Online. 2008;17:617-27.
94. Hammoud I, Boitrelle F, Ferfouri F, Vialard F, Bergere M, Wainer B, et al. Selection of normal spermatozoa with a vacuole-free head (6300) improves selection of spermatozoa with intact DNA in patients with high sperm DNA fragmentation rates. Andrologia. 2013;45:163-70.
95. Chelli MH, Albert M, Ray PF, Guthauser B, Izard V, Hammoud I, et al. Can intracytoplasmic morphologically selected sperm injection be used to select normal-sized sperm heads in infertile patients with macrocephalic sperm head syndrome? Fertil Steril. 2010;93:1347.
96. Cassuto NG, Le Foll N, Chantot-Bastaraud S, Balet R, Bouret D, Rouen A, et al. Sperm fluorescence in situ hybridization study in nine men carrying a Robertsonian or a reciprocal translocation: relationship between segregation modes and high-magnification sperm morphology examination. Fertil Steril. 2011;96:826-32.
97. Chelli MH, Ferfouri F, Boitrelle F, Albert M, Molina-Gomes D, Selva J, et al. High-magnification sperm selection does not decrease the aneuploidy rate in patients who are heterozygous for reciprocal translocations. J Assist Reprod Genet. 2013;30:525-30.
98. Figueira Rde C, Braga DP, Setti AS, Iaconelli Jr. A, Borges Jr. E. Morphological nuclear integrity of sperm cells is associated with preimplantation genetic aneuploidy screening cycle outcomes. Fertil Steril. 2011;95:990-3.
99. Engelmann U, Krassnigg F, Schatz H, Schill WB. Separation of human X and Y spermatozoa by free-flow electrophoresis. Gamete Res. 1988;19:151-60.
100. Chaudhuri AR, Datta H. A novel technique for isolation of pure sperm heads from disintegrated mammalian spermatozoa. Prep Biochem. 1994;24:185-92.
101. Ainsworth C, Nixon B, Aitken RJ. Development of a novel electrophoretic system for the isolation of human spermatozoa. Hum Reprod. 2005;20;2261-70.
102. Zarei-Kheirabadi M, Shayegan Nia E, Tavalaee M, Deemeh MR, Arabi M, Forouzanfar M, et al. Evaluation of ubiquitin and annexin v in sperm population selected based on density gradient centrifugation and zeta potential (DGC-Zeta). J Assist Reprod Genet. 2012;29:365-71.
103. Zahedi A, Tavalaee M, Deemeh MR, Azadi L, Fazilati M, Nasr-Esfahani MH. Zeta potential vs apoptotic marker: which is more suitable for ICSI sperm selection? J Assist Reprod Genet. 2013;30:1181-6.
104. Razavi SH, Nasr-Esfahani MH, Deemeh MR, Shayesteh M, Tavalaee M. Evaluation of zeta and HA-binding methods for selection of spermatozoa with normal morphology, protamine content and DNA integrity. Andrologia. 2010;42:13-9.
105. Esfahani MHN, Deemeh MR, Tavalaee M, Sekhavati MH, Gourabi H. Zeta sperm selection improves pregnancy rate and alters sex ratio in male factor infertility patients: a double-blind, randomized clinical trial. Int J Fertil Steril. 2016;10:253-60.
106. Plouffe BD, Murthy SK, Lewis LH. Fundamentals and application of magnetic particles in cell isolation and enrichment: a review. Rep Prog Phys. 2015;78:016601.
107. Elmore S. Apoptosis: a review of programmed cell death. Toxicol Pathol. 2007;35:495-516.
108. Vermes I, Haanen C, Steffens-Nakken H, Reutellingsperger C. A novel assay for apoptosis Flow cytometric detection of phosphatidylserine expression on early apoptotic cells using fluorescein labeled Annexin V. J Immunol Methods. 1995;184:39-51.
109. Gil M, Sar-Shalom V, Melendez Sivira Y, Carreras R, Checa MA. Sperm selection using magnetic activated cell sorting (MACS) in assisted reproduction: a systematic review and meta-analysis. J Assist Reprod Genet. 2013;30:479-85.
110. Grunewald S, Paasch U, Glander HJ. Enrichment of non-apoptotic human spermatozoa after cryopreservation by immunomagnetic cell sorting. Cell Tissue Bank. 2001;2:127-33.
111. Degheidy T, Abdelfattah H, Seif A, Albuz FK, Gazi S, Abbas S. Magnetic activated cell sorting: an effective method for reduction of spermDNA fragmentation in varicocele men prior to assisted reproductive techniques. Andrologia. 2015;47:892-6.
112. Tavalaee M, Deemeh MR, Arbabian M, Nasr-Esfahani MH. Density gradient centrifugation before or after magnetic-activated cell sorting: which technique is more useful for clinical sperm selection? J Assist Reprod Genet. 2012;29:31-8.

113. Nadalini M, Tarozzi N, Di Santo M, Borini A. Annexin V magneticactivated cell sorting versus swim-up for the selection of human sperm in ART: is the new approach better then the traditional one? J Assist Reprod Genet. 2014;31:1045-51.
114. Cakar Z, Cetinkaya B, Aras D, Koca B, Ozkavukcu S, Kaplanoglu I, et al. Does combining magnetic-activated cell sorting with density gradient or swim-up improve sperm selection? J Assist Reprod Genet. 2016;33:1059-65.
115. Berteli TS, Da Broi MG, Martins WP, Ferriani RA, Navarro PA. Magnetic-activated cell sorting before density gradient centrifugation improves recovery of high-quality spermatozoa. Andrology 2017;5(4):776-82.
116. Zhang, H, Xuan X, Yang S, Li X, Xu C, Gao X. Selection of viable human spermatozoa with low levels of DNA fragmentation from an immotile population using density gradient centrifugation and magnetic-activated cell sorting. Andrologia. 2018;50(1):e12821.
117. Esbert M, Pacheco A, Soares SR, Amorós D, Florensa M, Ballesteros A, et al. High sperm DNA fragmentation delays human embryo kinetics when oocytes from young and healthy donors are microinjected. Andrology. 2018;6:697-706.
118. Romany L, Garrido N, Motato Y, Aparicio B, Remohí J, Meseguer M. Removal of annexin V-positive sperm cells for intracytoplasmic sperm injection in ovum donation cycles does not improve reproductive outcome: a controlled and randomized trial in unselected males. Fertil Steril. 2014;102(6):1567-75.
119. García-Ferreyra J, Villegas L, Romero R, Zavala P, Hilario R, Dueñas-Chacón J. High pregnancy and implantation rates can be obtained using magnetic-activated cell sorting (MACS) to selection spermatozoa in patients with high levels of spermatic DNA fragmentation. JFIV Reprod Med Genet. 2014;3:133.
120. Stimpfel M, Verdenik I, Zorn B, Virant-Klun I. Magnetic activated cell sorting of non-apoptotic spermatozoa improves the quality of embryos according to female age: a prospective sibling oocyte study. J Assist Reprod Genet. 2018;35(9):1665-74.
121. Ziarati N, Tavalaee M, Bahadorani M, Nasr Esfahani MH. Clinical outcomes of magnetic activated sperm sorting in infertile men candidate for ICSI. Hum Fertil. 2019;22(2): 118-25.
122. Dandekar P, Aggeler J, Talbot P. Structure, distribution and composition of the extracellular matrix of human oocytes and cumulus masses. Hum Reprod. 1992;7(3):391-8.
123. Cayli S, Jakab A, Ovari L, Delpiano E, Celik-Ozenci C, Sakkas D, et al. Biochemical markers of sperm function: male fertility and sperm selection for ICSI. Reprod. Biomed. Online. 2003;7(4):462-8.
124. Huszar G, Ozkavukcu S, Jakab A, Celik-Ozenci C, Sati GL, Cayli S. Hyaluronic acid binding ability of human sperm reflects cellular maturity and fertilizing potential: selection of sperm for intracytoplasmic sperm injection. Curr Opin Obstet Gynecol. 2006;18(3):260-7.
125. Barak Y, Menezo Y, Veiga A, Elder K. A physiological replacement for polyvinylpyrrolidone (PVP) in assisted reproductive technology. Hum Fertil. 2001;4:99-103.
126. Parmegiani L, Cognigni GE, Bernardi S, Troilo E, Ciampaglia W, Filicori M. "Physiologic ICSI": hyaluronic acid (HA) favors selection of spermatozoa without DNA fragmentation and with normal nucleus, resulting in improvement of embryo quality. Fertil Steril. 2010;93:598-604.
127. Van den Bergh MJ, Fahy-Deshe M, Hohl MK. Pronuclear zygote score following intracytoplasmic injection of hyaluronan-bound spermatozoa: a prospective randomized study. Reprod Biomed Online. 2009;19(6):796-801.
128. Nasr-Esfahani MH, Razavi S, Vahdati AA, Fathi F, Tavalaee M. Evaluation of sperm selection procedure based on hyaluronic acid binding ability on ICSI outcome. J Assist Reprod Genet. 2008;25(5):197-203.
129. Yagci A, Murk W, Stronk J, Huszar G. Spermatozoa bound to solid state hyaluronic acid show chromatin structure with high DNA chain integrity: an acridine orange fluorescence study. J Androl. 2010;31(6):566-72.
130. Mongkolchaipak S, Vutyavanich T. No difference in highmagnification morphology and hyaluronic acid binding in the selection of euploid spermatozoa with intact DNA. Asian J Androl. 2013;15(3):421-4.
131. Huang MT, Kuo-Kuang Lee R, Lu CH, Chen YJ, Li SH, Hwu YM. The efficiency of conventional microscopic selection is comparable to the hyaluronic acid binding method in selecting spermatozoa for male infertility patients. Taiwan. J Obstet Gynecol. 2015;54(1):48-53.
132. Parmegiani L, Cognigni GE, Ciampaglia W, Pocognoli P, Marchi F, Filicori M. Efficiency of hyaluronic acid (HA) sperm selection. J Assist Reprod Genet. 2010;27(1):13-6.
133. Choe SA, Tae JC, Shin MY, Kim HJ, Kim CH, Lee JY, et al. Application of sperm selection using hyaluronic acid binding in intracytoplasmic sperm injection cycles: a sibling oocyte study. J Korean Med Sci. 2012;27(12):1569-73.
134. Parmegiani L, Cognigni GE, Bernardi S, Troilo E, Taraborrelli S, Arnone A, et al. Comparison of two ready-to-use systems designed for spermhyaluronic acid binding selection before intracytoplasmic sperm injection: PICSI vs. sperm slow: a prospective, randomized trial. Fertil Steril. 2012;98(3):632-7.
135. Majumdar G, Majumdar A. A prospective randomized study to evaluate the effect of hyaluronic acid sperm selection on the intracytoplasmic sperm injection outcome of patients with unexplained infertility having normal semen parameters. J Assist Reprod Genet. 2013;30(11):1471-5.
136. Mokánszki A, Tóthné EV, Bodnár B, Tándor Z, Molnár Z, Jakab A, et al. Is sperm hyaluronic acid binding ability predictive for clinical success of intracytoplasmic sperm injection: PICSI vs. ICSI? Syst Biol Reprod Med. 2014;60(6):348-54.
137. Worrilow KC, Eid S, Woodhouse D, Perloe M, Smith S, Witmyer J, et al. Use of hyaluronan in the selection of sperm for intracytoplasmic sperm injection (ICSI): significant improvement in clinical outcomes—multicenter, double-blinded and randomized controlled trial. Hum Reprod. 2013;28(2):306-14.
138. Erberelli RF, Salgado RM, Pereira DHM, Wolff P. Hyaluronan-binding system for sperm selection enhances pregnancy rates in ICSI cycles associated with male factor infertility. JBRA. Assist Reprod. 2017;21(1):2-6.
139. Miller D, Pavitt S, Sharma V, Forbes G, Hooper R, Bhattacharya S, et al. Physiological, hyaluronan-selected intracytoplasmic sperm injection for infertility treatment (HABSelect): a parallel, two-group, randomised trial. Lancet. 2019;393(10170):416-22.
140. Brody JP, Yager P. Diffusion-based extraction in a microfabricated device. Sensors and Actuators, Physical. 1997;58(1):13-8.

141. Wiegl BH, Yager P. Microfluidic diffusion-based separation and detection. Science.1999;283(5400):346-7.
142. Kenis PJA, Ismagilov RF, Whitesides GM. Microfabrication inside capillaries using multiphase laminar flow patterning. Science. 1999;285(5424):83-5.
143. Takayama S, Ostuni E, LeDuc P, Naruse K, Ingber DE, Whitesides GM, et al. Laminar flows: subcellular positioning of small molecules. Nature. 2001;411(6841):1016.
144. Shirota K, Yotsumoto F, Itoh H, Obama H, Hidaka N, Nakajima K, et al. Separation efficiency of a microfluidic sperm sorter to minimize sperm DNA damage. Fertil Steril. 2016;105(2):315-21.
145. Schulte RT, Chung YK, Ohl DA, Takayama S, Smith GD. Microfluidic sperm sorting device provides a novel method for selecting motile sperm with higher DNA integrity. Fertil Steril. 2007;88(Suppl 1):S76.
146. Jackson RE, Bormann CL, Hassun PA, Rocha AM, Motta EL, Serafini PC, et al. Effects of semen storage and separation techniques on sperm DNA fragmentation. Fertil Steril. 2010;94:2626-30.
147. Hughes CM, Lewis SE, McKelvey-Martin VJ, Thompson W. The effects of antioxidant supplementation during Percoll preparation on human sperm DNA integrity. Hum Reprod. 1998;13(5):1240-7.
148. Pérez-Cerezales S, Ramos-Ibeas P, Acuña OS, Avilés M, Coy P, Rizos D, et al. The oviduct: from sperm selection to the epigenetic landscape of the embryo. Biol. Reprod. 2018;98(3):262-76.
149. Miki K, Clapham DE. Rheotaxis guides mammalian sperm. Curr. Biol. 2013;23(6):443-52.
150. De Martin H, Cocuzza MS, Tiseo BC, Wood GJA, Miranda EP, Monteleone PAA, et al. Positive rheotaxis extended drop: a one-step procedure to select and recover sperm with mature chromatin for intracytoplasmic sperm injection. J Assist Reprod Genet. 2017;34(12):1699-708.
151. Nagata MPB, Endo K, Ogata K, Yamanaka K, Egashira J, Katafuchi N, et al. Live births from artificial insemination of microfluidic-sorted bovine spermatozoa characterized by trajectories correlated with fertility. Proc Natl Acad Sci USA. 2018;115(14):E3087-96.
152. Zhang Z, Liu J, Meriano J, Ru C, Xie S, Luo J, et al. Human sperm rheotaxis: a passive physical process. Sci Rep. 2016;6: 23553.
153. Oren-Benaroya R, Orvieto R, Gakamsky A, Pinchasov M, Eisenbach M. The sperm chemoattractant secreted from human cumulus cells is progesterone. Hum Reprod. 2008; 23(10):2339-45.
154. Gatica LV, Guidobaldi HA, Montesinos MM, Teves ME, Moreno AI, Uñates D, et al. Picomolar gradients of progesterone select functional human sperm even in subfertile samples. Mol Hum Reprod. 2013;19(9):559-69.
155. Bahat A, Tur-Kaspa I, Gakamsky A, Giojalas LC, Breitbart H, Eisenbach M. Thermotaxis of mammalian sperm cells: a potential navigation mechanism in the female genital tract. Nat Med. 2003;9:149-50.
156. Mondal MA, Takagi Y, Baba SA, Hamano K. Involvement of calcium channels and intracellular calcium in bull sperm thermotaxis. J Reprod Dev. 2016;63:143-8.

CHAPTER 102

# Semen Banking

*Guruprasad Kalthur, Sandhya Kumari, Satish Kumar Adiga*

## INTRODUCTION

Semen banking has become an integral part of reproductive medicine field, in which spermatozoa in the ejaculate are stored at subzero temperatures for future purpose. Theoretically, the spermatozoa can be maintained in its viable form for an indefinite period provided the storage conditions are good. The concept of semen banking has completely changed the infertility practice and cancer treatment in the recent years. This chapter gives an overview of various aspects of semen banking and the latest developments in the semen cryopreservation field.

## HISTORY OF SEMEN BANKING

The first observation of semen cryopreservation was made by an Italian physiologist Lazzaro Spallanzani in 1776. He observed that the spermatozoa from frog which were motionless when cooled by snow were able to regain their motility upon warming. Even though Montegazza was the first one to propose the concept of semen banking for soldiers as a method of having a legal heir with their frozen semen in mid 1800s itself, the first major breakthrough in semen cryopreservation was achieved only in 1949 by Polge, Smith and Parke1 using glycerol as cryoprotective agent. The first successful pregnancy from frozen-thawed spermatozoa was reported in 1953 by Bunge and Sherman. Their report also indicated that cryopreservation does not affect the fertilizing ability of the spermatozoa and development of embryos derived from such spermatozoa.[2] Ever since this report, in last five decades, a steady progress has been witnessed in the methodological approach to the cryobiology of human spermatozoa **(Table 1)**.

## PROTOCOLS

Despite the fact that semen cryopreservation is practiced since several years, we still do not have a gold standard method, which is universally accepted and induces minimum damage to spermatozoa. The currently employed semen cryopreservation techniques vary with respect to the components present in the freezing medium, type of sample used, and the freezing method followed.

### Media Composition

The conventional semen cryopreservation medium is usually composed of a penetrating cryoprotectant (glycerol), nonpenetrating cryoprotectant (sucrose), semen extender (egg yolk/serum albumin/lipoproteins), and buffer system

**TABLE 1:** Milestones in semen cryopreservation.

| *Year* | *Breakthrough* | *Group* |
|---|---|---|
| 1776 | Viable sperm recovered from dead man buried in ice | Lazzaro Spallanzani[34,38] |
| 1866 | Suggested that soldier could produce a legal heir with stored semen sample | Paolo Montegazza[35,39] |
| 1949 | Spermatozoa can be frozen and thawed without loss of motility by includingglycerol in the suspending medium | Polge et al.[1] |
| 1953 | Normal embryonic development from freeze-dried spermatozoa | Bunge and Sherman[2] |
| 1964 | First child born from sperm frozen in liquid nitrogen | Perloff et al.[36,40] |
| 1970s | Mandatory semen freezing for the United States military men | — |
| 1995 | First birth from frozen epididymal sperm | Devroey et al.[37,41] |
| 1996 | First birth from frozen testicular sperm | Gil-Salom et al.[38,42] |
| At present | Integral part of andrology lab/assisted reproductive technique clinic | — |

{Tris/2-[4-(2-Hydroxyethyl)-1-piperazinyl]ethanesulfonic acid (HEPES)/citrate buffer} and osmolytes (glycine). Egg yolk, though rich in membrane lipids such as cholesterol and phospholipids, the major drawbacks are its variability in composition based on the nutritional status and health conditions of hen, infectious microorganisms of avian origin and, possible risk of endotoxins. In this direction, efforts to cryopreserve the human spermatozoa in medium devoid of egg yolk have been successfully achieved.[3] Use of low density lipoprotein has been shown to enhance the cryosurvival of bull,[4] buffalo[5] and rabbit[6] spermatozoa. For short-term storage, electrolyte free medium has been successfully demonstrated in human spermatozoa at low temperature.[7] Further studies are necessary to confirm whether it is possible to store the spermatozoa in liquid nitrogen using electrolyte free medium

## Type of Sample

- *Cryopreservation of neat ejaculate:* In this approach, the liquefied semen samples are mixed with semen freezing medium and subjected to cryopreservation. The advantage with this approach is that the seminal plasma is very rich in some of the antioxidants, which can minimize the freeze-thaw-induced damage.[8] In addition, the decapacitation factors present in the seminal plasma prevent the spermatozoa from undergoing premature capacitation or acrosome reaction.[9] However, the disadvantage with this approach is that the neat ejaculate contains dead spermatozoa, abnormal spermatozoa, round cells, etc., which can increase the generation of reactive oxygen species (ROS) during the cryopreservation process, and thus can reduce the functional competence of the spermatozoa.
- *Cryopreservation of sorted spermatozoa:* To overcome the drawbacks of using neat ejaculate, sorting of the spermatozoa with respect to their quality prior to cryopreservation has been attempted earlier.[10] Extraction of motile spermatozoa fraction from the ejaculate and, elimination of apoptotic spermatozoa, leukocytes and abnormal spermatozoa by simple sperm preparation methods like swim up technique or density gradient separation methods have demonstrated considerable improvement in the outcome of semen cryopreservation.[10,11] However, the major drawback with this approach is that the loss of antioxidants and decapacitation factors present in the seminal plasma, which may lead to poor freeze-thaw outcome.

## Storage Devices

Semen samples can be stored in variety of devices. The initial experiments of semen cryopreservation were conducted with glass ampoules as storage materials. However, due to their low surface to volume ratio and fragile nature of the material, loss of precious stored samples due to breakage is most likely. Most popular storage devices currently used are high security plastic straws and cryovials with screw caps. To keep the samples secure and avoid any contact with liquid nitrogen, plastic straws require sealing after loading the semen samples either with any nontoxic adhesive materials, clay, polyvinyl plugs or by heat sealing method. To enable correct identification of the sample, the storage devices have to be labeled with proper patient details.

## Cooling and Storage

The storage device containing semen samples are usually exposed to gradual decrease in temperature instead of directly plunging into liquid nitrogen. There are two different protocols—rapid freezing, where the samples are kept at 4°C for 10 minutes followed by 10–15 minutes exposure to liquid nitrogen vapor and then finally placed in liquid nitrogen; in slow cooling protocol, the samples are gradually exposed to decreasing temperature with the help of a programmable freezer. Theoretically, the semen samples can be stored indefinitely provided the storage conditions are maintained properly. There are reports available in the literature indicating successful pregnancy from the semen samples cryopreserved for >20 years.[12,13]

## Semen Vitrification

Vitrification is an ultrarapid method of freezing. It is an alternative method of sperm cryopreservation based on the solidification of solution into glass-like state without formation of crystallization or expansion.[14] Increased rate of freezing and the concentration of cryoprotectant in freezing medium help in avoiding ice crystal formation. However, due to toxicity of high concentration of cryoprotectants and direct contact of liquid nitrogen this procedure did not find any advantage compared to conventional cryofreezing method.[15] Cryoprotectant-free technique of vitrification has advantage over other methods since it does not use any permeable cryoprotectants and therefore does not cause any osmotic shock. Birth of two healthy babies from spermatozoa vitrified in absence of permeating cryoprotectant has been reported by Isachenko et al.[16]

## Storage Duration

The semen samples can be cryopreserved for long duration provided the storage conditions such as liquid nitrogen level is maintained properly. Few studies have shown that long-term storage of semen sample does not lead to any adverse effects on the motility potential and chromatin integrity of the spermatozoa.[17,18] Clarke et al.[18] have shown that the ability of spermatozoa to undergo acrosome reaction and zona binding potential were retained even after prolonged storage period. Live births have been achieved following intrauterine insemination (IUI) and intracytoplasmic sperm injection (ICSI) with spermatozoa stored for 28 and 21 years, respectively[12,13] indicating that the storage duration may not have any adverse effect on the functional competence of the spermatozoa. However, genetic instability in spermatozoa due to cosmic radiation is a matter of concern.

*Thawing:* Like the cooling rate, thawing temperature is also very critical for achieving good post-thaw survival of the spermatozoa. Rapid thawing by incubating the cryovials or the high security straws in a water bath maintained at 37°C is most commonly followed. Once the frozen sample is completely thawed, it is very essential to remove the cryoprotectants completely by washing so that the toxicity exerted by the cryoprotectants can be minimized.

*Documentation:* A proper documentation system should be used for maintaining the details of the samples stored in liquid nitrogen. Location of each sample, date of semen freezing, number of samples stored from a particular person (donor/infertile man/man opting for fertility preservation), date of expiry of the legal agreement between semen bank and the party for the storage of semen sample, etc., has to be maintained safely. Loss of stored material due to loss of la beling, improper storage method, faulty sealing, etc., can be disastrous situation for the laboratory director. The number of semen samples stored from a particular donor, number of samples released for insemination, number of pregnancies achieved from that particular donor should be recorded. It is very essential to have a signed document that clearly states who will have the rights to access to the spermatozoa of the husband following his death. Usually, the wife becomes the legal heir, who can decide whether to discard the sample or donate it for research.

## Indications for Semen Cryopreservation

- *Donor semen samples:* Using donor semen samples for treating male factor infertility is widely accepted method. Since the fresh ejaculates cannot be used for insemination, it is mandatory to cryopreserve the semen samples and quarantine for at least 6 months. Repeated investigation during this quarantine period will help in identification and exclusion of the donor samples infected with sexually transmitted diseases (STDs). Cryopreservation of semen samples from suitable donors will help in creating a bank with wide variety of samples with different blood groups and phenotypes for achieving the best possible matching with recipient.

*Selection and recruitment of semen donor:* As per the current Indian guidelines,[19,20] semen donors should be anonymous to the recipient. The semen donor should be at least 21-years and not more than 55-years of age, free of any STDs and identifiable genetic disorders. Donor should produce Aadhar card as his proof of identity with a written consent from his wife. Ideally, the semen donor should not have any multiple sexual partners, with good educational background and with good lifestyle habits. The donor should be asked to provide his ejaculate preferably collected in the masturbatorium of the semen bank. As per the current ART (assisted reproductive technique) bill[19] a donor can donate maximum of 25 ejaculates. The ejaculates should be cryopreserved (quarantined) for at least 6 months prior to their release for insemination. The donor should be screened for serostatus once in every 6 months to rule out any sexually transmitted disease (STDs).

The semen bank, which can operate as an independent organization with professionally qualified and trained people, can store the ejaculates from donors with various phenotypic features and blood group. Donor can get a suitable financial remuneration from the bank. It is the responsibility of the semen bank to maintain complete details of the donor including height, weight, age, educational qualifications, profession, color of the skin and the eyes, record of major diseases including any psychiatric disorder, and the family background with respect to history of any familial disorder, number of samples used for insemination, details of blood investigation, etc. The donor should be giving a written consent for using his stored semen samples for insemination. He should be made aware that he will not know the identity of the recipients and the details of the child born through his spermatozoa and will not have any parental rights over the child. The do's and don'ts of semen banking is summarized in **Table 2**.

- *Convenient cryopreservation:* It has become a routine practice now to cryopreserve the semen sample of male partner well in advance of insemination time, whether it is for IUI, in vitro fertilization (IVF) or ICSI. Sometimes, male partner may fail to provide the ejaculate on demand due to psychological stress or anxiety, erectile dysfunction, unscheduled travelling, or poor quality ejaculate may be obtained on the day of the procedure. Cryopreservation of one or two ejaculates well in advance will avoid the cancellation of cycle due to the nonavailability of the spermatozoa, which will have huge psychological and financial burden on the infertile couple.
- *Pooling of ejaculates from men with severe oligozoospermia:* The sperm count and motility in the ejaculate can fluctuate, which can have an impact on the infertility treatment using assisted reproductive technology. Especially in ejaculates from severe oligoasthenoteratozoospermia (OAT), finding the motile spermatozoa on the day of the oocyte retrieval may be technically difficult. Therefore, in OAT, transient azoospermia and in virtual azoospermic cases, storage of multiple ejaculates from male partner can aid in increasing the number of motile spermatozoa fraction in the *safety pool* of the spermatozoa by pooling of many ejaculates. This will be beneficial in the management

**TABLE 2:** Summary of *do's* and *don'ts* of semen banking as per the recent Assisted Reproductive Technology [(ART) Regulation)] Act 2021, India.[43]

| *Do's* | *Don'ts* |
|---|---|
| • Registration or renewal of registration under the national ART board<br>• Screening of sperm donors, the collection, screening of semen sample, and storage of semen<br>• Recruiting the donor aged between 21 and 55 years<br>• Obtaining all necessary information about a sperm donor- name of donor, Aadhaar number, address, etc<br>• Taking undertaking in writing from donor about the confidentiality of information.<br>• After 10 years of storage period, allowing the sample to perish or donating to research organizations registered under the national ART Act for research purposes with the consent of the individual<br>• Submission of information about number of donors sample screened, maintained and supplied to the National Registry within a period of one month from the date of receipt of request for such information<br>• Maintaining the records of semen bank for at least 10 years<br>• Transferring the records to a central database of the National Registry upon expiry of the bank<br>• Ensuring the records are available for inspection to the National Board or the National Registry or the State Board or to any other person authorized by the National Board | • Storing donor sample for more than 10 years<br>• Treating woman with sperm derived from more than one man during any one treatment cycle<br>• Mixing the semen from two individuals for the ART procedures<br>• Supplying the sperm of a single donor to more than one commissioning couple<br>• The sale, transfer or use of sperm to any party within or outside India |

of ICSI for cryptozoospermic and oligozoospermic men to increase the number of progressively motile spermatozoa[20] and can avoid unnecessary testicular biopsy. In addition, pooling of ejaculates for IUI may be an option in men with borderline semen parameters who cannot afford to undergo expensive treatments like IVF or ICSI.

- *Preoperative and postoperative cryopreservation:* Semen samples can be cryopreserved prior to any surgical treatments such as varicocele ligation, vasectomy or orchidectomy, to protect against possible azoospermia due to any postoperative complication or any unforeseen postoperative course. It is advisable to cryopreserve the spermatozoa prior to planning transurethral resection of the ejaculatory ducts (TURED). This approach will give an opportunity for the men to have children through their cryopreserved spermatozoa with the help of ART in future, if situation make them to plan for a progeny. Spermatozoa collected at the time of surgical procedures (intraoperative cryopreservation) performed for unreconstructable obstructive azoospermia (OA), such as congenital bilateral absence of the vas deferens (CBAVD) can be cryopreserved and used later for ART. Various approaches such as microsurgical epididymal sperm aspiration (MESA), percutaneous epididymal sperm aspiration (PESA), electroejaculation (EE) and TURED have been followed for the sperm retrieval. In addition, it may be a wise option to store the spermatozoa obtained during surgical reconstructive procedures such as vasovasostomy and vasoepididymostomy.

It has become a routine practice now to cryopreserve the testicular spermatozoa obtained during diagnostic testicular biopsy or testicular sperm extraction (TESE). It avoids the pain and cost caused by repeated invasive procedures and, allows proper planning of ovarian stimulation of the female partner without leading to any situation of ICSI cycle getting cancelled with no spermatozoa available for microinjection after oocyte retrieval.

- *Cryopreservation prior to treatment for malignancies:* With advancement in diagnosis and understanding the biology of deadly diseases such as cancer, the disease-free survival rate has gone up. However, the cytotoxic treatments using chemotherapy and/or radiotherapy with other treatment modalities may lead to partial or complete arrest of spermatogenesis.[21] Even if the spermatogenesis is restored, the quality of the spermatozoa produced is known to be poor with high incidence of genetic and epigenetic defects.[22] Since it is difficult to predict the extent of testicular damage and the future fertility potential, it is recommended if the patient can store his semen sample before starting chemotherapy, which can be used by the cancer survivors to have the progeny from their own gametes at a later stage.
- *Cryopreservation prior to treatment for nonmalignant diseases:* Semen cryopreservation prior to any treatment is not only limited to malignant diseases. Men diagnosed with nonmalignant, systemic disease or undergoing any treatment which may have gonadotoxic disease can store their semen sample in advance. Patients undergoing immunosuppressive or cytotoxic therapy for treatment of autoimmune disorders, kidney disorders, diabetes, ulcerative colitis and heart transplants which has risk of loss of testicular function can also store their semen sample. For example, prolonged treatment with sulfasalazine has been shown to depress semen quality and cause reversible infertility.[23]

- *High-risk profession:* Spermatozoa from men involved in high-risk profession such as military services, nuclear reactor, pesticide or heavy metal industries, etc., can be encouraged to store their semen samples well in advance so that loss of fertility due to their high-risk profession can be avoided. However, still there is lack of awareness among people to make use of this option to retain their fertility potential. Even though the postmortem sperm collection and cryopreservation for the wife of the deceased to achieve pregnancy has been attempted in the past, there is a lot of legal and ethical issues involved. Written consent from wife for postmortem sperm retrieval is required and the following points may have to be taken into consideration.
  - Couple must have been planning for a family prior to the death of the husband
  - Death was sudden
  - Death was not due to any disease known to affect spermatogenesis
  - Death was not due to any infective disease that can cause transmission of disease
  - Spermatozoa should be retrieved from the dead man within 24 hours after death
  - Wife must consent for specimen quarantine.
- *Consequences of semen cryopreservation technique on functional competence of spermatozoa:* Studies have shown that at least 50% of spermatozoa are damaged or destroyed by freezing and thawing, due to chemical, physical, and oxidative stress as a result of changes in intracellular and extracellular environment.[24,25] Membrane damage, acrosome swelling, acrosome loss, damaged mitochondrial sheath, etc., are common ultrastructural changes reported. High polyunsaturated fatty acid content and limited cytoplasmic antioxidant defense system makes the spermatozoa highly susceptible to the oxidative stress generated during freeze-thaw process.[26-28] The lipid peroxides generated through oxidative stress and mitochondrial damage leads to high degree of DNA damage[25,29] and epigenetic changes in spermatozoa.[30] In spite of these ultrastructural, genetic and epigenetic changes induced by cryopreservation on spermatozoa, in humans no significant health problems was observed in the progenies born from frozen-thawed spermatozoa.[31]

## FUTURE DIRECTION

The goal of semen cryopreservation protocol is to prevent detrimental effects of freeze-thaw process on the sperm functional competence. However, the process is complicated due to biochemically and physically diverse compartments present in the spermatozoa (acrosome, nucleus, mitochondrial-flagellar network), all of which may respond quite differently to freezing and thawing. Since the detrimental effects are thought to be mainly mediated through oxidative stress, supplementation of various antioxidants is considered as future of research in the field of semen cryopreservation. Adding antioxidant enzymes and molecules such as catalase,[32] superoxide dismutase,[33] vitamin E,[34] vitamin C[35] to cryopreservation media has shown promising beneficial role in enhancing the post-thaw functional competence of spermatozoa. Trace elements with known biological functions such as copper, selenium, zinc, etc., have also been shown to prevent the freeze-thaw-induced damage to spermatozoa.[36,37]

## REFERENCES


1. Polge C, Smith AU, Parkes AS. Revival of spermatozoa after vitrification and dehydration at low temperatures. Nature. 1949;164(4172):666.
2. Bunge RG, Sherman JK. Fertilizing capacity of frozen human spermatozoa. Nature. 1953;172(4382):767-8.
3. Mutalik S, Salian SR, Avadhani K, Menon J, Joshi H, Hegde AR, et al. Liposome encapsulated soy lecithin and cholesterol can efficiently replace chicken egg yolk in human semen cryopreservation medium. Syst Biol Reprod Med. 2014;60(3):183-8.
4. Jiang ZL, Li QW, Hu JH, Li WY, Zhao HW, Zhang SS. Improvement of the quality of boar cryopreservation semen by supplementing with low density lipoprotein in diluents. Cryobiology. 2007;54(3):301-4.
5. Dalal J, Chandolia RK, Pawaria S, Kumar A, Kumar D, Selokar NL, et al. Low-density lipoproteins protect sperm during cryopreservation in buffalo: Unraveling mechanism of action. Mol Reprod Dev. 2020;87(12):1231-44.
6. Iaffaldano N, Di Iorio M, Rosato MP, Manchisi A. Cryopreservation of rabbit semen using non-permeable cryoprotectants: effectiveness of different concentrations of low-density lipoproteins (LDL) from egg yolk versus egg yolk or sucrose. Anim Reprod Sci. 2014;151(3-4):220-8.
7. Kanno H, Saito K, Ogawa T, Takeda M, Iwasaki A, Kinoshita Y. Viability and function of human sperm in electrolyte-free cold preservation. Fertil Steril. 1998 Jan;69(1):127-31.
8. Vernet P, Aitken RJ, Drevet JR. Antioxidant strategies in the epididymis. Mol Cell Endocrinol. 2004;216(1-2):31-9.
9. Begley AJ, Quinn P. Decapacitation factors in semen. Clin Reprod Fertil. 1982;1(3):167-75.
10. Said TM, Grunewald S, Paasch U, Rasch M, Agarwal A, Glander HJ. Effects of magnetic-activated cell sorting on sperm motility and cryosurvival rates. Fertil Steril. 2005;83(5):1442-6.
11. Grunewald S, Paasch U, Said TM, Rasch M, Agarwal A, Glander HJ. Magnetic-activated cell sorting before cryopreservation preserves mitochondrial integrity in human spermatozoa. Cell Tissue Bank. 2006;7(2):99-104.
12. Feldschuh J, Brassel J, Durso N, Levine A. Successful sperm storage for 28 years. Fertil Steril. 2005;84(4):1017.
13. Horne G, Atkinson AD, Pease EH, Logue JP, Brison DR, Lieberman BA. Live birth with sperm cryopreserved for 21 years prior to cancer treatment: case report. Hum Reprod. 2004;19(6):1448-9.
14. Katkov II, Isachenko V, Isachenko E. Low- and high-temperature vitrification as a new approach to biostabilization of reproductive and progenitor cells. Int J Refrig. 2006;29: 346-57.

15. Isachenko V, Maettner R, Petrunkina AM, Mallmann P, Rahimi G, Sterzik K, et al. Cryoprotectant-free vitrification of human spermatozoa in large (up to 0.5 mL) volume: a novel technology. Clin Lab. 2011;57(9-10):643-50.
16. Isachenko V, Isachenko E, Petrunkina AM, Sanchez R. Human spermatozoa vitrified in the absence of permeable cryoprotectants: birth of two healthy babies. Reprod Fertil Dev. 2012;24(2):323-6.
17. Kably-Ambe A, Carballo-Mondragón E, Roque-Sánchez AM. Evaluation of semen parameters in long term cryopreserved samples for over 10 years. Ginecol Obstet Mex. 2016;84(1):1-6.
18. Clarke GN, Liu DY, Baker HW. Recovery of human sperm motility and ability to interact with the human zona pellucida after more than 28 years of storage in liquid nitrogen. Fertil Steril. 2006;86(3):721-2.
19. ICMR. The Assisted Reproductive Technologies (Regulation) Rules. New Delhi: Indian Council of Medical Research; 2010.
20. Tur-Kaspa I, Dudkiewicz A, Confino E, Gleicher N. Pooled sequential ejaculates: a way to increase the total number of motile sperm from oligozoospermic men. Fertil Steril. 1990; 54(5):906-9.
21. Martin-du Pan RC, Campana A. Physiopathology of sperma togenic arrest. Fertil Steril. 1993;60(6):937-46.
22. Paoli D, Rizzo F, Fiore G, et al. Spermatogenesis in Hodgkin's lymphoma patients: a retrospective study of semen quality before and after different chemotherapy regimens. Hum Reprod. 2016;31(2):263-72.
23. Toovey S, Hudson E, Hendry WF, Pallotti F, Pulsoni A, Annechini G, et al. Sulfasalazine and male infertility: reversibility and possible mechanism. Gut. 1981;22(6):445-51.
24. Watson PF. Recent developments and concepts in the cryopreservation of spermatozoa and the assessment of their post-thawing function. Reprod Fertil Dev. 1995;7(4):871-91.
25. Gao DY, Liu J, Liu C, McGann LE, Watson PF, Kleinhans FW, et al. Prevention of osmotic injury to human spermatozoa during addition and removal of glycerol. Hum Reprod. 1995;10(5):1109-22.
26. Jones R, Mann T, Sherins R. Peroxidative breakdown of phospholipids in human spermatozoa, spermicidal properties of fatty acid peroxides, and protective action of seminal plasma. Fertil Steril. 1979;31(5):531-7.
27. Alvarez JG, Touchstone JC, Blasco L, Storey BT. Spontaneous lipid peroxidation and production of hydrogen peroxide and superoxide in human spermatozoa. Superoxide dismutase as major enzyme protectant against oxygen toxicity. J Androl. 1987;8(5):338-48.
28. Aitken RJ, Clarkson JS. Cellular basis of defective sperm function and its association with the genesis of reactive oxygen species by human spermatozoa. J Reprod Fertil. 1987;81(2):459-69.
29. Paasch U, Sharma RK, Gupta AK, Grunewald S, Mascha EJ, Thomas AJ Jr, et al. Cryopreservation and thawing is associated with varying extent of activation of apoptotic machinery in subsets of ejaculated human spermatozoa. Biol Reprod. 2004;71(6):1828-37.
30. Zeng C, Peng W, Ding L, He L, Zhang Y, Fang D, et al. A preliminary study on epigenetic changes during boar spermatozoa cryopreservation. Cryobiology. 2014;69(1): 119-27.
31. Lansac J, Royere D. Follow-up studies of children born after frozen sperm donation. Hum Reprod Update. 2001;7(1): 33-7.
32. Moghbeli M, Kohram H, Zare-Shahaneh A, Zhandi M, Sharafi M, Nabi MM, et al. Are the optimum levels of the catalase and vitamin E in rooster semen extender after freezing-thawing influenced by sperm concentration? Cryobiology. 2016;72(3):264-8.
33. Rossi T, Mazzilli F, Delfino M, Dondero F. Improved human sperm recovery using superoxide dismutase and catalase supplementation in semen cryopreservation procedure. Cell Tissue Bank. 2001;2(1):9-13.
34. Kalthur G, Raj S, Thiyagarajan A. Vitamin E supple-mentation in semen-freezing medium improves the motility and protects sperm from freeze-thaw-induced DNA damage. Fertil Steril. 2011;95(3):1149-51.
35. Martínez-Páramo S, Diogo P, Dinis MT, Herráez MP, Sarasquete C, Cabrita E. Incorporation of ascorbic acid and α-tocopherol to the extender media to enhance antioxidant system of cryopreserved sea bass sperm. Theriogenology. 2012;77(6):1129-36.
36. Kotdawala AP, Kumar S, Salian SR, Thankachan P, Govindraj K, Kumar P, et al. Addition of zinc to human ejaculate prior to cryopreservation prevents freeze- thaw-induced DNA damage and preserves sperm function. J Assist Reprod Genet. 2012;29(12):1447-53.
37. Dorostkar K, Alavi Shoushtari SM, Khaki A. Effects of In Vitro Zinc Sulfate Additive to The Semen Extender on Water Buffalo (Bubalusbubalis) Spermatozoa before and after Freezing. Int J Fertil Steril. 2014;8(3):325-32.
38. Royere D, Barthelemy C, Hamamah S, Lansac J. Cryopreservation of spermatozoa: a 1996 review. Hum Reprod Update. 1996;2(6):553-9.
39. Jensen JR, Morbeck DE, Coddington CC. Fertility preservation. Mayo Clin Proc. 2011;86(1):45-9.
40. Perloff WH, Steinberger E, Sherman JK. Conception with human spermatozoa frozen by nitrogen vapor technic. Fertil steril. 1964;15:501-4.
41. Devroey P, Silber S, Nagy Z, Liu J, Tournaye H, Joris H, et al. Ongoing pregnancies and birth after intracytoplasmic sperm injection with frozen-thawed epididymal spermatozoa. Hum Reprod. 1995;10(4): 903-6.
42. Gil-Salom M, Romero J, Minguez Y, Rubio C, De los Santos MJ, Remohí J, et al. Pregnancies after intracytoplasmic sperm injection with cryopreserved testicular spermatozoa. Hum Reprod. 1996;11(6):1309-13. Semen Banking

SECTION

# 15 Embryology

CHAPTER 103

# History of In Vitro Fertilization

*Neelima Gupta*

## INTRODUCTION

This chapter today would not have been written, rather I should say that there would have been no "history" in in vitro fertilization (IVF), had our pioneers in the field not thought of this innovation and breakthrough in science.

So, I would like to start this chapter by paying tribute to all of them, especially Sir Professor Bob Edwards (September 27, 1925–April 10, 2013), whose sad demise was a huge loss to the whole IVF fraternity.

Although research and great work were constantly happening on this subject, the history of which dates back to 1890 (details here), the world's first IVF baby, Louise Brown, was delivered in July 1978,[1] and the success and development in the field continue thereafter till date.

In 1973, the Monash University team reported in The Lancet, the first pregnancy achieved through IVF of a human oocyte.[2] This pregnancy lasted for only a few days and was a biochemical pregnancy. In the same year, Mr Landrum Shettles made an unsuccessful attempt to perform an IVF due to interdiction by the department chairman at the last minute.[3,4] In 1976, Patrick Steptoe and Robert Edwards reported an ectopic pregnancy. On July 25, 1978, Louise Brown was born in Oldham General Hospital, Greater Manchester, UK, who is the world's first baby to be conceived by IVF due to a successful procedure carried out by Steptoe and Edwards in 1977.[1,5,6] In October 1978, it was reported that Subhash Mukhopadhyay, a relatively unknown physician from Kolkata, India, was performing experiments on his own with primitive instruments and a household refrigerator and this resulted in a test tube baby, later named as "Durga" (alias Kanupriya Agarwal) who was born on October 3, 1978.[7] However, state authorities prevented him from presenting his work at scientific conferences,[8] and in the absence of scientific evidence, his work is not recognized by the international scientific community.

Steptoe and Edwards were responsible for the world's second (confirmed) baby conceived by IVF, Alastair Macdonald, born on January 14, 1979, in Glasgow.[9] A team led by Ian Johnston and Alex Lopata was responsible for Australia's first baby conceived by IVF, Candice Reed, born on June 23, 1980 in Melbourne.[10] It was the subsequent use of stimulated cycles with clomiphene citrate and the use of human chorionic gonadotropin (hCG) to control the time of oocyte maturation, thus controlling the time of collection, that converted IVF from a research tool to clinical treatment.

This was followed by a total of 14 pregnancies resulting in nine births in 1981 with the Monash University team. The Jones team[11] at the Eastern Virginia Medical School in Norfolk, Virginia, further improved stimulated cycles by incorporating the use of a follicle-stimulating hormone (FSH) [urinary human menopausal gonadotropin (uhMG)]. This then became known as controlled ovarian hyperstimulation (COH). Another step forward was the use of gonadotropin-releasing hormone (GnRH) agonists, thus decreasing the need for monitoring by preventing premature ovulation, and more recently, GnRH antagonists, which have a similar function. The additional use of the oral contraceptive pill has allowed the scheduling of IVF cycles, which has made the treatment far more convenient for both staff and patients.

The ability to freeze and subsequently thaw and transfer embryos has significantly improved the feasibility of IVF use.[12] The other very significant milestone in IVF was the development of the intracytoplasmic sperm injection (ICSI) of single sperm by André van Steirteghem and Paul Devroey in Brussels (UZ Brussel), 1992. This has enabled men with minimal sperm production to achieve pregnancies. ICSI is sometimes used in conjunction with sperm recovery, using a testicular fine needle or open testicular biopsy. Using this method, some men with Klinefelter's syndrome, and who would be otherwise infertile, have occasionally been able to achieve pregnancy.[12,13] Thus, IVF has become the final solution for most fertility problems, moving from tubal disease to male factor, idiopathic subfertility, endometriosis, advanced maternal age, and anovulation not responding to ovulation induction.

Robert Edwards was awarded the 2010 Nobel Prize in Physiology or Medicine "for the development of IVF."[14]

## HISTORY OF IN VITRO FERTILIZATION

### The Milestones

In the 1890s, Walter Heape, a professor and physician at the University of Cambridge, England, used to conduct research on reproduction in animal species. He reported the first case of embryo transplantation in rabbits. This was before the use of IVF and embryo transfer (ET) in human fertility.[15] "Brave New World," a science fiction novel, was published in 1932 by Aldous Huxley, which described the technique of IVF. Then in 1937, an editorial appeared in the New England Journal of Medicine (NEJM 1937, October 21), which is noteworthy.

Pincus and Enzmann first demonstrated successful pregnancy in unmated animals by isolating rabbit ovum and fertilizing and culturing it in a watch glass and later transferring it in a doe, following which they published a paper in 1934 from the Laboratory of General Physiology at Harvard University which was published in the Proceedings of National Academy of Sciences of the United States of America, indicating the possibility of in vitro development of mammalian eggs.

Later, Miriam Menken and John Rock published a paper almost 14 years later, in 1948, in the American Journal of Obstetrics and Gynecology, sharing their experience of IVF of human oocytes retrieved during operations for various medical conditions.

An indisputable evidence of the first successful birth of a mammal (rabbit) by Chang through IVF was published in Nature in 1959. He cultured the newly ovulated eggs with capacitated sperms for 4 hours in a small Carrel flask, paving the way for assisted conception.

Professionals from engineering, cell biology, and anatomy joined hands for further achievements in the field by improving the laboratory equipment quality, refinement of procedures, improved culture media, dishes, and embryo biopsy, which was supported by worldwide social and scientific interactions for further continuation.

Given here is a comprehensive list and review of the major milestones achieved in the field of IVF year-wise, in a chronological order, with relevant references, along with a few pictures of our pioneers.

*1965*

Robert Edwards along with Georgeanna and Howard Jones attempted in vitro human oocyte fertilization at Johns Hopkins Hospital in the USA **(Figs. 1 to 3)**.[16]

*1973*

Carl Wood and John Leeton from Monash, Australia, reported the first IVF pregnancy but it resulted in early miscarriage **(Figs. 4 to 6)**.[17]

*1976*

- First B2 culture medium was developed by Menezo, which was known as "French medium," composition of which reflects tubal and uterine environments of rabbits, sheep, and humans **(Fig. 7)**.

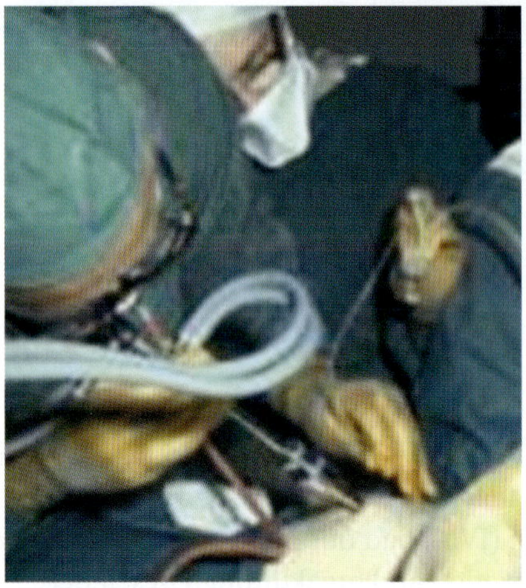

**Fig. 1:** Laparoscopic retrieval.

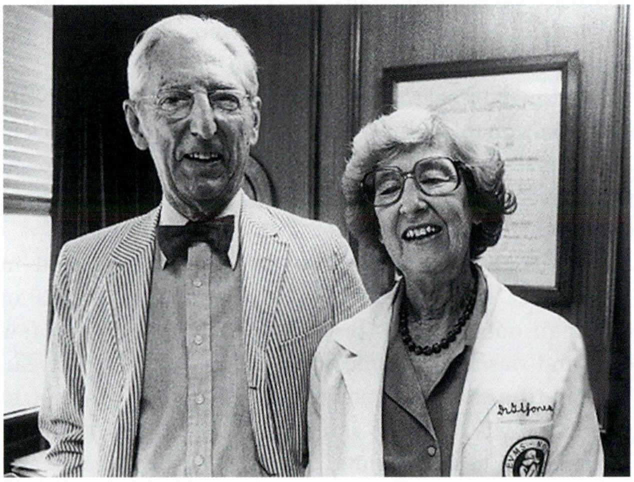

**Fig. 2:** Georgeanna and Howard Jones.

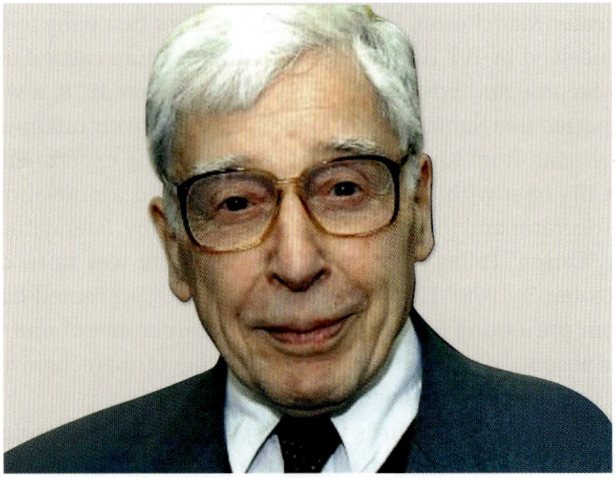

**Fig. 3:** Robert Edwards.

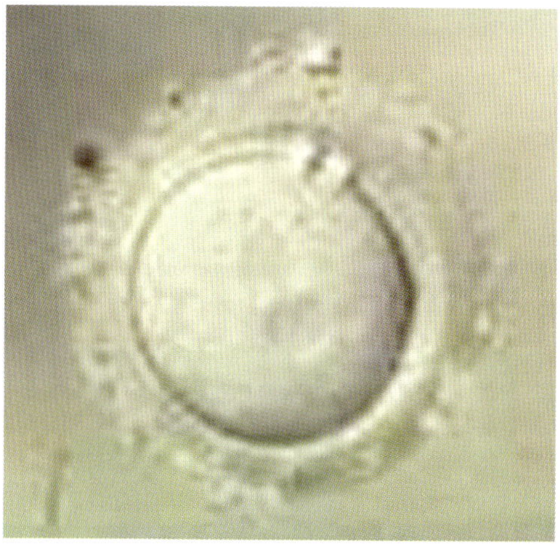

**Fig. 4:** Fertilized human oocyte.

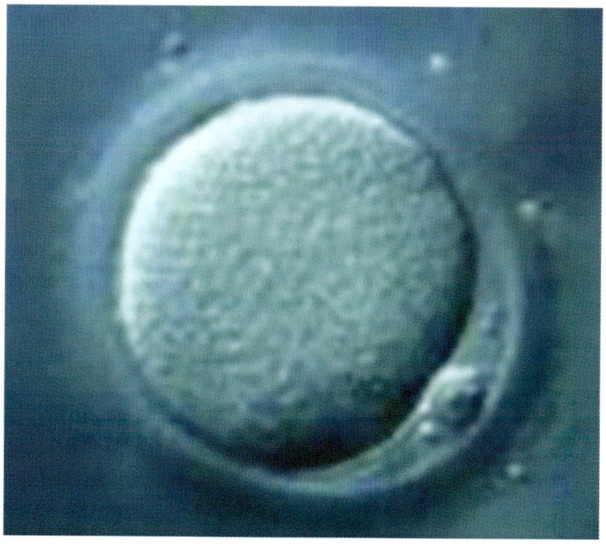

**Fig. 5:** Human oocyte.

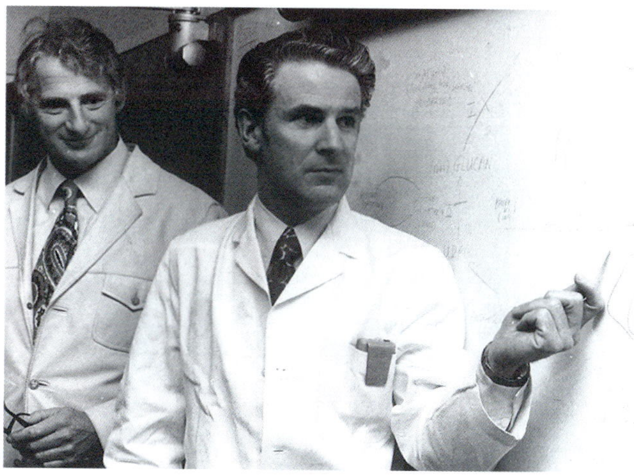

**Fig. 6:** Carl Wood and John Leeton.

- In the same year, Steptoe and Edwards published a report in "The Lancet" on an ectopic pregnancy following transfer of a human embryo.[18]

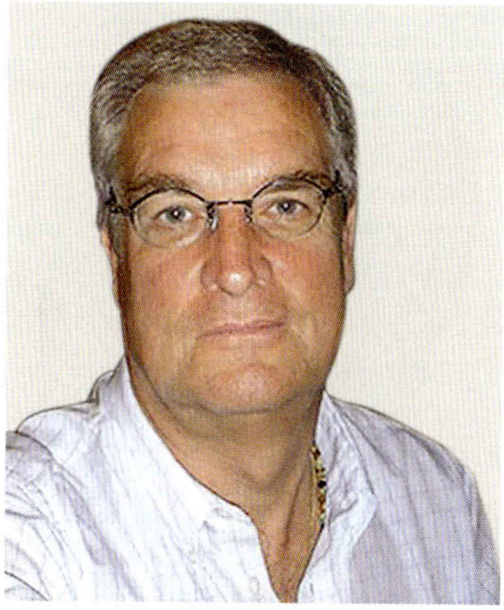

**Fig. 7:** Yves Menezo.

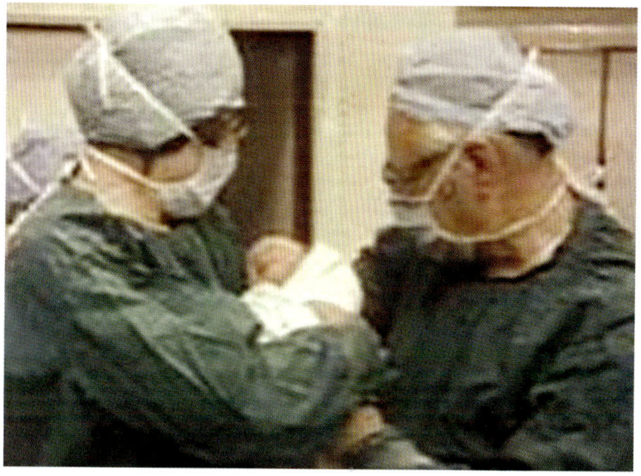

**Fig. 8:** Birth of Louise Brown.

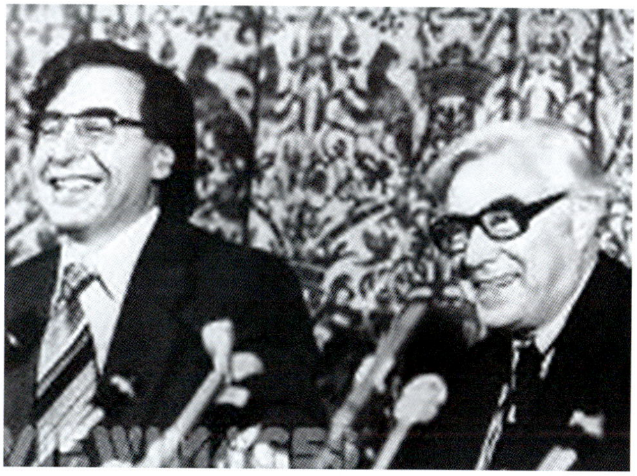

**Fig. 9:** Steptoe and Edwards.

*1978*

- Steptoe and Edwards reported the first ever IVF birth in Oldham, England, on July 25, 1978 **(Figs. 8 to 10)**.[19]
- First ever clomiphene citrate-stimulated cycle was reported by Lopata in Melbourne **(Fig. 11)**.[20]

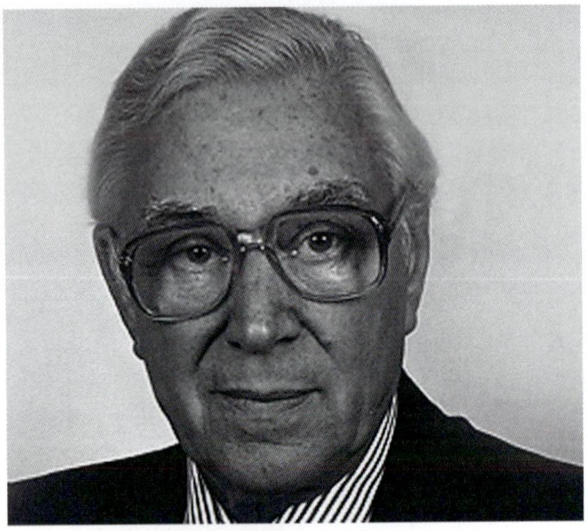

**Fig. 10:** Patrick Steptoe.

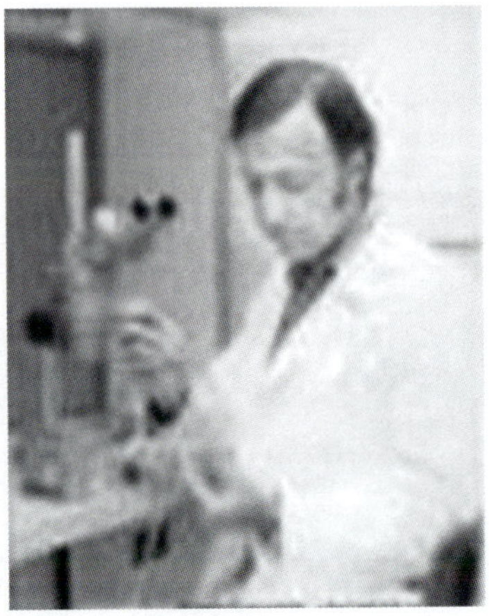

**Fig. 11:** Alex Lopata.

*1979*

- Pez et al. documented the first tracking of the growth of follicles by ultrasound and the relationship between the echographic and laparoscopic observations.[21]
- Use of ultrasound in identifying the growing follicles.[22]

*1980*

- A joint team by Monash–Melbourne reported the first IVF birth in Australia.[20]
- Introduction of culture medium.[23]

*1981*

- Delivery of the first IVF baby in the USA by using hMG by Howard and Georgeanna Seegar Jones.
- Introduction of a foot-controlled fixed aspiration pressure control by Wood et al.[24]
- Introduction of clomiphene citrate and human menopausal gonadotropin (hMG) in the IVF treatment protocol.[25]
- First luteinizing hormone (LH) assay to detect initial rise in LH to monitor accurate timing for oocyte retrieval developed by "The Clamart Group in France".[26]

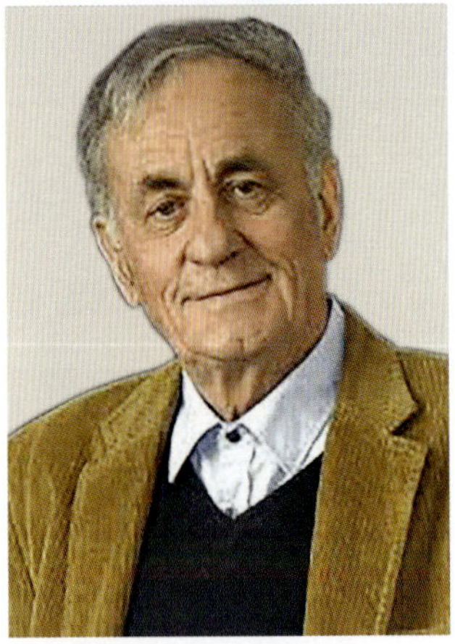

**Fig. 12:** Jacques Testart.

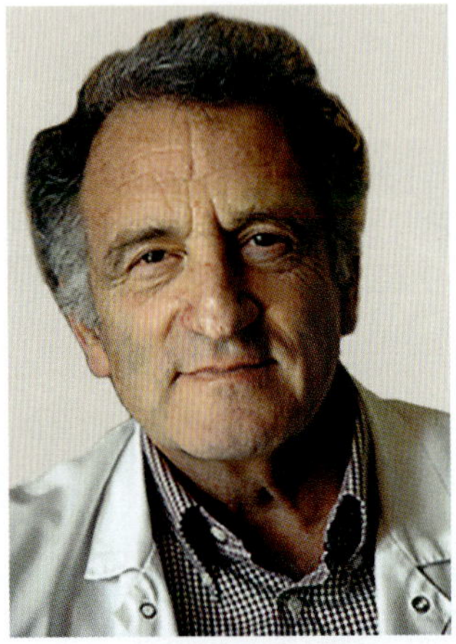

**Fig. 13:** Rene Frydman.

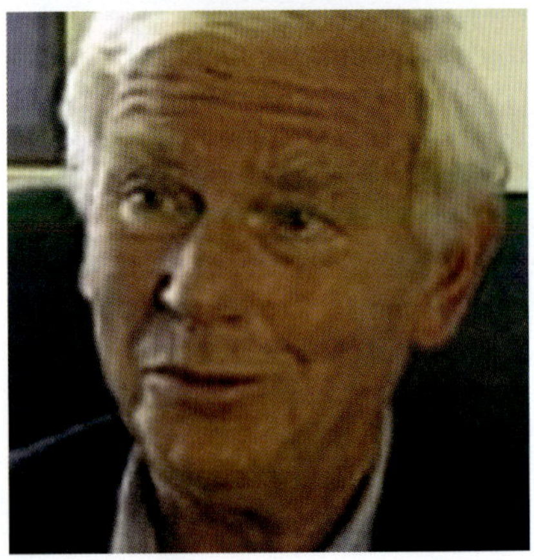

**Fig. 14:** Lars Hamberger.

*1982*

- The first French IVF birth occurred in Clamart, France, by the group of Frydman and Testart **(Figs. 12 to 14)**.
- The first IVF birth in Sweden.[27]
- Birth of first Austrian "test tube baby" (twin pregnancy)[28]

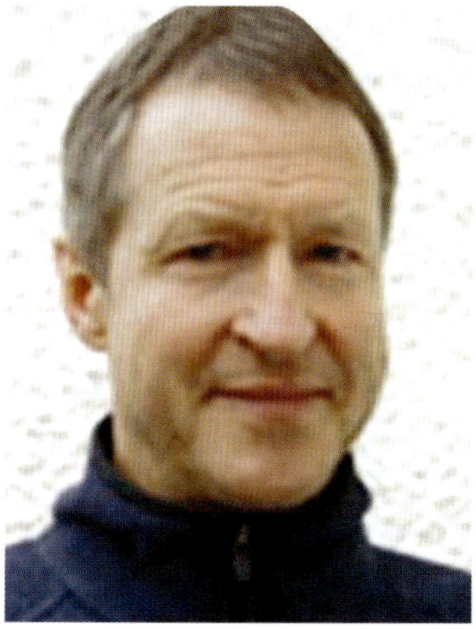

**Fig. 15:** Richard Fleming.

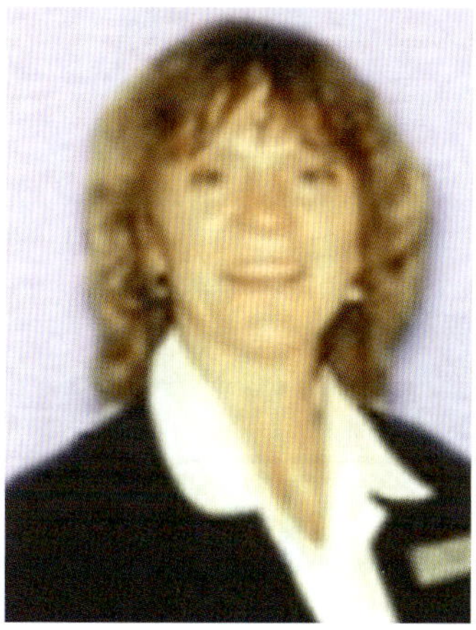

**Fig. 16:** Susan Lenz.

- In the same year, use of GnRH was introduced to avoid premature luteinization to get better control on ovarian stimulation **(Fig. 15)**.[29]
- The first publication on the need to delay insemination in order to allow the collected oocytes to complete their maturation over the next 2–4 hours.[30]
- Susan Lenz and Jurgen G. Lauritsen demonstrated transabdominal transvesical oocyte aspiration using an ultrasound-guided needle **(Fig. 16)**.[31]
- Ian Craft in London reported a pregnancy from transfer of gametes to the uterus **(Fig. 17)**.[32]

*1983*

- First pregnancy was reported by the Monash IVF team in women without ovaries using donor eggs and exogenous hormones to induce artificial menstruation and support the pregnancy for the first 10 weeks.[33]
- The same team reported the first human frozen ET delivered baby **(Fig. 18)** although Cambridge had already reported the same in cattle.[34]

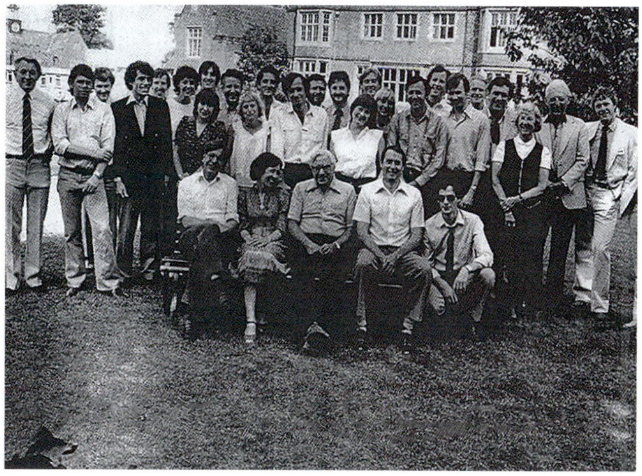

**Fig. 17:** World's first in vitro fertilization (IVF) conference at Bourn Hall. Front row, from left to right: Bob Edwards, Jean Purdy, Patrick Steptoe, John Webster, and Simon Fishel.

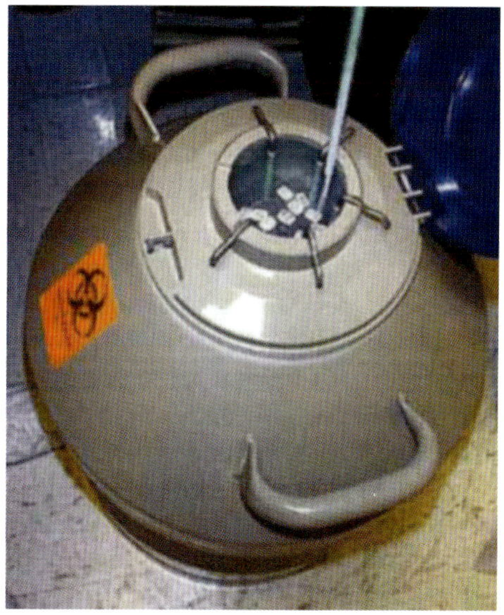

**Fig. 18:** Frozen embryos.

- In vitro maturation (IVM) of morphologically immature oocytes followed by fertilization of the same **(Fig. 19)**.[35]
- Embryo donation followed by pregnancy and successful delivery[33,36]
- Casper and his colleagues for the first time described the luteal phase support by using low-dose hCG in assisted reproductive technology (ART) cycle **(Fig. 20)**.[37]
- First time egg retrieval per vagina by Gleicher and his group by using abdominal ultrasound **(Fig. 21)**.[38]
- University of British Columbia reported its first Canadian IVF baby **(Fig. 22)**.
- Christopher Chen reported the world's first triplets through IVF.
- The first report on transfer of freeze-thaw eight-cell embryo, which led to pregnancy[34]
- First report on the use of follicular steroids as a prognostic indicator for successful IVF **(Fig. 23)**[39]

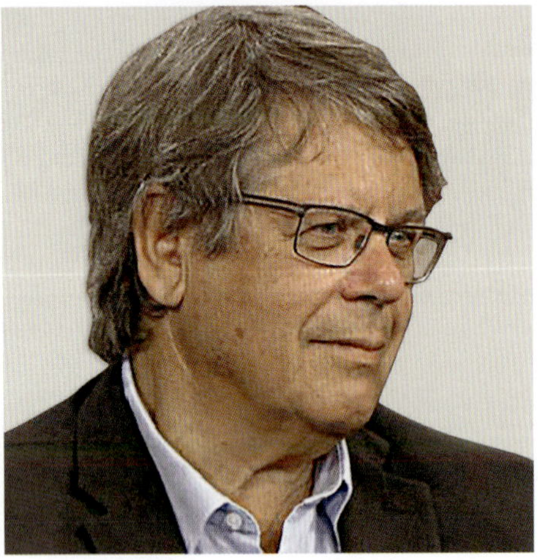

**Fig. 19:** Alan Trounson.

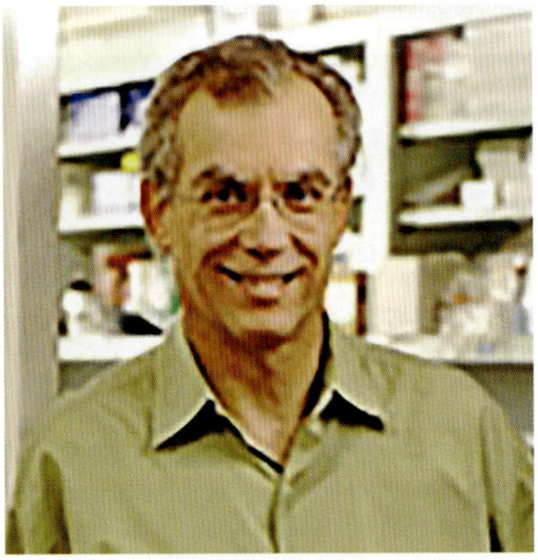

**Fig. 20:** Robert Casper.

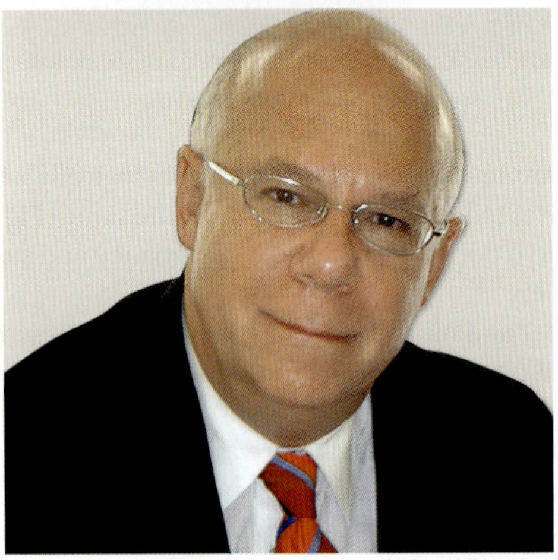

**Fig. 21:** Norbert Gleicher.

*1984*

- The Government of Victoria established the first legislation to regulate IVF and the research on human embryos, which led to the proclamation of Medical Procedures Act, 1984.

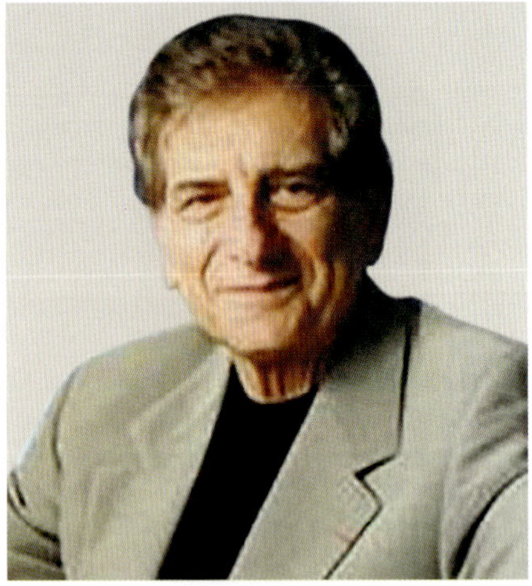

**Fig. 22:** Victor Gomel.

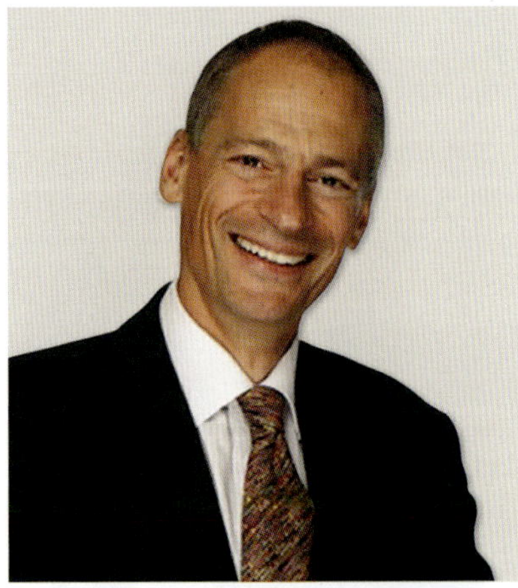

**Fig. 23:** Simon Fishel.

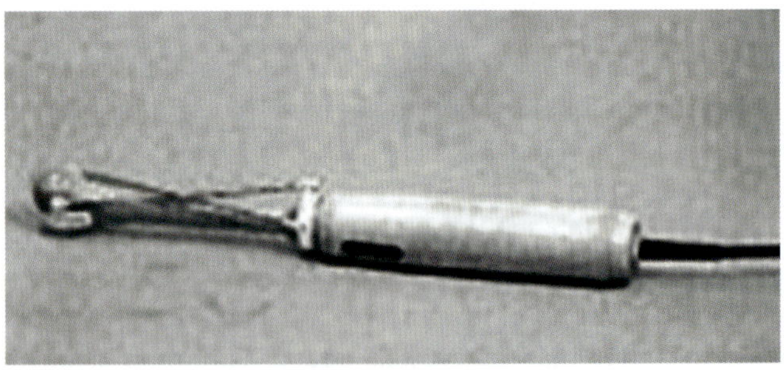

**Fig. 24:** Kretztechnik's mechanical rotary vaginal scanner in 1985 with puncture attachment.

- California reported its first baby born through surrogacy.
- First successful translaparoscopic gamete intrafallopian transfer (GIFT) procedure of pregnancy **(Fig. 24)**.[40]
- The first report on successful pregnancy in women with primary ovarian failure following egg donation.[41]
- GnRH agonists were introduced the first time for IVF protocol.[42]
- A report on the transfer of first intact frozen-thawed embryo followed by pregnancy.[43]

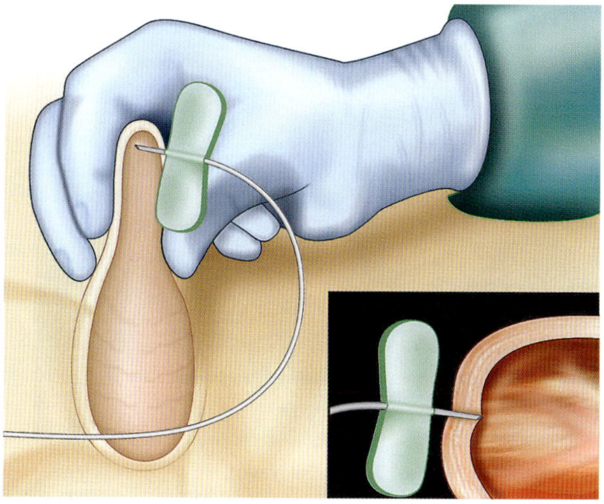

**Fig. 25:** Epididymis sperm aspiration.

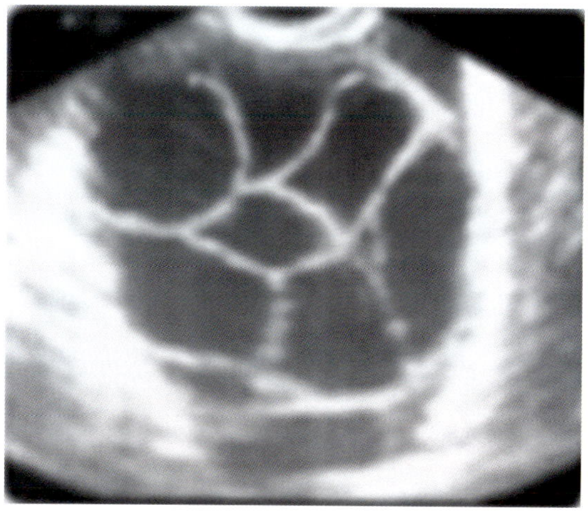

**Fig. 27:** Ultrasound image of follicles.

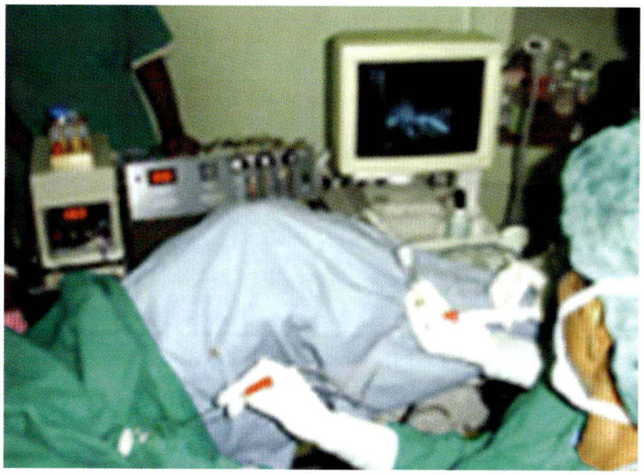

**Fig. 26:** Vaginal oocyte aspiration.

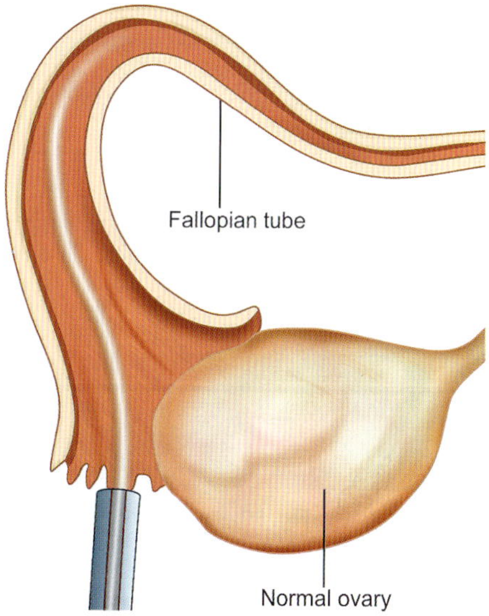


**Fig. 28:** Gamete intrafallopian transfer (GIFT) procedure.

- A novel work about the possibility that abnormal spermatozoa could be enriched and give rise to healthy babies were reported.[44]
- Demonstrating of hCG secretion by the human embryo.[45]
- The world's first quadruplets through IVF in Melbourne.

*1985*

- Human pregnancy by IVF using sperm aspirated from the epididymis **(Fig. 25)**.[46]
- Matts Wikland and associates for the first time described the possibility of oocyte aspiration using a vaginal sector scanner (transvaginal technique) **(Fig. 26)**.[47]
- First report on ET with the help of abdominal ultrasound guidance **(Fig. 27)**[48]
- Freeze-thaw transfer of hatched blastocyst followed by successful birth **(Fig. 28)**[49]
- Introduction of human tubal fluid (HTF) by Quinn and Warnes that mimics the in vivo environment[50]
- First delivery resulting from gestational surrogacy[51]
- First successful egg donation in Europe[52]
- Artificial induction of the endometrial cycle in the absence of ovaries was reported by Navot et al.,[53] although it was published 1 year later in 1986.

*1986*

- World's first pregnancy was reported by the Monash IVF team from surgical retrieval of sperm on a patient with a blocked sperm duct **(Fig. 29)**.
- First description of transvaginal sector scan sonography for needle-guided transvaginal follicle aspiration[54]
- First pregnancy, following IVF donated oocytes, in a nonovarian failure patient **(Fig. 30)**[55]
- First report on pregnancy after translaparoscopic zygote intrafallopian transfer.[56] In parallel, the group at the Royal Women's Hospital (RWH) was involved too in studies on GIFT **(Fig. 31)**.[57]

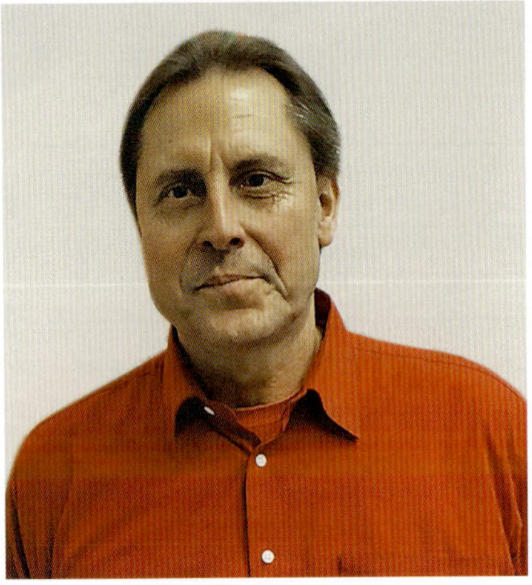

**Fig. 29:** W Feichtinger.

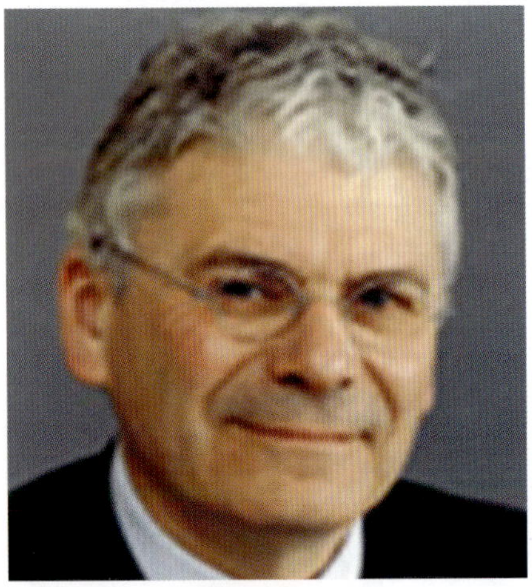

**Fig. 30:** Paul Devroey.

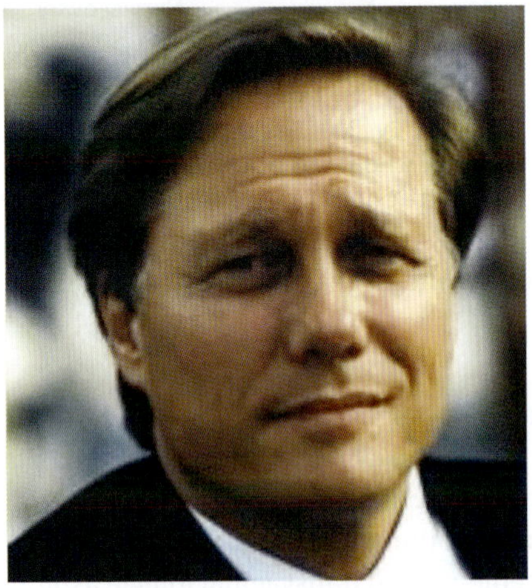

**Fig. 31:** Zev Rosenwaks.

- Delivery of twins from frozen human eggs **(Fig. 32)**.[58]
- Jacqueline Mandelbaum with Daniel Szollosi described the microstructures of the human oocyte, which came to be known as "oocyte dysmorphia."[59]

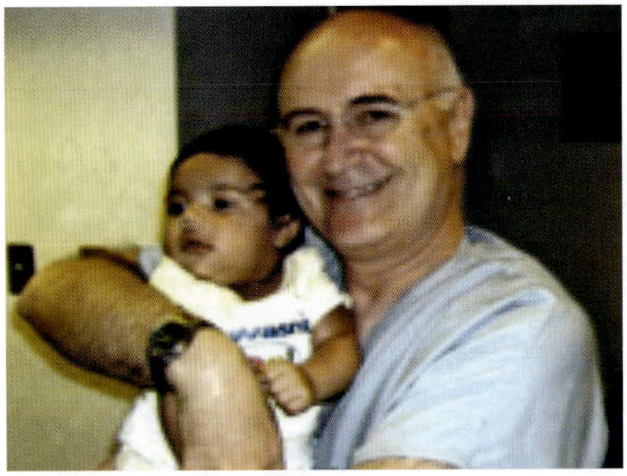

**Fig. 32:** Daniel Navot.

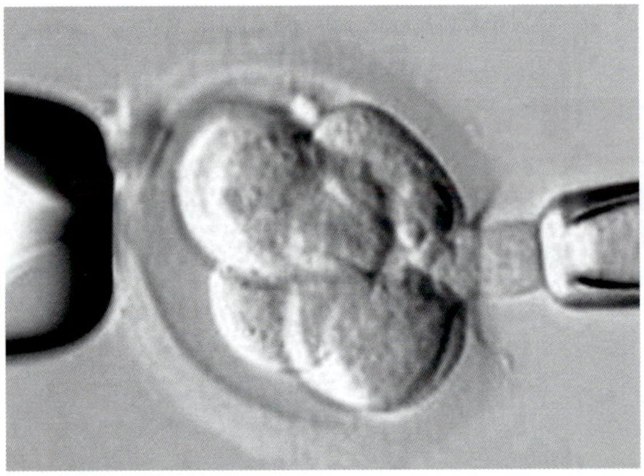

**Fig. 33:** Biopsy of an embryo.

*1987*

Fertilization of human oocytes by microinjection of a single sperm under the zona pellucida took place.[60]

*1988*

- First time epididymal sperm aspiration for men with absent vas or ejaculatory duct block. In the same year, two babies were born after this technique.[61]
- First IVF surrogate born in Australia.
- Successful subzonal insemination (SUZI) performed at the National University of Singapore.[62]
- Successful pregnancy obtained from zona drilling or partial zona dissection mechanically.[63]
- In the same year the pioneer Dr Patrick Steptoe left us forever—March 21, 1988.[64]
- The first preclinical evaluation of pronuclear formation by microinjection of human spermatozoa into human oocytes.[65]

*1989*

- First report on sexing of embryos by biopsy of human preimplantation embryos by deoxyribonucleic acid (DNA) amplification **(Fig. 33)**.[66]

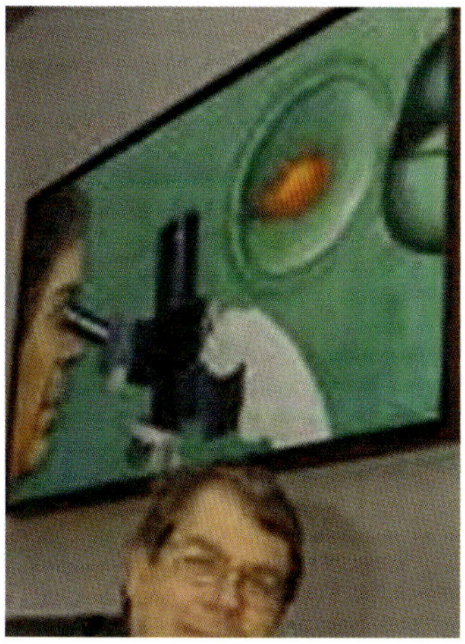

Fig. 34: Alan Trounson.

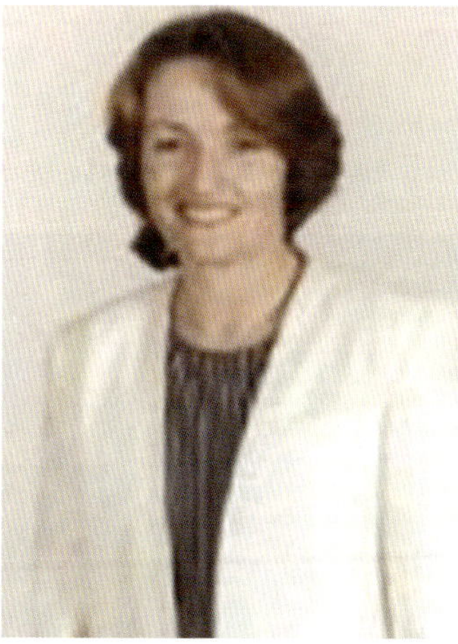

Fig. 35: Leeanda Wilton.

- First report on the implementation of laser in the field of assisted reproduction.[67]
- Ultrasound for endometrial quality for thickness and pattern was reported by Gonen and her colleagues in Toronto.[68]
- Embryo biopsy technique was developed in mice by Professor Alan Trounson and Leeanda Wilton **(Figs. 34 and 35)**.[69]

*1990*

- The first successful human cleavage-stage embryo vitrification followed by a successful delivery.[70]
- Biopsied embryos sexed for Y-chromosome-specific pregnancies.[71]
- First report on the use of assisted hatching on human embryos **(Fig. 36)**.[72]
- The first report on polar body biopsy, transfer of the embryo, and achieving pregnancy **(Fig. 37)**.[73]
- Gonen et al. proposed the use of GnRH agonist in place of hCG as a means to trigger the gonadotropic surge for IVF.[74]

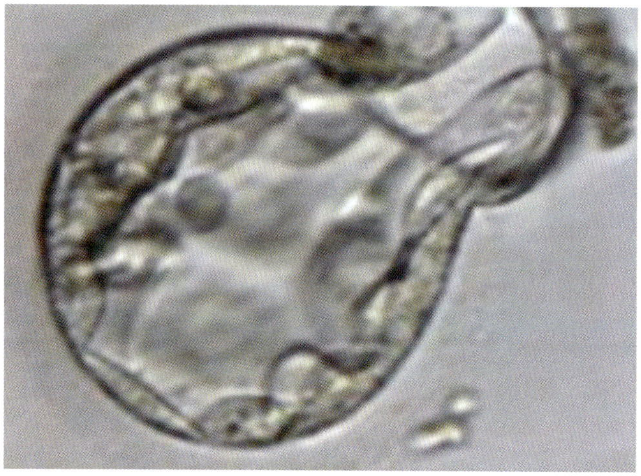

Fig. 36: Hatching of a blastocyst.

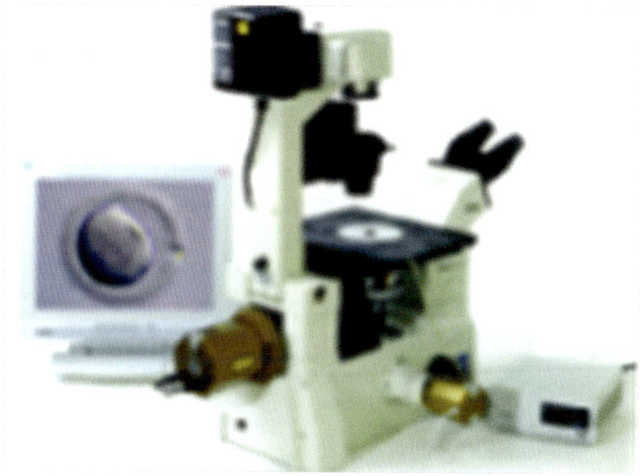

Fig. 37: Microscopic analysis of a blastocyst.

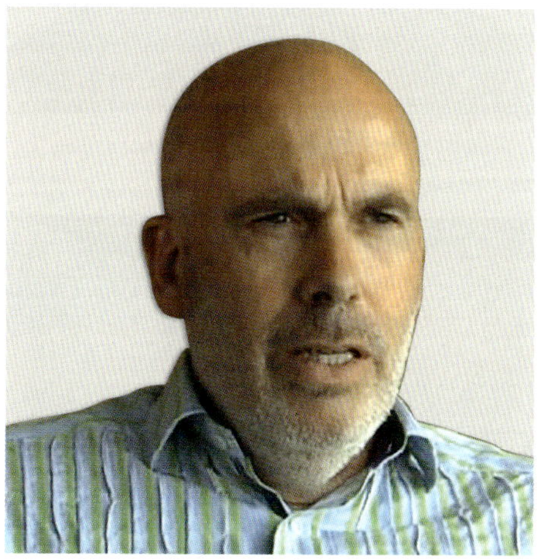

Fig. 38: Jacques Cohen.

- Gonen, Jacobson, and Casper pioneered the use of combined oral contraceptives for follicle synchronization and cycle scheduling in IVF **(Fig. 38)**.[75]
- Fishel et al. reported about twin birth after SUZI.[76]

*1991*

- IVM in an unstimulated cycle resulted in pregnancy in a donor oocyte program.[77]
- The first report on the prevention of premature LH rise of progesterone in COH treatment by using GnRH antagonist and Nal-Glue **(Fig. 39)**.[78]
- The first report on the use of a laser for zona pellucida drilling.[79]
- Navot et al. confirmed that the age-related decline in female fertility is attributable to oocyte quality.[80]
- ET catheter is visualized by vaginal ultrasound **(Fig. 40)**.[81]

*1992*

- Two groups simultaneously presented the report on the successful IVF followed by ET after treatment with recombinant human follicle-stimulating hormone (FSH) **(Figs. 41 to 43)**.[82,83]
- Assisted zona hatching was introduced in IVF programs to breach the zona pellucida and promote the natural process of hatching.[84]
- Report of the first pregnancy after ICSI by the group in Brussels **(Figs. 44 and 45)**.[85]
- Pregnancy after embryo biopsy and coamplification of DNA from X and Y chromosomes.[86]

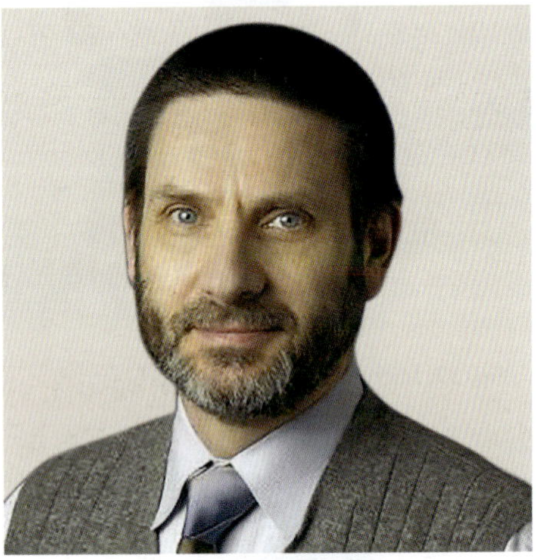

**Fig. 39:** Daniel Palanker.

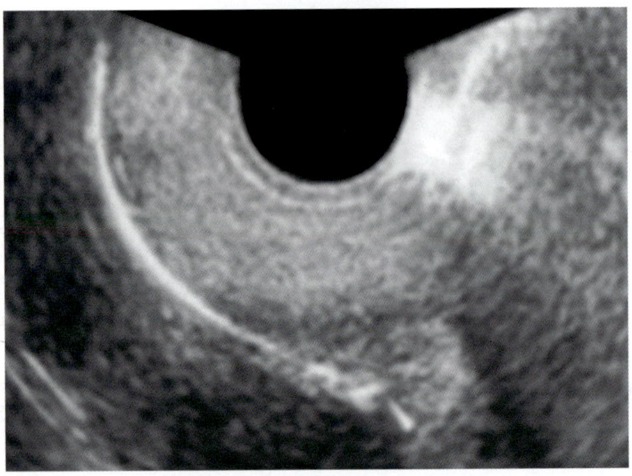

**Fig. 40:** Embryo transfer catheter.

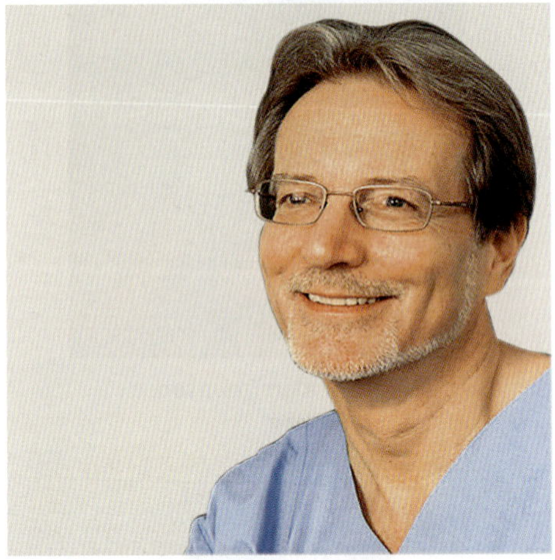

**Fig. 41:** Marc Germond.

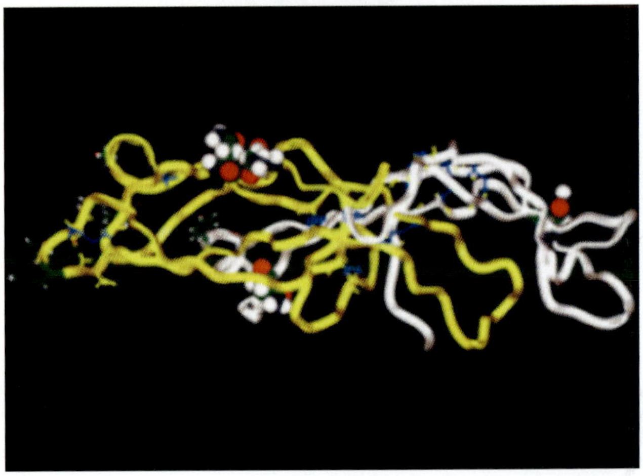

**Fig. 42:** Three-dimensional model structure of follicle-stimulating hormone (FSH).

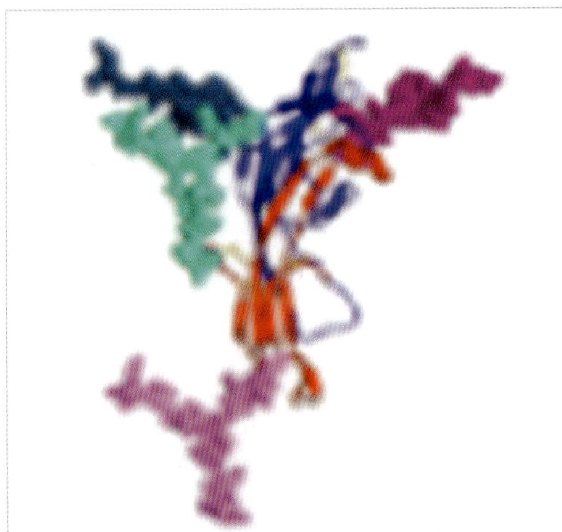

**Fig. 43:** Recombinant follicle-stimulating hormone (FSH).

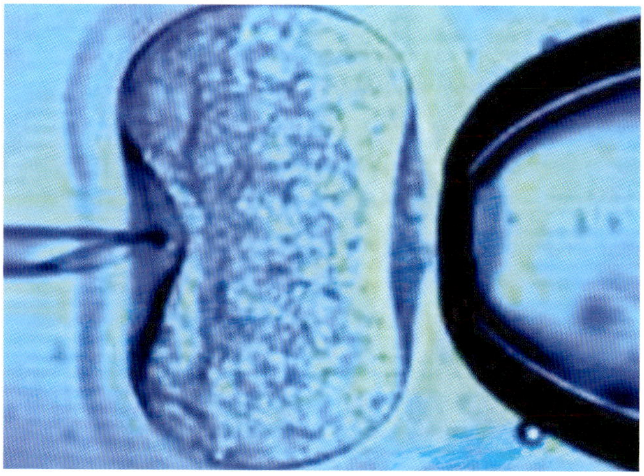

**Fig. 44:** Intracytoplasmic sperm injection (ICSI) process.

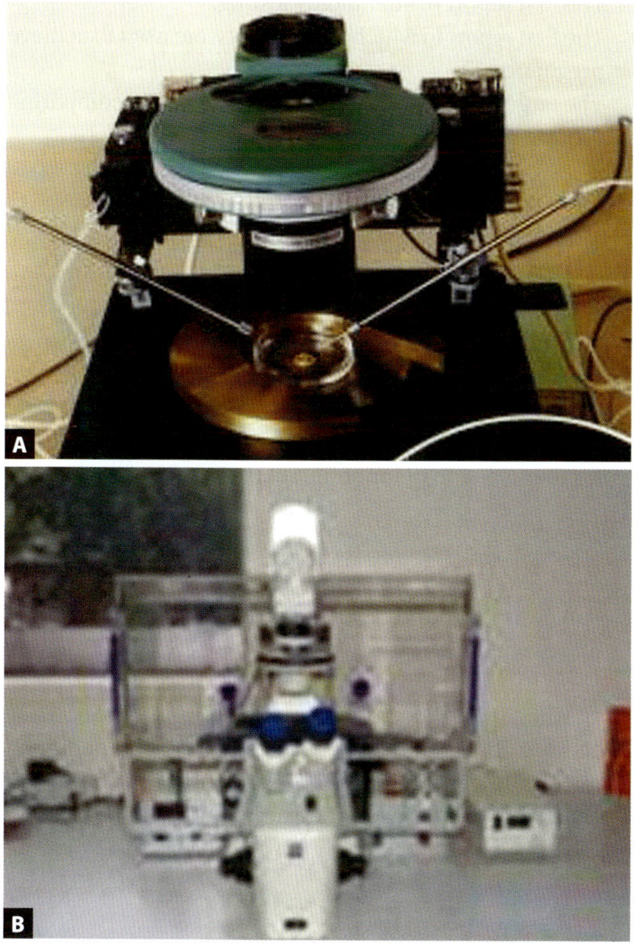

**Figs. 45A and B:** Intracytoplasmic sperm injection (ICSI) microscope.

- Ovulation induction by endogenous LH released by the administration of a luteinizing hormone-releasing hormone (LHRH) agonist after follicular stimulation for IVF.[87]
- First report on the cumulative conception and live-birth rates after IVF in relation to a patient's age and cause of infertility.[88]

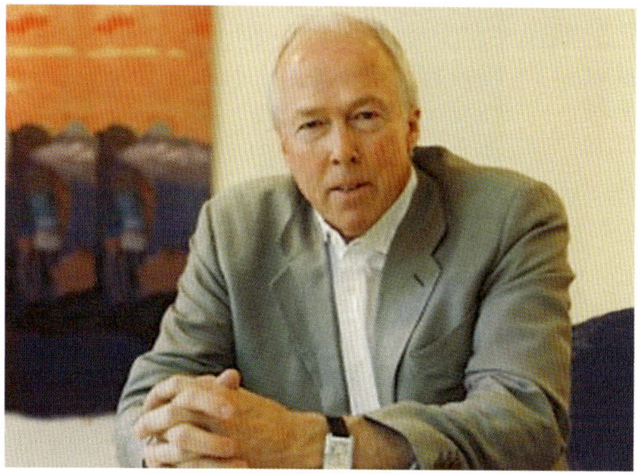

**Fig. 46:** Herjan JT Coelingh Bennink.

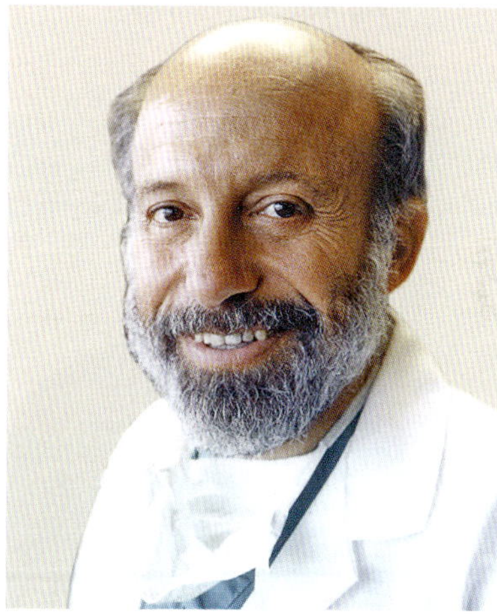

**Fig. 47:** Sherman Silber.

- First two births from the replacement of frozen embryos produced with epididymal sperm.[89]
- Report on using erbium yttrium aluminum garnet (YAG) laser for micromanipulation of oocytes and spermatozoa.[90]
- Investigating the role of FSH in hypogonadotropic women using the new recombinant FSH drug **(Fig. 46)**.[91]

*1993*

- The second-term pregnancy after ICSI reported by a group in Sweden.[92]
- Confirmation that men with congenital absence of the vas deferens have cystic fibrosis mutations, which can be transmitted to the offspring **(Fig. 47)**.[93]
- First report on the use of testicular sperm extraction (TESE) and ICSI.[94]
- First pregnancy and birth following treatment with recombinant FSH.[95]

*1994*

- The first live birth as a result of IVM following transvaginal ultrasound-guided oocyte collection **(Fig. 48)**.[96]

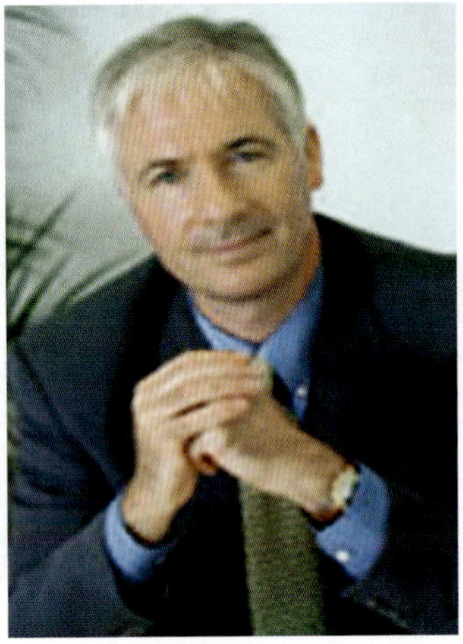

**Fig. 48:** Colin Howles.

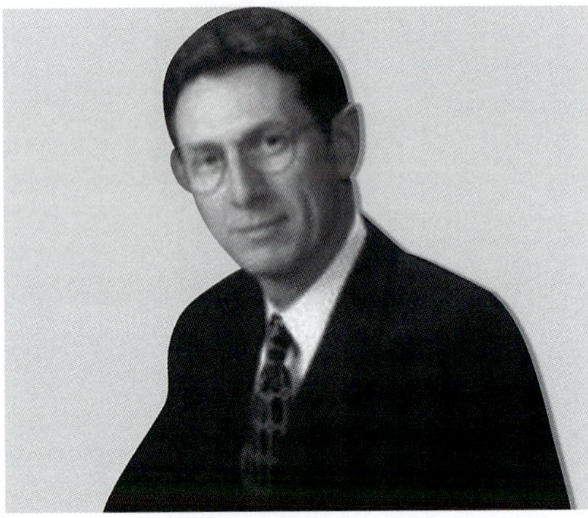

**Fig. 49:** Frank Barnes.

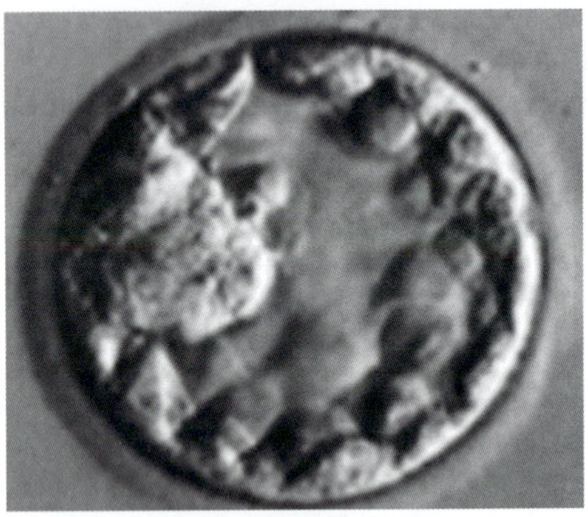

**Fig. 50:** Blastocyst.

- Development of the first highly purified FSH preparation for use in IVF.[97]

*1995*

- Pregnancies after TESE and ICSI in nonobstructive azoospermia.[98]
- Birth after blastocyst development from IVM oocyte plus ICSI plus assisted hatching **(Figs. 49 and 50)**.[99]

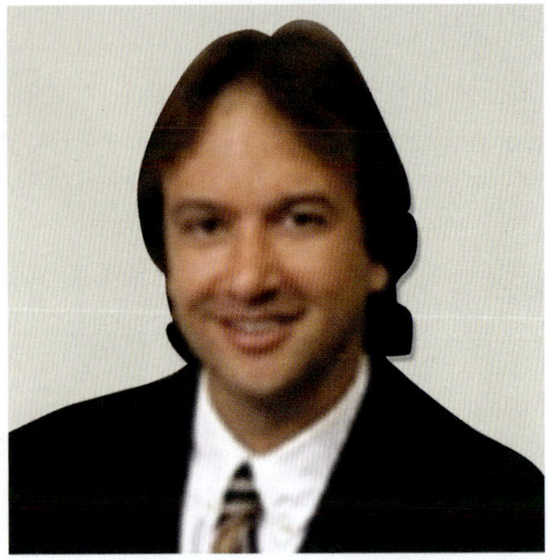

**Fig. 51:** David Gardner.

- The first report of aneuploidy testing.[100]
- The first report in which spermatids were used to achieve pregnancy.[101]
- The largest study was done in the field of IVF comparing urinary FSH with recombinant FSH.[102]

*1996*

- The Valencia group reported on the first pregnancy employing cryopreserved testicular sperm following IVF–ICSI.[103]
- Discovery that some men with severe oligoasthenospermia have deletions in the Y-chromosome.[104]
- Casper and his colleagues were the first to demonstrate and introduce the use of the hypo-osmotic swelling test for the selection of immotile sperm for ICSI.[105]

*1997*

- First report on cytoplasmic transfer.[106]
- Sun, Jurisicova, and Casper described the use of Terminal deoxynucleotidyl transferase dUTP Nick-End Labeling (TUNEL) for the detection of DNA fragmentation in sperm and its correlation with IVF outcome. They showed almost uniform presence of DNA fragmentation in round spermatids as the explanation for failure to achieve pregnancy with these immature gametes.[107]
- First births of babies from frozen oocytes following the use of ICSI.[108]

*1998*

- First established pregnancy using recombinant FSH and GnRH antagonist.[109]
- Gardner introduced sequential media and blastocyst transfer which now greatly assists in the move to single ET **(Fig. 51)**.[110]
- Births after intracytoplasmic injection of sperm obtained by testicular extraction from men with nonmosaic Klinefelter's syndrome.[111]

- The first pregnancies following embryo culture in sequential media and transfer at the blastocyst stage of development.[112]
- First ovum pick-up under three-dimensional (3D) ultrasound vision.[113]

### 1999

- First unaffected pregnancy using preimplantation genetic diagnosis (PGD) for sickle cell anemia.[114]
- Birth following vitrification of human oocyte[115]
- World's first IVF/ICSI pregnancy and live birth after successful air transport of oocytes reported by the McGill Reproductive Centre, enabling the creation of an air-transport IVF program in large countries with scattered populations or in areas remote from infertility centers.[116]
- *Cryopreserved oocytes and testicular sperm:* First ever birth.[117]

### 2000

- Oktay and Karlikaya were the first to report on ovarian tissue transplants after frozen storage **(Fig. 52)**.[118]
- The development of a completely chemically defined protein-free embryo culture medium and the births of the first batch of babies generated from the fertilization of eggs collected and inseminated in the said protein-free medium using spermatozoa also prepared in the same protein-free medium in both conventional IVF and ICSI.[119]

### 2001

- Birth of an infant from cryopreserved embryos (zygotes) produced by IVM oocytes derived from an unstimulated patient with polycystic ovary syndrome (PCOS).[120]
- Ongoing twin pregnancy after ICSI of percutaneous sperm aspiration (PESA)-retrieved spermatozoa into in vitro matured oocytes reported by the McGill group.[121]
- Live birth after sperm retrieval from a moribund man.[122]

### 2002

- First live birth following blastocyst biopsy and PGD analysis.[123]
- First clinical application of comparative genomic hybridization and polar body testing for PGD of aneuploidy.[124]

### 2003

- Live births after vitrification of oocytes in a stimulated IVF-ET program[125]
- First live birth after ovarian stimulation using a chimeric long-acting human recombinant follicle-stimulating hormone agonist (recFSH-CTP) for IVF **(Fig. 53)**.[126]
- Dr Barash and Professor Dekel showed an increasing implantation rate following endometrial injury, performed by Pipelle curettage as a simple outpatient procedure.[127]
- Normal birth after microsurgical enucleation of tripronuclear human zygotes.[128]

### 2004

- Successful pregnancy and delivery following combined treatment of IVM and TESE.[129]
- Jacques Donnez reported on the first live birth after orthotopic transplantation of cryopreserved ovarian tissue.[130]
- Gardner and colleagues performed the world's first prospective single blastocyst trial, which showed the feasibility of single blastocyst transfer (SBT) and in keeping high pregnancy rates.[131]
- First report of fertility preservation for cancer patients using IVM and oocyte vitrification.[132]

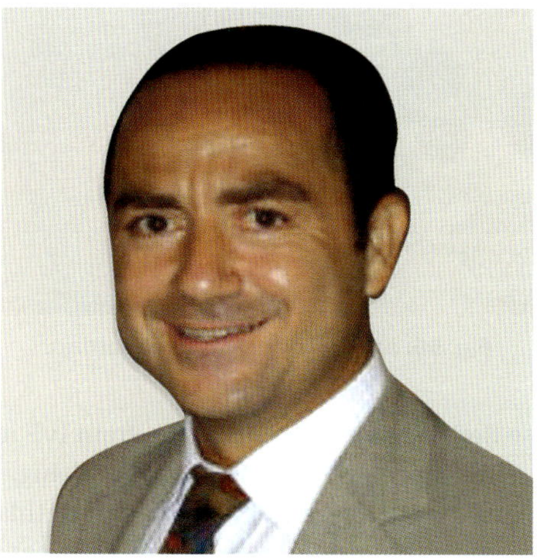

**Fig. 52:** Kutluk Oktay.

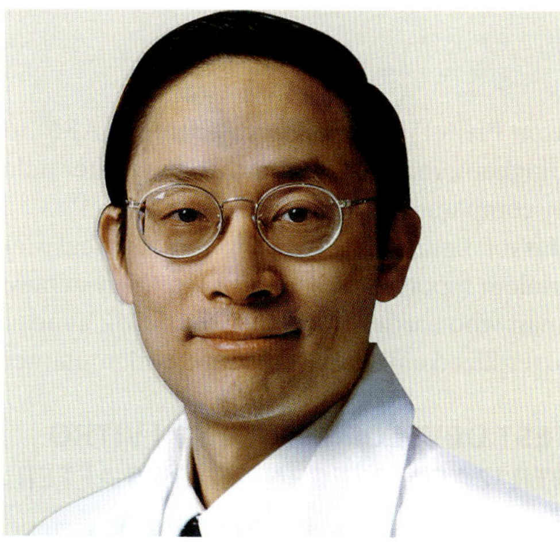

**Fig. 53:** Ren-He Xu.

- First report on a natural cycle in IVF combined with IVM as a potential approach to infertility treatment.[133]

*2005*

- Pregnancies and live births after trophectoderm biopsy and preimplantation genetic testing of human blastocysts.[134]
- First birth in Israel from thawed ovarian cortex retransplants.[135]
- The first live birth after trophectoderm biopsy and preimplantation genetic testing of human blastocysts for β-thalassemia **(Fig. 54)**.[136]

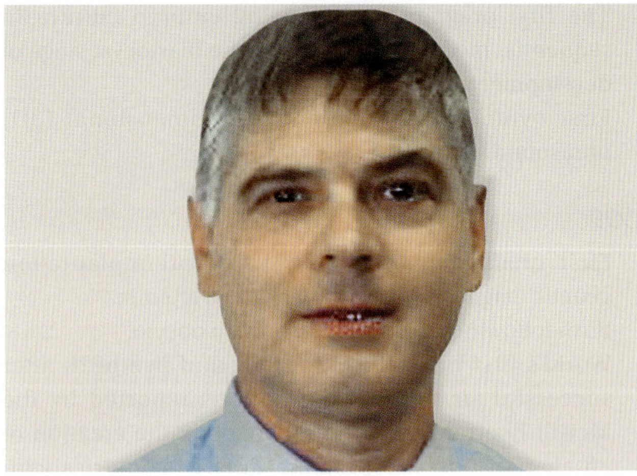

**Fig. 54:** Dror Meirow.

*2006*

- First successful pregnancy after PGD for aneuploidy screening in embryos generated from natural-cycle IVF combined with IVM, achieved at the McGill Reproductive Centre **(Figs. 55 and 56)**.[137]
- Cryopreservation of intact human ovary with its vascular pedicle.[138]

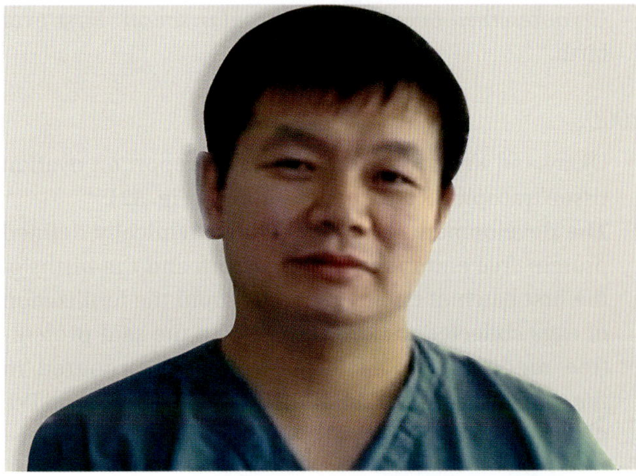

**Fig. 55:** Son Weon-Young.

*2007*

- Introducing the concept of mild treatment strategy for IVF.[139]
- A novel multigradient freezing technique for the cryopreservation of the whole ovary. Thawing the ovary resulted in normal ovarian architecture and no damage to the vascular wall or intima.[140]

*2008*

- The first report of DNA fingerprinting to identify the blastocyst of origin for live births and that gene expression profiles of biopsied trophectoderm can discriminate between viable and nonviable blastocysts.[141]
- *Cryopreserved oocytes in cancer patients*: First ever birth of healthy twins after oocyte cryopreservation and bilateral ovariectomy.[142]

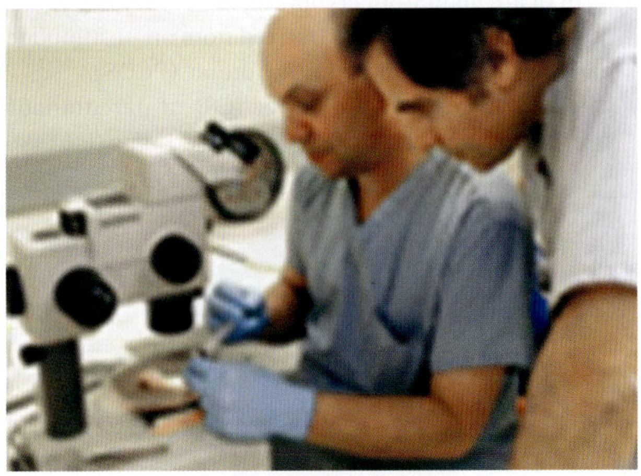

**Fig. 56:** Amir Arav and Pasquale Patrizio.

*2009*

- Simon Fishel and his group from CARE fertility, Nottingham, reported about a live birth after polar body array comparative genomic hybridization.[143]
- Professor Laufer at the Hadassah Medical Center in Jerusalem reported on a viable pregnancy achieved in a woman who carries the defective *BRCA2* genes after in vitro fertilized embryos were tested and implanted.[144]

## LATEST DEVELOPMENTS IN IN VITRO FERTILIZATION TECHNOLOGIES AFTER 2009

Since 1978, numerous advances in fertility science have granted prospective parents an increasing array of options to increase their chances of conception, from IVF to ovarian tissue freezing. Since, this field is rapidly evolving, there are many achievements that have happened after this chapter was last written. So, here is a list of major milestones achieved after the year 2009 in this field.

- *Time-lapse imaging (TLI)*: During the last decade, TLI has emerged as a novel technology that enables continuous evaluation of early embryo development by automated image acquisition every 5–20 minutes and accordingly does not rely on static observations to define a highly dynamic process. Furthermore, it is possible to score embryos without removing them from the incubator, so there is no exposure to changes in light, humidity, temperature, pH, or gas. The world's first embryoscope baby was born in Valencia in June 2010.

  A recent meta-analysis assessed whether TLI resulted in favorable outcomes for embryo incubation and selection compared with conventional methods in clinical IVF. This analysis included 10 randomized controlled studies and concluded that there is insufficient evidence to support TLI as a superior method compared to conventional methods for human embryo incubation and selection. A well-designed randomized controlled trial (RCT) is still needed to evaluate the effectiveness of the clinical use of TLI.
- *Stem cells research*: Ovaries of women in their 20s and early 30s contain a rare population of oogonial stem cells (OSCs) that generate oocytes in defined cultures in vitro and after introduction into human ovarian tissue in xenografts in vivo. The use of stem cell-based strategies as fertility treatment options are often viewed as being clinically applicable only in the distant future; however, these new findings in the area of human ovarian biology bring stem cell-based approaches for treating infertility in women one significant step closer to reality.

In May 2015, an extension of this theory was used to rejuvenate a woman's old eggs and so-called world's first stem cell baby—Zain Rajani—was born in Canada.

The idea was that the mitochondria—cellular energy generators—in young, primitive cells function much better than those in the mature eggs collected for IVF. Collecting these mitochondria and injecting them into the prospective mother's mature eggs are supposed to improve their quality. This whole procedure is now known as "autologous mitochondrial transfer."

Similarly, there have been several cases reported of endometrial regeneration using adult autologous stem cells derived from bone marrow and successful pregnancies thereafter.

- *Endometrial receptivity array (ERA)—molecular test of endometrial receptivity:* Search for an adequate marker of endometrial receptivity led to the development of a molecular diagnostic test—the ERA. ERA consists of a customized microarray based on the transcriptomic signature of human ER, specifically when the human endometrium is receptive to blastocyst adhesion. The test analyses 238 genes that are differentially expressed around the time of implantation. This array is coupled to a computational predictor that can diagnose the personalized endometrial window of implantation (WOI) of a given patient regardless of their endometrial histology.
- *Uterus transplantation:* In 1931 in Germany, Lili Elbe, a Danish transgender woman, died from organ rejection 3 months after receiving one of the world's earliest uterine transplants. With the availability of IVF in 1978, uterine transplantation research was deferred.

In Saudi Arabia in 2000, a uterine transplant was performed by Dr Wafa Fageeh from a 46-year-old hysterectomy patient into a 26-year-old recipient whose own uterus had hemorrhaged after childbirth. The transplanted uterus functioned for 99 days but ultimately needed to be removed after failure due to blood clotting. Within the medical community, there was some debate as to whether or not the transplant could truly be considered to have been successful.

In Turkey, on August 9, 2011, the world's first uterus transplant from a deceased donor was conducted by a team of doctors at Akdeniz University Hospital in Antalya. The 21-year-old Turkish woman, Derya Sert, who had been born without a uterus, was the first woman in history to receive a womb from a deceased donor. The operation, performed by Dr Ömer Özkan, Dr Munire Erman Akar, and their team, was the world's first uterus transplant surgery gaining long-term function as evident by the fact that Ms. Sert had six menstrual periods postsurgery and is said to have a fully functioning uterus. The Turkish medical team who performed the delicate surgery, however, is still cautious about declaring the operation a complete success. In April 2013, Akdeniz University announced that Derya Sert was pregnant, but she had to terminate her pregnancy in its 8th week, following a routine examination where doctors failed to detect a fetal heartbeat.

In October 2014, it was announced that, for the first time, a healthy baby had been born to a uterine transplant recipient, at an undisclosed location in Sweden. The British Medical Journal and The Lancet reported that the baby boy had been born in September, weighing 1.8 kg (3.9 lb). The baby had been delivered prematurely at about 32 weeks, by cesarean section, after the mother had developed preeclampsia. The Swedish woman, aged 36 years, had received a uterus in 2013, from a live 61-year-old donor, in an operation led by Dr Brännström, professor of obstetrics and gynecology at the University of Gothenburg.

The first uterine transplant performed in India took place on May 18, 2017, at the Galaxy Care Hospital in Pune, Maharashtra. The 26-year-old patient had been born without a uterus and received her mother's womb in the transplant.

## THE FUTURE

In this century, it is clear how much the new reproductive technologies have allowed and initiated advances in genetics. The ability to transfer embryos screened for chromosomal and single-gene defects has reduced the risk of many inherited diseases, while immunoassay technology has provided detailed insight into the cellular processes involved in gene expression. However, such developments, as well as the publicly perceived ability to select embryos for their sex and genetic characteristics, have raised the fear of "designer babies" and a move toward some kind of eugenics under the pressure of parents.

Since the birth of Dolly, the sheep in Scotland in 1996, the issue of reproductive or therapeutic cloning has been exposed. In therapeutics, the transplantation of human embryonic stem cells now holds a great promise for the treatment of diseases such as Parkinson's disease or diabetes, whereas developments in stem cell biology will lead to a better understanding of infertility, implantation failure, genomic imprinting, and meiosis.[15] However, the field poses a huge challenge including inefficient existing protocols for differentiation, epigenetic and genetic changes associated with extensive in vitro manipulation, and also ethical/regulatory constraints.

Although direct correlates between cancer and infertile epigenetic profiles are rare, the general similarities between the two disease processes offer insights into the study of both abnormalities. Foremost among them is the nature of these pathologies, where one disease (cancer) is categorized by an inability to control or inhibit cellular proliferation, and the other (male infertility) is caused by an inability to maintain the normally efficient extreme proliferation of the male germ cell. Based on this similarity alone, the study of epigenetics in both male fertility and cancer has the potential to offer intriguing insights in both fields. The creative application of harmonious studies of both infertility and cancer is likely to yield useful and informative data that may aid in both the understanding and treatment of both pathologies.

So this implies that, still, there is a lot more to explore, and increasingly, this field is becoming superspecialized with a team of doctors, scientists, geneticists, and the researchers aiming toward excellence and improving the outcome in ART.

Hope this collaborative effort keeps on adding more value to the work initiated by our pioneers already.

## CONCLUSION

In the 1960s and 1970s, our understanding of the events in human oocyte fertilization grew to the point that in vitro fertilization (IVF) of human oocytes became possible. Ultimately, this knowledge led to the widely acclaimed first live birth of a "test tube baby," Louise Brown, in England in 1978.

## REFERENCES


1. BBC Report. (1978). First test tube baby born. [online] Available from: http://news.bbc.co.uk/onthisday/hi/dates/stories/july/25/newsid_2499000/2499411.stm.
2. Monash IVF Team. (2017). History of IVF article. [online] Available from: https://embryo.asu.edu/pages/history-monash-ivf-research-program-1971-1989.
3. Shettles LB. (2014). Test tube ovaries: biography on the American Experience. [online] Available from: https://www.pbs.org/video/trailer-test-tube-babies-american-experience/.
4. Shettles LB, Heniq RB. The Lives They Lived. New York: New York Times Magazine; 2003.
5. Cole M. (2007). World's first test-tube baby Louise Brown has a child of her own. [online] Available from: https://www.independent.co.uk/life-style/health-and-families/health-news/world-s-first-testtube-baby-louise-brown-has-a-child-of-her-own-432080.html.
6. Johnson MH. Robert Edwards: the path to IVF. Reprod Biomed Online. 2011;23(2):245-62.
7. Schulman JD, Edwards RG. A personal viewpoint. New Sci. 1978;2:158.
8. The Telegraph. (2010). Test tube triumph and tragedy—Nobel for UK scientist stirs memory of a Bengal doctor. [online] Available from: https://www.telegraphindia.com/india/test-tube-triumph-tragedy-nobel-for-uk-scientist-stirs-memory-of-a-bengal-doctor/cid/472542.
9. The Daily Telegraph. London: Telegraph Press; 1979. p. 1.
10. The Times. London: Telegraph Press; 1980. p. 7.
11. The Eastern Virginia Medical School (EVMS). (2012). The Jones Institute for Reproductive Medicine. [online] Available from: www.evms.edu/patient_care/specialties/jones_institute_for_reproductive_medicine/.
12. Kyono K, Uto H, Nakajo Y, Kumagai S, Araki Y, Kanto S. Seven pregnancies and deliveries from non-mosaic Klinefelter syndrome patients using fresh and frozen testicular sperm. J Assist Reprod Genet. 2007;24:47-51.
13. Okada H, Goda K, Muto S, Maruyama O, Koshida M, Horie S. Four pregnancies in nonmosaic Klinefelter's syndrome using cryopreserved-thawed testicular spermatozoa. Fertil Steril. 2005;84:1508.
14. Edwards RG. (2010). The 2010 Nobel Prize in Physiology or Medicine—Press Release. [online] Available from: www.nobelprize.org/nobel_prizes/medicine/laureates/2010/press.html.
15. Cohen J, Howard JW. In vitro fertilization: The first three decades. In: Gardner DK (Ed). In Vitro Fertilization: A Practical Approach. New York: Taylor and Francis; 2006. pp. 1-15.
16. Edwards RG, Donahue RP, Baramki TA, Jones Jr HW. Preliminary attempts to fertilize human oocytes matured in vitro. Am J Obstet Gynecol. 1966;96:192-200.
17. De Kretzer D, Dennis P, Hudson B, Leeton J, Lopata A, Outch K, et al. Transfer of a human zygote. Lancet. 1973;2:728-9.
18. Steptoe PC, Edwards RG. Reimplantation of a human embryo with subsequent tubal pregnancy. Lancet. 1976;1:880-2.
19. Steptoe PC, Edwards RG. Birth after the reimplantation of a human embryo. Lancet. 1978;2:366.
20. Lopata A, Johnston IW, Hoult IJ, Speirs AI. Pregnancy following intrauterine implantation of an embryo obtained by in vitro fertilization of a preovulatory egg. Fertil Steril. 1980;33:117-20.
21. Pez JP, Cohen J, Hackeloer BJ, et al. Recherche d'une concordance entre l'e´chographie et l'observation par coelioscopie des follicules stimule´s par les inducteurs de l'ovulation. 178 soire´e gyne´co-obstricale de St Maurice le

9.10.79. Bagnolet: Milupa; 1979. Available from https://ivf-worldwide.com/ivf-history.html
22. Hackeloer BJ. The ultrasonic demonstration of follicular development during the normal menstrual cycle and after hormone stimulation. In: Kurjak A (Ed). Recent Advances in Ultrasound Diagnosis. Amsterdam: Oxford; 1977. p. 122.
23. Mohr LR, Trounson AO. The use of fluorescein diacetate to assess embryo viability in the mouse. J Reprod Fertil. 1980;58:189-96.
24. Wood C, Leeton J, Talbot JM, Trounson AO. Technique for collecting mature human oocytes for in vitro fertilization. Br J Obstet Gynaecol. 1981;88:756-60.
25. Trounson AO, Leeton JF, Wood C, Webb J, Wood J. Pregnancies in humans by fertilization in vitro and embryo transfer in the controlled ovulatory cycle. Science. 1981;212:681-2.
26. Testart J, Frydman R, Feinstein MC, Thebault A, Roger M, Scholler R. Interpretation of plasma luteinizing hormone assay for the collection of mature oocytes from women: definition of a luteinizing hormone surge-initiating rise. Fertil Steril. 1981;36:50-4.
27. Hamberger L, Wikland M, Nilsson L, Janson PO, Sjogren A, Hillensjo T. Methods for aspiration of human oocytes by various techniques. Acta Med Rom. 1982;20:370-8.
28. Feichtinger W, Szalay S, Kemeter P, Beck A, Janisch H. Twin pregnancy after laparoscopic oocyte recovery, in-vitro fertilization and embryotransfer (author's transl). Geburtshilfe Frauenheilkd. 1982;42:197-9.
29. Fleming R, Adam AH, Barlow DH, Black WP, MacNaughton MC, Coutts JR. A new systematic treatment for infertile women with abnormal hormone profiles. Br J Obstet Gynaecol. 1982;89:80-3.
30. Trounson AO, Mohr LR, Wood C, Leeton JF. Effect of delayed insemination on in-vitro fertilization, culture and transfer of human embryos. J Reprod Fertil. 1982;64:285-94.
31. Lenz S, Lauritsen JG. Ultrasonically guided percutaneous aspiration of human follicles under local anesthesia: a new method of collecting oocytes for in vitro fertilization. Fertil Steril. 1982;38:673-7.
32. Craft I, Djahanbakhch O, McLeod F, Bernard A, Green S, Twigg H, et al. Human pregnancy following oocyte and sperm transfer to the uterus. Lancet. 1982;1:1031-3.
33. Trounson A, Leeton J, Besanko M, Wood C, Conti A. Pregnancy established in an infertile patient after transfer of a donated embryo fertilised in vitro. Br Med J (Clin Res Ed). 1983;286:835-8.
34. Trounson A, Mohr L. Human pregnancy following cryopreservation, thawing and transfer of an eight-cell embryo. Nature. 1983;305:707-9.
35. Veeck LL, Wortham JW, Witmyer J, Sandow BA, Acosta AA, Garcia JE, et al. Maturation and fertilization of morphologically immature human oocytes in a program of in vitro fertilization. Fertil Steril. 1983;39:594-602.
36. Buster JE, Bustillo M, Thorneycroft IH, Simon JA, Boyers SP, Marshall JR, et al. Non-surgical transfer of in vivo fertilised donated ova to five infertile women: report of two pregnancies. Lancet. 1983;2:223-4.
37. Casper RF, Wilson E, Collins JA, Brown SF, Parker JA. Enhancement of human implantation by exogenous chorionic gonadotropin. Lancet. 1983;2:1191.
38. Gleicher N, Friberg J, Fullan N, Giglia R, Mayden K, Kesky T, et al. EGG retrieval for in vitro fertilisation by sonographically controlled vaginal culdocentesis. Lancet. 1983;2:508-9.
39. Fishel SB, Edwards RG, Walters DE. Follicular steroids as a prognosticator of successful fertilization of human oocytes in vitro. J Endocrinol. 1983;99:335-44.
40. Asch RH, Ellsworth LR, Balmaceda JP, Wong PC. Pregnancy after translaparoscopic gamete intrafallopian transfer. Lancet. 1984;2:1034-5.
41. Lutjen P, Trounson A, Leeton J, Findlay J, Wood C, Renou P. The establishment and maintenance of pregnancy using in vitro fertilization and embryo donation in a patient with primary ovarian failure. Nature. 1984;307:174-5.
42. Porter RN, Smith W, Craft IL, Abdulwahid NA, Jacobs HS. Induction of ovulation for in-vitro fertilisation using buserelin and gonadotropins. Lancet. 1984;2:1284-5.
43. Zeilmaker GH, Alberda AT, van Gent I, Rijkmans CM, Drogendijk AC. Two pregnancies following transfer of intact frozen-thawed embryos. Fertil Steril. 1984;42:293-6.
44. Cohen J, Fehilly CB, Fishel SB, Edwards RG, Hewitt J, Rowland GF, et al. Male infertility successfully treated by in-vitro fertilisation. Lancet. 1984;1:1239-40.
45. Fishel SB, Edwards RG, Evans CJ. Human chorionic gonadotropin secreted by preimplantation embryos cultured in vitro. Science. 1984;223:816-8.
46. Temple-Smith PD, Southwick GJ, Yates CA, Trounson AO, de Kretser DM. Human pregnancy by in vitro fertilization (IVF) using sperm aspirated from the epididymis. J In Vitro Fert Embryo Transf. 1985;2:119-22.
47. Wikland M, Enk L, Hamberger L. Transvesical and transvaginal approaches for the aspiration of follicles by use of ultrasound. Ann N Y Acad Sci. 1985;442:182-94.
48. Strickler RC, Christianson C, Crane JP, Curato A, Knight AB, Yang V. Ultrasound guidance for human embryo transfer. Fertil Steril. 1985;43:54-61.
49. Cohen J, Simons RF, Fehilly CB, Fishel SB, Edwards RG, Hewitt J, et al. Birth after replacement of hatching blastocyst cryopreserved at expanded blastocyst stage. Lancet. 1985;1:647.
50. Quinn P, Kerin JF, Warnes GM. Improved pregnancy rate in human in vitro fertilization with the use of a medium based on the composition of human tubal fluid. Fertil Steril. 1985;44:493-8.
51. Utian WH, Sheean L, Goldfarb JM, Kiwi R. Successful pregnancy after in vitro fertilization and embryo transfer from an infertile woman to a surrogate. N Engl J Med. 1985;313:1351-2.
52. Feichtinger W, Kemeter P. Pregnancy after total ovariectomy achieved by ovum donation. Lancet. 1985;2:722-3.
53. Navot D, Laufer N, Kopolovic J, Rabinowitz R, Birkenfeld A, Lewin A, et al. Artificially induced endometrial cycles and establishment of pregnancies in the absence of ovaries. N Engl J Med. 1986;314:806-11.
54. Feichtinger W, Kemeter P. Transvaginal sector scan sonography for needle guided transvaginal follicle aspiration and other applications in gynecologic routine and research. Fertil Steril. 1986;45:722-5.

55. Rosenwaks Z, Veeck LL, Liu HC. Pregnancy following transfer of in vitro fertilized donated oocytes. Fertil Steril. 1986;45: 417-20.
56. Devroey P, Braeckmans P, Smitz J, Van Waesberghe L, Wisanto A, Van Steirteghem A, et al. Pregnancy after translaparoscopic zygote intrafallopian transfer in a patient with sperm antibodies. Lancet. 1986;1:1329.
57. Molloy D, Speirs A, du Plessis Y, McBain J, Johnston I. A laparoscopic approach to a program of gamete intrafallopian transfer. Fertil Steril. 1987;47:289-94.
58. Chen C. Pregnancy after human oocyte cryopreservation. Lancet. 1986;1:884-6.
59. Szollosi D, Mandelbaum J, Plachot M, Salat-Baroux J, Cohen J. Ultrastructure of the human preovulatory oocyte. J In Vitro Fert Embryo Transf. 1986;3:232-42.
60. Laws-King A, Trounson A, Sathananthan H, Kola I. Fertilization of human oocytes by microinjection of a single spermatozoon under the zona pellucida. Fertil Steril. 1987;48:637-42.
61. Patrizio P, Silber S, Ord T, Balmaceda JP, Asch RH. Two births after microsurgical sperm aspiration in congenital absence of vas deferens. Lancet. 1988;2:1364.
62. Ng SC, Bongso A, Ratnam SS, Sathananthan H, Chan CL, Wong PC, et al. Pregnancy after transfer of sperm under zona. Lancet. 1988;2:790.
63. Cohen J, Malter H, Fehilly C, Wright G, Elsner C, Kort H, et al. Implantation of embryos after partial opening of oocyte zona pellucida to facilitate sperm penetration. Lancet. 1988;2:162.
64. The Washington Post. (1988). Dr. Patrick Steptoe, 74, Dies; Pioneered Test-Tube Baby Field. [online] Available from https://www.washingtonpost.com/archive/local/1988/03/23/dr-patrick-steptoe-74-dies/39a50fb4-5955-44c8-9c9c-18df7d6c0bbe/.
65. Lanzendorf SE, Maloney MK, Veeck LL, Slusser J, Hodgen GD, Rosenwaks Z. A preclinical evaluation of pronuclear formation by microinjection of human spermatozoa into human oocytes. Fertil Steril. 1988;49:835-42.
66. Handyside AH, Pattinson JK, Penketh RJ, Delhanty JD, Winston RM, Tuddenham EG. Biopsy of human preimplantation embryos and sexing by DNA amplification. Lancet. 1989;1:347-9.
67. Tadir Y, Wright WH, Vafa O, Ord T, Asch RH, Berns MW. Micromanipulation of sperm by a laser generated optical trap. Fertil Steril. 1989;52:870-3.
68. Gonen Y, Casper RF, Jacobson W, Blankier J. Endometrial thickness and growth during ovarian stimulation: a possible predictor of implantation in in vitro fertilization. Fertil Steril. 1989;52:446-50.
69. Wilton LJ, Trounson AO. Biopsy of preimplantation mouse embryos: development of micromanipulated embryos and proliferation of single blastomeres in vitro. Biol Reprod. 1989;40:145-52.
70. Gordts S, Roziers P, Campo R, Noto V. Survival and pregnancy outcome after ultrarapid freezing of human embryos. Fertil Steril. 1990;53:469-72.
71. Handyside AH, Kontogianni EH, Hardy K, Winston RM. Pregnancies from biopsied human preimplantation embryos sexed by Y-specific DNA amplification. Nature. 1990;344:768-70.
72. Cohen J, Elsner C, Kort H, Malter H, Massey J, Mayer MP, et al. Impairment of the hatching process following IVF in the human and improvement of implantation by assisting hatching using micromanipulation. Hum Reprod. 1990;5:7-13.
73. Verlinsky Y, Ginsberg N, Lifchez A, Valle J, Moise J, Strom CM. Analysis of the first polar body: preconception genetic diagnosis. Hum Reprod. 1990;5:826-9.
74. Gonen Y, Balakier H, Powell W, Casper RF. Use of gonadotropin-releasing hormone agonist to trigger follicular maturation for in vitro fertilization. J Clin Endocrinol Metab. 1990;71:918-22.
75. Gonen Y, Jacobson W, Casper RF. Gonadotropin suppression with oral contraceptives before in vitro fertilization. Fertil Steril. 1990;53:282-7.
76. Fishel S, Antinori S, Jackson P, Johnson J, Lisi F, Chiariello F, et al. Twin birth after subzonal insemination. Lancet. 1990;335:722-3.
77. Cha KY, Koo JJ, Ko JJ, Choi DH, Han SY, Yoon TK. Pregnancy after in vitro fertilization of human follicular oocytes collected from nonstimulated cycles, their culture in vitro and their transfer in a donor oocyte program. Fertil Steril. 1991;55:109-13.
78. Frydman R, Cornel C, de Ziegler D, Taieb J, Spitz IM, Bouchard P. Prevention of premature luteinizing hormone and progesterone rise with a gonadotropin-releasing hormone antagonist, Nal-Glu, in controlled ovarian hyperstimulation. Fertil Steril. 1991;56:923-7.
79. Palanker D, Ohad S, Lewis A, Simon A, Shenkar J, Penchas S. Technique for cellular microsurgery using the 193-nm excimer laser. Lasers Surg Med. 1991;11:580-6.
80. Navot D, Bergh PA, Williams MA, Garrisi GJ, Guzman I, Sandler B, et al. Poor oocyte quality rather than implantation failure as a cause of age-related decline in female fertility. Lancet. 1991;337:1375-7.
81. Hurley VA, Osborn JC, Leoni MA, Leeton J. Ultrasound-guided embryo transfer: a controlled trial. Fertil Steril. 1991;55:559-62.
82. Germond M, Dessole S, Senn A, Loumaye E, Howles C, Beltrami V. Successful in-vitro fertilisation and embryo transfer after treatment with recombinant human FSH. Lancet. 1992;339:1170.
83. Devroey P, van Steirteghem A, Mannaerts B, Bennink HC. Successful in-vitro fertilisation and embryo transfer after treatment with recombinant human FSH. Lancet. 1992;339:1170.
84. Cohen J, Alikani M, Trowbridge J, Rosenwaks Z. Implantation enhancement by selective assisted hatching using zona drilling of human embryos with poor prognosis. Hum Reprod. 1992;7:685-91.
85. Palermo G, Joris H, Devroey P, Van Steirteghem AC. Pregnancies after intracytoplasmic injection of single spermatozoon into an oocyte. Lancet. 1992;340:17-8.
86. Grifo JA, Tang YX, Cohen J, Gilbert F, Sanyal MK, Rosenwaks Z. Pregnancy after embryo biopsy and coamplification of DNA from X and Y chromosomes. JAMA. 1992;268:727-9.
87. Emperaire JC, Ruffié A, Audebert AJ. Ovulation induction by endogenous LH released by the administration of an LHRH agonist after follicular stimulation for in vitro fertilization. J Gynecol Obstet Biol Reprod (Paris). 1992;21:489-94.
88. Tan SL, Royston P, Campbell S, Jacobs HS, Betts J, Mason B, et al. Cumulative conception and livebirth rates after in-vitro fertilisation. Lancet. 1992;339:1390-4.
89. Patrizio P, Silber S, Ord T, Marello E, Balmaceda JP, Asch RH. Replacement of frozen embryos generated from epididymal

spermatozoa: the first two pregnancies. Hum Reprod. 1992;7:652-3.
90. Feichtinger W, Strohmer H, Radner KM. Erbium YAG laser for micromanipulation of oocytes and spermatozoa. Lancet. 1992;340:115-6.
91. Schoot DC, Coelingh Bennink HJ, Mannaerts BM, Lamberts SW, Bouchard P, Fauser BC. Human recombinant follicle-stimulating hormone induces growth of preovulatory follicles without concomitant increase in androgen and estrogen biosynthesis in a woman with isolated gonadotropin deficiency. J Clin Endocrinol Metab. 1992;74:1471-3.
92. Hamberger B. Micromanipulation. In: Gordts S (Ed). Proceedings of European Symposium on Micromanipulation. Belgium: Drukkerij Nauwelaerts Leuven; 1993. p. 85.
93. Patrizio P, Asch RH, Handelin B, Silber SJ. Aetiology of congenital absence of vas deferens: genetic study of three generations. Hum Reprod. 1993;8:215-20.
94. Silber SJ, Nagy ZP, Liu J, Godoy H, Devroey P, Van Steirteghem AC. Conventional in-vitro fertilization versus intracytoplasmic sperm injection for patients requiring microsurgical sperm aspiration. Hum Reprod. 1994;9:1705-9.
95. Devroey P, Mannaerts B, Smitz J, Coelingh Bennink H, Van Steirteghem A. First established pregnancy and birth after ovarian stimulation with recombinant human follicle stimulating hormone (Org 32489). Hum Reprod. 1993;8:863-5.
96. Trounson A, Wood C, Kausche A. In vitro maturation and the fertilization and developmental competence of oocytes recovered from untreated polycystic ovarian patients. Fertil Steril. 1994;62:353-62.
97. Howles CM, Loumaye E, Giroud D, Luyet G. Multiple follicular development and ovarian steroidogenesis following subcutaneous administration of a highly purified urinary FSH preparation in pituitary desensitized women undergoing IVF: a multicentre European phase III study. Hum Reprod. 1994;9:424-30.
98. Devroey P, Liu J, Nagy Z, Goossens A, Tournaye H, Camus M. Pregnancies after testicular sperm extraction and intracytoplasmic sperm injection in non-obstructive azoospermia. Hum Reprod. 1995;10:1457-60.
99. Barnes FL, Crombie A, Gardner DK, Kausche A, Lacham-Kaplan O, Suikkari AM. Blastocyst development and birth after in-vitro maturation of human primary oocytes, intracytoplasmic sperm injection and assisted hatching. Hum Reprod. 1995;10:3243-7.
100. Munné S, Sultan KM, Weier HU, Grifo JA, Cohen J, Rosenwaks Z. Assessment of numeric abnormalities of X, Y, 18, and 16 chromosomes in preimplantation human embryos before transfer. Am J Obstet Gynecol. 1995;172:1191-9.
101. Fishel S, Green S, Bishop M, Thornton S, Hunter A, Fleming S. Pregnancy after intracytoplasmic injection of spermatid. Lancet. 1995;345:1641-2.
102. Out HJ, Mannaerts BM, Driessen SG, Bennink HJ. A prospective, randomized, assessor-blind, multicentre study comparing recombinant and urinary follicle stimulating hormone (Puregon versus Metrodin) in in-vitro fertilization. Hum Reprod. 1995;10:2534-40.
103. Gil-Salom M, Romero J, Minguez Y, Rubio C, De los Santos MJ, Remohí J, et al. Pregnancies after intracytoplasmic sperm injection with cryopreserved testicular spermatozoa. Hum Reprod. 1996;11:1309-13.
104. Reijo R, Alagappan RK, Patrizio P, Page DC. Severe oligozoospermia resulting from deletions of azoospermia factor gene on Y chromosome. Lancet. 1996;347:1290-3.
105. Casper RF, Meriano JS, Jarvi KA, Cowan L, Lucato ML. The hypo-osmotic swelling test for selection of viable sperm for intracytoplasmic sperm injection in men with complete asthenozoospermia. Fertil Steril. 1996;65:972-6.
106. Cohen J, Scott R, Schimmel T, Levron J, Willadsen S. Birth of infant after transfer of anucleate donor oocyte cytoplasm into recipient eggs. Lancet. 1997;350:186-7.
107. Sun JG, Jurisicova A, Casper RF. Detection of deoxyribonucleic acid fragmentation in human sperm: correlation with fertilization in vitro. Biol Reprod. 1997;56:602-7.
108. Porcu E, Fabbri R, Seracchioli R, Ciotti PM, Magrini O, Flamigni C. Birth of a healthy female after intracytoplasmic sperm injection of cryopreserved human oocytes. Fertil Steril. 1997;68:724-6.
109. Itskovitz-Eldor J, Kol S, Mannaerts B, Coelingh Bennink H. First established pregnancy after controlled ovarian hyperstimulation with recombinant follicle stimulating hormone and the gonadotrophin-releasing hormone antagonist ganirelix (Org 37462). Hum Reprod. 1998;13:294-5.
110. Gardner DK, Schoolcraft WB, Wagley L, Schlenker T, Stevens J, Hesla J. A prospective randomized trial of blastocyst culture and transfer in in-vitro fertilization. Hum Reprod. 1998;13:3434-40.
111. Palermo GD, Schlegel PN, Sills ES, Veeck LL, Zaninovic N, Menendez S, et al. Births after intracytoplasmic injection of sperm obtained by testicular extraction from men with nonmosaic Klinefelter's syndrome. N Engl J Med. 1998;338:588-90.
112. Jones GM, Trounson AO, Gardner DK, Kausche A, Lolatgis N, Wood C. Evolution of a culture protocol for successful blastocyst development and pregnancy. Hum Reprod. 1998;13:169-77.
113. Feichtinger W. Follicle aspiration with interactive three-dimensional digital imaging (Voluson): a step toward real-time puncturing under three-dimensional ultrasound control. Fertil Steril. 1998;70:374-7.
114. Xu K, Shi ZM, Veeck LL, Hughes MR, Rosenwaks Z. First unaffected pregnancy using preimplantation genetic diagnosis for sickle cell anemia. JAMA. 1999;281:1701-6.
115. Kuleshova L, Gianaroli L, Magli C, Ferraretti A, Trounson A. Birth following vitrification of a small number of human oocytes: case report. Hum Reprod. 1999;14:3077-9.
116. Buckett WM, Fisch P, Dean NL, Biljan MM, Tan SL. In vitro fertilization and intracytoplasmic sperm injection pregnancies after successful transport of oocytes by airplane. Fertil Steril. 1999;71:753-5.
117. Porcu E, Fabbri R, Petracchi S, Ciotti PM, Flamigni C. Ongoing pregnancy after intracytoplasmic injection of testicular spermatozoa into cryopreserved human oocytes. Am J Obstet Gynecol. 1999;180:1044-5.
118. Oktay K, Karlikaya G. Ovarian function after transplantation of frozen, banked autologous ovarian tissue. N Engl J Med. 2000;342:1919.
119. Ali J, Shahata MA, Al-Natsha SD. Formulation of a protein-free medium for human assisted reproduction. Hum Reprod. 2000;15:145-56.
120. Chian RC, Gülekli B, Buckett WM, Tan SL. Pregnancy and delivery after cryopreservation of zygotes produced by in-vitro

matured oocytes retrieved from a woman with polycystic ovarian syndrome. Hum Reprod. 2001;16:1700-2.

121. Abdul-Jalil AK, Child TJ, Phillips S, Dean N, Carrier S, Tan SL. Ongoing twin pregnancy after ICSI of PESA-retrieved spermatozoa into in-vitro matured oocytes: case report. Hum Reprod. 2001;16:1424-6.
122. Belker AM, Swanson ML, Cook CL, Carrillo AJ, Yoffe SC. Live birth after sperm retrieval from a moribund man. Fertil Steril. 2001;76:841-3.
123. De Boer K, McArthur S, Murray C, Jansen RPS. First live birth following blastocyst biopsy and PGD analysis. Reprod Biomed Online. 2002;4:35.
124. Wells D, Escudero T, Levy B, Hirschhorn K, Delhanty JD, Munné S. First clinical application of comparative genomic hybridization and polar body testing for preimplantation genetic diagnosis of aneuploidy. Fertil Steril. 2002;78:543-9.
125. Yoon TK, Kim TJ, Park SE, Hong SW, Ko JJ, Chung HM, et al. Live births after vitrification of oocytes in a stimulated in vitro fertilization-embryo transfer program. Fertil Steril. 2003;79:1323-6.
126. Beckers NG, Macklon NS, Devroey P, Platteau P, Boerrigter PJ, Fauser BC. First live birth after ovarian stimulation using a chimeric long-acting human recombinant follicle-stimulating hormone (FSH) agonist (recFSH-CTP) for in vitro fertilization. Fertil Steril. 2003;79:621-3.
127. Barash A, Dekel N, Fieldust S, Segal I, Schechtman E, Granot I. Local injury to the endometrium doubles the incidence of successful pregnancies in patients undergoing in vitro fertilization. Fertil Steril. 2003;79:1317-22.
128. Kattera S, Chen C. Normal birth after microsurgical enucleation of tripronuclear human zygotes: case report. Hum Reprod. 2003;18:1319-22.
129. Fuchinoue K, Nakajo Y, Yagi A, Takeda M, Kyono K. Successful pregnancy and delivery following combined treatment of in vitro maturation (IVM) and testicular sperm extraction (TESE): a case report. J Assist Reprod Genet. 2004;21:371-3.
130. Donnez J, Dolmans MM, Demylle D, Jadoul P, Pirard C, Squifflet J, et al. Livebirth after orthotopic transplantation of cryopreserved ovarian tissue. Lancet. 2004;364:1405-10.
131. Gardner DK, Surrey E, Minjarez D, Leitz A, Stevens J, Schoolcraft WB, et al. Single blastocyst transfer: a prospective randomized trial. Fertil Steril. 2004;81:551-5.
132. Rao GD, Chian RC, Son WS, Gilbert L, Tan SL. Fertility preservation in women undergoing cancer treatment. Lancet. 2004;363:1829-30.
133. Chian RC, Buckett WM, Abdul Jalil AK, Son WY, Sylvestre C, Rao D, et al. Natural-cycle in vitro fertilization combined with in vitro maturation of immature oocytes is a potential approach in infertility treatment. Fertil Steril. 2004;82:1675-8.
134. McArthur SJ, Leigh D, Marshall JT, de Boer KA, Jansen RP. Pregnancies and live births after trophectoderm biopsy and preimplantation genetic testing of human blastocysts. Fertil Steril. 2005;84:1628-36.
135. Meirow D, Levron J, Eldar-Geva T, Hardan I, Fridman E, Zalel Y, et al. Pregnancy after transplantation of cryopreserved ovarian tissue in a patient with ovarian failure after chemotherapy. N Engl J Med. 2005;353:318-21.
136. Kokkali G, Vrettou C, Traeger-Synodinos J, Jones GM, Cram DS, Stavrou D, et al. Birth of a healthy infant following trophectoderm biopsy from blastocysts for PGD of beta-thalassaemia major. Hum Reprod. 2005;20:1855-9.
137. Ao A, Jin S, Rao D, Son WY, Chian RC, Tan SL. First successful pregnancy outcome after preimplantation genetic diagnosis for aneuploidy screening in embryos generated from natural-cycle in vitro fertilization combined with an in vitro maturation procedure. Fertil Steril. 2006;85:1510.e9-11.
138. Bedaiwy MA, Hussein MR, Biscotti C, Falcone T. Cryopreservation of intact human ovary with its vascular pedicle. Hum Reprod. 2006;21:3258-69.
139. Heijnen EM, Eijkemans MJ, De Klerk C, Polinder S, Beckers NG, Klinkert ER, et al. A mild treatment strategy for in-vitro fertilisation: a randomised non-inferiority trial. Lancet. 2007;369:743-9.
140. Arav P, Pasquale P. Yale practice by Yale Medical Group. Yale Pract. 2007;12:2.
141. Jones GM, Cram DS, Song B, Kokkali G, Pantos K, Trounson AO. Novel strategy with potential to identify developmentally competent IVF blastocysts. Hum Reprod. 2008;23:1748-59.
142. Porcu E, Venturoli S, Damiano G, Ciotti PM, Notarangelo L, Paradisi R, et al. Healthy twins delivered after oocyte cryopreservation and bilateral ovariectomy for ovarian cancer. Reprod Biomed Online. 2008;17:265-7.
143. Fishel S, Gordon A, Lynch C, Dowell K, Ndukwe G, Kelada E, et al. Live birth after polar body array comparative genomic hybridization prediction of embryo ploidy-the future of IVF? Fertil Steril. 2010;93:1006.e7-10.
144. Sagi M, Weinberg N, Eilat A, Aizenman E, Werner M, Girsh E, et al. Preimplantation genetic diagnosis for BRCA1/2—a novel clinical experience. Prenat Diagn. 2009;29:508-13.

CHAPTER 104

# In Vitro Fertilization and Embryo Transfer

*Alex C Varghese, Shrey Balani, Kannamannadiar Jayaprakasan*

## INTRODUCTION

Since the birth of Louise Brown at Oldham, Cambridge by the pioneering works of Edwards and Steptoe in vitro fertilization (IVF) and embryo transfer (ET) techniques, many developments in the field have occured and resulted so far, in the birth of >8 million babies worldwide. The active research in both the clinical side (new drugs and regimens for stimulation, advanced ultrasonography, and ET techniques) and the laboratory (preimplantation genetic testing (PGT), sperm selection methods, and novel embryo culture systems) in the last three decades has dramatically increased the take home baby rates. Although newer technologies and methods have definitely improved the pregnancy rate the risks associated with assisted reproductive technologies (ART) have also surfaced concurrently. Current ART practices are trying to minimize the risks by offering mild stimulation protocols, elective single ET (SET), and PGT using high throughput molecular and genetic platforms to select the euploid embryos for transfer, offering donor gametes or embryos in unavoidable conditions. The success of an IVF program should always be measured by the live birth (LB) of healthy babies. To achieve this level of success, many aspects of assisted reproduction play an important role. Artificial intelligence (AI) and machine learning are rapidly changing the practice of medicine. AI has remarkable potential to overcome the barriers of low success rate, cost and accessibility of IVF. There is a huge scope of robotics or automation in IVF lab systems. The IVF laboratory process is very complex and needs high level of accuracy and errors close to zero, along with proper documentation. This chapter tries to give an insight on these areas.

## IMPORTANCE OF TOTAL QUALITY

### Management in Assisted Reproductive Technologies

The absence of a strict program control can cause potential compromise in the IVF success due to the extreme sensitivity of the gametes and the early embryos to the physical and environmental factors. The attention to the general components of a quality control (QC) and quality assurance program are necessary for a repeatable process and as such the total quality management (TQM) of the program must be stressed. The implementation of TQM involves satisfying customers, controlling the changes in the system or process, managing personnels and quality improvement tools. These are further identified as the five pillars of TQM—(1) Product (service), (2) Process, (3) Organization, (4) Leadership, and (5) Commitment.

Such an undertaking requires an organizational culture change involving a major staff learning and training program followed by pilot quality initiatives in a number of major areas including human, financial, technological, and natural resources.

Quality management is a culture that needs to be implemented at different levels in an organization to yield fruitful results. Merely introducing few QC gadgets does not suffice to obtain the desired. Proper staff training, continuous education, internal and external auditing of the process, implementation of ideal QC strategies, etc., will yield the desired outcomes.

## IN VITRO FERTILIZATION LABORATORY AND CULTURE SYSTEMS

### In Vitro Fertilization Laboratory

Unlike other pathological, biological, or tissue culture laboratories, the design and layout of IVF laboratories need proper planning since these laboratories are going to deal with human gametes, which are sensitive to external environmental conditions. Sites near significant point sources of contaminants should be avoided or evaluated carefully. A detailed site review is done by environmental firms and includes an onsite inspection, baseline analysis of the prospective location, and a review of public documents. The inspection must include baseline sampling for toxic organics (as listed by the USEPA). The baseline samples should be done by recognized analytical methods [USEPA toxic organics (TO)15 and USEPA TO11] providing both identity and concentrations at the microgram/cubic meter ($\mu g/m^3$) level by an accredited environmental laboratory. Measurements at milligram/cubic meter ($mg/m^3$) are not sufficiently rigorous because of the potentially high detection limits. Avoid handheld analysis by photoionization detectors (PIDs) as the investigation tool as PIDs use highenergy photons, typically in the ultraviolet (UV) range. The use of UV light to excite the molecules results in the ionization of gas molecules. The energy of the photons is typically in the range of 10 eV, so that only gases with low ionization energy, e.g., organic vapor, can be ionized. The main air constituents, oxygen and nitrogen, do not form ions at this photon energy. The resulting ions produce an electric current proportional to the signal output of the detector. More molecules are present in the air, more ions are produced, and higher will be the resulting current. Finally, the ions recombine after the detector to reform the original molecules.

The major factor to be taken care while designing such units is the clean room facility especially for the laboratory and the ovum recovery or ET units. These rooms should be maintained at a higher pressure compared to adjacent rooms for exchange of air. A dedicated air handling unit specific for these rooms can definitely be a good investment. These units ideally should have air handling units having prefilters, high efficiency particulate air (HEPA) filters, and activated volatile organic compounds (VOC) filters to trap all chemically active compounds (CAC) sweeping into the rooms or generated in the clean rooms. The existing unit can also opt for standalone VOC filtration units but these are less efficient. Timely changing of filters ensures their optimal functioning. This is also true for the VOC inline filters connected to gas cylinders supplying "medical grade gases" to IVF incubators.

## In Vitro Fertilization Culture Systems

The earliest stages of human development, until day 5 or 6 after fertilization, normally occur in the woman's fallopian tube (or oviduct). However, after IVF, much of this period of early development occurs in the laboratory. The conditions under which the preimplantation embryos are cultured have been carefully formulated in the form of culture media and systems to provide an environment that mimics—as closely as possible—that of the fallopian tube.

Commercially prepared culture (sequential or single step) media support embryo development in the laboratory for up to 6 days. By allowing the embryo to reach the blastocyst stage, one can make a more stringent selection of those to be transferred during an IVF cycle. This paves the way for elective single or double ETs. However, the extended culture of preimplantation embryos requires the use of hypoxic conditions. Ideally, the use of benchtop incubators with low oxygen concentration achieves the required gas concentration. In vivo, oocytes and embryos are exposed to a maximum of ~5–8% $O_2$ in the reproductive system. Atmospheric $O_2$ may lead to supraphysiologic reactive oxygen species levels, potentially causing oxidative stress [damage to cell organelles, lipids, membranes, deoxyribonucleic acid (DNA), and gene expression] and ultimately poor embryo development.[1]

There are many variables in an IVF laboratory affecting the pregnancy rates, from the air filters to the culture media and the incubators. Only when all the processes are fine-tuned, products of high quality are used, pH and temperature are closely monitored, all equipment are maintained, the results will be optimal. There is a tendency in the running IVF units to procure a single "small" benchtop incubator and culture the embryos from just the zygote stage onward. The preequilibration of culture media, fertilization, and incubation up to zygote stage still performed in the large $CO_2$ incubators (20% $O_2$). Hence, gametes and embryos are exposed to 20% $O_2$ and 5% $O_2$ consecutively. Data obtained using timelapse incubation strongly supports the notion that at no time during the preimplantation period the embryos should be exposed to 20% oxygen. In a study by Wale, et al., (2010), timelapse microscopy was performed with imaging of individual mouse embryos at 15 minutes intervals. Compared with embryos cultured in 5% oxygen, embryos cultured in 20% oxygen were delayed at the first cleavage by 0.45 hours ($p < 0.05$), at the second cleavage by 0.84 hours ($p < 0.01$), and at the third cleavage by 3.19 hours ($p < 0.001$). Switching from 20 to 5% oxygen after 48 hours did not completely alleviate the earlier induced perturbations. Partial or complete culture in atmospheric oxygen resulted in significantly fewer blastocyst cell numbers compared with control ($p < 0.05$). Oxygen can influence mouse embryo development at both the cleavage and postcompaction stages. This must be true for human embryos too.

The introduction of timelapse imaging (TLI) systems in clinical human IVF, however, has stirred discussions about how new technologies should be implemented in the daily clinical routine. Many reviews and observational studies have discussed the value of timelapse monitoring in routine laboratory practice. It is as yet unclear, however, whether the observed benefits came from the undisturbed culture or improved selection based on continuous timelapse images. In short—what is the weight of these benefits in the added value of timelapse? The recent (Csaba Pribenszky, et al., 2017) metaanalysis of five randomized controlled trials (RCT) (n = 1,637) showed that the application of time-lapse monitoring was associated with a significantly higher ongoing clinical pregnancy rate (51.0% versus 39.9%), with a pooled odds ratio of 1.542 ($p < 0.001$), significantly lower early pregnancy loss (15.3% versus 21.3%; or 0.662; $p = 0.019$), and a significantly increased LB rate (44.2% versus 31.3%; or 1.668; $p = 0.009$). Difference in stillbirth was not significant between groups (4.7% versus 2.4%). Quality of the evidence was moderatetolow owing to inconsistencies across the studies.[2] Comparison of LB rates and the perinatal outcomes after fresh and frozen ET between TLI and standard culture (SC) incubators were done by Mascarenhas, et al., (2018). The fresh ET LB rate was noted to be higher for TLI cycles [TLI 36.8% versus SC 33.9%, adjusted odds ratio (aOR) 1.28, 95% confidence interval (CI) 1.05–1.57], but the frozen ET LB rates were not significantly different. The mean birth weight was higher in the TLI group after both fresh [adjusted mean difference (aMD) 174.78 g, 95% CI 64.80–284.77] and frozen ETs (aMD 175.91 g, 95% CI 16.98–334.84). After a fresh ET, there was a lower risk of early preterm birth (PTB) and very low birth weight (LBW) in the TLI group. Among frozen ETs, there was a lower risk of early PTB and LBW in the TLI group. TLI incubators are associated with improved perinatal outcomes and higher mean birth weight after fresh and frozen ET.[3]

Air quality, particle count, and sterility are extremely important in an IVF laboratory to ensure the best clinical outcomes. Human embryos are extremely sensitive to the presence of any VOC and CAC. Globally, a class 10,000 laboratory is recommended for IVF, that is, 10,000 ppm in air. The best way to achieve this is by building a modular clean room. This is done with a combination of various panels (Steel, Bioclad, etc.), medical grade vinyl flooring, and high efficiency heating, ventilation, and air conditioning (HVAC) air system that control air temperature and particulate matter, as well as filter harmful VOC. Moreover, incorporation of UVC light enables the elimination of the build-up of any fungal or bacterial colonization in the air handling system or ducts. The modular clean room concept facilitates ease in building of partitions, ease of cleaning, curving of joints, and provision for electrical and gas pipelines, with proper esthetic looks. Hence, proper laboratory design and quality assurance and control can prevent compromises. Burnin, validation, and commissioning of new laboratories are very important before starting the new IVF cycles.

## Workstations

Tissue handling directives generally recommend the use of laminar air flow workstations whenever cell or tissue material is manipulated. The aim of the laminar filtration is to mitigate the dramatic particle contamination that can be found in any room—even a state of the art clean room—when it has been transformed into a busy laboratory. The first sweep in the room with a high-grade particle counter will astonish most as the particle levels will usually be beyond their wildest expectation. Inside the air curtain of the laminar air flow workstation this is reduced to almost zero.

The challenge with the use of workstations is to integrate them so that their benefits do not become liabilities for the embryos.

The workstation must be equipped with heating systems sophisticated enough to maintain the correct temperature of the specimens during handling under all circumstances. Especially some kind of heated glass stage is vital as the manipulations take place mostly under the microscope.

The most advanced workstations incorporate temporary storing facilities for the dishes where they can be kept in like incubator conditions when they are in between procedures or handling.

The biggest challenge to handle in workstations is open culture conditions as the heat applied below will cause immediate evaporative cool down of the liquid in the dish. There is no way to avoid this other than adding high humidity or some kind of provisions for heat from above to slow down the evaporative cooling. The overall aim is to reduce the total temperature drop during handling. Increasing the heat which seems the logical way to avoid the drop actually have the opposite effect as it increases the evaporative cooling. Only careful testing can reveal what the best method is for keeping the best possible temperature in open culture conditions and what average handling times can be allowed before the temperature drop becomes critical.

Working under oil it is essential to have the correct temperature as oil is not very forgiving for too high temperature.

The laminar air flow can have a cooling effect—but if the workstation has been designed correctly it is possible to maintain a stable and correct temperature in the dish under oil. A possibility that can be utilized successfully with open culture is working in humidified environments. They do, however, have the drawback of risk of contamination or at least being quite difficult to maintain a suitable aseptic state.

A regulatory caused delusion occurred in some countries within IVF when a widespread adoption of Class II (biological safety cabinets) was introduced for IVF work. This type of safety cabinet, designed to protect the operator as well as the specimens being handled, are the least suited laminar air flow workstations for IVF. They are designed to adhere to certain standards as they are meant for biological contaminated work. This means that the mandatory high airflow and design of flow in the tabletop makes it not suited for IVF work. The possible benefit of the operator protection when there is really nothing to protect against is not worth the extra risk to the embryos. Even the best designs of the Class II workstations will never be better than the most average designs of a vertical laminar air flow workstation.

Horizontal laminar air flow workstations offer no benefits over vertical and should be avoided alone because of the extra discomfort they provide for the operator by blowing directly into their face.

The future will surely bring better systems that can offer a more natural environment with both filtration of the air, temperature control, and gas mixture. These systems will allow for safely working with bicarbonatebuffered media without the risk of rapid pH changes. They will also provide better solutions to the afore-mentioned temperature challenges. Furthermore, they will serve as small clean rooms inside the laboratory so that any moving around in the laboratory does not interfere with the aseptic conditions like it can happen even with good vertical laminar air flow workstations.

Future embodiments might even make it possible to do the complicated procedures such as intracytoplasmic sperm injection (ICSI) and biopsies in a controlled environment instead of manipulations taking place in the open rooms on big microscopes placed on antivibration tables. Thus, offering both a safe environment and also space saving which is so critical in the modern laboratory where space is at a premium.

Ideally a 6 foot cabinet with heated workbench and high-quality stereo zoom microscope is an ideal option anticipating the future workload. One can install a second stereo zoom microscope in these 6 foot cabinets which enables simultaneous work by two embryologists in busy laboratories. Otherwise, an inverted microscope such as Primo Vert (with integrated monitor, Carl Zeiss) can be integrated on the other end which can be used for embryo grading. Using a low magnification stereo microscope can sometimes lead to misleading embryo scoring grades, as the image may not reveal fine details of the embryos. Modern laboratories opt for closed workstations such as Incu chamber (KSystem, Denmark), active IVF (UK), Vitrosafe (UK), or IVF chamber (ORIGIO, Denmark). These workstations offer the ideal physiological environments for gametes and embryos while being manipulated outside the incubator.

The laboratory should also have a dedicated warming incubator (150 L or above, Forma, USA; Binder, Germany or Memert, Germany). This can be of utmost help for warming up the culture dishes and other disposables used in IVF cycles. Moreover, this type of large warming incubators can be used to offgas the VOCs from culture dishes before use. Special care should be done while selecting tissue culture wares or disposables for gamete or embryo culture. The dishes should be IVF or mouse embryo tested.

Since, male factor infertility is becoming increasingly responsible for the couple infertility, the unit should have a dedicated ICSI workstation and a proper training by laboratory personal on micromanipulation techniques. The ICSI workstation requires a vibrationfree heavy table (either commercially available one or a modified heavy table with granite table top). The options are Nikon Narishige (Japan), Olympus Narishige (Japan), Eppendorf (Germany), and Integra (RI, UK). The ICSI workstation should have a dedicated inverted microscope (Leica, Carl Zeiss, Nikon, or Olympus) with optional intracytoplasmic morphology selection (IMSI) attachment for sperm organellar morphology assessment and IMSI. Several sperm selection methods are available which include magnetic activated cell sorting (MACS), microfluidic sperm selection, IMSI, and physiological intracytoplasmic sperm injection (PICSI). Interferometric phase microscopy (IPM), also called digital holographic microscopy, for labelfree sperm imaging in fertility clinics, is also getting explored by Israeli scientists. According to recent studies, epigenetic modifications of sperm could be evaluated by noninvasive Raman spectroscopy by analyzing DNA and ribonucleic acid (RNA), as well as histones and protamines. Label-free optical spectroscopy and imaging techniques, based on the combination of Raman spectroscopy or imaging with holographic imaging, which are able to noninvasively measure the biochemistry and morphology of sperm cells is also being explored.[1]

## OOCYTE ABNORMALITIES AND PREGNANCY OUTCOMES

Oocytes retrieved after ovarian stimulation have not undergone the integral process of natural selection. These oocytes may be developmentally defective and would have been pushed to grow by the supraphysiologic gonadotropins. This can have serious impact on the developmental potential of the embryo as well as on the health of the offspring. The morphological examination of the oocyte, documentation of the findings, and segregation of abnormal oocytes which are inseminated is essential. Few important oocyte abnormalities and their pregnancy outcomes are being discussed.

### Smooth Endoplasmic Reticulum Oocytes

This abnormality is characterized by disk-like accumulation of the smooth endoplasmic reticulum (SER) due to dilatation and fusion of saccules during maturational process. Since, SER has a major role in calcium homeostasis, it is postulated that the calcium balance in SER + oocytes is abnormal. Studies have shown that SER oocytes are associated with decreased fertilization rates, cleavage rates, and blastulation. Few congenital malformations and genetic abnormalities are also reported. Hence, Alpha Scientists and European Society of Human Reproduction and Embryology (ESHRE) advised against the insemination of SER + oocytes,[4] but there are studies after that reporting delivery of healthy babies.[5,6] Hence, centers inseminating SER oocytes should report their outcomes so that the exact data will be known.

### Central Granulation

It is characterized by the appearance of numerous cytoplasmic pits of about 1.5 μ. Studies have divided opinions about the presence of granularity; few suggesting no role in in vitro developmental outcome,[7] while a study suggested that cases of extreme granularity may lead to early pregnancy loss.[8]

### Cytoplasmic Vacuolation

This is one of the most common oocyte dysmorphisms. These membrane-bound cytoplasmic inclusions vary in size and number. It had been demonstrated that vacuoles of >14 µ diameter can block fertilization. There are few case reports in the literature showing successful pregnancies in vacuolated oocytes with vacuoles of average diameter of 52.2 µm.[9]

## EFFECT OF OVARIAN STIMULATION ON OOCYTE QUALITY

Oocyte quality impacts early embryonic survival, the establishment and maintenance of pregnancy, fetal development, and even adult disease. Quality, or developmental competence, is acquired during folliculogenesis as the oocyte grows and during the period of oocyte maturation.

The interaction between granulosa cells and the oocyte is controlled by gonadotropins and the oocyte itself. Both gonadotropins influence oocyte competence through the two main local growth factor systems—(1) the bone morphogenetic protein system and (2) the insulin-like growth factors (IGF) system.

It has been observed in the animal model that modification of these systems influences ovulation rates, oocyte competence, and resulting embryo quality.[10]

Inevitably, controlled ovarian stimulation (COS) for IVF necessitate variations in theca and granulosa cell functions that may affect oocyte quality. Multiple follicular development causes the growth of follicles of different sizes and functional activity that will contain oocytes at different maturation stages.[11]

On the other hand, success of IVF is clearly dependent on the size and quality of the oocyte cohort.[12-14] Effects of ovarian stimulation on oocyte and embryo quality have been well-characterized in animals, showing that aggressive stimulation leads to poorer embryo development potential and could increase the rate of chromosomal abnormalities.[15-17] Later studies in animals suggested that embryo development seems to be adversely affected in a dose-dependent manner.[18,19]

In humans though, studies are limited and less conclusive. In fact, when natural and stimulated cycles are compared, no differences have been observed in terms of embryo cleavage capacity,[20] oocyte,[21] and embryo aneuploidy rate,[22] or incidence of aneuploidy in aborted fetuses[23] or in chorionic villus sampling in the late first trimester of pregnancy.[24]

A significantly different follicular endocrine milieu has been detected when natural cycle mature follicles and stimulated follicles have been compared,[25] although another group could not detect a relationship between this modification in follicular physiology and embryo morphology or even oocyte meiotic spindle structure.[26]

Most of the studies in humans designed to evaluate the impact of gonadotropins on oocyte quality have compared different doses of gonadotropins. When mild and conventional stimulation are compared, a higher proportion of good morphologic quality embryos is observed in the former.[27,28]

Additionally, a positive relationship between doses of gonadotropins and aneuploidy rate was found, both in the embryo[29] and in granulosa cells.[30]

Another study concluded that ovarian stimulation does not significantly raise the embryo aneuploidy rate in IVF-derived human embryos when compared with an unstimulated cycle and that ovarian response was not positively related to aneuploidy.[31]

The proportion of euploid oocytes is directly related to the number of mature oocytes, and inversely related to the number of units of follicle-stimulating hormone (FSH) per oocyte and per mature oocyte obtained.[32,33]

This is in-line with recent studies, which do not support the idea that ovarian stimulation is so detrimental to oocyte and embryo quality. In fact, it has been shown that high ovarian response to conventional ovarian stimulation does not increase embryo aneuploidy rates in PGT cycles using array comparative genomic hybridization (aCGH), either in infertile patients or in oocyte donors.[34,35]

Moreover, the more euploid blastocysts that are available, the higher the clinical pregnancy rate, even in fresh cycles[36,37] and the higher the ovarian response, the higher the cumulative pregnancy rate after the thawed ETs.[15,38] This is consistent with the recently introduced concept of "ovarian sensitivity index"[39] which is the ratio between the total dose of gonadotropins used during COS and the number of oocytes retrieved. It was shown that the higher this index is, the higher the pregnancy rates, reflecting that healthier ovaries that display a good response with low doses of gonadotropins also provide the best oocyte quality.

A review of a very large series of patients (>650,000) supports this concept. The authors observed that gonadotropin dose, as an independent factor, correlated negatively with the probability of LB.[40]

## INDIVIDUALIZED OR PATIENT-TAILORED STIMULATION STRATEGIES

The main objective of individualization of treatment in IVF is to offer every single woman the best treatment tailored to her specific characteristics, thus maximizing success, eliminating iatrogenic risks, such as ovarian hyperstimulation syndrome (OHSS), and minimizing the risk of cycle cancellation.

A key factor determining the outcome of COS and subsequent IVF outcome is selection of the gonadotropin starting dose. The need for individualizing gonadotropin dosage comes from the assumption that variability in the functional ovarian reserve (the pool of recruitable follicles) is very wide[41-45] and consequently a standard fixed dose of gonadotropin may not be suitable for all women. Correct individualization of the gonadotropin start dose is an extremely important clinical decision.

The correct individualization of treatment protocols in IVF should be based on the correct estimation of ovarian response especially the extremes, namely poor and hyper response. The aim is then to choose the ideal treatment protocol according to this prediction. The prediction of ovarian response allows clinicians to give women more accurate information regarding the likelihood of these scenarios occurring during their IVF cycle.

Patients may receive more accurate information on possible protracted treatment, cycle cancellation OHSS, treatment burden, and reduced success. If personalization is based on the accurate prediction of ovarian response, then the prediction of ovarian response should be based on the most sensitive markers of ovarian reserve.[46,47]

Lan, et al., compared the efficacy and safety of two simple dosing algorithms, one based on anti-Müllerian hormone (AMH) and the other on the antral follicle count (AFC), to determine the starting dose recombinant follicle stimulating hormone (rFSH) for ovarian stimulation in 348 women. This pilot study, concluded that, with subtle differences, both AMH and AFC appear to have the ability to predict poor ovarian response and guide the starting dose of rFSH.[48]

Oliveira, et al., presented a new ovarian response prediction index (ORPI), based on AMH levels, AFC, and age, and set-up a study to verify whether it could be a reliable predictor of the ovarian stimulation response. The ORPI might be used to improve cost-benefit ratio of ovarian stimulation regimens by guiding the selection of medication and by modulating the doses and regimens according to the actual needs of the patients.[49]

The availability of new markers of ovarian reserve, the improvement in methodology for their measurement, and the huge amount of clinical data has supported the view that individualization in IVF is the way forward. The correct measurement of markers of ovarian reserve allows a scientific estimate of the pool of follicles that potentially respond to ovarian stimulation.

Published studies indicate an important role for both AFC and AMH in the prediction of the extremes of ovarian response and for enabling the subsequent individualization of a therapeutic strategy.

This is the basis for the correct selection of women for use of the different GnRH (gonadotropin-releasing hormone) analogs and, for the fine-tuning of the gonadotropin dose.

The ultimate goal would be the selection of an effective protocol for ovarian stimulation which has to be well-balanced between the risk of maximal and suboptimal ovarian response. The benefits of a personalized therapy may include reduced incidence of risks and dropouts as well as a reduced treatment burden.

## Mild Stimulation In Vitro Fertilization

In 1996, Edwards, et al., were the first to express concern with regard to contemporary ovarian stimulation approaches for IVF and called for the use of milder stimulation protocols.[50] The aim of mild stimulation is to develop safer and more patient-friendly protocols in which the risks of treatment are minimized.[51-54] The protocols are considered to be patient-friendly as they include fewer injections and days of injections and less monitoring. There is reduced risk of OHSS, discomfort, and stress, all documented in literature.

In addition, there is accumulating evidence that milder stimulation protocols result in better quality embryos and a lower percentage of aneuploid embryos when compared to embryos from conventional or high dose gonadotropin stimulation protocols.

The challenges in mild stimulation remain that cancellation rates are higher and per cycle pregnancy rates are lower with fewer embryos frozen from mild stimulation protocols compared to conventional stimulation. However, if one looks at accumulative cycles over a similar time period the percentage of couples becoming pregnant from the two protocols is similar, with one or more additional IVF cycles required for those couples having low dose protocols.

Studies suggest that ovarian stimulation affects embryo quality as assessed by morphology as well as the chromosomal constitution of the embryos.[29,55]

This phenomenon could be the result of interference with the natural selection of good quality oocytes or the exposure of growing follicles to the potentially negative effects of ovarian stimulation. Supporting this evidence comes from various human and animal studies reporting detrimental effects of ovarian stimulation on oocyte and embryo quality. An increased incidence of morphology and chromosomal abnormalities have been observed in oocytes after exposure to high doses of gonadotropins during in vitro maturation of mouse oocytes.[56,57]

Mild stimulation approaches, aiming at a more physiological response, might therefore improve embryo quality. A randomized trial concerning the chromosomal competence of human embryos as assessed by preimplantation aneuploidy screening by fluorescence in situ hybridization (FISH) showed a significantly higher proportion of euploid embryos following mild ovarian stimulation compared with conventional stimulation, suggesting that through maximal stimulation the surplus of obtained oocytes and embryos are of lower quality.[29]

A meta-analysis combining the results of three separate RCTs suggests that the retrieval of a modest number of oocytes following mild stimulation is associated with a distinctly higher implantation rate compared with patients where the same number of oocytes is retrieved following conventional stimulation.[58]

These observations have led to the contention that when few oocytes are obtained following mild ovarian stimulation, they are more likely to represent a more homogenous group of good quality oocytes instead of a pathological reduction in the ovarian response.

These findings suggest that the fear of obtaining low numbers of oocytes following mild ovarian stimulation is unjustified thereby contradicting the assumption that an increased quantity of oocytes leads to better outcomes.[59]

In fact, in most of the studies investigating the relationship between oocyte numbers and pregnancy rates, the positive effect on pregnancy rates with a growing number of oocytes eventually levels off.[59,60] A potential disadvantage of the development of lower numbers of oocytes might be the reduction of supernumerary embryos for cryopreservation to transfer in subsequent cycles.

The number of good quality embryos resulting from mild ovarian stimulation was found to be similar to that following a conventional stimulation protocol and should therefore lead to equal total number of pregnancies.[29]

Evidence in favor of mild ovarian stimulation for IVF is accumulating in recent literature. Young, poor responders, estrogen sensitive cancer patients, and hyper responders to conventional IVF may benefit from mild stimulation.

However, an important concern regarding the use of a mild treatment strategy remains the reduction in the per cycle chance of pregnancy. Again, chances for IVF success should be balanced against patient discomfort, chances for complications, and costs.

Mc Donald, et al., designed a computer algorithm for day-to-day decision making in IVF. It shows that the use of AI technology in day-to-day IVF decision making is feasible, at least as an adjunct tool, and it should be explored further with big data. The authors conclude that as new data and images are added to the repository, metadata, and outcomes can be extended to improve algorithm precision. Ultimately, it would be interesting to see if machine learning platforms outperform physicians in decision making during ovarian stimulation.

## OOCYTE RETRIEVAL

Oocyte retrieval is performed 36 hours after the trigger injection of human chorionic gonadotropin (hCG) or GnRH agonist. Methods of egg collection have improved considerably since the introduction of ART. At first, all egg collections were performed laparoscopically. This is now rarely used and is reserved for women if their ovaries are inaccessible through the transvaginal route. With the introduction of endovaginal transducers, the transvaginal ultrasound-guided approach became the predominant method for egg collection. In this, the specially designed transducer is used to visualize the follicles and the aspirating needle is passed alongside it. This method is generally well-tolerated when carried out under light intravenous sedation, can be learnt by clinicians very quickly and is associated with minimal morbidity.

Several designs of aspiration needles are available. They may have a single or double lumen to enable aspiration and flushing through different routes. The needle is usually 16-gauge and must have a very sharp tip to enable easy puncture of mobile ovaries and its distal 2 cm should be roughened to enhance ultrasound visualization **(Fig. 1)**. The needle is connected to a test tube by tubing and suction is applied either from a foot-operated pump **(Fig. 2)** or manually. The ultrasound transducer **(Fig. 3)** is enclosed in a special sterile condom and plastic sleeve prior to insertion into the vagina and should be thoroughly cleaned with a damp cloth after each procedure.

It is important to provide effective anesthesia and analgesia for transvaginal oocyte recovery as they are painful. No technique of anesthesia, analgesia, or sedation is free from side effects. Whatever technique is used, recognized standards of practice should be adhered to and all IVF professionals should follow the safe practice of administering sedative drugs. Conscious sedation should be offered to all women having the procedure as it is safe and acceptable method of providing analgesia.

Generally, very few technical difficulties are encountered during vaginal egg collections. The main risks of transvaginal oocyte recovery are pelvic infection (0.6%) and bleeding (>100 mL in 0.8% cases) (Bennett, et al., 1993), which may be serious, sometimes even fatal. Appropriate preoperative vaginal preparation and minimizing the number of repeated vaginal penetrations may serve to lower the risk of infection. While there is no evidence that routine antibiotics reduce the risk of infection, the administration of an intravenous bolus of antibiotics is generally recommended to women

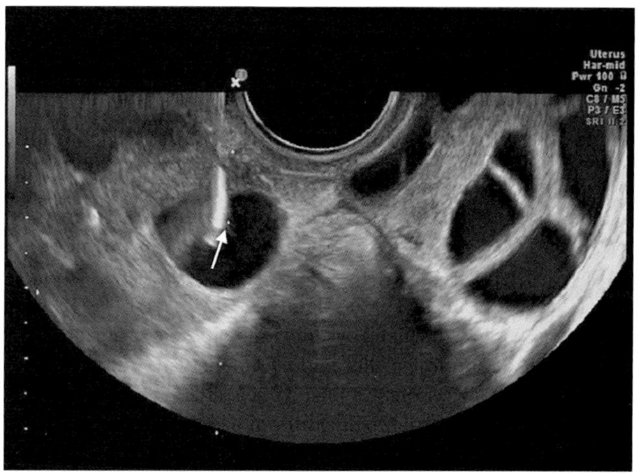


**Fig. 1:** Ultrasound picture during vaginal egg recovery. The tip of the needle (arrow) is seen within the follicle (F).

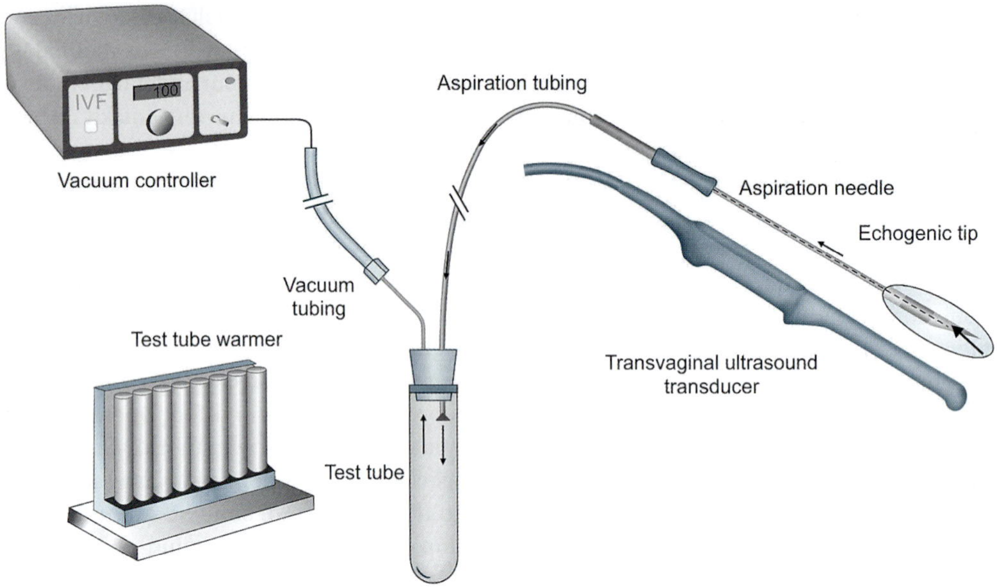


**Fig. 2:** Follicle aspiration equipment. An assembled follicle aspiration single lumen needle connected to a test tube. The test tube is in turn connected to a suction pump. The needle is attached to the transvaginal ultrasound transducer through needle guide and bracket.

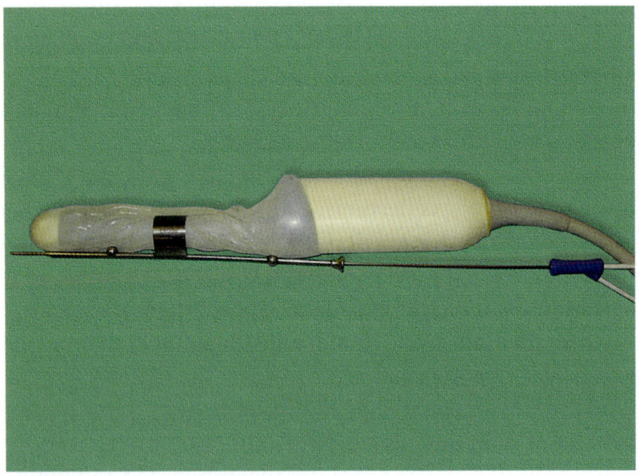

**Fig. 3:** Vaginal ultrasound transducer enclosed in a sterile condom with needle guide attached. The needle tip is protruding from the proximal end of the probe.

with history of severe pelvic inflammatory disease or if an endometrioma is punctured. Intestinal, vascular, uterine, and tubal injuries with the aspiration needle have also been reported. Bleeding and infections may be serious, sometimes even fatal complications.[61]

## IN VITRO FERTILIZATION VERSUS INTRACYTOPLASMIC SPERM INJECTION INSEMINATION

The editor-in-chief of human reproduction has criticized the overuse of ICSI, following a world report into the use of ART.

The report, published in the same journal, finds that ICSI—a technique used during IVF for men with very low sperm counts—is used in almost 100% of IVF cycles in the middle East and some parts of Latin America. This is not different in India where an increase trend in ICSI practice is noted (based on a survey done by lifeinvitro.com).

In an editorial in the journal, Professor Hans Evers of Maastricht University wrote: "Unless the majority of couples" infertility in the world today is determined by severe male causes, the report offers a sobering confrontation with modern reproductive medicine practice".

He added that there has been "unjustified enthusiasm for ICSI on the part of patients and doctors" and that "we have arrived in a situation of therapeutic illusion on a grand scale".

The oldest ICSI offspring cohort worldwide has recently reached adulthood. In a large follow-up project at UZ Brussels focused on reproductive and metabolic health of young adults, between 18 and 22 years, conceived after ICSI with ejaculated sperm. Results of both physical examination and semen analysis were compared between young ICSI men being part of a longitudinally followed cohort and spontaneously conceived controls who were recruited cross-sectionally. Young ICSI adults had a lower median sperm concentration (17.7 million/mL), lower median total sperm count (31.9 million), and lower median total motile sperm count (12.7 million) in comparison to spontaneously conceived peers (37.0 million/mL; 86.8 million; 38.6 million, respectively). The median percentage progressive and total motility, median percentage normal morphology, and median semen volume were not significantly different between these groups. These first results in a small group of ICSI men indicate a lower semen quantity and quality in young adults born after ICSI for male infertility in their fathers.

Many studies have compared the efficacy of conventional insemination versus ICSI—for all. The results from a similar study by Eftekhar, et al., (2012) show that in IVF group, fertilization and implantation rates were significantly higher than ICSI group (66.22 and 16.67% in IVF group versus 57.46% and 11.17% in ICSI group, respectively). Chemical and clinical pregnancy rates were statistically higher in IVF group as compared with the ICSI group (42.9% versus 27.3% and 35.7% versus 21.5%, respectively). According to these authors, the routine use of ICSI is not improved fertilization, implantation, and chemical pregnancy rates and is not recommended in nonmale factor, normozoospermic patients.[62]

A recent study aimed to compare the clinical outcomes between IVF and ICSI in sibling oocytes. A total of 571 cycles in 555 couples undergoing split insemination cycles were included in this study. The clinical outcomes did not differ between IVF and ICSI in split insemination cycles. Split insemination can decrease the risk of total fertilization failure. However, the authors conclude that unnecessary ICSI is carried out in most split insemination cycles and the use of split insemination might make ICSI more common.[63]

In a study by Hershlaq, et al., (2002) found superiority of ICSI over conventional insemination in cases of unexplained infertility cases. In couples with unexplained infertility, a higher fertilization rate was achieved through ICSI compared with conventional IVF. No such benefit could be demonstrated for couples with borderline semen parameters. The use of ICSI rescued 12 of 110 cycles (10.9%) where IVF failed. Adoption of the ICSI–IVF insemination split in cases of unexplained infertility may help eliminate fertilization failures.[64]

A recent meta-analysis looked as if ICSI, compared with conventional insemination, improves fertilization rates, and prevents total failed fertilization (TFF) in couples with unexplained infertility. The pooled relative risk (RR) of TFF was significantly higher with conventional insemination than with ICSI (RR 8.22, 95% CI 4.44–15.23). The number of subjects needed to treat with ICSI to prevent one case of TFF was five. This meta-analysis favors the use of ICSI to increase fertilization rates and decrease the risk of TFF in couples with well-defined unexplained infertility.[65]

Some studies show preference of ICSI over conventional inseminations in cases such as endometriosis-associated infertility, unexplained infertility, with regard to better fertilization status. A recent study provides strong evidences that the conventional IVF exhibits advantages over the ICSI method in non-male factor infertility for advanced age patients with five or fewer oocytes retrieved.[66] Studies have shown that in the USA there is an increasing usage of ICSI for non-male factor infertility despite a lack of evidence-based benefit. The study by Grimstad, et al., (2016) corroborates this increasing use over the last 8 years, specifically in the tubal ligation only patient population. Even after adjusting for multiple confounders, the patients who underwent ICSI had no statistically significant improvement in fertilization rate and actually had a lower likelihood of achieving a clinical pregnancy and LB. Therefore, their data suggest that the use of ICSI in tubal ligation patients has no overall benefit. This study contributes to the body of evidence that the use of ICSI for non-male factor diagnosis does not improve ART outcomes over conventional IVF.[67]

American Society for Reproductive Medicine (ASRM) committee concludes that ICSI without male factor infertility may be of benefit for selected patients undergoing IVF such as with PGT and cryopreserved oocytes. In other conditions additional cost-burden of ICSI must be considered.[68]

## Transfer of Euploid Embryos by Preimplantation Genetic Testing–Next-generation Sequencing

Embryonic aneuploidy is one of the most common cause attributed for IVF failures. The quoted rates of aneuploidy being 40% in younger women and 80% in women older than 43. PGT was proposed as a method to screen the embryos and to select for transfer only the chromosomally normal ones. Also, this strategy would ease the selection of embryos for single ET. The PGS version 1 used FISH to screen polar body and day 3 embryos. FISH could screen 3–12 chromosomes with a specificity of ~90% in detecting aneuploidy when compared to the newer comprehensive chromosome screening. A meta-analysis of PGS version 1 by Mastenbroek, et al., showed that there is no benefit in younger women and in older women it may actually reduce the pregnancy rates attributed to the fact that the loss of genetic material from a lesser cell stage of day 3 embryo may reduce the implantation potential.

Comprehensive chromosome screening technologies which can assess all 24 chromosomes and advances in embryo culture systems led to the introduction of PGS version 2. This is characterized by blastocyst culture and biopsy of the trophectoderm after breaching zona pellucida and in most cases followed by frozen ET. Single nucleotide polymorphism microarrays (SNP arrays), micro aCGH, and quantitative polymerase chain reaction (qPCR) were the earlier used and validated methods. Advantages of next-generation sequencing (NGS) over these methods are—it allows the analysis of chromosomes for aneuploidies, inversions, deletions, the detections of point mutations, copy number variations, and even the mitotic chromosomal abnormalities in a single run. NGS can also evaluate the mitochondrial genome in the same sample.[69]

Next-generation sequencing uses massive parallel sequencing of small DNA fragments until required depth of reads to analyze the copy numbers of the chromosome. The advantage in NGS is that the read depth can be increased even to cover the whole genome. SNP arrays and microarray

CGH are also equipped for processing high sample volumes but as the volume of sample increases the number of array slides required and the cost also increase.

Criticisms on PGS version 2 are that the standards of a day 5 biopsy itself can lead to a lot of embryo wastage considering the blastulation rates to be around 50% even in ideal scenarios. Given the higher degree of prevalence of mosaicism in trophectoderm and the lesser representation of inner cell mass by trophectoderm biopsy the accuracy of PGS in determining the embryo ploidy is questioned. The evidence of benefits for the indications which PGS was initially proposed—indications such as recurrent implantation failures, recurrent pregnancy loss, and advanced maternal age are still lacking.[70]

Preimplantation genetic screening—NGS have given promising results.[71-73] The results of the ongoing trials and more well-conducted studies would clear the controversies and PGS would make its way to standard of care in ART. Several RCTs have demonstrated an improvement in implantation rates and pregnancy rates with reduced time to conception

## FREEZE ALL STRATEGY

The routine procedure after IVF or ICSI is the transfer of embryo in the same cycle and freezing the available embryos. With the advent of advanced laboratory techniques and improved embryo survival rate postvitrification, the pregnancy rate following frozen ET also improved. One of the lessons learned from donor oocyte programs is that the pregnancy rates were better when compared to the fresh transfer counterparts. This led to the identification of the causes for lesser implantation in a fresh transfer cycle: (1) exposure to the supraphysiological doses of estrogen and (2) premature elevation of progesterone in the late follicular phase—both these leading to functional dysregulation of the endometrium. Also, the GnRH antagonist cycle with agonist trigger have been increasingly used in the predicted hyper responders to prevent OHSS. The GnRH agonist trigger causes significant luteal phase defect due to the intense luteolysis. Freeze all strategy refers to electively freezing all the available embryos and transfer later on in an unstimulated cycle, thereby bypassing the untoward effect of elevated hormones and allowing segmentation of IVF procedure thereby reducing the OHSS risk. Also, in the need for embryo accumulation for preimplantation genetic diagnosis (PGD) or PGS and in cases of embryo endometrial asynchrony as in the case of a day 6 blastocyst, freeze all strategy is of utmost benefit.

Chen, et al., in a RCT of 1,508 polycystic ovary syndrome (PCOS) patients demonstrated that freeze all strategy helped in achieving significantly better pregnancy rates, lower risk of OHSS, and reduced miscarriage rates. The 2017 Cochrane review on fresh versus frozen ET in ART suggested a moderate quality evidence that there is no significant increase in the LB rate and a low-quality evidence in reducing the OHSS risk.[74] The recent meta-analysis done by Dieamant, et al., 2017 concluded that freeze all strategy is not helpful when the mean number of retrieved oocytes is <15 but it may be advantageous when there is an increased response.[75]

In the absence of a grade A evidence to adopt freeze all strategy, Blockeel, et al., 2017, conducted a SWOT analysis and the increased pregnancy rates, better perinatal out-comes, reduced ectopic pregnancy, and very importantly OHSS free clinics were identified as the strengths of this strategy. The weaknesses highlighted were the lack of robust evidence and the cost increment. The birth of large for gestational age babies and the need for optimization of cryopreservation techniques were cited as weaknesses. However, this strategy provided the opportunity for scheduling and any day start of stimulation.[76]

The recent multicenter randomized controlled trial in the UK (E-Freeze) although limited by sample size, provides no evidence to support the adoption of a routine policy of elective freeze in preference to fresh ET in order to improve IVF effectiveness in obtaining a healthy baby.[77] No significant increase in the LB rates or the miscarriage rates between fresh or frozen cycles were noted in properly chosen patients. The decision for freeze all or to go ahead with fresh transfer should ideally be patient or cycle oriented, limiting freeze all policy to hyper responders. The one important complication which can be prevented by freeze all strategy is late OHSS.

## EMBRYO TRANSFER

Embryo transfer is a critical step in determining the final outcome of the treatment. The convention has been to replace embryos on the second or third day postinsemination, when the embryos are usually 2–8 cell stage of cleavage. With improvements in culture media, there is an increasing tendency for delaying ET with an aim to improve the implantation rates. While there is no improvement in LB rates (1.07, 95% CI 0.84–1.37) with delaying ET from day 2 to day 3 (Oatway, et al., 2004), transfer of embryos at blastocyst stage (day 5/6) has shown significant increase in LB rate (OR 1.35, 95% CI 1.05–1.74) when compared with day 2–3 transfers (Blake, et al., 2007). It is a more physiological approach, allowing synchronization of the embryo with the endometrium and the selection of viable embryos for transfer will be more efficient. However, the rates of embryos freezing are lower and the treatment cancellation rates are higher with blastocyst transfer. But in selected group of couples, the practice of blastocyst transfer has the potential to favor single ET without compromising the overall success rates but can significantly reduce the occurrence of multiple pregnancies. The most favored group for blastocyst transfer are those having high numbers of eight cell embryos on day 3, in whom the cycle cancellation is not increased.

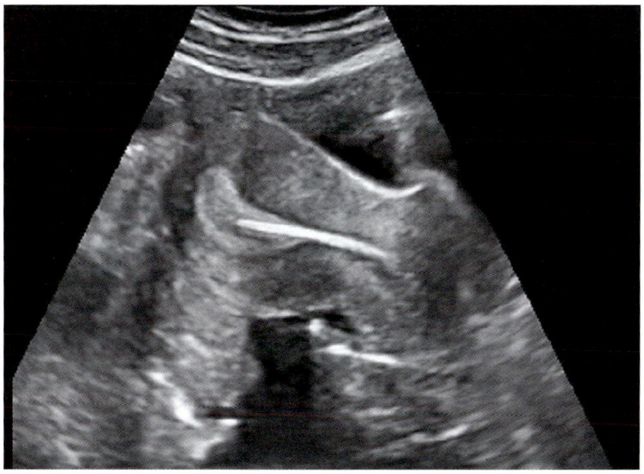

**Fig. 4:** Embryo transfer: The echogenic tip of the catheter is placed approximately 1–1.5 cm from the uterine fundus so that the embryo/s are expelled gently into the midcavity of the uterus.

Transcervical embryo replacement into the uterine cavity is a relatively simple procedure, which must be carried out meticulously to ensure appropriate placement of the embryos. Variations among clinicians in the technique of ET may influence the pregnancy rate. Avoidance of blood, mucus, bacterial contamination, excessive uterine contractions, and trauma to the endometrium is associated with optimal pregnancy and implantation rates after transcervical ET. Transabdominal ultrasonographic guidance to determine the precise depth of embryo placement within the uterus appears to facilitate successful ET and is preferred (Brown, et al., 2010). The tip of the catheter is placed approximately 1-1.5 cm from the uterine fundus **(Fig. 4)** so that the embryo/s are expelled gently into the midcavity of the uterus. Soft catheters are preferred over rigid ones as they are less likely to traumatize the cervix and endometrium and to invoke any uterine contractions. The commonly used soft catheters (Wallace) **(Fig. 5)** have a softer inner cannula and a stiffer outer sheath. Occasionally, resistance to pass the soft inner cannula into the uterus usually at the level of internal OS is encountered and in these cases the stiffer outer sheath is advanced in the cervical canal to negotiate the resistance with the inner cannula can now be advanced into the uterine cavity. A firmer malleable catheter with a stylet and an outer sheath is another option in difficult cases, where the catheter is advanced up to the level of the internal OS. The inner stylet is then removed and the softer cannula with embryos loaded in and it is fed through the outer sheath to advance into the uterine cavity for transfer. The outer sheath or the malleable catheter should never be advanced beyond the internal OS.[78]

Following ET, women are often advised to continue their normal daily activities as prolonged bed rest has not shown to improve the IVF outcome. Luteal support is usually required as ART is associated with inadequate luteal function, possibly because of the feedback inhibition of LH due to the supraphysiological hormonal milieu, the removal of the granulosa cells surrounding the oocytes while performing the oocyte retrieval and of the use of GnRH agonists. hCG or progesterone is traditionally used to provide luteal support during conventional IVF cycles. However, the routine use of hCG is not recommended because of the increased likelihood of OHSS and no benefit over progesterone in terms of IVF success. The progesterone can be administered either 200–800 mg/day vaginally or 50–100 mg/day intramuscularly and is continued for 14–16 days, when pregnancy test is performed.

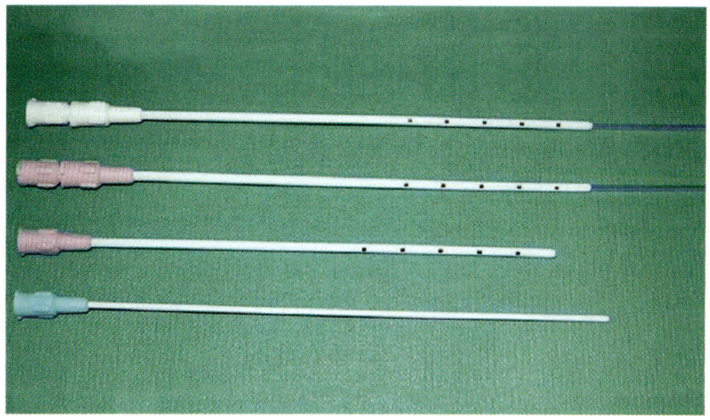

**Fig. 5:** Embryo transfer catheters. From top to bottom—Trial Wallace (no lumen), Wallace, outer sheath, and stylet of malleable catheter.

## TRAINING IN OPU AND ET BY SIMULATORS

The value of training and certification in fellowship programs in reproductive medicine is most evident in the remarkable and consistent improvement in the success of ART procedures, particularly IVF. For both patient and physician, the final step of IVF—the transfer of the embryo into the uterine cavity for implantation— is often stressful. This anxiety is often attributed to the high-cost and time-associated with IVF treatment, the potential difficulty of the transfer due to individual patient anatomy, and the delicate nature of the embryo itself. It is said that nearly 50% of fellows training to be IVF specialists have historically received little or no training in ET because of the importance of this final step in the IVF process and the difficulty in allowing trainees to perform it on patients for the first time. The simulator provides in training physicians the opportunity to practice simulated transfers with varying degrees of difficulty in a safe, risk-free environment, and with unlimited repetitions under supervision by experts. They receive real-time simulation feedback of their metrics that, when combined with structured debriefing with expert faculty, further facilitates development of motor and cognitive skills required to attain proficiency in ET.

**TABLE 1:** Innovative/AI based platforms currently introduced in in-vitro fertilization.

| *Company name* | *Website* | *Overview* |
|---|---|---|
| *Preconception* | | |
| *Ovaterra* | https://myovaterra.com/ | Ovaterra is the the first intelligent fertility content and commerce platform focused on optimizing fertility naturally |
| *IMMA health* | https://www.imma.health/ | At home ovarian stimulation monitoring system for IVF |
| *Hertility health* | https://hertilityhealth.com/ | At-home hormone and fertility testing |
| *Béa fertility* | https://beafertility.com/ | The first intracervical insemination kit designed for home use |
| *Apricity* | https://www.apricity.life/ | Fertility prediction |
| *Infertility workflow* | | |
| *MIM solutions* | https://www.mim-solutions.ai/en/ | FOLLISCAN: Intelligent algorithms supporting the doctor in the ultrasound diagnosis of a woman's ovarian reserve |
| *Ferty U* | https://www.f6s.com/assistant-in-human-reproduction-and-ivf | Service for ovarian response prediction in IVF infertility treatment |
| *FertilAI* | https://fertilai.com/ | AI and big data-based platform for automating protocol management in the IVF clinic |
| *Improving stimulation* | | |
| *OptIVF* | | A software package for predicting optimal drug dosage customized for each patient for IVF cycles, marketed by Stochastic Research Technologies LLC., USA |
| *Choosing the best oocyte* | | |
| *Future fertility* | https://futurefertility.com/ | A novel, non-invasive oocyte scoring system using AI applied to 2D images |
| *AIVF* | https://www.aivf.co/ | provide the IVF clinic with a proprietary fertility OS™ platform that changes the "art" of IVF into a more data-driven and predictable science |
| *Choosing the best embryo* | | |
| *Life whisperer* | https://www.lifewhisperer.com/ | Using deep learning and computer vision, it identifies embryo features for selection |
| *Amplexa genetics* | https://amplexa.dk/ | Noninvasive PGT-A and NGS for optimizing IVF treatments |
| *Fairtility* | https://fairtility.com/ | Novel AI and computer vision algorithms enabling accurate classification and prediction of the best embryos |
| *Embryonics* | https://www.embryonics.me/ | Ubar: Next generation<br>Embryo selection |
| *iDAScore* | https://www.vitrolife.com/our-products/idascore-intelligent-data-analysis-for-embryo-evaluation/ | Intelligent data analysis for embryo evaluation-vitrolife |
| *Choosing the best sperm for fertilization* | | |
| *QART medical* | https://www.qart-medical.com/ | Quantitative, morphometric sperm cell selection in ICSI |
| *Baibys* | https://www.baibys.com/ | Artificial intelligence system for autonomous sperm selection before ICSI |
| *IVF 2.0 Ltd* | https://www.ivf20.ai/ | SiD: AI enabled real-time sperm selection based on morphology, speed, and motility patterns |

(AI: artificial intelligence; ICSI: intracytoplasmic sperm injection; IVF: in vitro fertilization; NGS: nextgeneration sequencing)

## ARTIFICIAL INTELLIGENCE AND AUTOMATION

Many innovative systems and products are in either clinical trial/developmental phase for ART **(Table 1)**. In recent times, the use of AI has gained popularity in its ability to predict clinical outcomes using routinely obtained information, such as patient attributes, medical images, and blood results. AI may help embryologists in selecting the best oocyte and sperm combination as well as predicting embryo quality. Furthermore, AI may assist the infertility specialists in developing an optimal patient-specific treatment regimen to improve treatment success.

Recent studies using AI to predict embryo developmental competence are on the rise and show promise in improving the accuracy of manual grading and predicting development to blastocyst and pregnancy.[79] Interestingly, AI is able to use cellular textures to accurately discern between the inner cell mass and trophectoderm of the blastocyst. The use of AI to accurately identify cell lineages may lead to improved embryo classification and IVF success. AI will likely aid clinicians in devising patient-specific treatment regimens, before and after oocyte collection, as well as improving gamete and embryo selection.

Even though medical/tissue culture laboratories embraced advanced automation workflow systems, the IVF laboratories still lag behind in introducing new technologies. Unlike any other clinical/cell culture laboratories, IVF labs need an error-free system as it deals with creation of human embryos.[80]

Microfluidics platforms hold high promise for embryo culture. Integration of microfluidics into the ART laboratory may give rise to several foreseeable advantages: (1) precisely controlled fluidic manipulations of gametes/embryos; (2) contribute biomimetic environments for in vitro culture; (3) facilitating genetic and molecular bioassays at microscale level; and (4) making miniaturization and automation a reality. The basic utility and advantages of individual microfluidic devices/systems for gamete and preimplantation embryo isolation, manipulation, and assessment have been demonstrated by many research groups. Current efforts are focused on integrating individualized microfluidic procedural components into a future IVF lab-on-a-chip. Presently, two startups are doing the clinical trials—one in Europe (https://www.overture.life/) and another one in Australia (https://www.fertil.is/).

The IVF embryo culture has already been partially automated with use of time-lapse incubators which helps continuous monitoring of embryo development in a closed environment. Data generated from time-lapse incubators can be analyzed with machine learning/AI to aid in the selection of embryos with the highest implantation potential. Additional information about embryo viability may be gleaned from other omics technologies which can either sample the embryo directly or indirectly via its culture media.

Vitrification has become the dominant method for oocyte and embryo cryopreservation. While semiautomated/automated systems for oocyte/embryo vitrification have been reported and are now in early stages of clinical adoption.

Furthermore, automation will likely significantly decrease the staffing requirements and alter the type of skills required to operate fertility centers.[81] It is likely that the technical aspects of IVF will be gradually assumed by machines.

## REFERENCES


1. Štiavnická M, Abril-Parreño L, Nevoral J, Králíčková M, García-Álvarez O.. Non-invasive approaches to epigenetic-based sperm selection. Med Sci Monit. 2017;23:4677-83.
2. Pribenszky C, Nilselid AM, Montag M. Time-lapse culture with morphokinetic embryo selection improves pregnancy and live birth chances and reduces early pregnancy loss: a meta-analysis. Reprod Biomed Online. 2017;35(5):511-20.
3. Mascarenhas M, Fox SJ, Thompson K, Balen AH. Cumulative live birth rates and perinatal outcomes with the use of time lapse imaging incubators for embryo culture: a retrospective cohort study of 1882 ART cycles. BJOG. 2019;126(2):280-6.
4. Sa R, Cunha M, Silva J, Luís A, Oliveira C, Teixeira da Silva J, et al. Ultrastructure of tubular smooth endoplasmic reticulum aggregates in human metaphase II oocytes and clinical implications. Fertil Steril. 2011;96(1):143-9.
5. Alpha Scientists in Reproductive Medicine and ESHRE Special Interest Group of Embryology. The Istanbul consensus workshop on embryo assessment: proceedings of an expert meeting. Hum Reprod. 2011;26:1270-83.
6. Mateizel I, Van Landuyt L, Tournaye H, Luís A, Oliveira C, Teixeira da Silva J, et al. Deliveries of normal healthy babies from embryos originating from oocytes showing the presence of smooth endoplasmic reticulum aggregates. Hum Reprod. 2013;28(8):2111-7.
7. Itoi F, Asano Y, Shimizu M, Nagai R, Saitou K, Honnma H, et al. Clinical outcomes after IVF or ICSI using human blastocysts derived from oocytes containing aggregates of smooth endoplasmic reticulum. Reprod Biomed Online. 2017;34(4):337-44.
8. Wilding M, Di Matteo L, D'Andretti S. An oocyte score for use in assisted reproduction. J Assist Reprod Genet. 2007;24:350-8.
9. Ebner T, Moser M, Sommergruber M, Gaiswinkler U, Shebl O, Jesacher K, et al. Occurrence and developmental consequences of vacuoles through-out preimplantation development. Fertil Steril. 2005;83:1635-40.
10. Fancsovits P, Murber A, Gilan ZT. Human oocytes containing large cytoplasmic vacuoles can result in pregnancy and viable offspring. Reprod Biomed Online. 2011;23(4):513-6.
11. Webb R, Garnsworthy PC, Campbell BK, Hunter MG. Intra-ovarian regulation of follicular development and oocyte competence in farm animals. Theriogenology. 2007;68 (Suppl 1):S22-9.
12. Lindner C, Lichtenberg V, Westhof G, Braendle W, Bettendorf G. Endocrine parameters of human follicular fluid and fertilization capacity of oocytes. Horm Metab Res. 1988;20:243-6.
13. Sunkara SK, Rittenberg V, Raine-Fenning N, Bhattacharya S, Zamora J, Coomarasamy A. Association between the number of eggs and live birth in IVF treatment: an analysis of 400 135 treatment cycles. Hum Reprod. 2011;26:1768-74.
14. Fatemi HM, Doody K, Griesinger G, Witjes H, Mannaerts B. High ovarian response does not jeopardize ongoing pregnancy rates and increases cumulative pregnancy rates in a GnRH-antagonist protocol. Hum Reprod. 2013;28:442-52.
15. Ji J, Liu Y, Tong XH, Luo L, Ma J, Chen Z. The optimum number of oocytes in IVF treatment: an analysis of 2455 cycles in China. Hum Reprod. 2013;28:2728-34.

16. Chang MC. Digynic triploidy after superovulation. Nature. 1977;266:382-3.
17. Ertzeid G, Storeng R. The impact of ovarian stimulation on implantation and fetal development in mice. Hum Reprod. 2001;16:221-5.
18. Van der Auwera I, D'Hooghe T. Superovulation of female mice delays embryonic and fetal development. Hum Reprod. 2001;16:1237-43.
19. Edwards LJ, Kind KL, Armstrong DT. Effects of recombinant human follicle-stimulating hormone on embryo development in mice. Am J Physiol Endocrinol Metab. 2005;288:E845-51.
20. Lee ST, Kim TM, Cho MY. Development of a hamster superovulation program and adverse effects of gonadotropins on microfilament formation during oocyte development. Fertil Steril. 2005;83(Suppl 1):1264-74.
21. Ziebe S, Bangsboll S, Schmidt KL, Loft A, Lindhard A, Nyboe Andersen A. Embryo quality in natural versus stimulated IVF cycles. Hum Reprod. 2004;19:1457-60.
22. Gras L, McBain J, Trounson A, Kola I. The incidence of chromosomal aneuploidy in stimulated and unstimulated (natural) uninseminated human oocytes. Hum Reprod. 1992;7:1396-401.
23. Labarta E, Bosch E, Alama P, Rubio C, Rodrigo L, Pellicer A. Moderate ovarian stimulation does not increase the incidence of human embryo chromosomal abnormalities in in vitro fertilization cycles. J Clin Endocrinol Metab. 2012;97:E1987-94.
24. Qin JZ, Pang LH, Li MQ, Xu J, Zhou X. Risk of chromosomal abnormalities in early spontaneous abortion after assisted reproductive technology: a meta-analysis. PLoS One. 2013; 8:e75953.
25. Conway DA, Patel SS, Liem J, Fan KJ, Jalian R, Williams J 3rd, et al. The risk of cytogenetic abnormalities in the late first trimester of pregnancies conceived through assisted reproduction. Fertil Steril. 2011;95:503-6.
26. von Wolff M, Kollmann Z, Fluck CE, Stute P, Marti U, Weiss B, et al. Gonadotrophin stimulation for in vitro fertilization significantly alters the hormone milieu in follicular fluid: a comparative study between natural cycle IVF and conventional IVF. Hum Reprod. 2014;29:1049-57.
27. de los Santos MJ, Garcia-Laez V, Beltran-Torregrosa D, Horcajadas JA, Martínez-Conejero JA, et al. Hormonal and molecular characterization of follicular fluid, cumulus cells and oocytes from pre-ovulatory follicles in stimulated and unstimulated cycles. Hum Reprod. 2012;27:1596-605.
28. Hohmann FP, Macklon NS, Fauser BC. A randomized comparison of two ovarian stimulation protocols with gonadotropin-releasing hormone (GnRH) antagonist cotreatment for in vitro fertilization commencing recombinant follicle-stimulating hormone on cycle day 2 or 5 with the standard long GnRH agonist protocol. J Clin Endocrinol Metab. 2003;88:166-73.
29. Baart EB, Martini E, Eijkemans MJ, Van Opstal D, Beckers NG, Verhoeff A, et al. Milder ovarian stimulation for in-vitro fertilization reduces aneuploidy in the human preimplantation embryo: a randomized controlled trial. Hum Reprod. 2007;22:980-8.
30. Kaleli S, Yanikkaya-Demirel G, Erel CT, Senturk LM, Topçuoğlu A, Irez T. High rate of aneuploidy in luteinized granulosa cells obtained from follicular fluid in women who underwent controlled ovarian hyperstimulation. Fertil Steril. 2005;84:802-4.
31. Labarta E, Bosch E, Pellicer A. Impact of ovarian stimulation with gonadotrophins on embryo aneuploidy. Hum Reprod Update. 2014;20:964.
32. Haaf T, Hahn A, Lambrecht A, Grossmann B, Schwaab E, Khanaga O, et al. A high oocyte yield for intracytoplasmic sperm injection treatment is associated with an increased chromosome error rate. Fertil Steril. 2009;91:733-8.
33. Gianaroli L, Magli MC, Cavallini G, Crippa A, Capoti A, Resta S, et al. Predicting aneuploidy in human oocytes: key factors which affect the meiotic process. Hum Reprod. 2010;25:2374-86.
34. Ata B, Kaplan B, Danzer H, Glassner M, Opsahl M, Tan SL, et al. Array CGH analysis shows that aneuploidy is not related to the number of embryos generated. Reprod Biomed Online. 2012;24:614-20.
35. Labarta E, Bosch E, Mercader A. Relationship between ovarian response and number of euploid embryos in oocyte donor cycles. Fertil Steril. 2012;98:S282.
36. Morin S, Melzer-Ross K, McCulloh D, Grifo J, Munné S. A greater number of euploid blastocysts in a given cohort predicts excellent outcomes in single embryo transfer cycles. J Assist Reprod Genet. 2014;31:667-73.
37. Gleicher N, Kim A, Weghofer A, Barad DH. Lessons from elective in vitro fertilization (IVF) in, principally, non-infertile women. Reprod Biol Endocrinol. 2012;10:48.
38. Fatemi HM, Doody K, Griesinger G, Witjes H, Mannaerts B. High ovarian response does not jeopardize ongoing pregnancy rates and increases cumulative pregnancy rates in a GnRH-antagonist protocol. Hum Reprod. 2013;28:442-52.
39. Huber M, Hadziosmanovic N, Berglund L, Holte J. Using the ovarian sensitivity index to define poor, normal, and high response after controlled ovarian hyperstimulation in the long gonadotropin-releasing hormone agonist protocol: suggestions for a new principle to solve an old problem. Fertil Steril. 2013;100:1270-6.
40. Baker VL, Brown MB, Luke B, Smith GW, Ireland JJ. Gonadotropin dose is negatively correlated with live birth rate: analysis of more than 650,000 assisted reproductive technology cycles. Fertil Steril. 2015;104:1145-52.e5.
41. Gougeon A, Lefèvre B. Evolution of the diameters of the largest healthy and atretic follicles during the human menstrual cycle. J Reprod Fertil. 1983;69:497-502.
42. Gougeon A. Ovarian follicular growth in humans: ovarian ageing and population of growing follicles. Maturitas. 1998;30:137-42.
43. Almog B, Shehata F, Shalom-Paz E, Tan SL, Tulandi T. Age-related normogram for antral follicle count: McGill reference guide. Fertil Steril. 2011;95:663-66.
44. La Marca A, Spada E, Sighinolfi G, Argento C, Tirelli A, Giulini S, et al. Age-specific nomogram for the decline in antral follicle count throughout the reproductive period. Fertil Steril. 2011;95:684-88.
45. Monget P, Bobe J, Gougeon A. The ovarian reserve in mammals: a functional and evolutionary perspective. Mol Cell Endocrinol. 2012;356:2-12.
46. Fauser BC, Van Heusden AM. Manipulation of human ovarian function: physiological concepts and clinical consequences. Endocr Rev. 1997;18(1):71-106.

47. La Marca A, Argento C, Sighinolfi G. Possibilities and limits of ovarian reserve testing in ART. Curr Pharm Biotechnol. 2012;13(3):398-408.
48. Lan VT, Linh NK, Tuong HM. Anti-Müllerian hormone versus antral follicle count for defining the starting dose of FSH. Reprod Biomed Online. 2013;27:390-9.
49. Oliveira JBA, Baruffi RLR, Petersen CG. A new ovarian response prediction index (ORPI): implications for individualised controlled ovarian stimulation. Reprod Biol Endocrinol. 2012;10:94.
50. Edwards RG, Lobo R, Bouchard P. Time to revolutionize ovarian stimulation. Hum Reprod 1996;11:917-9.
51. Diedrich K, Felberbaum R. New approaches to ovarian stimulation. Hum Reprod. 1998;13(Suppl 3):1-13.
52. Olivennes F. GnRH antagonists: do they open new pathways to safer treatment in assisted reproductive techniques? Reprod Biomed Online. 2002;5(Suppl 1):20-5.
53. Ubaldi F, Rienzi L, Baroni E, Ferrero S, Iacobelli M. Hopes and facts about mild ovarian stimulation. Reprod Biomed Online. 2007;14:675-81.
54. Pennings G, Ombelet W. Coming soon to your clinic: patient-friendly ART. Hum Reprod. 2007;22:2075-9.
55. Katz-Jaffe MG, Trounson AO, Cram DS. Chromosome 21 mosaic human preimplantation embryos predominantly arise from diploid conceptions. Fertil Steril. 2005;84: 634-43.
56. Eppig JJ, O'Brien MJ, Pendola FL, Watanabe S. Factors affecting the developmental competence of mouse oocytes grown in vitro: follicle-stimulating hormone and insulin. Biol Reprod. 1998;59:1445-53.
57. Roberts R, Iatropoulou A, Ciantar D, Stark J, Becker DL, Franks S, et al. Follicle-stimulating hormone affects metaphase I chromosome alignment and increases aneuploidy in mouse oocytes matured in vitro. Biol Reprod. 2005;72:107-18.
58. Verberg MF,4, Eijkemans MJ, Macklon NS, Heijnen EM, Baart EB, Hohmann FP, et al. The clinical significance of the retrieval of a low number of oocytes following mild ovarian stimulation for IVF: a meta-analysis. Hum Reprod Update. 2009;15(1):5-12.
59. Devreker F, Pogonici E, De Maertelaer V, Revelard P, Van den Bergh M, Englert Y. Selection of good embryos for transfer depends on embryo cohort size: implications for the 'mild ovarian stimulation' debate. Hum Reprod. 1999;14:3002-8.
60. van der Gaast MH, Eijkemans MJ, van der Net JB. Optimum number of oocytes for a successful first IVF treatment cycle. Reprod Biomed Online. 2006;13:476-80.
61. Bennett SJ, Waterstone JJ, Cheng WC, Parsons J. Complications of transvaginal ultrasound-directed follicle aspiration: a review of 2670 consecutive procedures. J Assist Reprod Genet. 1993;10:72-7.
62. Eftekhar M, Mohammadian F, Yousefnejad F, Molaei B, Aflatoonian A. Comparison of conventional IVF versus ICSI in non-male factor, normoresponder patients. Iran J Reprod Med. 2012;10(2):131-6.
63. Lee SH, Lee JH, Park YS, Yang KM, Lim CK. Comparison of clinical out-comes between in vitro fertilization (IVF) and intracytoplasmic sperm injection (ICSI) in IVF-ICSI split insemination cycles. Clin Exp Reprod Med. 2017;44(2):96-104.
64. Hershlag A, Paine T, Kvapil G, Feng H, Napolitano B. In vitro fertilization-intracytoplasmic sperm injection split: an insemination method to prevent fertilization failure. Fertil Steril. 2002; 77(2):229-32.
65. Johnson LN, Sasson IE, Sammel MD, Dokras A. Does intracytoplasmic sperm injection improve the fertilization rate and decrease the total fertilization failure rate in couples with well-defined unexplained infertility? A systematic review and meta-analysis. Fertil Steril. 2013;100(3):704-11.
66. Liu H, Zhao H, Yu G, Li M, Ma S, Zhang H, et al. Conventional in vitro fertilization (IVF) or intracytoplasmic sperm injection (ICSI): which is preferred for advance age patients with five or fewer oocytes retrieved? Arch Gynecol Obstet. 2018.
67. Grimstad FW, Nangia AK, Luke B, Stern JE, Mak W. Use of ICSI in IVF cycles in women with tubal ligation does not improve pregnancy or live birth rates. Hum Reprod. 2016;31(12):2750-5.
68. ICSI for non-male factor indications: A committee opinion. Practice committees of the American Society for Reproductive medicine and the Society for Assisted Reproductive Technology. Fertil Steril 2020;114(2):239-45.
69. Handyside AH. 24-chromosome copy number analysis: a comparison of available technologies. Fertil Steril. 2013;100:595-602.
70. Gleicher N, Orvieto R. Is the hypothesis of preimplantation genetic screening (PGS) still supportable? A review. J Ovarian Res. 2017;10:21.
71. Martin J, Cervero A, Mir P, Martinez-Conejero JA, Pellicer A, Simón C. The impact of next-generation sequencing technology on preimplantation genetic diagnosis and screening. Fertil Steril. 2013;99:1054-61.
72. Rubio C. Next-generation sequencing: challenges in reproductive genetics. Fertil Steril. 2014;101:1252-3.
73. Wells D. Next-generation sequencing: the dawn of a new era for preimplantation genetic diagnostics. Fertil Steril. 2014; 101:1250-1.
74. Wong K, van Wely M, Mol F. Fresh versus frozen embryo transfers in assisted reproduction. Cochrane Database Syst Rev. 2017;(3):CD011184.
75. Dieamant FC, Petersen CG, Mauri AL. Fresh embryos versus freeze-all embryos-transfer strategies: nuances of a meta-analysis. JBRA Assist Reprod. 2017;21(3):260-72.
76. Blockeel C, Drakopoulos P, Santos-Ribeiro S. A fresh look at the freeze-all protocol: a SWOT analysis. Hum Reprod. 2016;31(3):491-7.
77. Maheshwari A, Bell JL, Bhide P, Brison D, Child T, Chong HY, et al. Elective freezing of embryos versus fresh embryo transfer in IVF: a multicentre randomized controlled trial in the UK (E-Freeze). Hum Reprod. 2022;37(3):476-87.
78. Brown J, Buckingham K, Abou-Setta AM, Buckett W. Ultrasound versus 'clinical touch' for catheter guidance during embryo transfer in women. Cochrane Database Syst Rev. 2010;(1):CD006107.
79. Erlich I, Ben-Meir A, Har-Vardi I. Pseudo contrastive labeling for predicting IVF embryo developmental potential. Sci Rep. 2022;12:2488.
80. Varghese AC, Siristatidis CS. Automation, Artificial Intelligence and Innovations in the Future of IVF. In: Nagy Z, Varghese A, Agarwal A (Eds) In Vitro Fertilization. Cham: Springer; 2019.
81. Bori L, Meseguer M. Will the introduction of automated ART laboratory systems render the majority of embryologists redundant? Reprod Biomed Online. 2021;43(6):979-81.

CHAPTER 105

# Intracytoplasmic Sperm Injection

*Alex C Varghese, Kenichiro Hiraoka*

## INTRODUCTION

In the 1980s, several micromanipulation procedures were adopted from animal husbandry to facilitate gamete interaction, and this resulted in the development of intracytoplasmic sperm injection (ICSI), a procedure through which an oocyte can be fertilized independent of the morphology and/or motility of the single spermatozoon injected. The procedure was first used in cases of fertilization failure after standard in vitro fertilization (IVF) or when an inadequate number of sperm cells were available. The consistency of fertilization independent of the functional quality of the spermatozoon has extended the application of ICSI to immature spermatozoa retrieved surgically from the epididymis and testis.[1] Moreover, the need to denude the oocyte has allowed assessment of the nuclear maturity of the oocyte. ICSI **(Fig. 1)** is also preferred in conjunction with preimplantation genetic diagnosis (PGT) and recently has been used to treat human immunodeficiency virus (HIV) discordant couples, where there is a pressing need to minimize the exposure of the oocyte to a large number of spermatozoa. For all ages and with all the different sperm types used, fertilization after ICSI is at approximately 70–80% and it ensures a clinical pregnancy rate of up to 45%. These results have made ICSI a procedure comparable in popularity with conventional IVF and have minimized the need for couples suffering from all forms of male infertility to resort to adoption or the use of donor sperm.[2]

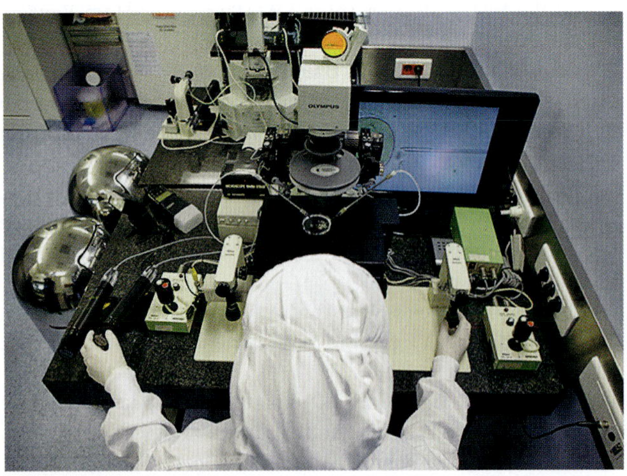

**Fig. 1:** Two intracytoplasmic sperm injection (ICSI) workstations in opposite direction—a space-saving placement in a busy laboratory. *Courtesy:* Giles Palmer, Mitera Hospital, Greece.

The first gamete micromanipulation techniques date back to the late 1990s. In Rome, in 1990, there was the first birth by injection of the sperm into the perivitelline space [subzonal insemination (SUZI)] obtained by the team Simon Fishel, Severino Antinori, and Franco Lisi. The technique was developed by Gianpiero Palermo in 1991 at the Vrije Universiteit Brussel in the Center for Reproductive Medicine headed by Paul Devroey and Andre Van Steirteghem.[3] It has been estimated that approximately 40% of sterility in couples can be attributed to male subfertility. ICSI has raised hopes that these couples can have children of their own. This method of treating predominantly male-factor patients has achieved a breakthrough, and it has established itself as the preferred method of treatment in the field of assisted reproduction.

In recent years, researchers have been working to produce a more effective ICSI protocol, from introducing novel sperm selection techniques to evaluating how appropriate ICSI may be for an infertile couple. These include techniques such as physiological ICSI (PICSI) and intracytoplasmic morphologically selected sperm injection (IMSI).[4] Moreover, oocyte activation has also been tried to alleviate failed fertilization cases in ICSI cycles.[5]

## INDICATIONS FOR INTRACYTOPLASMIC SPERM INJECTION

The indications for ICSI are:

- Oligozoospermia
- Severe asthenozoospermia
- Teratozoospermia (≤4% normal morphology)
- Fertilization failure in previous cycles
- Surgically retrieved spermatozoa

- High titers of antisperm antibodies
- Frozen-thawed spermatozoa with compromised motility
- Unexplained infertility
- Patients with immotile cilia syndrome
- PGT/noninvasive PGT (niPGT) cases.

## INDICATIONS FOR INTRACYTOPLASMIC SPERM INJECTION WITH SURGICALLY RETRIEVED SPERMATOZOA

### Intracytoplasmic Sperm Injection with Epididymal Sperms

- Congenital bilateral absence of the vas deferens (CBAVD)
- Failed vasoepididymostomy
- Failed vasectomy reversal
- Obstruction of ejaculatory duct
- An ejaculation due to spinal cord injuries
- Young syndrome.

### Intracytoplasmic Sperm Injection with Testicular Sperms

- Hypospermatogenesis
- Sertoli cell-only syndrome
- Incomplete maturation arrest
- Klinefelter syndrome.

### Factors Influencing Intracytoplasmic Sperm Injection Results

- Intrinsic changes in oocyte
- Fragmentation of deoxyribonucleic acid (DNA) in sperm.

## LOCATION OF INTRACYTOPLASMIC SPERM INJECTION SETUP

The ICSI workstation should preferably be near a structural frame or wall to minimize vibration interference and must be kept dust free. The equipment must be installed on a substantial bench top, away from distractions of traffic such as people or trolleys. Any vibration will seriously interfere with the injection procedure, and it is essential to make sure that the equipment is completely stable, using antivibration equipment if necessary, situated on a stable floor. Subdued lighting is helpful for microscopy. The proper visibility of specimens in the inverted microscope should be checked well in advance of any ICSI procedures. Ensure that the tool holders and all other parts of the micromanipulation system are correctly fitted and adjusted for optimal range of movement and that the microtools can be accurately aligned (the angle of the tool holder to the microscope stage should be set at 30–35°).

## INTRACYTOPLASMIC SPERM INJECTION

Intracytoplasmic sperm injection involves several micromanipulation procedures that involve delicate maneuvers using glass microtools operated by joysticks. The operator has control over movements in three dimensions (X, Y, and Z directions) with a resolution of up to 1 µm. Common hurdles to be overcome when using micromanipulators include long setup times, visualizing the tip of the microtool under the microscope, and moving the tools without inadvertently breaking them in the dish. Most suppliers provide a "home" function where microtools are returned to their setup position to enable faster changeover of culture dishes and to allow users to locate pipette tips if they should "lose" them in the field of view. With such delicate instruments and the need for precise positioning, the microscope used for micromanipulation procedures should be protected from any vibration which could disturb the system and/or compromise focus. Magnifications of 200–400× are generally required to visualize procedures. Quality optics with high numerical apertures and long working distances are also essential. Contrast optics, such as Nomarski differential interference contrast (DIC) (with glass culture dishes) or Hoffman modulation contrast (suitable for both glass and plastic), are commonly used. Apodized phase contrast objectives can help to overcome the halo effects common in phase contrast techniques to provide sharper edges, enhanced specimen detail, and a greater apparent depth of field. A correction collar that compensates for the effects of working at physiological temperatures is also useful. The warming stage should be calibrated and frequently checked. Traditionally, many laboratories use the ones with hole but nowadays many embryologists prefer thin glass warming stages which give a better and uniform heating of ICSI dishes. The configuration of the ICSI setup may vary from laboratory to laboratory.

### Materials

#### *Equipment*

Intracytoplasmic sperm injection demands a high level of skill and careful manipulation of cells under a microscope. An important determining factor to the success of this procedure is the performance of the manipulation set. Each micromanipulation set consists of the following equipment:

- Inverted microscope equipped with Hoffman modulation contrast or DIC and 4×, 10×, 20×, and 40× objectives
- Two micromanipulators (one for moving the holding capillary and another for transferring the sperm)
- Adapter for inverted microscope
- Air microinjector for holding the oocyte
- Oil microinjector for transferring the sperm.

There are many systems available in the market. **Figures 2A to D** show different models of ICSI work station.

Inverted microscope equipped with heated stage allows work to be carried out without fluctuation in temperature. Consistency of temperature is important as transient cooling

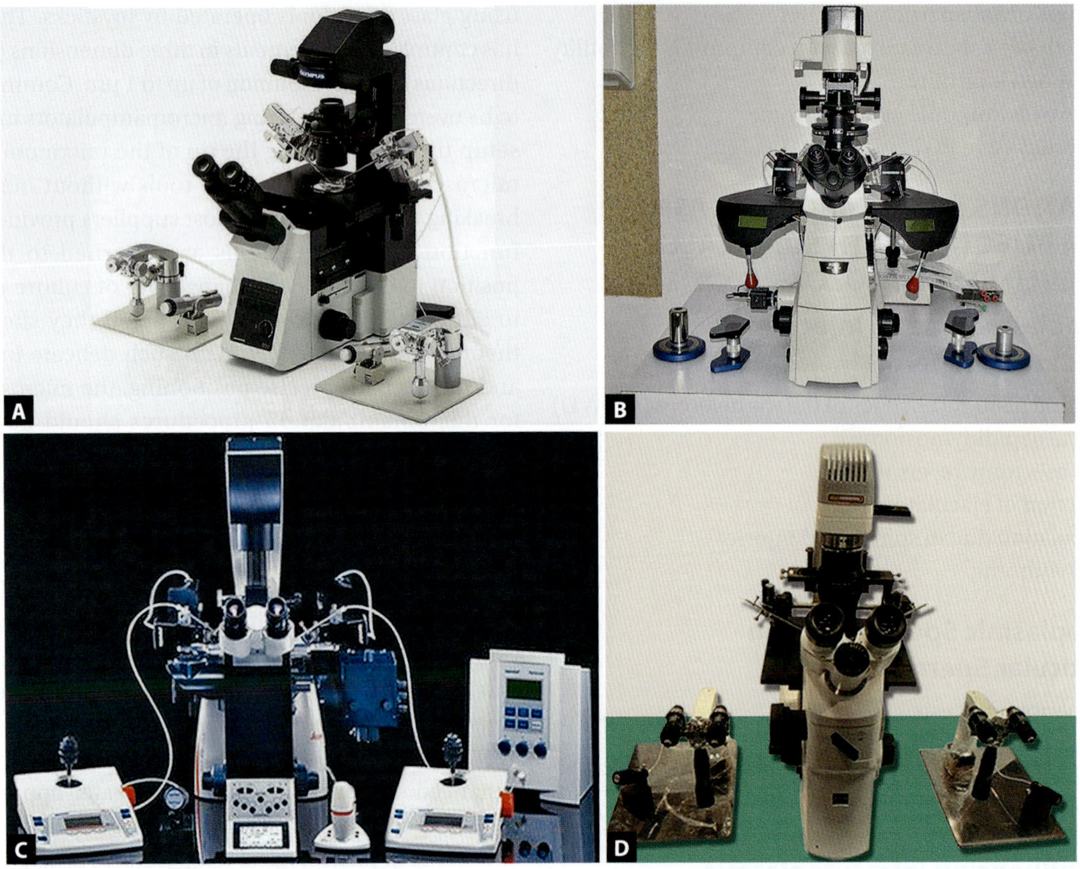

**Figs. 2A to D:** Different models of intracytoplasmic sperm injection (ICSI) workstations. (A) Olympus inverted microscope with Narishige (Takanome) micromanipulator; (B) Integra workstation (ORIGIO, CooperSurgical); (C) Leica microscope with Eppendorf micromanipulator; (D) Carl Zeiss microscope with S-micromanipulator.

can cause irreversible spindle damage. Narishige, Olympus, Integra, Leica, and Carl Zeiss are different types of inverted microscopes.

Micromanipulators are devices intended to translate macroscopic movement of human hand into microscopic movement of a fine tool held in its grasp. Two identical sets of two manipulators are mounted on the microscope: One set for coarse movements and another set for fine movements. One on the left side is for manipulation of the holding side and one on the right side is for manipulation of the injection side.

Each manipulation set is completed with a microinjector. Microinjectors are used either to fix or to release the oocyte with holding pipette or to aspirate and inject a spermatozoon with injection pipette. The injectors consist of airtight glass syringes which are connected to the steel pipette holders with Teflon tubing. They are filled with mineral oil or air. The plunger of the syringe is controlled by micrometer. Since movements in oil-filled syringes are fine, they are usually used for the injection side. But it has drawbacks such as oil leakage, oil breakdown due to ultraviolet (UV) exposure, and air bubble entrapment. Pneumatic injector, on the other hand, can be used on the holding side owing to its robust control. Upright pneumatic injector is referred to as mushroom due to its upright handle and large base design. The positioning of the injectors is up to the embryologist.

Some prefer both on the left side while some prefer injection on left and holding on right side.

### *Consumables*

- Shallow Petri dishes, tissue culture grade (e.g., 351006 Petri dishes: BD Falcon, NUNC 0150265, Oosafe ICSI dish, Vitrolife ICSI dish 16006)
- Holding pipettes
- ICSI injection needles (either 30 or 35° bevel tips).

In the early years, each unit used to make its own microtools from capillary tubes with the use of commercially available microtool pullers, grinders, and forges. Nowadays, there are many companies making microtools, many with computer-generated automation. ICSI pipettes may differ in ways of packaging to facilitate the handling before installation on the microscope, some with spike or non-spike and differences in the bevel (angle) at the tip (30–21°). The choice is entirely up to the preference of the operator and the procedure. For procedures such as spermatid injection, wider bore needles can be used (Humagen MIC-9-35).

### Media

- 4-(2-hydroxyethyl)-1-piperazineethanesulfonic acid (HEPES)/3-(N-morpholino) propanesulfonic acid (MOPS)/HEPES–MOPS combination
- Polyvinylpyrrolidone (PVP) or SpermCatch
- Light mineral oil/paraffin oil (Vitrolife, Vitromed, LifeGlobal, Lite Oil).

Many laboratories use flushing medium (HEPES-buffered, supplemented with antibiotics and protein) or sperm preparation media to make the ICSI droplets. Some laboratories even use the cleavage media as the oocyte holding droplets. However, there is a chance of drastic shift of pH while using such bicarbonate buffered media, especially when the injection process takes longer duration. Currently, there are many commercially available formulations having the chemical composition of cleavage stage media, but buffered by HEPES (global total HEPES). Since oocytes are stripped off the cumulus mass, the gamete is prone to changes in the surrounding microenvironment including the pH and osmolarity.

Polyvinylpyrrolidone is used as a medium to reduce motility prior to immobilization before ICSI. Since PVP contains synthetic plastic which cannot be digested by the lysosomal enzymes in the oocyte, it can cause a deleterious effect on post-zygote development. Another physiologic alternative is "sperm catch" [current Good Manufacturing Practice (cGMP), Nidacon International AB], which contains hyaluronate-containing product.

## Microinjection Preparation and Procedure

- Microinjection dish preparation
- Setting up and alignment of microinjection pipettes
- Transfer of gametes to injection dish
- Sperm selection and immobilization.

### Microinjection Dish Preparation

It is essential to heat all media and oil to 37°C prior to use.

Prepare injection dishes with 4–8 droplets of 5–10 µL of HEPES-buffered culture medium (global total with HEPES) for each individual oocyte and a 5 µL droplet of PVP for the sperm. The droplets can be arranged in a circle with sperm or PVP in the center or in parallel groups, but must be positioned so that they are not too close to the edge of the dish, where manipulation will be difficult. Some embryologists make river-like flat and long spreads of PVP which makes the sperm tail immobilization easier **(Figs. 3A to C)**. The oocyte droplets should not be too close to the sperm or PVP in order to avoid mixing—use an arrangement that allows quick and easy distinction between sperm and oocyte droplets, with numbers etched on the bottom of the dish. Small volumes of media evaporate very quickly and they should be covered immediately with a layer of oil. Light mineral oil also maintains the stability of droplets as well as the temperature and osmolarity. Equilibrate the dishes in the incubator for at least 20–30 minutes and keep them in the incubator until you are ready to begin the procedure. If Falcon 1006 dishes are being used with HEPES-buffered medium, the lid must be tightly fixed if they are to equilibrate in a $CO_2$ incubator. Dishes with HEPES medium and no lids should be warmed to 37°C without $CO_2$ atmosphere.

A prepared and preequilibrated traditional culture dish should be available to transfer and further culture the oocytes after injection **(Figs. 3A and B)**.

For surgically retrieved samples which will have sperms mixed with red blood cells (RBC) and tissue and for samples with very poor count and motility (no motility in PVP), conventional ICSI dish will pose a technical problem. In such cases "sperm fishing dish can be prepared," wherein the sample will be loaded in the HEPES river in the middle from where the sperms can be picked and moved to adjacent PVP drop where it can be immobilized and subsequently proceed with oocyte injection. Additionally, in this dish, one

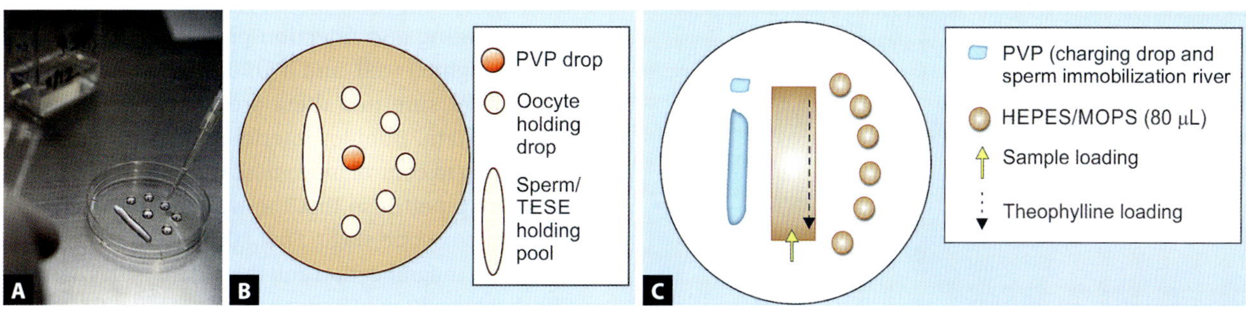


**Figs. 3A to C:** Two different types of fishing dish preparation for surgically retrieved samples (A and B) polyvinylpyrrolidone (PVP) in drop form (C) PVP spread like a river. Prepared testicular sperm extraction (TESE) suspension is placed in 4-(2-hydroxyethyl)-1-piperazineethanesulfonic acid (HEPES)/3-(N-morpholino)propanesulfonic acid (MOPS) pool having added theophylline (GM501 SpermMobil, Gynemed, Germany). The intracytoplasmic sperm injection (ICSI) pipette is slightly raised from dish floor to avoid debris. Spermatozoa wakes up and swims through the edges which can be picked, placed in PVP for immobilization (tail crushing). TESE/micro-TESE (mTESE)/SOAT sample loading dish.

also has a provision to add sperm motility adjuvants such as pentoxifylline or theophylline in the HEPES river.

### Setting Up and Alignment of the Microinjection Pipettes

The micropipettes have to be fitted, aligned, and equilibrated (charges) before starting the ICSI procedure. Since the holding pipette is much bigger than the injection pipette, it can be used as a guide for positioning and equilibrating. First, the micropipettes have to be fitted into the universal capillary holder, which is connected to the microinjector via a tube. When working with oil-filled systems, please make sure that no air bubbles are in the system. Gently push the pipettes past the sealing rings inside the tool holder. After attaching the universal capillary holder, check the alignment. The injection angle can be adjusted independently.

To align the capillary in the vertical position, the universal capillary holder can be rotated, even when the pipette is tightly gripped in place. Both pipettes have to appear straight in the field of view. The end of the holding pipette should be flat, that is, at 90° **(Fig. 4)**.

The alignment in the horizontal plane has to be done with great care. The following points must be taken into account—the holding pipette has to be aligned without tilt as it needs to lie flat on the bottom of the dish in order to aspirate the oocyte in a controlled manner. In contrast, the injection pipette needs to tilt downward slightly so that the tail of the spermatozoon can be broken properly. It is also necessary to prime micropipettes with medium (ideally PVP) before use so that the manipulated gametes never come into contact with air or oil.

*Cumulus-corona removal (denudation):* There are many hyaluronidase solutions in the market—Cumulase, SynVitroHyadase, etc.; the preferred one is 80 IU.

1. Prepare a culture dish containing one drop of hyaluronidase solution and five wash drops of a HEPES-buffered medium (global total HEPES), covered with an overlay of equilibrated mineral oil (denudation may also be carried out in BD, center-well organ culture dishes). Incubate at 37°C for 30–60 minutes. *Note:* HEPES-buffered medium has been adjusted to pH 7.4 and usually 5 mM bicarbonate, and exposure to a $CO_2$ atmosphere will cause the pH to drop; therefore, culture dishes that contain HEPES-buffered media should be warmed to 37°C in a warming oven and not in a $CO_2$ incubator.
2. Prepare a thin glass probe and select denudation pipettes or use the commercially available denuding pipettes (140/150 µm diameter, 175 µm to start with).
3. Remove the oocyte and hyaluronidase dishes from the incubator. Place 1–4 oocytes together into the enzyme drop, agitating gently until the cells start to dissociate. Do not leave them in the enzyme for >1 minute. Carefully aspirate the oocytes, leaving as much cumulus as possible behind. Wash by transferring them through at least five drops of culture medium and change to a fine-bore tip for aspiration in order to remove all of the coronal cells. The remaining coronal cells may help in getting better-quality embryos or blastocysts.[6]
4. Assess the quality and maturity of each oocyte under an inverted microscope. Use the glass probe to roll the oocytes around gently in order to identify the polar body and examine the ooplasm.[7]

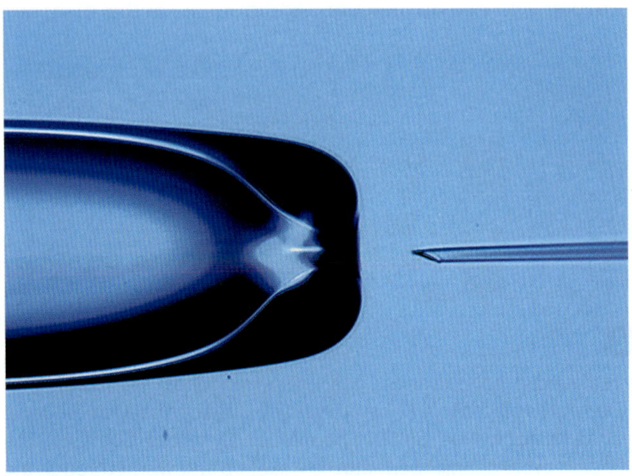

**Fig. 4:** Alignment of micropipettes.

### Micromanipulator

1. Make sure that the microscope heating stage is at a temperature that will maintain droplet temperature in the dishes at 37°C and ensure that all controls are set to neutral (adjusted to zero in Narishige system) and can be comfortably operated and that you are confident that all parts function smoothly before you begin. It is essential to check that you can smoothly carry out very small movements. Ensure that the pipettes are operating smoothly and are in field of view. This involves not only the equipment itself, but also its position on the bench in relation to your (comfortable) seating position.
2. Insert holding and injection pipettes into the pipette holders, tighten well, and if an oil-filled system is being used, make sure that there are no air bubbles in the tubing system. Bubbles interfere with sensitivity when attempting to control movement with fine precision.
3. Align the pipettes so that the working tips are parallel to the microscope stage. First, align the holding pipette under low magnification and then at high magnification. Check the position of both under high magnification. It is important to begin with pipettes in accurate alignment, with both working tips sharply in focus. If a part of the length is out of focus, the pipette is probably not parallel to the stage, but pointing upward or downward.

4. *Adjust the injection controls:* If using an oil system, the oil should just reach the distal end of the pipette, do not try to fill the needle with oil; this will work only if you leave a tiny 5 mm gap of air between the oil and the medium. Briefly touch the tips of both pipettes in oil and then in medium (ideally PVP drop, which gives better control) so that the ends fill by capillary action (a drop of oil behind the drop of medium/PVP will act as a buffer). The injection dish is still in the incubator, so you should be using a "blank" dish for this. Align the injection pipette again under low magnification.

### Transfer of Gametes to the Injection Dish

1. Carefully add a small aliquot of sperm suspension (3–4 μL, depending on the concentration of prepared sperm) to the edge of the central PVP droplet. The viscous solution should facilitate sperm handling by slowing down their motility and also prevents the sperm cells from sticking to the injection pipette during the procedure. Be careful of sperm density—too many sperm will make selection and immobilization more difficult.
2. After the sperm droplet has been carefully examined for the presence of debris or any other factors that might cause technical difficulties, examine all the denuded oocytes again for the presence of a first polar body; wash them gently with HEPES-buffered medium and transfer one oocyte into each oocyte dropleton the injection dish, taking care to avoid too much handling or cooling of the oocytes. Keep the oocytes in the incubator until you are confident that the injection procedure can proceed smoothly. Until sufficient experience of the procedure has been gained, it may be advisable to keep sperm and oocyte dishes separate, avoiding overexposure of the oocytes while selecting and immobilizing sperm.
3. Place the injection dish with central sperm droplet on the microscope stage. Using the coarse controls of the manipulator, lower the injection pipette into the drop.
4. In case of samples with very low motility and surgically retrieved samples, the sample can be loaded in the HEPES river (80 μL). Before loading, remove 40 μL of HEPES from the river. This will prevent bulging of the edge of the river, thus making visualization of sperm easy. To the HEPES river, one can add sperm motility enhancers such as theophylline (1:3 ratio theophylline: HEPES + sample) or pentoxifylline (1:1 ratio) half an hour before fishing for sperms.

### Sperm Selection and Immobilization

1. Select sperm that appears morphologically normal. Sperm can be selected and stored in the PVP drop for a limited period of time (be aware that prolonged exposure to PVP can cause damage to sperm membranes) before starting the injection procedure; this is an advantage in cases of extreme cryptozoospermia, and reduces oocyte exposure time. If SpermSlow is being used for immobilization, the sperm becomes rigid and sticks to the dish after approximately 30 minutes.
2. At 200× magnification, immobilize motile spermatozoa by crushing their tails: select the sperm to be aspirated and lower the tip of the injection needle (by mechanical joystick) onto the mid-piece of the sperm, striking down and across, and crushing the tail against the bottom of the dish. This "tail crushing" impairs motility and destabilizes the cell membrane; the latter may be required for sperm head decondensation. If the resulting sperm has a "bent" tail, it will be difficult to aspirate into the needle and will stick inside it. When this happens, abandon that sperm and repeat the procedure with another sperm. Do not strike too hard, or the sperm will stick to the bottom of the dish, also making aspiration into the needle difficult and sometimes causes sperm head decapitation, especially in testicular sperm. After some practice, sperm immobilization in routine ICSI cases can be carried out quite quickly. If the preparation contains only a few sperm with barely recognizable movement and a large amount of debris, this part of the procedure can be very tedious and require great patience. Do not hesitate to change the injection needle if you find that it is blocked. There is no hard and fast rule that one has to use only a single set of needle for each patient. The patient always comes before the price of a pipette. Increased disruption of sperm plasma membrane at sperm immobilization promotes dissociation of perinuclear theca from sperm chromatin after ICSI as shown in some animal models.
3. Aspirate the selected immobilized sperm into the injection pipette by rotating the knob of the injector anticlockwise. Sperm were traditionally aspirated into the pipette tailfirst, but they can be aspirated headfirst.[8] Position the sperm approximately 20 μm from the tip.
4. Lift the injection needle slightly. If the sperm moves up the pipette (due to the difference in density between culture medium and PVP), bring it back near the tip before beginning the injection procedure. If ever the sperm sticks to the pipette, better choose another sperm as it has a tendency to stick during injection. Before injection, when the injection pipette is ready to inject into the oocyte, try to move up and down the sperm inside the pipette. This "flushing" might help dispel any PVP around the sperm.

### Microinjection

1. Move the Petri dish until you can see an oocyte in one of the surrounding drops and bring it into focus. Move the holding capillary to the oocyte droplet. The oocyte is attached gently but firmly to the holding capillary with

the help of negative pressure created by the air device. The pressure should be great enough to hold the oocyte in place but not so strong that it causes the oolemma to bulge outward. Occasionally, embryologists experience a kinking in the oocyte during injection due to improper angle of injection. This can be avoided by slight upward or downward rotation of joystick (oocyte holding side) knob so as to allow the injection pipette to go smoothly into the oocyte. Polar body positioning at 6 or 12 o'clock in order to minimize the possibility of damaging the meiotic spindle was thought to be important, but later evidence using polarized microscopy to visualize the spindle itself suggests that polar body positioning is of less benefit than minimizing the duration of the ICSI procedure.[8] Some embryologists keep the position of polar bodies at either 7 or 11 o'clock position to avoid the damage to spindle.

2. Make sure that the oocyte is slightly elevated from the bottom of the Petri dish to facilitate the easy injection process. Otherwise, one may find difficulty while the injection needle is penetrated to the oocyte and it may slide away from the direction of the injection needle.
3. Then, focusing on the ICSI pipette and the oocyte, move the spermatozoon along the capillary and bring it to rest at its very tip by rotating the knob of the injector. Move the injection pipette close to the oocyte, and check that it is in the same plane as the right outer border of the oolemma on the equatorial plane at the 3 o'clock position. Check that the sperm can be moved smoothly within the injection needle and position it near the beveled tip.
4. By moving the joystick slightly, carefully push the injection pipette through the zona pellucida (ZP) and the oolemma into the ooplasm at 3 o'clock. The oocyte should be pricked in the middle so that the oolemma membrane is gently and atraumatically broken. Advance the injection pipette to the ooplasm into the injection capillary to be sure that the membrane is ruptured. Deposit the aspirated ooplasm and the spermatozoon toward the center of the oocyte. To introduce a minimal volume of the medium and PVP solution into the cytoplasm, gently withdraw the injection pipette after the head of the sperm cell has left the pipette tip. Release the injected oocyte from the holding capillary and raise both pipettes by pressing the joystick button.

If the pipette is in the wrong plane, entry into the cell will be difficult. The membrane may rupture spontaneously or may require negative pressure, sucking the membrane into the pipette before expelling the sperm. When it breaks, there will be a sudden flux of cytoplasm into the pipette. For many embryologists, failed fertilization in ICSI happens in their early days of ICSI practice just because of improper cytoplasmic aspiration and lack of proper membrane rupture while injection. Many times, it has been observed that sperm gets ejected once the pipette is withdrawn from the oocyte. To avoid this, make sure that there is a sudden flux of ooplasm into the injection needle. However, care should be exercised not to aspirate too much ooplasm. This happens if the injection needle is not properly installed or if there are air columns in the oil tubing, which causes abrupt movement of fluid in the ICSI needle. Inject the sperm slowly into the oocyte with a minimal amount of fluid (1–2 pL). The sperm should be ejected past the tip of the pipette, to ensure a tight insertion among the organelles, which will hold it in place while the pipette is withdrawn. Some surplus medium may be reaspirated to reduce the size of the breach created during perforation. If the plasma membrane is elastic and difficult to break, it may be necessary to withdraw the pipette from the first membrane invagination and slowly repeat the procedure **(Figs. 5A to I)**. Occasionally, some maneuvering of pipette tip (to different directions inside the ooplasm) may be required in cases of ooplasm which are viscous and prevent the smooth entry into the pipette.

Yanaihara et al.[9] studied sperm retention site and its influence on cleavage rate and early development following ICSI cases involving 336 ICSI patients (age 27–44 years; average 37.4), where 1,545 oocytes were observed. An oocyte was divided into nine sites and the sperm retention site was observed microscopically after injection. The polar body was placed at either the 12 or the 6 o'clock position. The injection pipette was introduced at the 3 o'clock position and oolemma rupture was ascertained by mild suction. The main outcome measures were the relationship of sperm remaining in position in the oocyte to fertilization rate and embryo quality.

When the injection pipette was introduced at the 3 o'clock position, about 80% of the sperm remained in the center or left of center. The fertilization rate was significantly lower ($p < 0.05$) when the sperm remained near the site of introduction. Embryo quality was not significantly affected by the sperm retention site. About 12–14% of the spermatozoa remained near the introducing position, and in these cases, the fertilization rate was low. However, once fertilization occurred, the sperm retention site had minimal impact on embryo quality. The study indicates that injecting sperm near the spindle site may improve embryo quality.

5. Gently remove the injection pipette, and examine the breach area. The membrane should be funnel-shaped, pointing in toward the center. If the border of the oolemma is everted, cytoplasm may leak out and the oocyte may subsequently cytolyze. Release the oocyte from the holding pipette.

If several oocytes are obtained, only three to four oocytes are injected as a rule. They are first washed in cleavage medium and placed there for long-term culture, and the remaining oocytes are then injected.

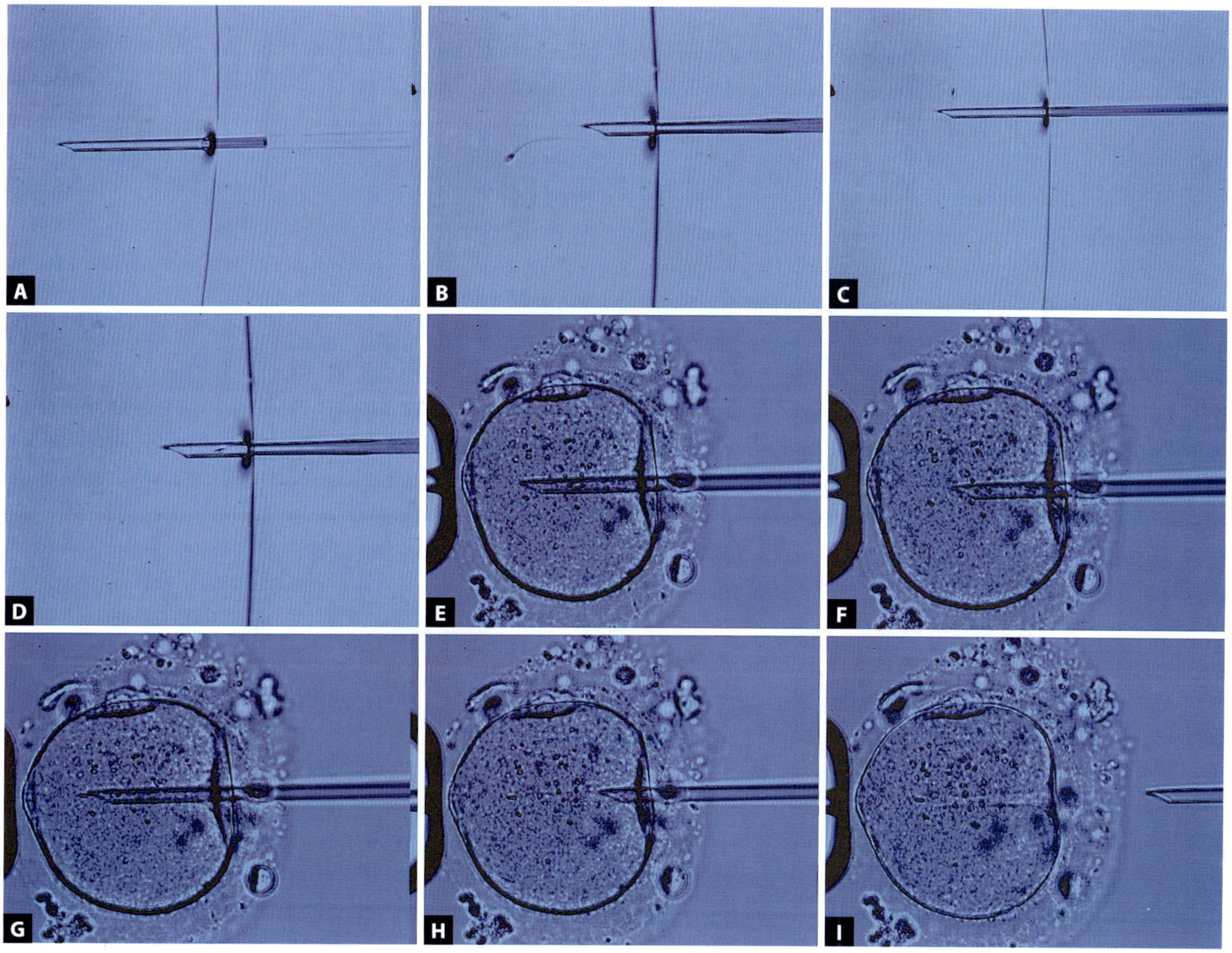

**Figs. 5A to I:** Intracytoplasmic sperm injection procedure stepwise.

### *Injection Procedure: Important Points*

1. *All conditions must be stable*: Temperature, pH, equipment properly set up, adjusted, aligned, and checked for leaks and air bubbles. Check everything, including secure and comfortable operating position, before you begin.
2. Correct immobilization of sperm.
3. Advance far enough into the ooplasm with the injection pipette.
4. Ensure that the plasma membrane is broken (immediate membrane rupture after introducing the injection needle results in a lower probability of fertilization). Fertilization failure in many cases is due to improper aspiration (confirmation of a sudden gushing in of ooplasm) of cytoplasm and thereby deposition of sperm outside.
5. Inject a minimal volume.
6. If the sperm comes out of the ooplasm into the perivitelline space, reinject.
7. If there is debris sticking to the injection pipette surface, move the microscope stage so that injection needle passes through the media droplet-oil interface to wipe out the debris.
8. After injection, if pressure builds up in the holding pipette making it difficult to dislodge the egg, move the holding pipette along with the attached egg to the media–oil interface by moving the microscope stage (not into oil). It automatically gets dislodged from the pipette.
9. There is a tendency by some embryologists to pick up 10 or even more sperms into injection pipettes and do the consecutive injection of multiple oocytes. Sometimes, this can lead to injection of more than one spermatozoa into oocytes.
10. Make sure that one changes the injection and holding pipettes after each patient's injection cycles. It has been noticed that some embryologists retain the holding pipette, some do not change the either needle to save time and simply clean it before the next injection process. Both these practices should be avoided and should not be encouraged.
11. Pneumatic syringe is ideal for the holding side of the micromanipulator and hassle-free compared to the oil syringes (IM-11-2, Narishige) **(Figs. 6A to E)**.

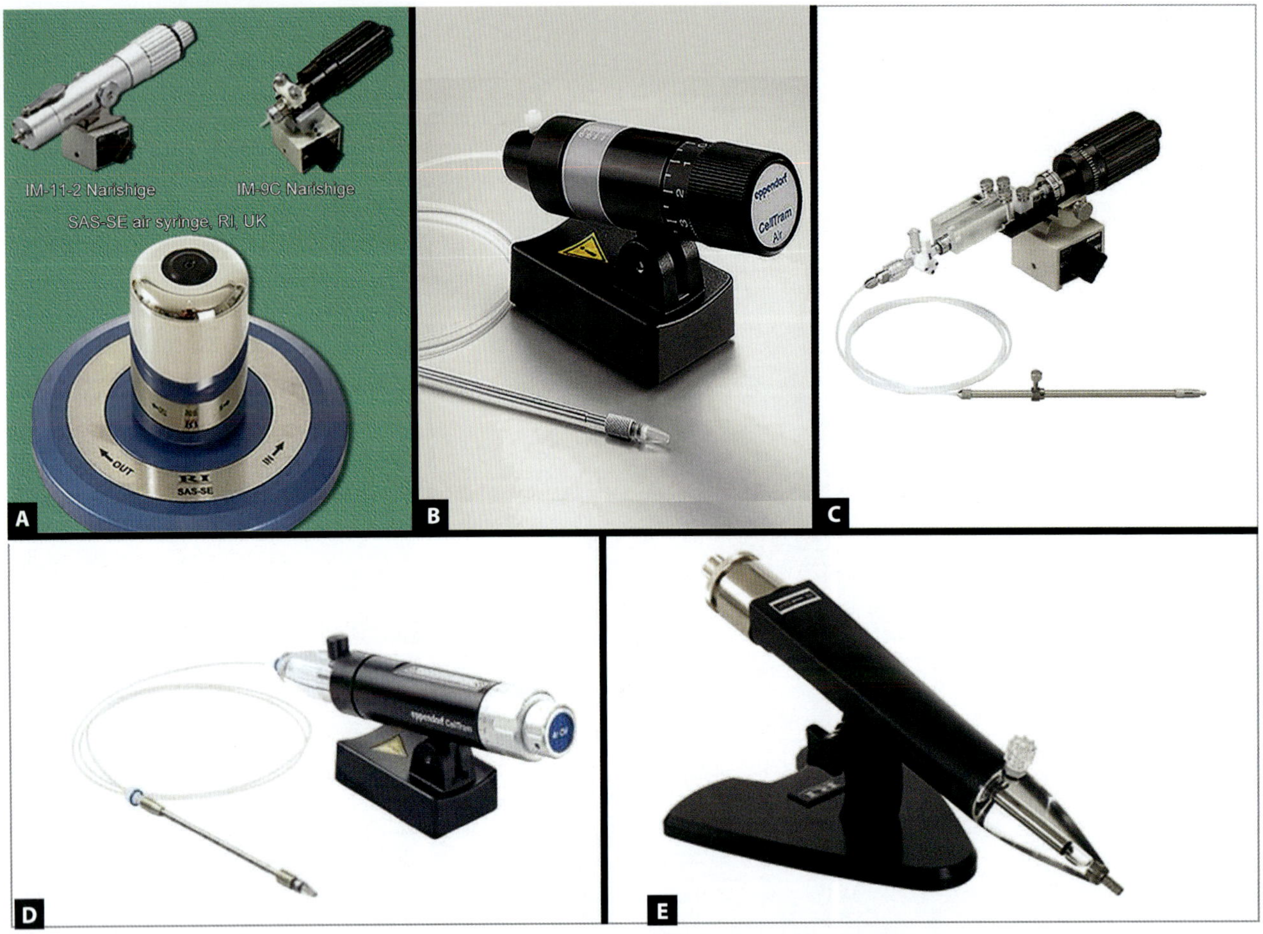


**Figs. 6A to E:** Narishige, ORIGIO (A) and Eppendorf (B), pneumatic syringes and oil syringes from Narishige (C), Eppendorf (D), and ORIGIO (E).

12. Four-axis hanging joystick oil hydraulic micromanipulator (Narishige) spares the laborious work of pipette alignment with optical axis (***see* Fig. 2A**). The injection holder is provided with a special clamp which memorizes the length of the pipette from injection holder, thus exchanging and repositioning the pipette more accurately at a shorter time (**Fig. 7**).
13. The newly launched TrakJector micromanipulators (**Fig. 8**) from Hamilton Thorne offer a new standard in smooth, fine control, and precision (tolerance <1 μm), and this allows one-handed operation using the all-in-one trackball (AIO$^{\text{trackball}}$) in conjunction with the motorized oil injection unit (MIU$^{\text{mot}}$Oil). The system can easily control both the injection holding pressure and the motorized movement using the trackball and the two buttons. The integrated, ergonomic gel pillow allows hands to stay relaxed during extended operating sessions. An adjustable velocity setting permits balancing between operators and different magnifications.

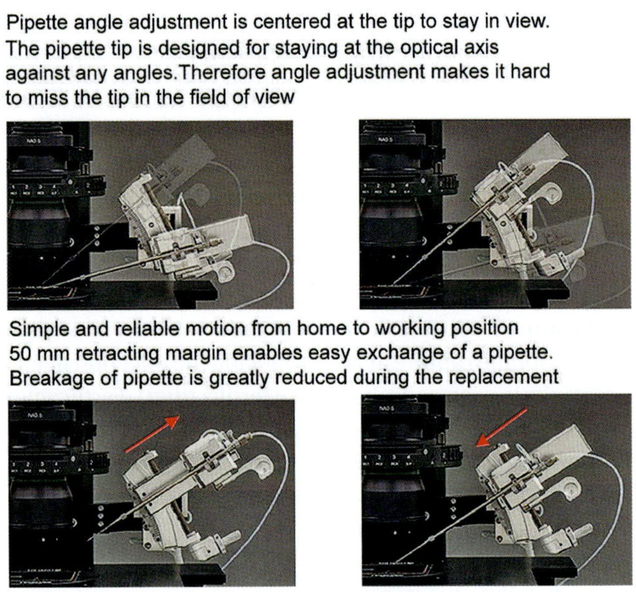


**Fig. 7:** Home positioning function in Takanome (Narishige).

### *Assessment of Fertilization*

About 16–18 hours after microinjection, check the oocytes for the presence of pronuclei and polar bodies. After another 24 hours, score the embryos (e.g., equal size of blastomeres) and transfer them into the uterus.

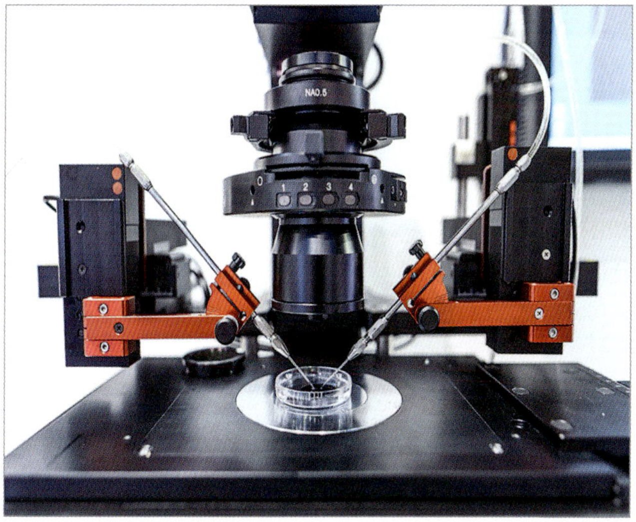


**Fig. 8:** TrakJector micromanipulators from Hamilton Thorne (USA).

## CONVENTIONAL INSEMINATION VERSUS INTRACYTOPLASMIC SPERM INJECTION

Though many clinics opt for 100% ICSI for insemination of oocytes irrespective of semen quality, the debate is on for the risks associated with this invasive procedure. Recent studies show that assessment of sperm function prior to actual cycles can discriminate the mode of insemination required for each couple.

Wiser et al.,[10] in a prospective study, analyzed if hyperactivated motility (HAM) and acrosome reaction (AR) can be useful tests for evaluating semen quality during male infertility evaluations and to help the clinician decide whether regular insemination or ICSI is preferable during IVF. Patients with normal sperm, according to World Health Organization guidelines, who underwent IVF treatment and planned regular insemination were asked to participate and a portion of sperm sample was evaluated for HAM and AR on the day of ovum pickup. In HAM assessment, 93.3% of patients with increased HAM had a high fertilization rate compared with 64% in the group without increased HAM ($p = 0.059$). For the AR evaluation, 91.7% of samples with a low rate of spontaneous AR had a high fertilization rate compared with 39.3% in the group with a high rate of spontaneous AR ($p = 0.004$).

The same group in another study evaluated the post-wash sperm characteristics as a tool to discriminate the insemination procedure by either conventional method or ICSI. They evaluated 112 cycles fertilized with both regular and ICSI insemination during the same cycle. In 62 cycles, fertilization was obtained with both ICSI and IVF, and in 50 cycles, fertilization was obtained by ICSI alone. The sperm samples were reevaluated after the preparation process. The mean initial total motile sperm count (TMSC) was 66.3 × 106 ± 47.5 in the group that underwent both methods and $23.1 \times 10^6 \pm 20.4$ in the ICSI-only group ($p < 0.05$). After sperm preparation, the mean post-wash TMSC was $4.4 \times 10^6 \pm 3.4$ and $1.06 \times 10^6 \pm 0.9$, respectively ($p < 0.05$). They found a cutoff of $1.5 \times 10^6$ or fewer sperm after preparation as an indicator for ICSI has a sensitivity of 80% and a specificity of 77%. Reevaluation of TMSC can prevent unexpected fertilization failure. The study shows that fewer than 1.5 million TMSC after wash should be considered an indication for ICSI fertilization.[11]

Breznik et al.[12] studied the diagnostic value of the following sperm function tests in predicting the fertilizing ability of spermatozoa in conventional IVF and ICSI—hyaluronan binding assay (HBA), DNA fragmentation (Halosperm), and hyperactivity. Both fertilization rate and embryo quality in IVF cycles negatively correlated with sperm DNA fragmentation. Furthermore, a positive correlation was observed between fertilization rate and hyaluronan-binding ability or induced hyperactivity. The semen samples from the IVF cycles with low fertilization rate (group 1) were characterized by statistically significantly higher sperm DNA fragmentation and lower hyaluronan-binding ability in comparison with semen samples from the group with high levels of fertilization (group 2). In ICSI cycles, no relationship was found between sperm function tests and fertilization rate or embryo quality. This study also proves that the Halosperm test, the HBA test, and induced hyperactivity are useful in predicting the ability of spermatozoa to fertilize oocytes in IVF and are helpful in distinguishing semen samples suitable for IVF or ICSI.

### Key Performance Indicators For Intracytoplasmic Sperm Injection

Key performance indicators (KPIs) are essential for evaluating the introduction of a process in the IVF laboratory, establishing minimum standards for proficiency, monitoring ongoing performance within a quality management system, benchmarking, and quality improvement. The Vienna consensus jointly developed by European Society of Human Reproduction and Embryology (ESHRE) and Alpha Society of Reproductive Scientists focuses on the four most important performance indicators: (1) normal fertilization rate, (2) oocyte degeneration rate, (3) poor fertilization rate, and (4) failed fertilization rate in ICSI.[13] The definition used most often for the ICSI normal fertilization rate is the proportion of injected oocytes with 2 pronuclei (2PN) the day after injection. ICSI damage rate is defined as the number of oocytes damaged during ICSI and/or observed at fertilization check over the number of injected oocytes. It is useful to monitor this indicator for operator competence, oocyte quality, and laboratory performance. The damage rate can also be indicative of technical problems (e.g., cumulus cell removal stress, vibration) **(Table 1)**.

**TABLE 1:** PI and KPI for the ICSI

| *Performance indicator (PI)* | *Calculation* | *Competence (%)* | *Benchmark value (%)* |
|---|---|---|---|
| 1 PN rate (ICSI) | $\frac{\text{no. 1 PN oocytes} \times 100}{\text{no. MII oocytes injected}}$ | <3 | |
| *KPI* | | | |
| ICSI damage rate | $\frac{\text{no. damaged or degenerated} \times 100}{\text{all oocytes injected}}$ | ≤ 10 | ≤ 5 |
| ICSI normal fertilization rate | $\frac{\text{no. oocytes with 2 PN and 2 PB} \times 100}{\text{no. MII oocytes injected}}$ | ≤ 65 | ≤ 80 |

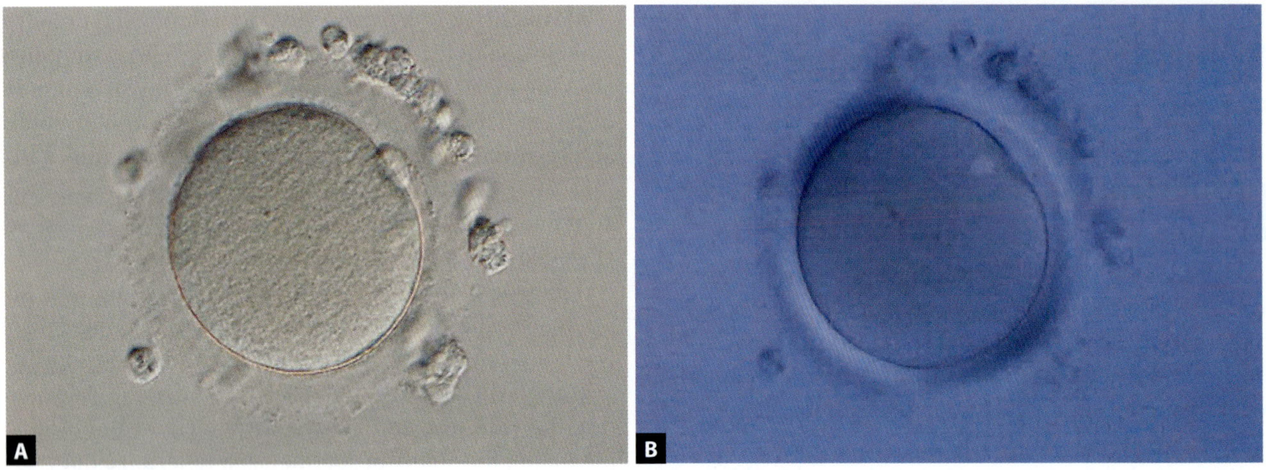

**Figs. 9A and B:** Oocyte with a visible meiotic spindle. (A) Oocyte positioned with polar body located at 1.5 o'clock position for better facilitating spindle observation under the bright-field; (B) Meiotic spindle appears bright white in the oocyte under the polarized light microscopy.

Oocyte degeneration is a common phenomenon experienced by all embryologists who perform ICSI. Generally observed after withdrawal of the injection needle, it is characterized by lysis of the oocyte but also may follow normal injection, being noted the following day by a darkened ooplasm. In severe cases, the degeneration rate may be as high as 30–50% and the potential implications are concerning to both the physician and the embryologist. Data suggest that oocyte degeneration is not technician- or physician-dependent. Some reports suggested that the rate of oocyte degeneration is operator-dependent and a smaller injection needle can minimize the incidence of degeneration.

Degeneration is likely a function of the inherent oocyte quality in women who underwent ovarian stimulation. However, the remaining cohort of retrieved oocytes appears to be unaffected by virtue of an uncompromised implantation rate. The first author of this manuscript has noted higher ICSI degeneration in centers where higher recombinant gonadotropin is used for controlled ovarian stimulation (COS) without any human menopausal gonadotropin (hMG), hence less luteinizing hormone (LH).

## AUTOMATION OF INTRACYTOPLASMIC SPERM INJECTION

Gamete micromanipulation requires an experienced and highly skilled embryologist and the process is labor-intensive. The laboratory outcomes of this manual operation are susceptible to human factors such as volume of work, stress, and fatigue as well as variations in performance between operators. Is it possible for this most sophisticated of all assisted reproductive technologies (ART) to ultimately be automated? In the first report of robotic ICSI (RICSI), using a hamster oocyte or human sperm model, the robotic system demonstrated a high (90%) survival rate.[14] Human trials are already under way for RICSI (Yu Sun personal communication), and it may only be a matter of time before automation, in some form, gains confidence among the IVF community.

### Meiotic Spindle Imaging by Using a Polarized Microscope

The presence of the first polar body is a sign of oocyte maturation **(Figs. 9A and 10A)**. However, actual nuclear

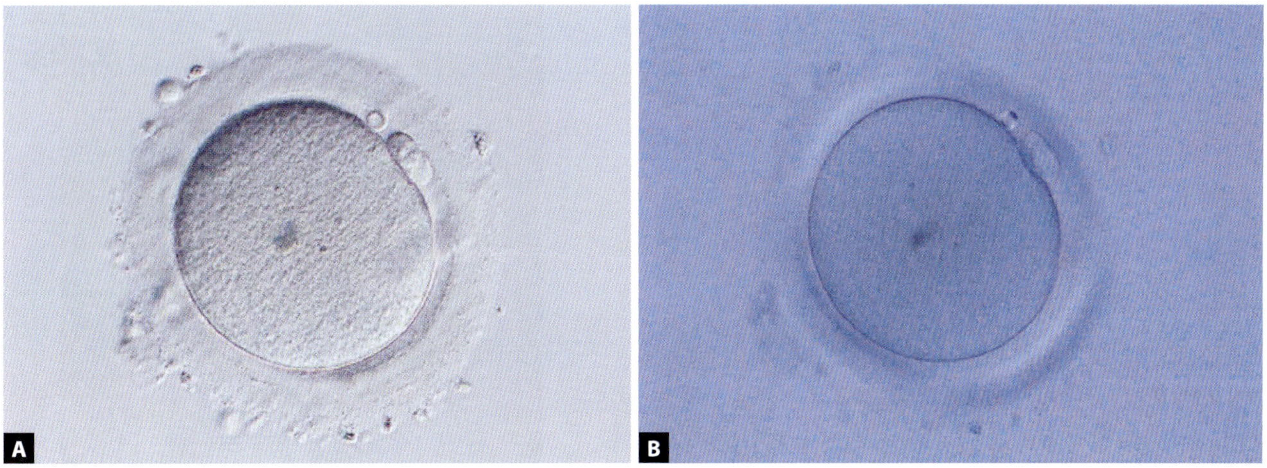

**Figs. 10A and B:** Oocyte with not observed meiotic spindle. (A) Oocyte positioned with polar body located at 1.5 o'clock position for better facilitating spindle observation under the bright-field; (B) Meiotic spindle does not appear in the oocyte under the polarized light microscopy.

maturity is unclear. The technique of assessing the actual nuclear maturity of oocytes before sperm injection is meiotic spindle imaging. A polarized microscope combined with a glass bottom dish enables one to observe the status of the meiotic spindle. The oocyte with a visible meiotic spindle **(Fig. 9B)** means the oocyte is metaphase II and is ready for sperm injection. But the oocyte with no visible meiotic spindle **(Fig. 10B)** means the oocyte is telophase I (immature) or overmatured.[16,17] The visible or no visibility of the meiotic spindle affects oocyte fertilization and embryo development. Petersen et al. compared fertilization and embryo development after standard ICSI between oocytes with visible meiotic spindle and oocytes with no visible meiotic spindle in a meta-analysis.[18] The fertilization rate of spindle-positive oocytes was significantly higher (75.6%) as compared with that of spindle-negative oocytes (61.5%). The blastocyst rate of spindle-positive oocytes was also significantly higher (50.7%) as compared with that of spindle-negative oocytes (28.6%). Recently, Hiraoka et al. assessed the effect of meiotic spindle visuality on ICSI results after Piezo-ICSI.[19] The authors used polarized light microscopy (Olympus IX73 inverted microscope equipped with IX3 ICSI/IMSI, Olympus, Life Science Solutions, Tokyo, Japan) and a glass bottom dish (87-453, NIPRO, Osaka, Japan), and then first positioned with the polar body located at 1.5 o'clock positions because this position facilitates better spindle observation under the bright field **(*see* Figs. 1 and 2A)**. The fertilization rate of spindle-positive oocytes **(*see* Fig. 1)** was significantly higher (92.0%) as compared with that of spindle-negative oocytes **(*see* Fig. 2B)** (70.0%). The blastocyst rate of spindle-positive oocytes was significantly higher (53.7%) as compared with that of spindle-negative oocytes (32.1%). These results show the importance of meiotic spindle imaging for better timing of sperm injection and predicting embryo development.

## Piezo-Intracytoplasmic Sperm Injection

Piezo-ICSI is one of the ICSI techniques that uses a piezo actuator. A piezo actuator can make it possible to do sperm immobilization, zona opening, and membrane breakage semiautomatically. Therefore, Piezo-ICSI can contribute to standardizing the ICSI technique. In this section, we describe the equipment, preparation, and procedures.

### *Equipment*

- Piezo-ICSI system (operation box, controller, footswitch, and drive unit)
- Inverted microscope
- Air injectors.

### *Microtool*

- Glass bottom dish
- Operation liquid
- Flat tip micropipette
- Holding pipette.

### *Media*

- 7% PVP
- MOPS-buffered medium
- Mineral oil.

### *Preparation*

Piezo-ICSI system is composed of an operation box **(Fig. 11A)**, controller **(Fig. 11B)**, footswitch **(Fig. 11C)**, and drive unit **(Fig. 11D)**. Attach the drive unit to the pipette holder **(Fig. 11D)** and put the footswitch on the floor **(Fig. 12)**. Footswitch drives the piezo pulse. Put an operation box and controller inside the clean bench appropriately **(Fig. 12)**.

Place three drops (two PVP drops and one MOPS-buffered medium drop) on the glass bottom dish and cover

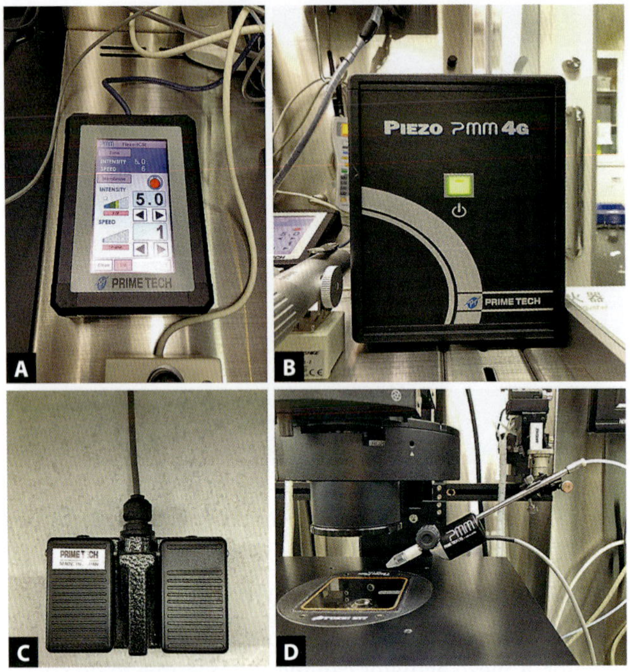


**Figs. 11A to D:** Four types of equipment of Piezo-ICSI. (A) Operation box; (B) Controller; (C) Footswitch; (D) Drive unit.

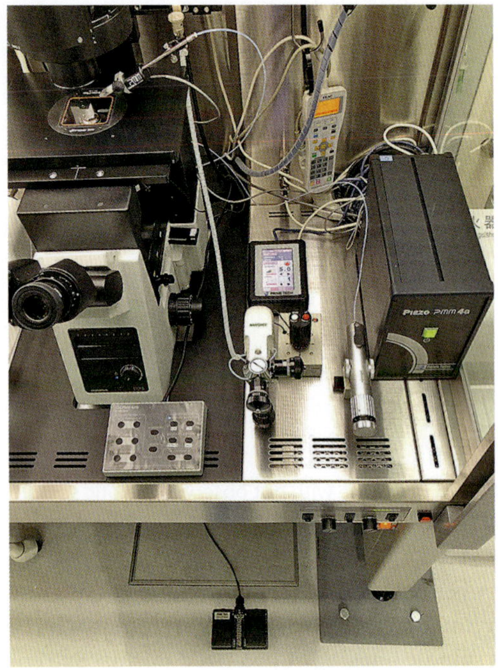

**Fig. 12:** Piezo-ICSI system.

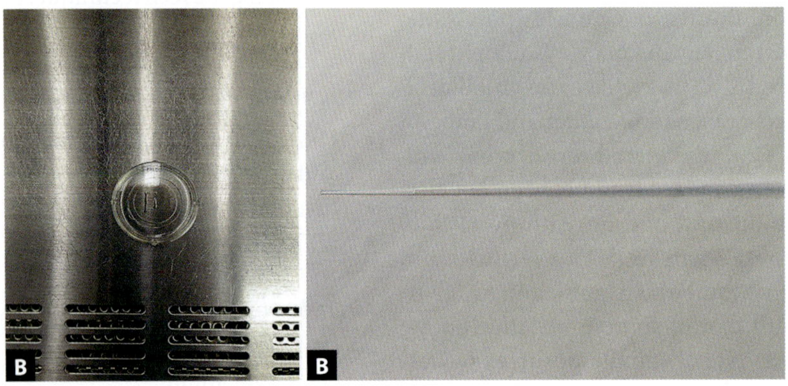


**Figs. 13A and B:** ICSI dish and micropipette preparation for Piezo-ICSI. (A) Place three drops (two PVP drops and one MOPS buffered medium drop) on the glass bottom dish and cover these drops with the mineral oil; (B) PVP is aspirated at the tip of the micropipette next to the operation liquid.

these drops with the mineral oil **(Fig. 13A)**. Inject the sperm suspension into the lower of the longer PVP drop.

Inject the operation liquid **(Fig. 14A)** inside the micropipette 2.0 cm **(Figs. 14B and C)**. Avoid the air getting mixed in the line of operation liquid. The specific gravity of operation liquid is about 1.8, colorless, transparent, and nonwater soluble. Attach the micropipette to the pipette holder and twist the holder cap firmly. The micropipette used for Piezo-ICSI has a flat tip **(Fig. 14D)**. Expel the operation liquid inside the micropipette toward the micropipette tip. Immerse the micropipette tip into the smaller PVP drop and aspirate PVP into the micropipette. Try to keep the volume aspirated into the micropipette 300 µm during procedures for stable operation **(Fig. 13B)**.

### *Sperm Immobilization*

After selecting the sperm upper of longer PVP drop **(Fig. 13A)**, attach the micropipette tip to the sperm's tail and apply a piezo pulse **(Figs. 15A and B)**. Repeat this procedure one to two times until the complete stopping of the tail motion is confirmed. Then aspirate the immobilized sperm into the micropipette tailfirst **(Figs. 15C and D)**.

### *Microinjection*

Transfer the oocyte to the MOPS-buffered medium drop **(Fig. 13A)**. Observe the spindle by polarized microscope and rotate the oocyte as avoiding the spindle is at 3 o'clock. Hold the oocyte keeping the spindle location away at

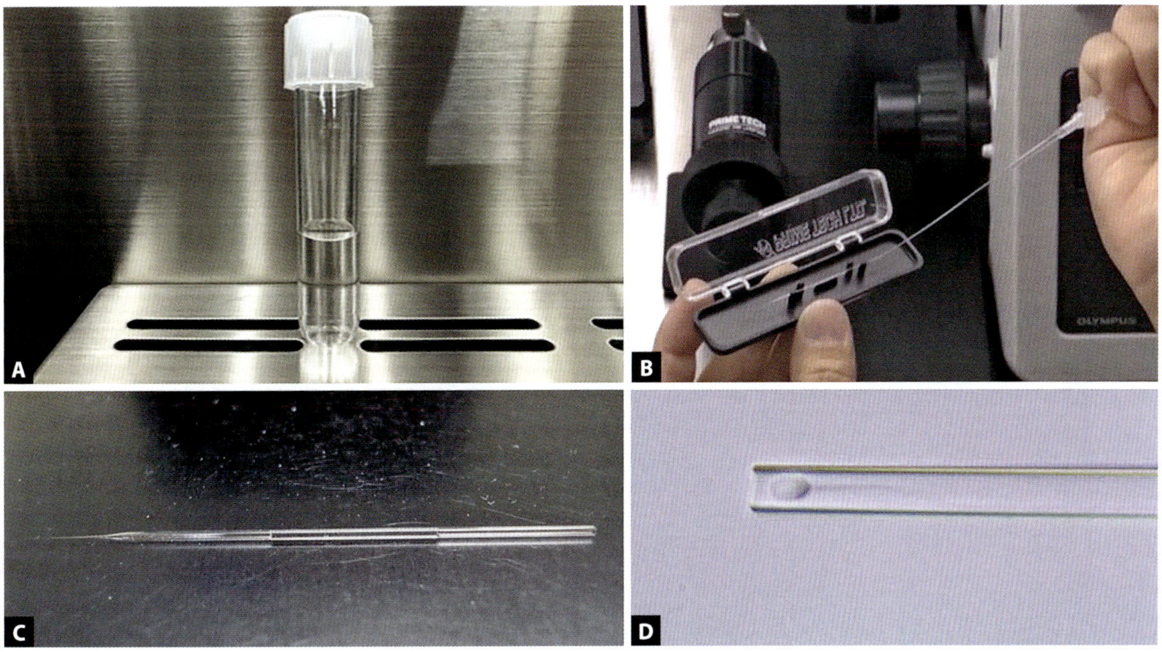

**Figs. 14A to D:** Micropipette preparation for Piezo-ICSI. (A) Operation liquid. The specific gravity of operation liquid is about 1.8, colorless, transparent, and non-water soluble; (B) Inject the operation liquid inside the micropipette; (C) The operation liquid is injected inside the micropipette 2.0 centimeters; (D) The micropipette used for Piezo-ICSI has a flat tip.

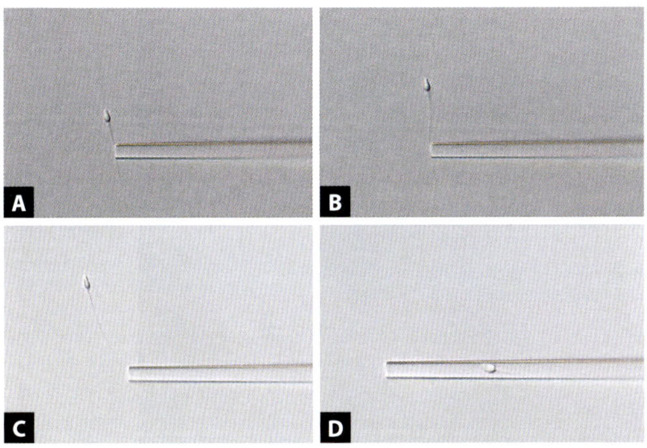

**Figs. 15A to D:** Sperm immobilization. (A and B) Attaching the micropipette tip to the sperm's tail and applying a piezo pulse; (C and D) Aspirating the immobilized sperm into the micropipette tail first.

3 o'clock. Attach the micropipette tip to the surface of ZP **(Fig. 16A)**. While applying the piezo pulses, move the micropipette tip slowly toward the oocyte without zona deformation **(Fig. 16B)**. When the micropipette tip reaches the inner layer of the ZP, aspirate the piece of ZP **(Fig. 16C)**. Remove the micropipette tip outside of the ZP and expel the ZP piece from the micropipette **(Fig. 16D)**. Pass through the micropipette tip via opened ZP and move deep inside the oocyte (about 90% of oocyte diameter) **(Fig. 16E)**. After stopping the movement of the micropipette, apply one piezo pulse to break the membrane. After confirming the membrane breakage by observing the rebounding of the membrane **(Fig. 16F)**, inject the sperm head into the oocyte **(Fig. 16G)**. Remove the micropipette tip outside of the ZP **(Fig. 16H)**.

## Standard-Intracytoplasmic Sperm Injection Versus Piezo-Intracytoplasmic Sperm Injection

To the best of our knowledge, seven papers compared the clinical results between Standard-ICSI and Piezo-ICSI. All of the seven papers reported higher fertilization rates of Piezo-ICSI than the Standard-ICSI.[15,20-25] Hiraoka and Kitamura assessed the average volume of aspirated cytoplasm into the micropipette at membrane breakage. These authors reported significantly more volume of Standard-ICSI (2746 ± 940 $\mu m^3$) than the Piezo-ICSI (0 ± 0 $\mu m^3$).[15] Cytoplasmic aspiration procedure might cause damage to the cytoplasm. Piezo-ICSI could avoid this damage by getting rid of cytoplasmic aspiration. More studies would be needed to assess the clinical efficiency of Piezo-ICSI.

## KEY POINTS

- Currently, however, ICSI is also being performed for infertile couples with normozoospermic males, even if the less-invasive IVF would likely produce a similar outcome. Some clinics even utilize ICSI in all instances of treatment with IVF. This could be problematic since several studies have advised against routinely using ICSI for all cases of IVF treatment. ICSI undoubtedly can be a

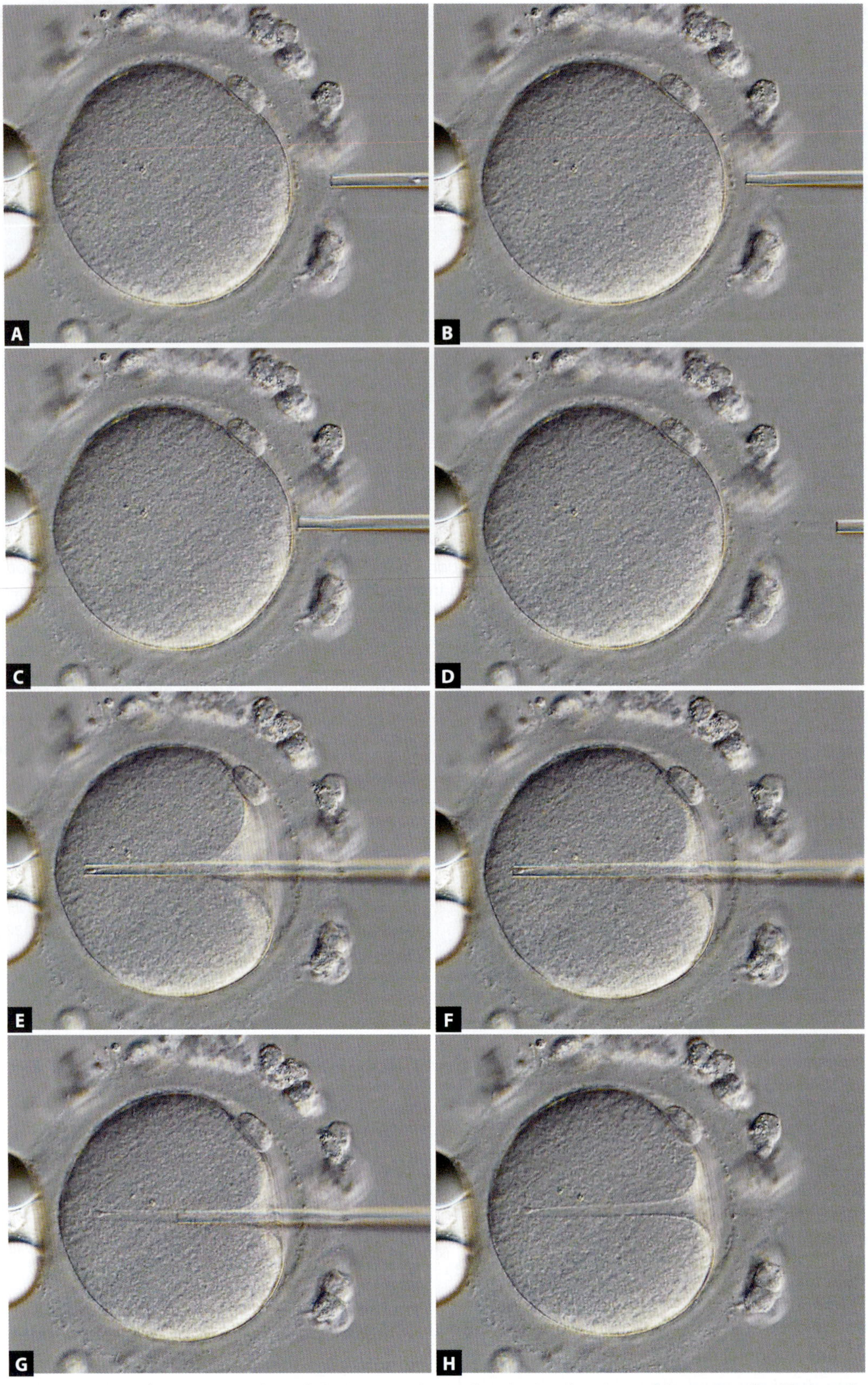


**Figs. 16A to H:** Piezo-ICSI procedure stepwise. (A to C) During opening and aspirating the piece of the zona pellucida into the micropipette; (D) Expelling the piece of the zona pellucida. (E) Moving the micropipette tip deep inside the oocyte (about 90% of oocyte diameter); (F) After applying the piezo pulse to break the membrane; (G) Injecting the sperm head into the oocyte; (H) Removing the micropipette outside the zona pellucida.

blessing for those men suffering from severe male factor infertility. However, due to the invasive nature of the procedure, there is great potential for complications of all degrees of severity.

- Additionally, the long-term consequences of this procedure on the resulting embryos and children remain largely unknown since the first successful ICSI-conceived child was born in 1992, and most long-term ICSI studies have not yet completed data collection. A number of factors could affect the ICSI outcome, including poor embryonic genetic health and failure of germ cells to properly execute vital biological events such as fertilization.
- In some instances, success with ICSI is compromised because of the technical limitations of ICSI instruments, clinicians, and laboratory technicians. In other failed cases, solutions cannot be proposed until more knowledge is gained about the underlying pathology of infertility.
- Proposed techniques which need more dedicated work and extensive studies are:
  - Use of round spermatid (ROSI) from men with no elongated spermatid or spermatozoa in testes
  - In vitro culture of immature germ cells to more mature stages
  - But the possibility of genetic and epigenetic risks to offspring cannot be ruled out in these cases.
- As new studies on the subject, especially on sperm physiology and molecular biology, continue to be published, it is important that the established protocol for ICSI is revised on a regular basis and that its role in infertility therapy is continually reevaluated.

## REFERENCES


1. Palermo GD, Neri QV, Monahan D, Takeuchi T, Schlegel PN, Rosenwaks Z. Intracytoplasmic sperm injection. In: Nagy ZP, Varghese AC, Agarwal A (Eds). Practical Manual of In Vitro Fertilization: Advanced Methods and Novel Devices. New York: Springer; 2012.
2. Varghese AC, Goldberg E, Agarwal A. Current and future perspectives on intracytoplasmic sperm injection: a critical commentary. Reprod Biomed Online. 2007;15(6):719-27.
3. Palermo G, Joris H, Devroey P, Van Steirteghem AC. Pregnancies after intracytoplasmic injection of single spermatozoon into an oocyte. Lancet. 1992;340(8810):17-8.
4. Varghese AC, Arsalan A, Agarwal A. An update on developments and future prospects of ICSI. Arch Med Sci. 2009;5(1A):S109-14.
5. Dozortsev D, Nasr-Esfahani MH. Mechanism of human oocyte activation during ICSI and methodology for overcoming low or failed fertilization. In: Nagy ZP, Varghese AC, Agarwal A (Eds). Practical Manual of In Vitro Fertilization: Advanced Methods and Novel Devices. New York: Springer; 2012.
6. Ebner T. Oocyte treatment and preparation for microinjection. In: Nagy ZP, Varghese AC, Agarwal A (Eds). Practical Manual of In Vitro Fertilization: Advanced Methods and Novel Devices. New York: Springer; 2012.
7. Maggiulli R, Ubaldi F, Rienzi L. Oocyte denuding. In: Nagy ZP, Varghese AC, Agarwal A (Eds). Practical Manual of In Vitro Fertilization: Advanced Methods and Novel Devices. New York: Springer; 2012.
8. Woodward BJ, Montgomery SJ, Hartshorne GM, Campbell KH, Kennedy R. Spindle position assessment prior to ICSI does not benefit fertilization or early embryo quality. Reprod Biomed Online. 2008;16(2):232-8.
9. Yanaihara A, Iwasaki S, Negishi M, Okai T. Sperm retention site and its influence on cleavage rate and early development following intracytoplasmic sperm injection. J Assit Reprod Genet. 2006;23(2):63-7.
10. Wiser A, Sachar S, Ghetler Y, Shulman A, Breitbart H. Assessment of sperm hyperactivated motility and acrosome reaction can discriminate the use of spermatozoa for conventional in vitro fertilisation or intracytoplasmic sperm injection: preliminary results. Andrologia. 2014;46(3):313-5.
11. Wiser A, Ghetler Y, Gonen O, Piura E, Berkovits A, Itskovich A, et al. Re-evaluation of post-wash sperm is a helpful tool in the decision to perform in vitro fertilisation or intracytoplasmic sperm injection. Andrologia. 2012;44(2):73-7.
12. Pregl Breznik B, Kovačič B, Vlaisavljević V. Are sperm DNA fragmentation, hyperactivation, and hyaluronan-binding ability predictive for fertilization and embryo development in in vitro fertilization and intracytoplasmic sperm injection? Fertil Steril. 2013;99:1233-41.
13. ESHRE Special Interest Group of Embryology, Alpha Scientists in Reproductive Medicine. The Vienna consensus: report of an expert meeting on the development of art laboratory performance indicators. Hum Reprod Open. 2017;2017(2):hox011.
14. Lu Z, Liu X, Zhang X, Leung C, Esfandiari N, Casper RF, et al. Automated robotic intracytoplasmic sperm injection. In: Nagy ZP, Varghese AC, Agarwal A (Eds.) Practical Manual of In Vitro Fertilization: Advanced Methods and Novel Devices. New York: Springer; 2012. pp. 353-9.
15. Hiraoka K, Kitamura S. Clinical efficiency of Piezo-ICSI using micropipettes with a wall thickness of 0.625 μm. J Assist Reprod Genet. 2015;32:1827-33.
16. Kilani S, Cooke S, Chapman M. Time course of meiotic spindle development in MII oocytes. Zygote. 2011;19:55-62.
17. Montag M, Schimming T, van der Ven H. Spindle imaging in human oocytes: the impact of the meiotic cell cycle. Reprod Biomed Online. 2006;12:442-6.
18. Petersen CG, Oliveira JBA, Mauri AL, Massaro FC, Baruffi RLR, Pontes A, et al. Relationship between visualization of meiotic spindle in human oocytes and ICSI outcomes: a meta-analysis. Reprod Biomed Online. 2009;18:235-43.
19. Hiraoka K, Uchida N, Ishikawa T, Kawai K. Value of meiotic spindle imaging on fertilization and embryo development following human oocyte Piezo-ICSI. Fertil Reprod. 2022;4:26-31.
20. Fujii Y, Endo Y, Mitsuhata S, Hayashi M, Motoyama H. Evaluation of the effect of piezo-intracytoplasmic sperm injection on the laboratory, clinical, and neonatal outcomes. Reprod Med Biol. 2020;19:198-205.

21. Furuhashi K, Saeki Y, Enatsu N, Iwasaki T, Ito K, Mizusawa Y, et al. Piezo-assisted ICSI improves fertilization and blastocyst development rates compared with conventional ICSI in women aged more than 35 years. Reprod Med Biol. 2019;18:357-61.
22. Hiraoka K, Isuge M, Kamada Y, Kaji T, Suhara T, Kuga A, et al. Piezo-ICSI for human oocytes. J Vis Exp. 2021;(170).
23. Takeuchi S, Minoura H, Shibahara T, Shen X, Futamura N, Toyoda N. Comparison of piezo-assisted micromanipulation with conventional micromanipulation for intracytoplasmic sperm injection into human oocytes. Gynecol Obstet Invest. 2001;52:158-62.
24. Yanagida K, Katayose H, Yazawa H, Kimura Y, Konnai K, Sato A. The usefulness of a piezo-micromanipulator in intracytoplasmic sperm injection in humans. Hum Reprod. 1999;14:448-53.
25. Zander-Fox D, Lam K, Pacella-Ince L, Tully C, Hamilton H, Hiraoka K, et al. PIEZO-ICSI increases fertilization rates compared with standard ICSI: a prospective cohort study. Reprod Biomed Online. 2021;43(3):404-12.

CHAPTER 106

# Analysis of Fertilization

Shailaja Gada Saxena, Ritu Gada, Dhiraj Gada

## INTRODUCTION

History was created on July 25th 1978, when Louise Brown was born to John and Lesley Brown in United Kingdom through in vitro fertilization (IVF). Since then, the field of assisted reproductive technology (ART) has witnessed huge stride toward finding suitable, cost-effective, and easily acceptable treatment options for infertile couples. There have been several technological advances in the stimulation protocols, oocyte retrieval procedure, embryo culture, and transfer technique to improve the success rate in ART. Despite all these technological advances, the success of IVF still faces many obstacles, especially recurrent implantation failure and multiple pregnancies and its associated complications, which are mainly related to selection of appropriate embryos for implantation. There are many different techniques and approaches used worldwide for evaluation of fertilization and selection of best embryo for transfer. Most commonly used method is to assess the developmental potential and morphological characteristics of the gametes and the embryos. In addition, morphokinetic evaluation and time-lapse imaging have also been attempted by various IVF centers. However, studies have revealed that genetic studies of gametes and embryos reveal chromosomal aberrations, which in turn are an important factor in developmental arrest of preimplantation embryos and the concomitant higher implantation failures, and early first-trimester pregnancy losses. Genetic evaluation of the embryos can be done through preimplantation genetic diagnosis/screening (PGD/PGS). However, these studies are invasive in nature. Apart from these, evaluation of embryo metabolism through metabolomic profiling to assess the growth and viability potential of the embryo is another method, which has been attempted. This chapter focuses on various techniques used for analysis of fertilization and embryo selection.

## MORPHOLOGICAL EVALUATION OF GAMETES AND EMBRYOS

Morphological evaluation of gametes and embryos currently is the most easily available and widely used method for embryo selection, with the advantage that it is cost-effective and can be easily implemented in all ART laboratories. However, this technique has its inherent drawbacks. The visual grading of embryos is static and requires training and is best carried out by experienced embryologists. Being a subjective assessment, accuracy is always questionable. The morphological evaluation can be carried out at various stages of embryo development right from the gamete stage to the blastocyst stage.

### Evaluation of the Quality of Gametes

The impact of assessment of the gamete quality and the success of the treatment has not been well established. However, oocyte quality affects the pronucleus (PN) stage and early cleavage-stage embryo development. Abnormalities in the form of shape, color of cytoplasm, size of polar body (PB), and perivitelline space affect the viability and developmental potential of embryos.[1] Recent studies have shown that the morphology and structure of the zona pellucida can also be considered as a predictor of oocyte quality and embryos.[2] Likewise, sperm quality also affects the early 4–8-cell stage embryo development when the embryonic genome is activated.[3]

### Evaluation of Pronucleus-stage Embryos

Scott and Smith (1998) and Tessarik et al. (2000) had developed assessment of pronuclear morphology, a pronuclear scoring system, Embryo development markers as well as patients status determine the number of resulting good quality embryos. Successful fertilization is visible as early as 4–5 hours post insemination. Various groups have attempted various scoring system. Pronuclear stage embryos are evaluated at 16–18 hours after fertilization. The key parameters monitored at this stage include pronuclei (size and symmetry), nucleoli (size, number, and distribution), and cytoplasmic appearance.[4-7] Presence of two fully formed PN, two PB and an intact zona pellucida is an indicator of proper fertilization. Fertilization failure is when there is absence of pronuclei and presence of only one PB, whereas presence of two or more pronuclei and two PB suggest polyspermy.[8] Pronuclear morphology is also considered as an indicator of embryo development. Failure of the two pronuclei to become completely opposed is an abnormality. Other features such as position of the second PB in relation to the first as well as the position of the polar bodies in relation to axis of the pronuclei has also been evaluated as an indicator for embryo quality.[9] In a retrospective study carried out by Balaban et al. (2001), they concluded that ideal pronuclear score was associated with better quality embryos both at cleavage stage and blastocyst stage, which are demonstrated by higher implantation potential.[10]

## Evaluation of Cleavage Stage Embryos

The second criterion of assessment is the cleavage stage at 23–27 hours after insemination. The criteria evaluated at this stage of embryo development include the rate of cell division in blastomeres, their shape and size, the cytoplasmic features in terms of vacuoles and granularity, the thickness of the zona pellucida, etc. If the embryo has two blastomeres present at this stage, it is labeled as an early cleavage embryo.

Giorgetti et al. (1995) suggest evaluation of embryo morphology 48 hours after insemination, when the embryos that have cleaved, have no fragmentation or irregularities, and have reached the 4-cell stage are considered to have the best potential for implantation.[11] On the other hand, Lucinda Veeck has laid down embryo grading on day 3 based on the size of the blastomere and fragmentation. **Table 1** gives the details of the scoring pattern as per Veeck et al. (1991).[12] Several other scoring systems have been proposed by different groups.

Fisch et al. (2001) introduced the concept of graduated embryo score (GES).[13] They recommended scoring of the embryos successively at 16–18 hours, 25–27 hours, and 64–67 hours postinsemination, respectively. They are given an aggregate score out of 100 as detailed in **Table 2**. An aggregate score >70 was found to be associated with 30% implantation rate, whereas the implantation rate dropped down to 24%, if the total score was <65.

**TABLE 1:** Cleavage stage embryo scoring (Day 3).

| *Grade* | *Description* |
|---|---|
| Grade 1 | Embryo with blastomeres of equal size, no cytoplasmic fragments |
| Grade 2 | Embryo with blastomeres of equal size, minor cytoplasmic fragments or blebs |
| Grade 3 | Embryo with blastomeres of distinctly equal size, none or few cytoplasmic fragments |
| Grade 4 | Embryo with blastomeres of equal or unequal size, significant cytoplasmic fragmentation |
| Grade 5 | Embryo with blastomeres of any size, severe or complete fragmentation |

*Source:* Adapted from Veeck LL. Atlas of the human oocyte and early conceptus. Baltimore: Williams and Wilkins; 1991. pp. 427-44.

## Evaluation of Blastocyst (Figs. 1 to 6)

From the morula, the embryo develops into a blastocyst and undergoes the first cell-fate division forming two layers the trophoblast and inner cell mass. Blastocyst stage embryo transfer has been shown to be associated with improved pregnancy rate, as it helps in natural selection of embryo, eliminating cleavage stage embryos without implantation potential. However, some studies have reported that the success of blastocyst transfer depends on the quality of early cleavage-stage embryos.[14] In addition, growing embryos in

**TABLE 2:** Graduated embryo score.

| *Evaluation* | *Hours after insemination* | *Developmental milestone* | *Score* |
|---|---|---|---|
| 1 | 16–18 | Nucleoli aligned | 20 |
| 2 | 25–27 | Cleavage regular and symmetrical | 30 |
| | | Fragmentation absent | 30 |
| | | Fragmentation <20% | 25 |
| | | Fragmentation >20% | 0 |
| 3 | 64–67 | Cell number and grade | 20 |
| | | 7, I; 8, I; 8, II; 9, I | |
| | | 7, II; 9, II; 10, I; 11, I; compacting I | 10 |
| | | Total score | 100 |

*Source:* Adapted from Fisch JD, Rodriguez H, Ross R, Overby G, Sher G. The Graduated Embryo Score (GES) predicts blastocyst formation and pregnancy rate from cleavage-stage embryos. Hum Reprod. 2001;16:1970-5.

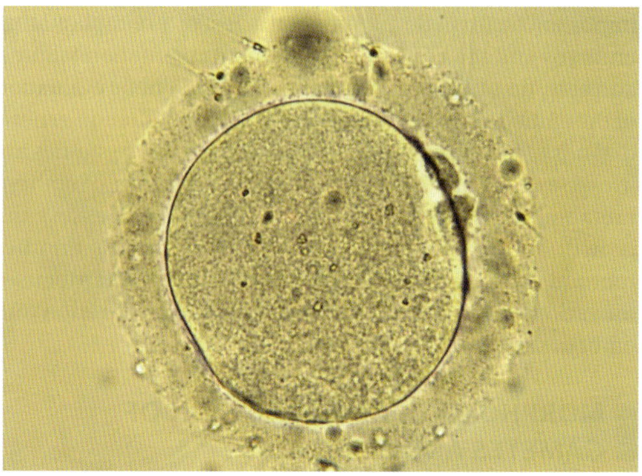

**Fig. 1:** A oocyte depicting 0PN after ICSI and two polar bodies separated distinctly.

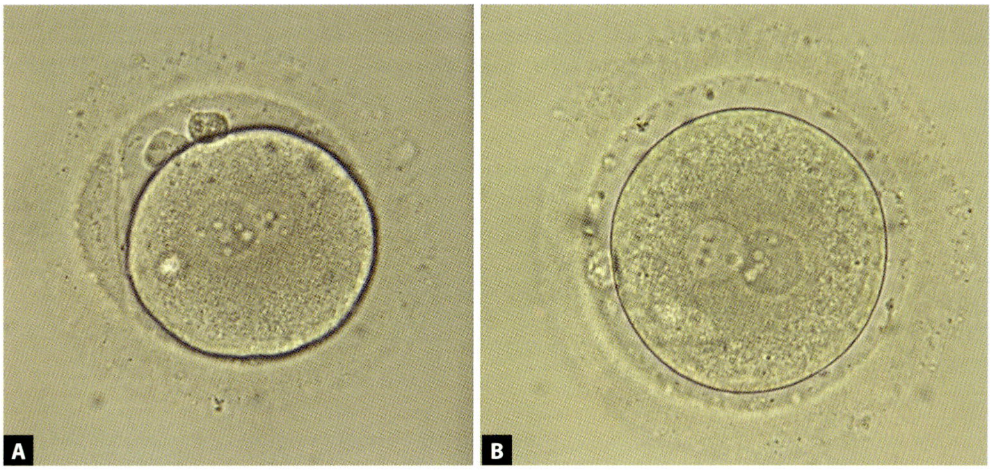


**Figs. 2A and B:** A zygote checked 16.5 h post-ICSI, having PNs with scattered NPBs with two visible polar bodies (400X magnification). The zona pellucida (ZP) appears regular; minimal debris is present in the perivitelline space (PVS) and the cytoplasm is homogeneous.

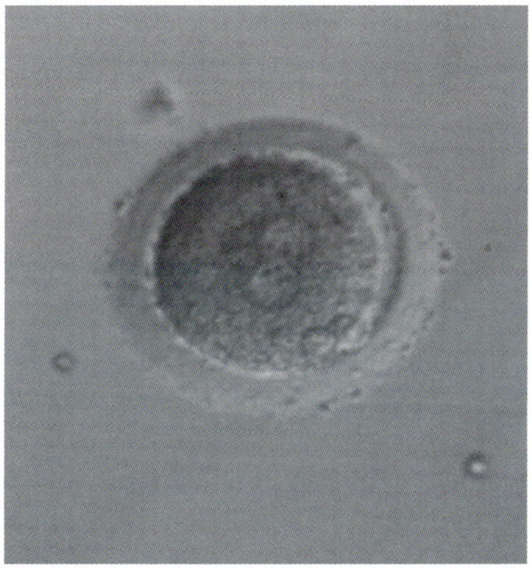

**Fig. 3:** A zygote produced by ICSI with NPBs exactly aligned at the junction of centrally located and juxtaposed PNs (400X magnification). Fragmented polar bodies are in the longitudinal axis of the PNs. PVS appears to include debris.

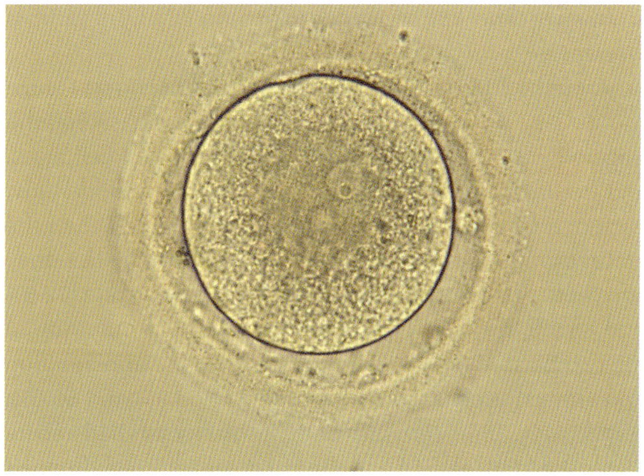

**Fig. 4:** A zygote 17 h post-ICSI depicting a single PN with an NPB (bull's eye) and two polar bodies.

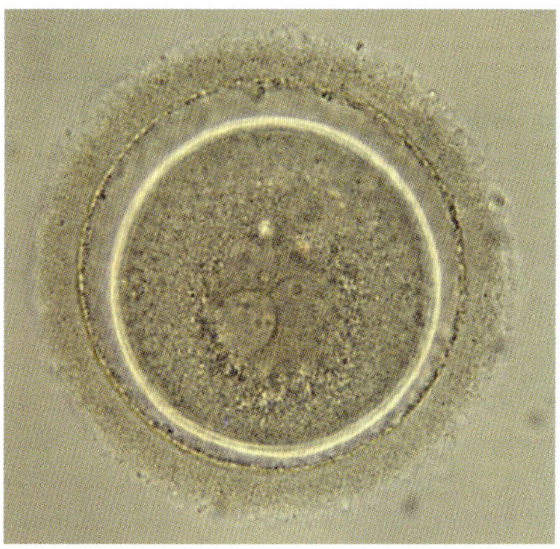

**Fig. 5:** A zygote displaying 3PNs with small-sized NPBs (400X magnification). One of the three PNs is slightly greater in size than the other two. The zygote was produced by ICSI.

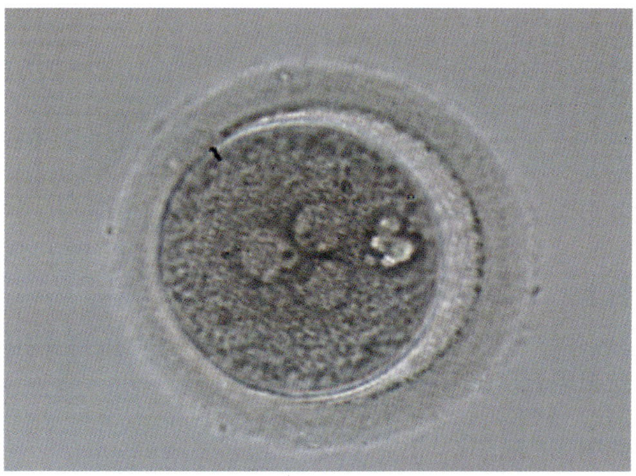

**Fig. 6:** A zygote formed by ICSI displaying three PNs of approximately the same size.

**TABLE 3:** Scoring of blastocyst.

| *Expansion and hatching* | | *Inner cell mass (ICM) score* | | *Trophectoderm (TE) score* | |
|---|---|---|---|---|---|
| 1. | Blastocoel cavity less than half the volume of the embryo | A | Many cells, tightly packed | A | Many cells, forming a cohesive layer |
| 2. | Blastocoel cavity more than half the volume of the embryo | B | Several cells, loosely grouped | B | Few cells, forming a loose epithelium |
| 3. | Full blastocyst, cavity completely filling the embryo | C | Very few cells | C | Very few large cells |
| 4. | Expanded blastocyst, cavity larger than the embryo, with thinning of the shell | | | | |
| 5. | Hatching out of the shell | | | | |
| 6. | Hatched out of the shell | | | | |

*Source:* Adapted from Gardner DK, Lane M, Stevens J, Schlenker T, Schoolcraft WB. Blastocyst score affects implantation and pregnancy outcome: towards a single blastocyst transfer. Fertil Steril. 2000;73(6):1155-8.

vitro to blastocyst stage may be associated with inherent problem of cancelled cycles due to nonavailability of embryo for transfer.

A method for grading embryos at the blastocyst stage was devised by Gardner et al. (2000), which is based on the stage of blastocyst development, quality of inner cell mass, and trophectoderm as detailed in **Table 3.**[15] In their study, each patient received transfer of two blastocyst. When the embryo grade of both the embryos was more than 3AA, they have better implantation and clinical pregnancy rate (72.8% and 86.5%, respectively). When the score of only one of the two blastomeres was more than 3AA, the implantation and clinical pregnancy rate dropped to 54.3% and 69.6%, respectively. Similarly, when both the blastocysts had a score <3AA, the implantation and clinical pregnancy rate dropped further to 28.1% and 43%, respectively.

## TIME-LAPSE IMAGING

Time-lapse monitoring (TLM) helps in identification the morphokinetics of cultured oocytes as well as embryos, and it can majorly prevent missed PN observations by enabling the continuous observation of the oocyte morphology as well as PN appearance. The above listed methods of embryos selection are based on observing the embryo morphology at different time points, which is subjective and static evaluation. The training of the embryologist and interpersonal variations in grading are likely to be present. In addition, embryos thus chosen are based on the growth at various fixed time points of development, which may not necessarily always be informative of various cellular events and kinetic events occurring between any two observations. This is likely to be one important reason that the technological developments for assessing embryo competence have not been able to translate into corresponding increase in implantation and pregnancy rates. In addition, removing the embryos from the incubators once per day or at fixed time intervals to assess the morphology and development, disturbs the embryo development as there is change in the temperature, pH, and carbon dioxide levels, which may be harmful.

Time-lapse technology offers a solution to many of problem listed earlier, as it allows embryos to be monitored dynamically in their controlled culture environment.[16] This newly developed technology allows monitoring of the embryos throughout the developmental stages without removing them from the incubator repeatedly. This automated technology eases the work of the embryologist and also aids in selection of embryo with maximum implantation potential, as it provides more information on the correlation of morphological development to embryo viability. Various time-lapse techniques are currently used of which the three available systems currently used in the clinical practice include Primo Vision, EmbryoScope, and Eeva. These systems take image of the embryo at fixed time intervals, which can then be converted to a video for the ease of viewing. The EmbryoScope is compact incubator with an in-built camera, while the Eeva and Primo Vision systems consist of only the camera, which is placed in the regular incubator. Since, EmbryoScope and Primo Vision use bright-field imaging, they are useful for assessing both the morphology of the embryo and the associated kinetic event.

On the other hand, Eeva uses dark-field imaging and is thus, not good for assessing the embryo morphology. All systems need the embryos to be cultured in microwell dishes and necessarily require an oil overlay.[17] The advantage of this technique is that the embryos are not exposed to repeat changes in the environmental milieu in terms of gas composition, pH, or temperature shifts, or to the movements as needed for periodic embryo evaluated.[18] Another major advantage is that this technique gives information about additional developmental morphokinetic changes, i.e,. by analyzing their complex patterns of cell division and cell movement and phenotypic markers as against the standard and static morphological grading.

It has known earlier cleaving embryos have a better chance of developing into blastocysts.[19] In a retrospective time-lapse video observational study conducted by Meseguer et al. (2011), they observed that direct cleavage from 1 to 3 cells, presence of unequal sized blastomeres at the 2-cell stage and multinucleation at the 4-cell stage were associated with low implantation potential and they suggest to exclude these embryos from the selection process for embryo transfer.[20] On the other hand, embryos reaching 5-cell stage by 48.8–56.6 hours, time for 3–4- cell division of <76 hours and that of two to three division of <11.9 hours, have maximum chance of implantation and hence should be included in the selection criteria for embryo transfer. A randomized controlled trial (RCT) conducted by Rubio et al. (2014) that monitoring of embryo using time-lapse monitoring was associated with an improved the implantation potential and ongoing pregnancy rates and reduced abortion rate.[21]

## METABOLOMICS

Another method of embryo selection is based on metabolomic profiling of embryo. This involves testing of the culture media using various techniques. Alteration in pyruvate and/or glucose concentration in the culture medium has been attempted to predict the energy metabolism of the embryo.[22,23] It is believed that oxygen consumption and amino acid turnover may be more accurate indicators of viability of the embryo. Many metabolic parameters of developing embryos have been studied using a variety of noninvasive methods.[24] Various studies have been conducted to evaluate the differences in metabolomics profile of embryos that result in a pregnancy in contrast to the embryos that do not result in pregnancy, with a focus on studying the pyruvate, carbohydrate, and amino acid metabolism. Gardner et al. (2001) suggested that better pyruvate uptake on day 4 is associated with more chances that the embryo will develop to blastocyst. Studies have also demonstrated that similar to pyruvate, the capacity of embryo to metabolize glucose increases significantly, as the embryo progresses to blastocyst from the morula stage. Thus, increased glucose metabolism capacity also reflects better developmental potential and viability. However, other studies have not been able to conclusively prove correlation between glucose uptake or the role of pyruvate uptake to blastocyst development or as a predictor for embryo development and viability.[25] Brison et al. (2004) evaluated the changes in concentration of amino acids (glycine, leucine, and asparagine) and noted that embryos with greater viability have a lower amino acid metabolism compared to the embryos that arrest.[26]

Various different technologies have been tried to evaluate the different analytes in the culture medium. However, widespread use of metabolomics in clinical setting has remained limited due to need of complex equipment and dedicated staff to carry out the assay trained in using the special equipment. Also in some cases, the testing is cumbersome and results may not be available in the limited timeframe of an IVF cycle to allow fresh embryo transfer.

## PREIMPLANTATION GENETIC DIAGNOSIS/SCREENING

Morphological evaluation of embryos requires expertise. Yet, as discussed earlier, it is not always accurate as many times embryos labeled as low grade on morphological evaluation have shown to have high-developmental potential. Chromosomal aberrations occur due to errors in meiosis and mitosis both at the time of formation of the gamete and during embryonic development. These chromosomal aberrations are a major obstacle to achieving a healthy pregnancy. Preimplantation genetic diagnosis (PGD) involves testing the embryo for a specific genetic condition likely to be inherited from the parents to the offspring, while preimplantation genetic screening (PGS) is used to screen the embryo prior to implantation for any chromosomal aberrations, i.e., for establishing chromosomal normalcy. PGS, thus, seems to be a logical step for evaluating the embryo quality. For PGS, the embryos are subjected to biopsy, which can be performed at different stages of embryo development. The commonly used techniques include PB biopsy from unfertilized and fertilized oocytes,[27-29] blastomere biopsy from day 3 cleavage-stage embryos[30,31] and trophectoderm biopsy from blastocyst stage embryos.[32,33] The genetic testing can then be performed on the cell thus obtained. Fluorescence in situ hybridization (FISH) and polymerase chain reaction (PCR) are the two commonly used first-generation technologies in PGD. Generally, PCR-based methods are used for DNA-based analysis for monogenic disorders and FISH is used for numerical and structural chromosomal aberrations. In recent times, these first generation tests are being replaced by more advanced tests such as comparative genomic hybridization (CGH), microarrays, array CGH (a-CGH), next generation sequencing (NGS), single nucleotide polymorphism (SNP) array, etc.

The classical form of PGS involved removal of one or two blastomeres from day 3 embryo and analysis of this cell by FISH for aneuploidies, for a limited number of chromosomes helping in selection of euploid embryos.[34] Initial studies using FISH testing on cleavage stage embryos revealed favorable ongoing pregnancy rate with PGS, but the later studies could not reproduce the results.[35] The increase in the number of chromosomes analyzed using FISH from routine 9 chromosomes to 15 aneuploid embryos, however, it showed a marked increase in the number of mosaic embryos.[36] The reason for low success using single-cell preimplantation FISH testing includes technical limitations like overlapping FISH signals, hybridization failure, nonspecific hybridization, and errors in interpretation. Other problems associated with FISH include mosaicism. Additionally in routine FISH testing, only 33% of chromosomes are tested, thus missing out on aneuploidy for the remaining chromosomes.

In an attempt to overcome the pitfalls associated with FISH based using carried on day 3 embryos, newer methods to determine the ploidy status of a single cell are developed, such as CGH, a-CGH, and SNP arrays.[37] In addition, to avoid the confounding effects of chromosomal mosaicism, PB biopsy and blastocyst biopsy have gained popularity.[38] CGH and a-CGH have gained more popularity in testing of all 24 chromosomes simultaneously in the same assay. The technique reveals gains or losses of genome segments, which may be related to a chromosomal segment or the entire chromosome by picking up changes in the hybridization ratio of target to control.[39,40] The advantage of the a-CGH over FISH is that preclinical validation is not required.[41] Like any technique, this technique is also associated with some inherent drawbacks. a-CGH fails to detect balanced chromosomal rearrangements or the ploidy status of the embryo.[42] SNP arrays and NGS are also commonly used for PGS.

The cost-effectiveness of PGS has always been a topic of controversy, as the technologies used for establishing the diagnosis are currently expensive. However, we need to keep in mind that the technique overall has cost-effective result, as it potentially helps to reduce the number of ART cycles plus it enables single embryo transfer[43-46] and helps to lower miscarriage rates.

## CONCLUSION

The test for a successful IVF cycle is successful implantation and pregnancy. In IVF, the selection of embryos for transfer is generally based on the morphology of the available embryos, which has been attempted at various stages of embryo development starting with assessing the quality of gamete and going up to the blastocyst stage. Each laboratory has their own algorithms for the same. Time-lapse imaging holds promise for aiding the embryologist in determining which embryos are most suitable for transfer, as it gives dynamic information about the embryo through various stages of cell division. Various groups have tried this technique with variable success. Hence, the adoption any new technique for selection of embryo or to analyze fertilization should be based on thorough scientific evaluation and validation in clinical scenario. Evaluation of numerous metabolic markers at various stages of embryo development to evaluate their development and implantation potential has also been attempted by many groups with limited success in clinical scenario in view of the time required for reporting of the results. Testing methodologies, which are less cumbersome and have better turnaround time, can help to improve the area of metabolomics. Apart from these noninvasive methods of embryo selection, the quest for selection on chromosomally normal embryo has led to introduction of PGS. This technology has seen various advances in the form of better test modalities. Hence, analysis of fertilization in selection of the best embryo continues to remain a challenging task with more and more ongoing research in this area to improve the success rate with IVF.

## REFERENCES


1. Alikani M, Palermo G, Adler A, Bertoli M, Blake M, Cohen J. Intracytoplasmic sperm injection in dysmorphic human oocytes. Zygote. 1995;3(4):283-8.
2. Shi W, Xu B, Wu L, Jin RT, Luan HB, Luo LH, et al. Oocytes with a Dark Zona pellucida demonstrate lower fertilization and clinical pregnancy rates. PLOS One. 2014;9(2):e89409.
3. Alvarez Sedó C, Bilinski M, Lorenzi D, Uriondo H, Noblía F, Longobucco V, et al. Effect of sperm DNA fragmentation on embryo development: clinical and biological aspects. JBRA Assist Reprod. 2017;21(4):343-50.
4. Brezinova J, Oborna I, Svobodova M, Fingerova H. Evaluation of day one embryo quality and IVF outcome—a comparison of two scoring systems. Reprod Biol Endocrinol. 2009;7:9.
5. Scott LA, Smith S. The successful use of pronuclear embryo transfers the day following oocyte retrieval. Hum Reprod. 1998;13:1003-13.
6. Senn A, Urner F, Chanson A, Primi MP, Wirthner D, Germond M. Morphological scoring of human pronuclear zygotes for prediction of pregnancy outcome. Hum Reprod. 2005;21(1):234-9.
7. Tesarik J, Greco E. The probability of abnormal preimplantation development can be predicted by a single static observation on pronuclear stage morphology. Hum Reprod. 1999; 14:1318-23.
8. Flaherty SP, Payne D, Swann NJ, Matthews CD. Assessment of fertilization failure and abnormal; fertilization after intracytoplasmic sperm injection. Reprod Fertil Dev. 1995;7(2):197-210.
9. Gardner DK, Lane M, Stevens J, Schoolcraft WB. Noninvasive assessment of human embryo nutrient consumption as a measure of developmental potential. Fertil Steril. 2001; 76:1175- 80.
10. Balaban B, Urman B, Isiklar A, Alatas C, Aksoy S, Mercan R, et al. The effect of pronuclear morphology on embryo quality parameters and blastocyst outcome. Hum Reprod. 2001;16(11):2357-61.
11. Giorgetti C, Terriou P, Auquier P, Hans E, Spach JL, Salzmann J, et al. Embryo score to predict implantation after in-vitro fertilization: based on 957 single embryo transfers. Hum Reprod. 1995;10: 2427-31.
12. Veeck LL. Atlas of the human oocyte and early conceptus. Baltimore: Williams and Wilkins; 1991. pp. 427-44.
13. Fisch JD, Rodriguez H, Ross R, Overby G, Sher G. The Graduated Embryo Score (GES) predicts blastocyst formation and pregnancy rate from cleavage-stage embryos. Hum Reprod. 2001;16:1970-5.

14. Wang SS, Sun HX. Blastocyst transfer ameliorates live birth rate compared with cleavage-stage embryos transfer in fresh in vitro fertilization or intracytoplasmic sperm injection cycles: reviews and meta-analysis. Yonsei Med J. 2014;55(3):815-25.
15. Gardner DK, Lane M, Stevens J, Schlenker T, Schoolcraft WB. Blastocyst score affects implantation and pregnancy outcome: towards a single blastocyst transfer. Fertil Steril. 2000;73(6):1155-8.
16. Cruz M, Garrido N, Herrero J, Ruberti A, Casciani V, Scarselli F, et al. Timing of cell divisions in human cleavage stage embryos correlates with blastocyst formation and quality. Reprod Biomed Online. 2012;25:371-81.
17. Racowsky C, Kovacs P, Martins WP. A critical appraisal of time-lapse imaging for embryo selection: where are we and where do we need to go? J Assist Reprod Genet. 2015;32(7):1025-30.
18. Armstrong S, Arroll N, Cree LM, Jordan V, Farquhar C. Time-lapse systems for embryo incubation and assessment in assisted reproduction. Cochrane Database Syst Rev. 2015; 27(2): CD011320.
19. Salumets A, Hydén-Granskog C, Mäkinen S, Suikkari AM, Tiitinen A, Tuuri T. Early cleavage predicts the viability of human embryos in elective single embryo transfer procedures. Hum Reprod. 2003;18(4):821-5.
20. Meseguer M, Herrero J, Tejera A, et al. The use of morphokinetics as a predictor of embryo implantation. Hum Reprod. 2011;10:2658-71.
21. Rubio I, Galan A, Larreategui Z, Ayerdi F, Bellver J, Herrero J, et al. Clinical validation of embryo culture and selection by morphokinetic analysis: a randomized, controlled trial of the EmbryoScope. Fertil Steril. 2014;102(5):1287-94.
22. Ajduk A, Zernicka-Goetz M. Advances in embryo selection methods. F1000 Biol Rep. 2012;4:11.
23. Gardner DK, Lane M, Stevens J, et al. Noninvasive assessment of human embryo nutrient consumption as a measure of developmental potential. Fertil Steril. 2001;76:1175-80.
24. Sakkas D, Gardner DK. Noninvasive methods to assess embryo quality. Curr Opin Obstet Gynecol. 2005;17(3):283-8.
25. Hardy K, Hooper MA, Handyside AH, Rutherford AJ, Winston RM, Leese HJ. Non-invasive measurement of glucose and pyruvate uptake by individual human oocytes and preimplantation embryos. Hum Reprod. 1989;4(2):188-91.
26. Brison DR, Houghton FD, Falconer D, Roberts SA, Hawkhead J, Humpherson PG, et al. Identification of viable embryos in IVF by non-invasive measurement of amino acid turnover. Hum Reprod. 2004;19(10):2319-24.
27. Montag M, van der Ven K, Dorn C, van der Ven H. Outcome of laser-assisted polar body biopsy. Reprod Biomed Online. 2004;9:425-9.
28. Munne S, Dailey T, Sultan KM, Grifo J, Cohen J. The use of first polar bodies for preimplantation diagnosis of anueuploidy. Hum Reprod. 1995;10(4):1014-20.
29. Verlinksy Y, Ginsberg N, Lifchez A, Valle J, Moise J, Strom CM. Analysis of the first polar body: preconception genetic diagnosis. Hum Reprod. 1990;5(7):826-9.
30. Boada M, Carrera M, De La Iglesia C, Sandalinas M, Barri PN, Veiga A. Successful use of a laser for human embryo biopsy in preimplantation genetic diagnosis: a report of two cases. J Assist Reprod Genet. 1998;15:302-7.
31. Joris H, De Vos A, Janssens R, Devroey P, Liebaers I, Van Steirteghem A. Comparison of the results of human embryo biopsy and outcome of PGD after zona drilling using acid Tyrode medium or a laser. Hum Reprod. 2003;18(9):1896-902.
32. Kokkali G, Vrettou C, Traeger-Synodinos J, Jones GM, Cram DS, Stavrou D, et al. Birth of a healthy infant following trophectoderm biopsy from blastocysts for preimplantation diagnosis of beta-thalassaemia major. Hum Reprod. 2005;20:1855-9.
33. Veiga A, Sandalinas M, Benkhalifa M, Boada M, Carrera M, Santaló J, et al. Laser blastocyst biopsy for preimplantation diagnosis in the human. Zygote. 1997;5:351-4.
34. Wilton L. Preimplantation genetic diagnosis for aneuploidy screening in early human embryos: a review. Prenat Diagn. 2002;22:512-8.
35. Mastenbroek S, Twisk M, Van Echten-Arends . Preimplantation genetic screening in women of advanced maternal age. N Engl J Med. 2007;357:9-17.
36. Baart EB, van den Berg I, Martini E, Eussen HJ, Fauser BC, Van Opstal D. FISH analysis of 15 chromosomes in human day 4 and 5 preimplantation embryos: the added value of extended aneuploidy detection. Prenat Diagn. 2007;27:55-63.
37. Wells D, Alfarawati S, Fragouli E. Use of comprehensive chromosomal screening for embryo assessment: microarrays and CGH. Mol Hum Reprod. 2008;14(12):703-10.
38. Geraedts J, Montag M, Magli MC, Repping S, Handyside A, Staessen C, et al. Polar body array CGH for prediction of the status of the corresponding oocyte. Part I: clinical results. Hum Reprod. 2009;26:3173-80.
39. Voullaire L, Slater H, Williamson R, Wilton L. Chromosome analysis of blastomeres from human embryos by using comparative genomic hybridization. Hum Genet. 2000; 106:210-7.
40. Wells D, Delhanty JD. Preimplantation genetic diagnosis: applications for molecular medicine. Trends Mol Med. 2001;7:23-30.
41. Fiorentino F, Spizzichino L, Bono S, Biricik A, Kokkali G, Rienzi L, et al. PGD for reciprocal and Robertsonian translocations using array comparative genomic hybridization. Hum Reprod. 2011;26:1925-35.
42. Harper JC, Harton G. The use of arrays in preimplantation genetic diagnosis and screening. Fertil Steril. 2010;94: 1173-7.
43. Polinder S, Heijnen E, Macklon N, Habbema JD, Fauser BJ, Eijkemans MJ.. Cost-effectiveness of a mild compared with a standard strategy for IVF: a randomized comparison using cumulative term live birth as the primary endpoint. Hum Reprod. 2008;23:316-23.
44. Chambers GM, Lee E, Hansen M, Hansen M, Sullivan EA, Bower C, et al. Hospital costs of multiple-birth and singleton-birth children during the first 5 years of life and the role of assisted reproductive technology. JAMA Pediatr. 2014;168:1045-53.
45. Depa-Martynow M, Jedrzejczak P, Pawelczyk L. Pronuclear scoring as a predictor of embryo quality in in vitro fertilization program. Histochem Cytobiol. 2007;45(Suppl 1):S85-9.
46. Kobayashi T, Ishikawa H, Ishii K, Sato A, Nakamura N, Saito Y, et al. Time-lapse monitoring of fertilized human oocytes focused on the incidence of 0PN embryos in conventional in vitro fertilization cycles. Sci Rep. 2021;11(1):18862.

CHAPTER 107

# Morphological Assessment of Oocyte and Embryo

*Vijay Mangoli, Ranjana Mangoli*

## INTRODUCTION

It is really fascinating to observe how male and female gametes unite together, transform themselves into beautiful embryos and one day, they come to you as a complete human being. While performing assisted reproductive technology (ART) procedures, these preimplanting embryos are with us for only 3–5 days. But even at this early stage, they are as unpredictable as toddlers. We have to pamper them with all their demands and day-to-day requirements to get best out of them. It is a period of rapid transition where foundations of all further embryonic growth are established. And apart from different stimulation protocols and laboratory techniques adapted, selecting best embryos plays crucial role in getting optimum results.[1]

Now, the million dollar question is—how to select an implantable embryo? And as of today, even after 44 years of human in vitro fertilization (IVF), there is no straight answer to this. The situation is complicated because even if the laboratory creates and selects a viable embryo, it requires an equally competent and receptive endometrium for a successful implantation. An embryo which is not implanted in one uterus might have implanted in another uterus but obviously one cannot transfer a single embryo in different uteri to test its implantation potential. We generally do not have choice of uterus, but we can select oocytes and embryos based upon certain morphological assessment and nuclear criteria.

Most commonly applied evaluation method is morphological selection because it is noninvasive, does not require any additional instruments, takes less time, and often—though not always—correlates with outcome. Recent times have seen methods of assessing oocytes and embryos through technical advances such as time-lapse monitoring, proteomics, and through genetic evaluation of blastomeres or trophectoderm cells as discussed in Section 17.

## OOCYTE

At birth, a baby girl has about two million oocytes in her ovaries. All these oocytes are arrested at the prophase of first meiotic division and they remain dormant until onset of puberty. During each menstrual cycle, one of these "sleeping beauties" is being kissed by "Prince" luteinizing hormone (LH), awakening it to continue its meiotic division. After completion of maturation, the oocyte is released into the fallopian tube and if it meets with the sperm, fertilization may occur. Though the whole process appears romantically simple, practically, not all the oocytes released are capable of getting fertilized. A large variation is seen in the sibling oocyte quality when retrieved after controlled ovarian stimulation.

These are some of the morphological aspects deciding potential of an oocyte to become a viable embryo:

- *Cellular and nuclear assessment:* Immediately after ovum pickup (OPU), oocyte can be grossly categorized as mature, immature, postmature, or atretic on the basis of cellular investments around it. A mature oocyte typically displays expanded cumulus with radiant or "sunburst" corona **(Figs. 1A and B)**. A densely packed cumulus-corona complex is generally associated with immaturity **(Figs. 2A to C)**. Loosely spreaded layers of cumulus with scanty corona indicate post maturity **(Figs. 3A and B)**, and one without any cellular investments indicates atretic oocyte **(Figs. 4A and B)**. Though this assessment closely approximates maturity status of oocytes, it can be imprecise and therefore it has to be co-assessed with nuclear status.
- *Size and shape of oocytes:* A mature, healthy meiosis II (MII) oocyte is spherical having diameter of about 120 µm. Rarely giant oocytes of >200 µm diameter with multiple polar bodies are observed which are generally associated with markedly reduced viability **(Fig. 5)**. Most giant oocytes are reported to be associated with aneuploidy.[2] Occasionally, elongated oocytes are retrieved which are usually result of increased aspiration pressure during OPU and do not exhibit altered fertilization, cleavage, or pregnancy rate **(Fig. 6)**.[3] Rarely, oocytes without zona are reported. Even such oocytes have potential to get

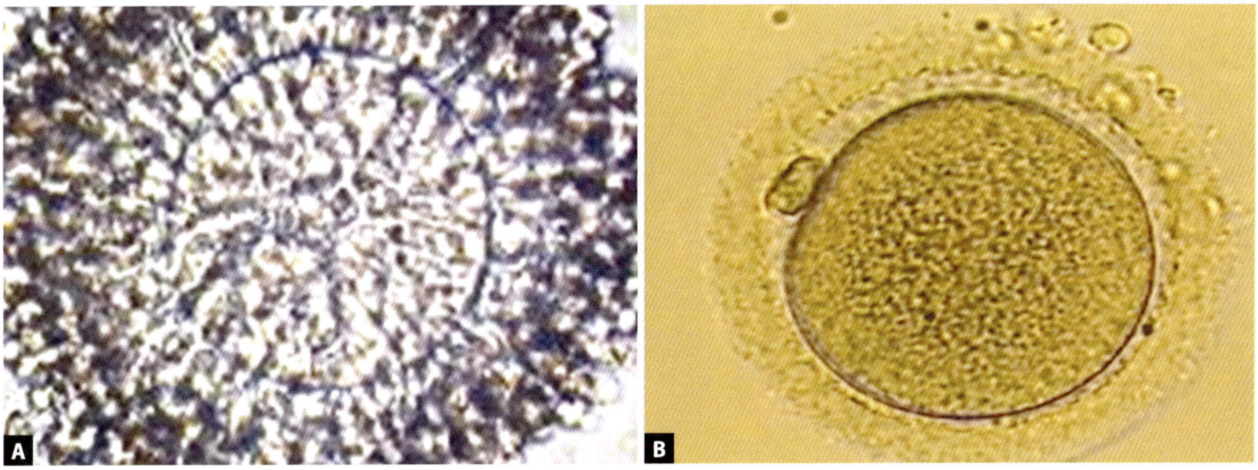

**Figs. 1A and B:** Mature oocyte.

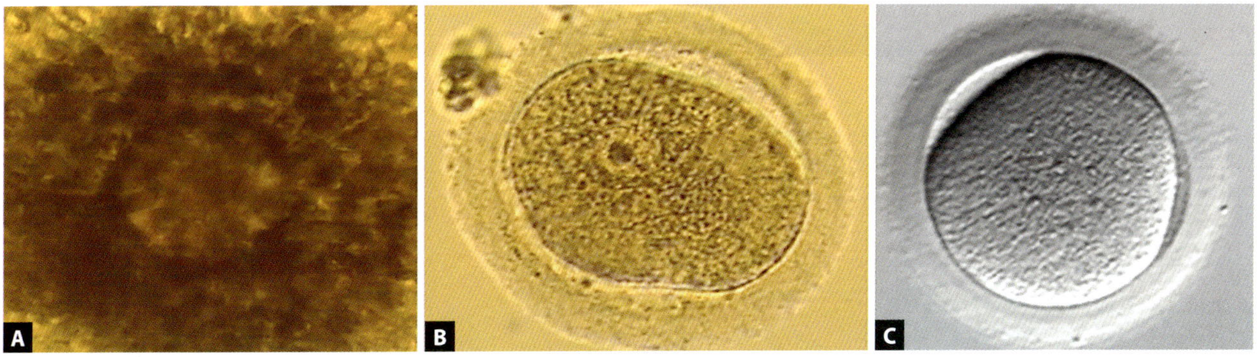

**Figs. 2A to C:** Immature oocyte. (A and B) Germinal vesicle; (C) Metaphase I oocyte.

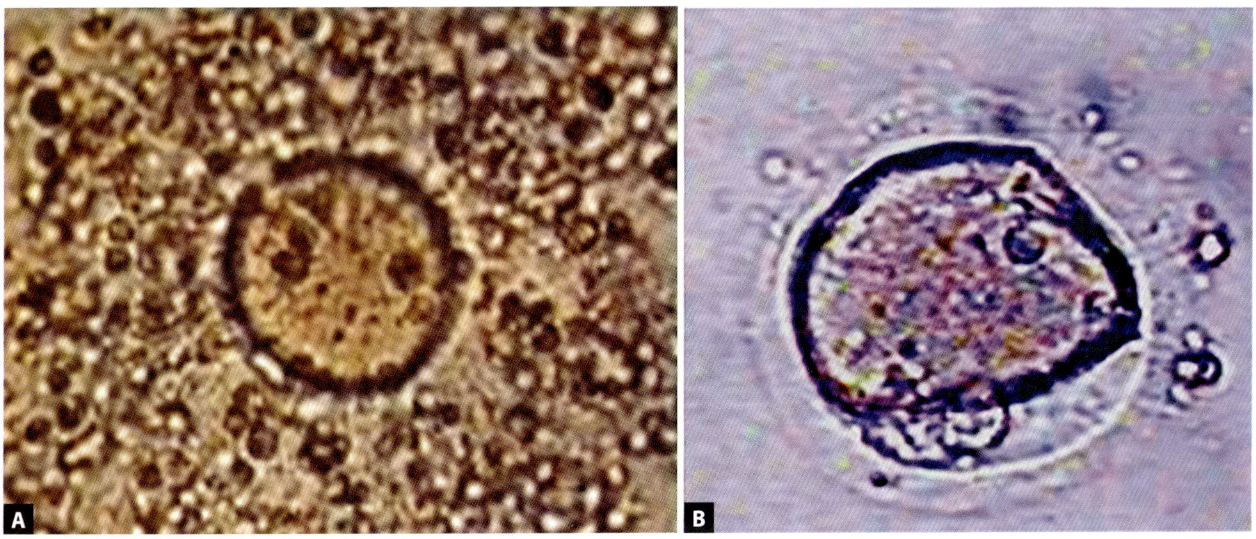

**Figs. 3A and B:** Postmature oocyte.

fertilized. They may display 2PN or polyploidy and are usually associated with hampered further embryonic growth.[4]

- *Zona pellucida (ZP):* It is a matrix of three intermediate filament proteins, ZP1, ZP2, and ZP3, laid down during folliculogenesis. ZP is a dynamic multifunctional structure at different stages of embryogenesis. At oocyte stage, it prevents polyspermy; at cleavage stage, it promotes selective permeability to maintain optimum concentration of nutrients; and at blastocyst stage, it thins out to facilitate hatching. A healthy zona is about 16–18 μm in width with a smooth, even, spongy, and

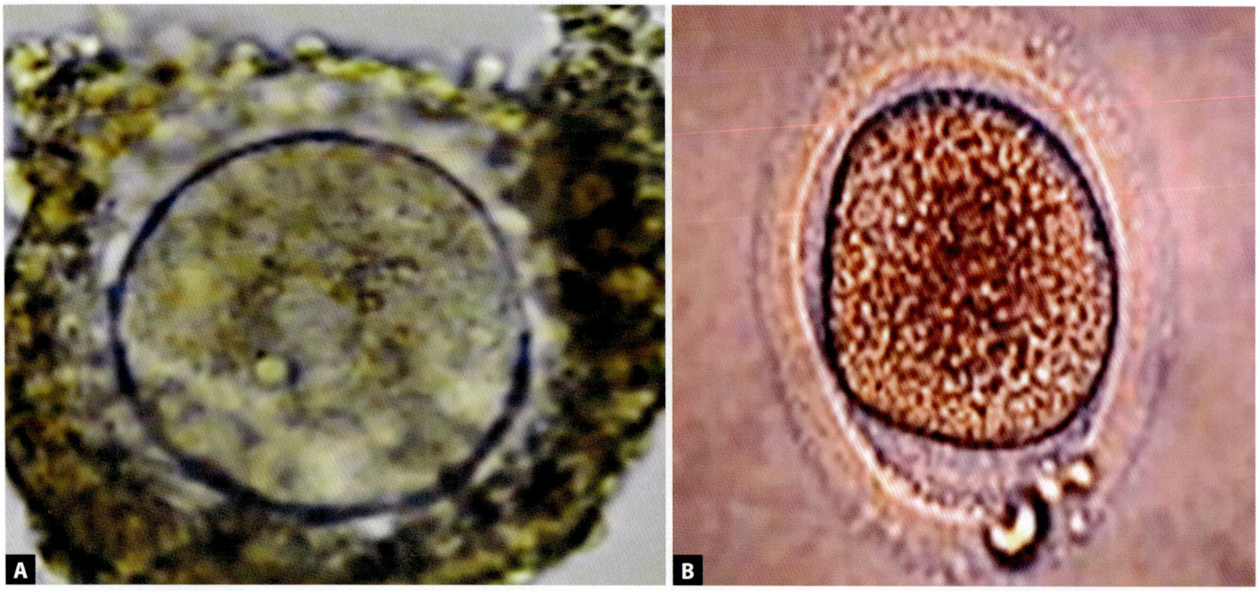


**Figs. 4A and B:** Atretic oocyte.

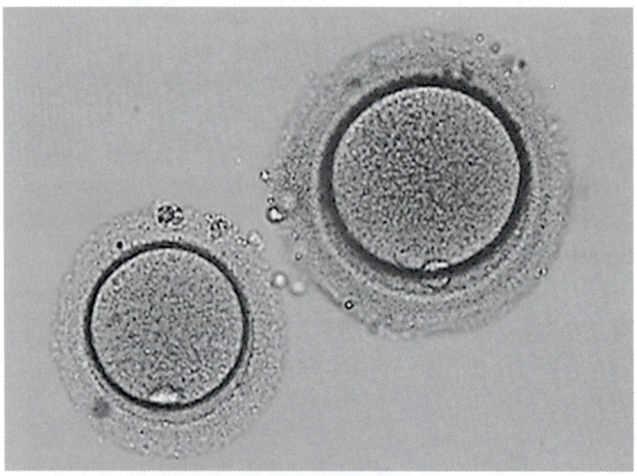

**Fig. 5:** Normal and giant oocytes.

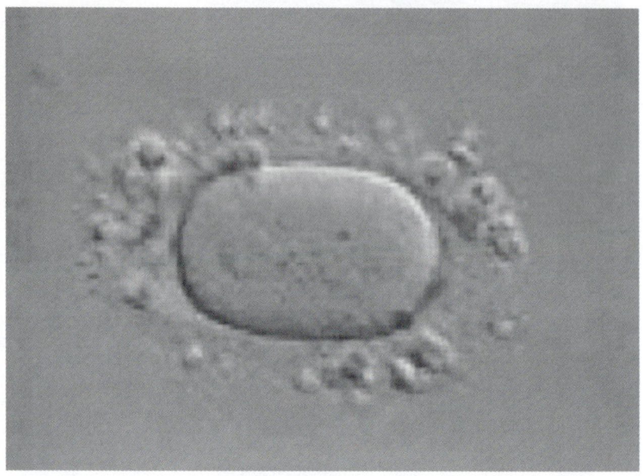

**Fig. 6:** Elongated oocyte.

flexible texture. Makiko et al. reported that the zona thickness in the range of 15–17 µm gives good fertilization rate with normal IVF using normozoospermic sample whereas, those with zona thickness between 17 and 21 µm results in drastically low fertilization rate. Those oocytes having zona thickness of >22 µm certainly requires intracytoplasmic sperm injection (ICSI). Such papers give us an idea about selecting mode of insemination to get good fertilization.[5] ZPs 2 and 3 also serve as receptors for sperm binding and help activate the sperm acrosome reaction **(Fig. 7)**. Sometimes oocytes with uneven zona are observed with controversial reports about their viability **(Fig. 8)**.

- *Cytoplasm:* A healthy oocyte displays translucent cytoplasm with evenly distributed fine granularity. It contains mitochondria, peroxisomes, endoplasmic reticulum, Golgi complex, vacuoles, and other organelles.

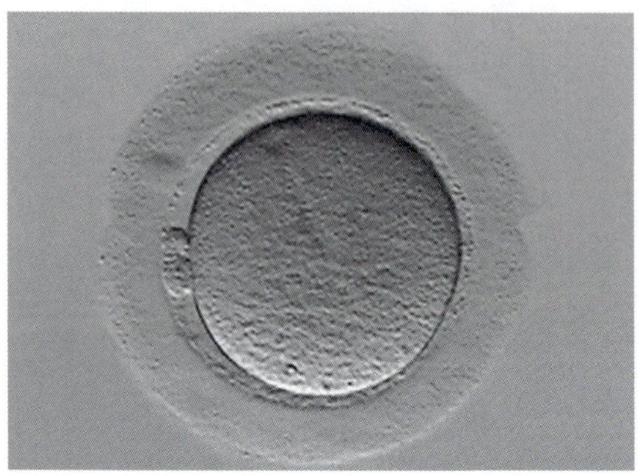

**Fig. 7:** Oocyte with thick zona.

Patchy or localized dark and granular cytoplasm has been associated with decreased fertilization, particularly in IVF, presumably related to atresia[6] **(Fig. 9)**.

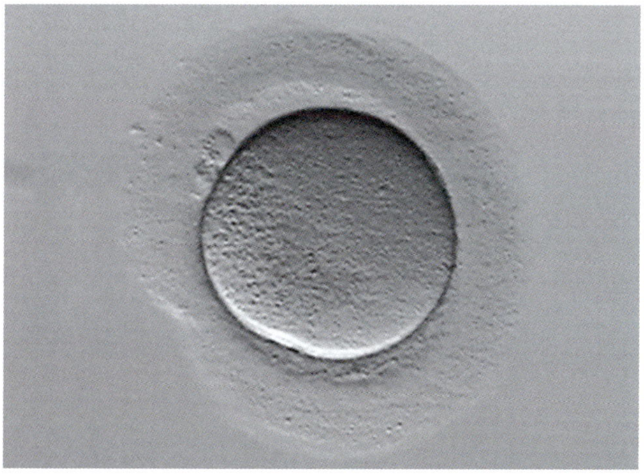

**Fig. 8:** Oocyte with uneven zona.

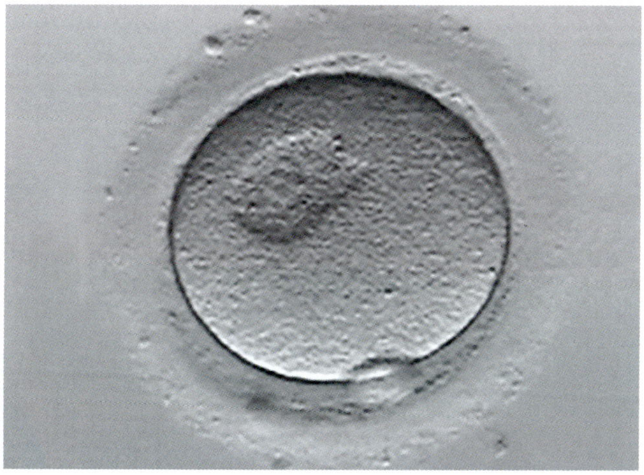

**Fig. 9:** Oocyte with eccentric granular ooplasm.

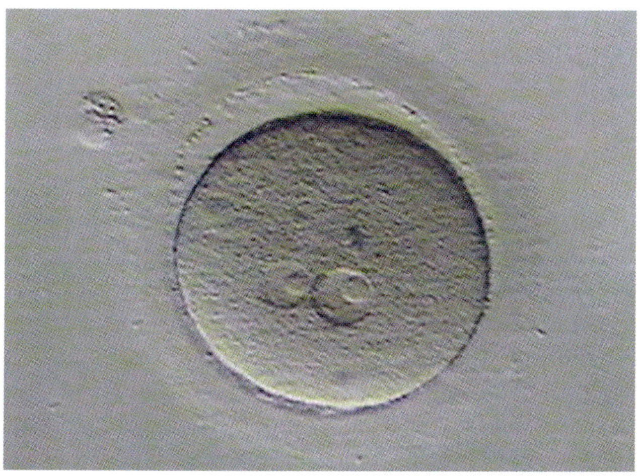

**Fig. 10:** Oocyte with two germinal vesicles.

Very rarely, an oocyte may display two germinal vesicles. Possible explanation for this is fusion of two primordial follicles during oogenesis resulting in creating single oocyte that shares common cytoplasm. Such oocytes do not have potential to continue maturation **(Fig. 10)**.

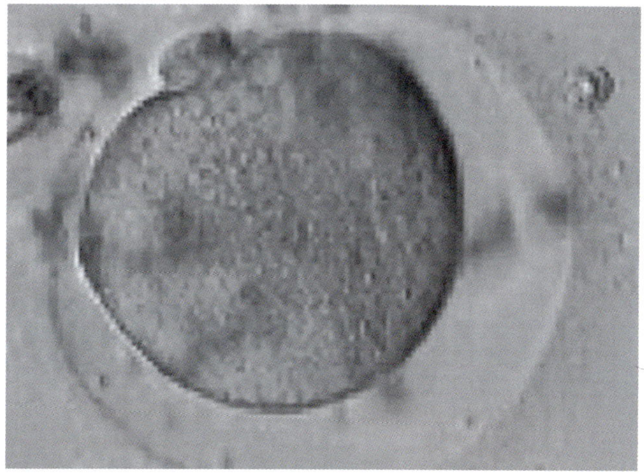

**Fig. 11:** Oocyte with large perivitelline space.

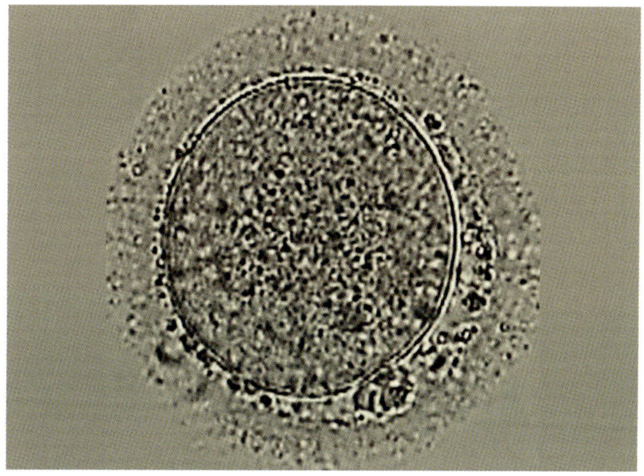

**Fig. 12:** Granules in perivitelline space.

- *Perivitelline space:* It is the space between the oolemma and ZP. Normally, the gap is almost invisible throughout the contact area, except near polar body. Occasionally, varying degree of gaps between the two is observed **(Fig. 11)**. Effect of such gap space has unclear effects on fertilization, preimplantation embryo development, and pregnancy rates. Granules may appear within this space, but they also do not appear to influence oocyte or embryo development.[7] Stimulation protocol can influence oocyte quality, e.g., exposure to high dosage of human menopausal gonadotropin (hMG) has been shown to be associated with granularity of the perivitelline space[8] **(Fig. 12)**.
- *Polar body:* Human chorionic gonadotropin (hCG) or the LH surge resumes meiosis, resulting in extrusion of the first polar body. The second polar body separates only after fertilization or activation. The timing of the first polar body extrusion varies among aspirated oocytes, presumably because of variations in the timing of meiotic maturation.[9]

Oocytes with incomplete cytokinesis, which leave the polar body attached to the oocyte, exhibit low fertilization

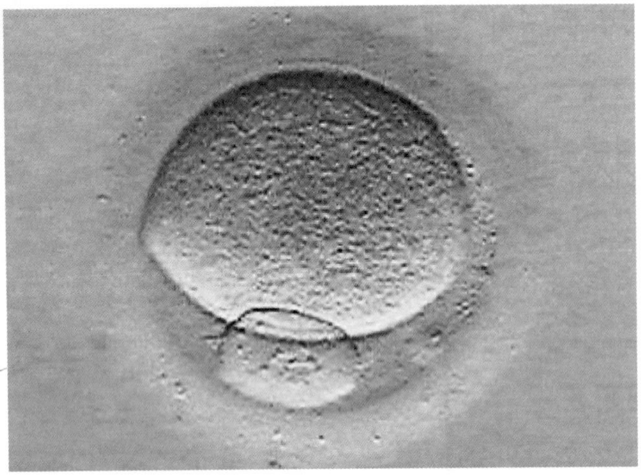

**Fig. 13:** Oocyte with large polar body.

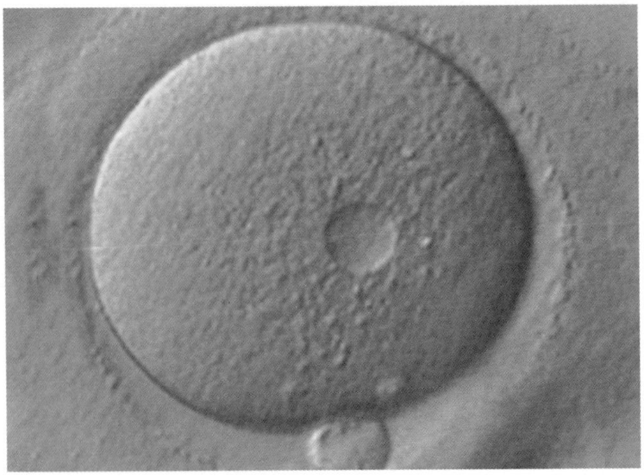

**Fig. 15:** Oocyte with vacuole.

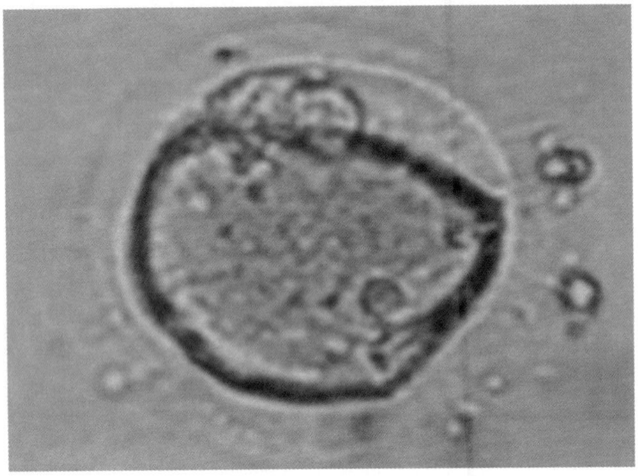

**Fig. 14:** Fragmented polar body.

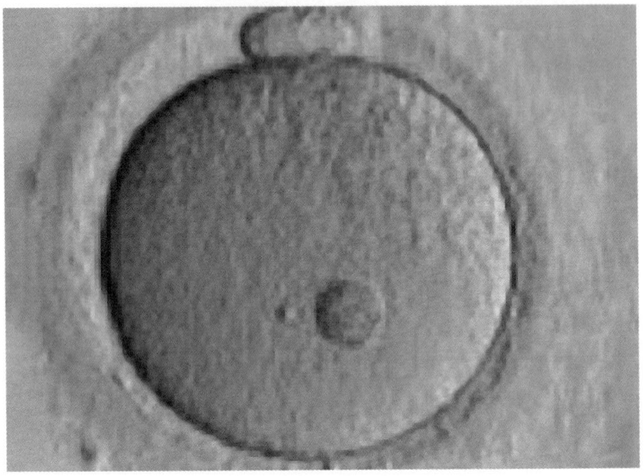

**Fig. 16:** Oocyte with refractile body.

and poor embryo cleavage rates, presumably because of their impaired meiotic competence.

A healthy oocyte has spherical or oval polar body. Occasionally, larger polar bodies are observed posing risk of aneuploidy, if inseminated **(Fig. 13)**. A fragmented polar body at OPU indicates postmature nature of the oocyte **(Fig. 14)**.

- *Vacuoles:* Some oocytes may display circular cytoplasmic inclusions either single or in clusters. Though their cellular basis is presumably of endocytotic origin, they are postulated to be associated with atresia with decreased fertilization rate and adversely affected cleavage pattern.[10] A few small, transparent, fluid-filled vacuoles (<5 μm diameter) are unlikely to be of consequence, whereas large vacuoles (>6 μm diameter) are associated with fertilization failure, and if fertilized, results in poor embryo development **(Fig. 15)**.
- *Refractile bodies:* These are dense, insoluble protein bodies that are produced within the cells presumably as a result of accumulated lipofuscin. They are called refractile bodies because their greater density (than the rest of the cell's body mass) causes light to be refracted (bent) when it is passed through them causing appearance of very bright and dark areas around them visible under a microscope. It is observed that refractile bodies are the single largest cause of failed fertilization even after ICSI[11] **(Fig. 16)**.
- *Smooth endoplasmic reticulum (sER):* It is an interconnected network of membranes without ribosomes. Normally, when evenly distributed, they are not prominently visible. When aggregated, they are visible either in small bunches, or seen as a large structure distinctly noticeable. Formation of sER is seen only in MII oocytes and is generally associated with high E2 levels. sER aggregation may be associated with early fetal demise and, in newborns, with certain imprinting disorders (e.g., Beckwith-Wiedemann syndrome)[12,13] **(Fig. 17)**.
- *Meiotic spindle:* Meiosis consists of two reduction steps. Meiosis I (MI), where homologous chromosomes

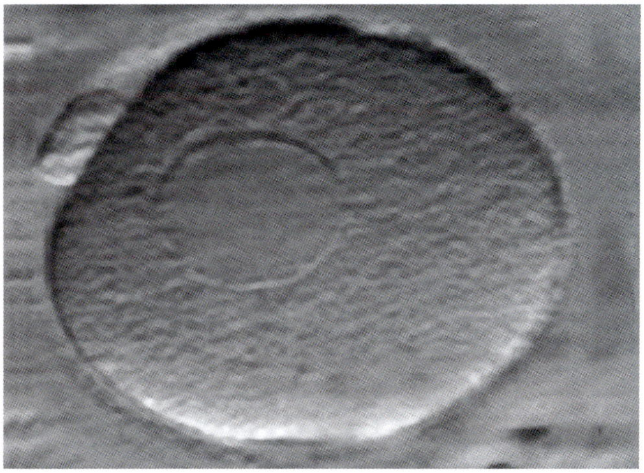

**Fig. 17:** Oocyte showing single cluster of aggregated smooth endoplasmic reticulum.

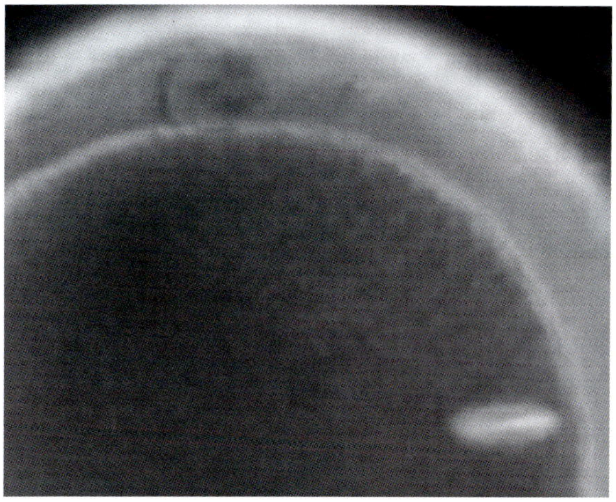

**Fig. 19:** Spindle away from polar body.

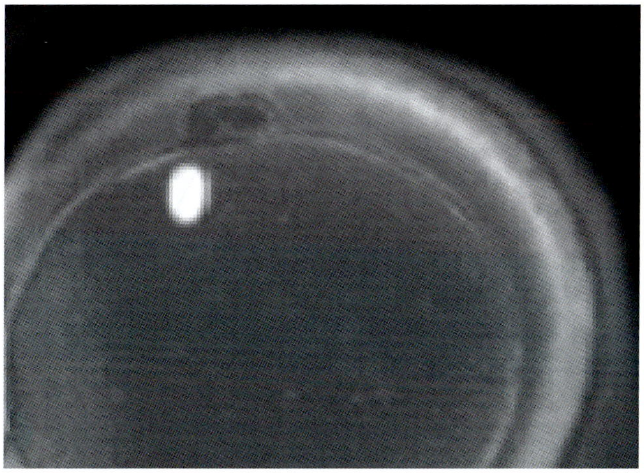

**Fig. 18:** Spindle near the polar body.

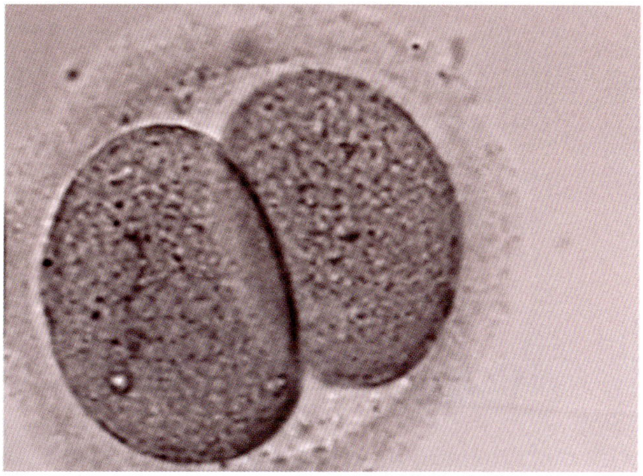

**Fig. 20:** Parthenogenetically activated oocyte.

separate, and metaphase II (MII), where chromatids separate. Mature oocytes are arrested in MII, with the MII spindle tethering chromatids, and a single extruded polar body. It is not possible to view meiotic spindle with commonly used contrasting systems like Hoffman modulation or differential interference contrast (DIC). However, they can be visualized using polarized microscopy because of a special property possessed by macromolecular tubules of spindle, called anisotropy.

Polscope helps to locate spindle in the oocyte. Though generally spindle is located near the first polar body **(Fig. 18)**, on some occasions, it is observed to be farther away from it **(Fig. 19)**. Under such circumstances, it is possible to disrupt it during ICSI.[14]

- *Parthenogenetically activated oocyte:* Occasionally, either immediately post-OPU or at the time of denudation, one can see oocyte with two to three blastomeres like structures. This can be a parthenogenetic activity caused due to excessive handling or sudden influx of $Ca^{++}$ during removal of cumulus corona investments around the oocyte. Insemination at this stage is not recommended due to increased probability of chromosomal imbalance in resulting embryo **(Fig. 20)**.

## ZYGOTE

A zygote is formed as a result of fertilization through sexual reproduction between two haploid cells—an ovum and a sperm. For a successful fertilization to occur, several events must follow in a disciplined manner, as under:

- Sperm penetration through cumulus oophorus
- Binding of sperm to the zona
- Sperm-oocyte fusion
- Oocyte activation
- Sperm nucleus decondensation nucleus
- Development and migration of male and female pronuclei
- Association of the parental chromosomes on spindle of first cleavage division.

Morphologically, optimal fertilized oocyte displays two spherical polar bodies and two centrally-located and

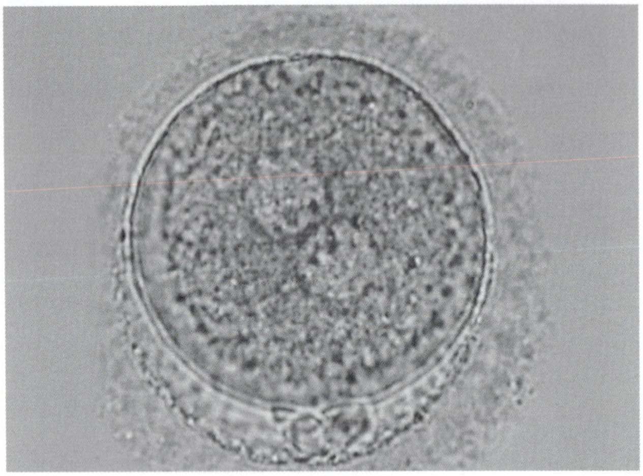

**Fig. 21:** Polarized zygote.

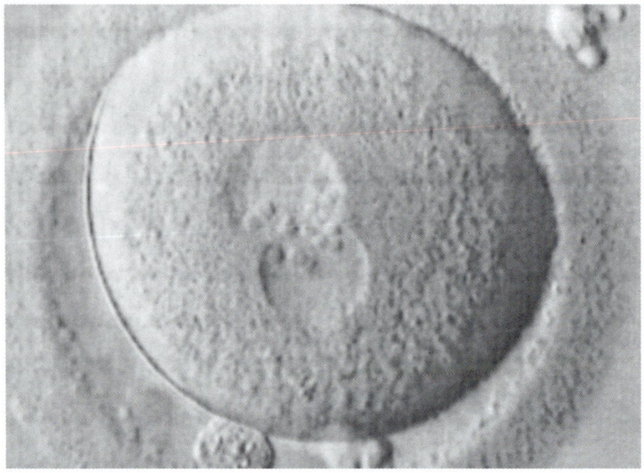

**Fig. 23:** Halo around pronuclei.

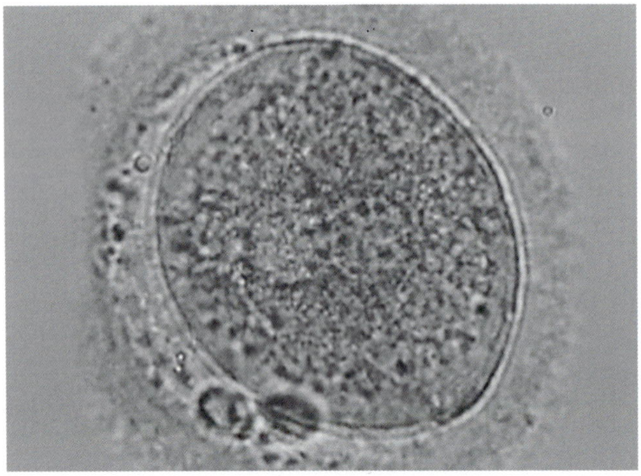

**Fig. 22:** Nonpolarized zygote.

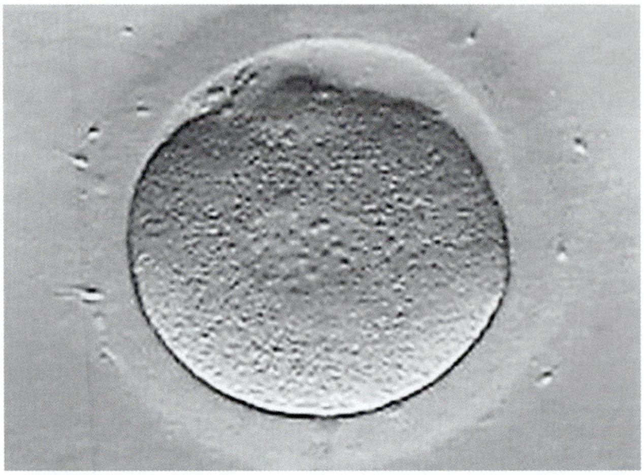

**Fig. 24:** Oocyte with single pronucleus (17 hours postinsemination).

juxta-posed pronuclei that are even-sized with distinct membranes. The pronuclei containing nucleolar precursor bodies equivalent in number and size, equatorially aligned at the region of membrane juxtaposition are called as polarized pronuclei **(Fig. 21)**. When pronuclei contain uneven number or uneven distribution of precursor bodies, they are known as nonpolarized pronuclei **(Fig. 22)**. The positive predictive value of pronuclear scoring has been the subject of some debate, with some papers showing a prognostic effect,[15-18] while others identified a correlation with aneuploidy,[19,20] and still others found no positive predictive value.[21,22]

Some zygotes display a characteristic halo appearance in the ooplasm. This phenomenon is thought to be the manifestation of a microtubule-organized translocation of mitochondria and other cytoplasmic components to the center of the oocyte due to their increased activities. This is a promising sign of getting good and implantable embryo **(Fig. 23)**.

Occasionally, oocyte displays single pronucleus post ICSI. This is because of suppressed oocyte activation. Terada et al. reported acceptable fertilization rate using Ca ionophore and ionomycin to induce cytoplasmic activation[23] **(Fig. 24)**.

## EARLY CLEAVAGE

Sign of syngamy **(Fig. 25)** and early cleavage **(Fig. 26)** (26 hours ± 1 post ICSI, 28 ± 1 post IVF) is predictive of further even cleavage pattern, and reported to have lower incidence of chromosomal errors.[24]

However, embryos with cleavage earlier than 20 hours postinsemination or those directly entering three or more cell stage have been shown to be associated with chromosomal abnormalities[24] **(Fig. 27)**.

## CLEAVAGE STAGE EMBRYOS

From day 2 onward, the number of blastomeres keeps on dividing at regular intervals. It is necessary that this division is stage specific. Mitosis in blastomeres should produce two equally sized daughter cells. When the division is

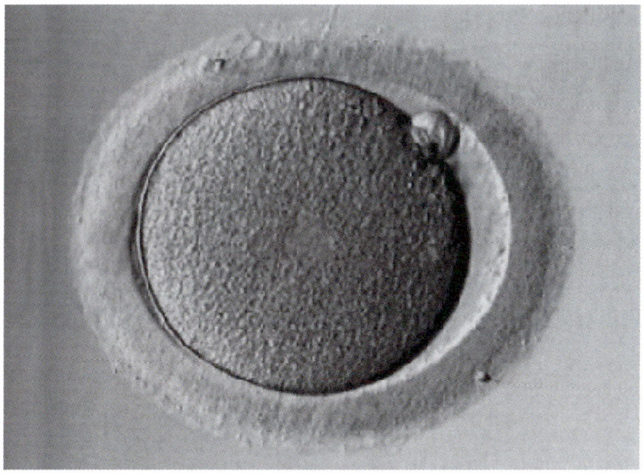

**Fig. 25:** Syngamy—21 hours postinsemination.

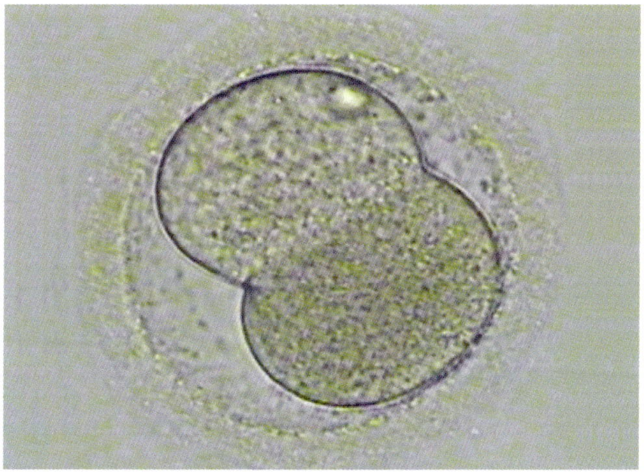

**Fig. 26:** Early cleavage (23 hours postinsemination).

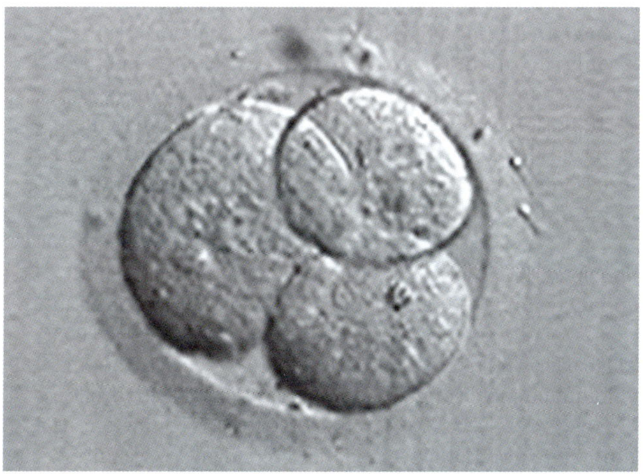

**Fig. 27:** 3-cell embryo.

asymmetric, one of the blastomeres of the next generation will inherit less than half the amount of cytoplasm from the parent blastomere, leading to a defective lineage in the embryo. 4- and 8-cell embryos with equal cell sizes have

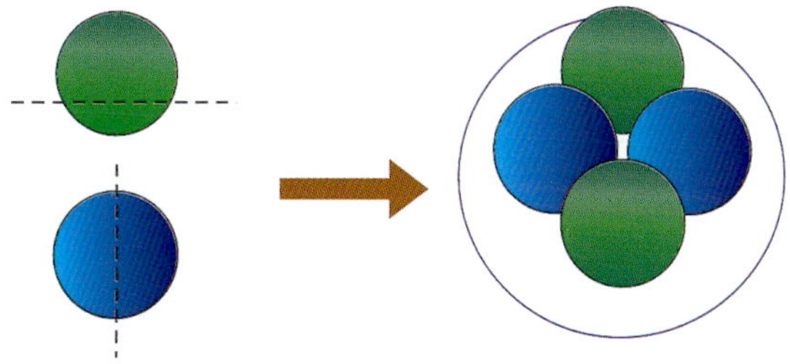

**Fig. 28:** Dividing planes of second mitotic cleavage. One cell cleaves equatorially and other cleaves meridionally resulting in four daughter cells with different polarity.

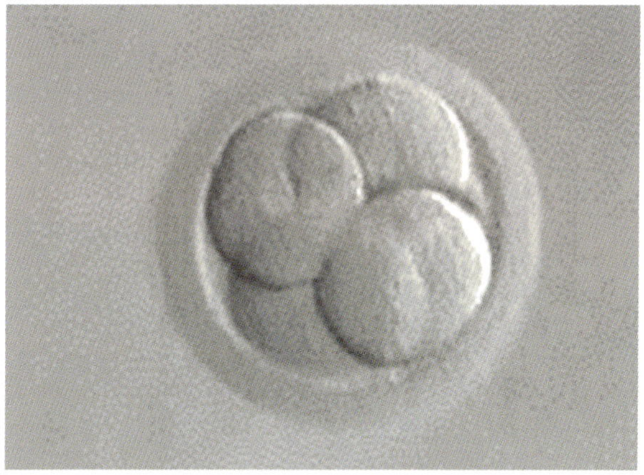

**Fig. 29:** Day 2: 4-cell grade I embryo.

been shown to have lower multinucleation and aneuploidy rates and increased implantation rates.[25,26]

Human oocytes are polarized from their earliest stages of formation and consist of an animal and vegetal pole.[27-29] This animal and vegetal gradient is distributed differently to specific 4-cell blastomeres via the combination of meridional and equatorial cleavage divisions.[30]

The first cleavage occurs meridionally and results in two nearly identical daughter blastomeres each inheriting similar polarities of animal and vegetal cytoplasm. In the second cleavage, one cell divides meridionally while the other cell divides equatorially which results in four cells with different polarity **(Fig. 28)**. The two daughter cells resulting from the meridional cleavage have inherited full polarity, while the two daughter cells from the equatorial cleavage differ in polarity with one cell containing mostly animal cytoplasm and the other cell containing mostly vegetal cytoplasm.[31,32]

## Day 2

At 44 ± 1 hours postinsemination, a healthy embryo display four equally sized mononucleated blastomeres in a 3-dimensional tetrahedral arrangement, with preferably nil or <10% fragmentation **(Fig. 29)**.

## Day 3

At 68 ± 1 hours postinsemination, a healthy embryo displays six to eight equally sized mononucleated blastomeres with

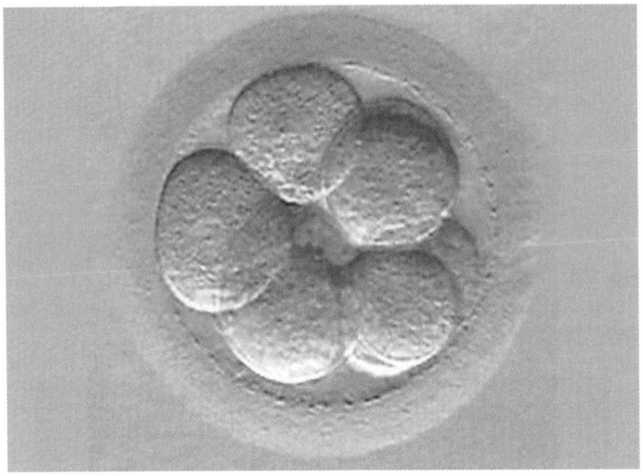

**Fig. 30:** Day 3: 8-cell grade I embryo.

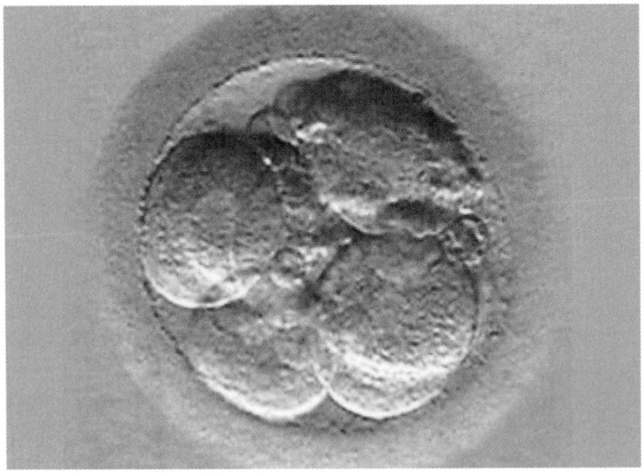

**Fig. 32:** Day 3: 6-cell grade II embryo with 15% fragmentation.

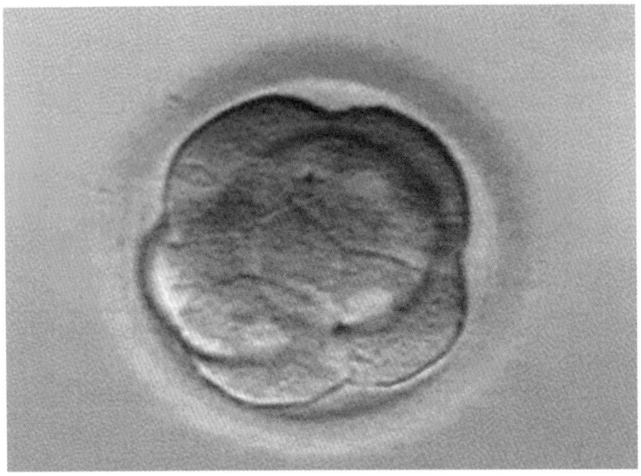

**Fig. 31:** Day 3: Beginning of compaction in 8-cell embryo.

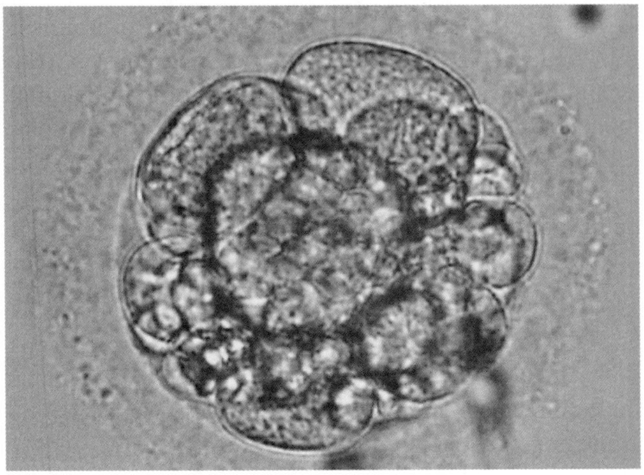

**Fig. 33:** Day 3: A 6-cell grade III embryo with >50% fragments, uneven blastomeres.

nil or <10% fragmentation **(Fig. 30)** and a sign of beginning of compaction **(Fig. 31)**. This is an important stage from embryogenesis point of view, as paternal genome is activated at this point that decides effect of genetic filiation on embryo development. Embryos with >15% fragmentation are categorized as grade II **(Fig. 32)**. Those with >50% fragments are termed as grade III and are not selected for transfer **(Fig. 33)**.

## Day 4

At 92 ± 2 hours postinsemination, one can observe a structure called "morula", where it is not possible to count number of blastomeres that range from 8 to 32 **(Fig. 34)**.

At this point, it is also not possible to assess presence of multinucleation, if any. Immediately after morula within 2–4 hours, a healthy embryo displays stage of compaction where intercellular junctions of blastomeres fuse to form an uneven, irregular ball-like structure. Such embryo almost always results in a blastocyst **(Fig. 35)**.

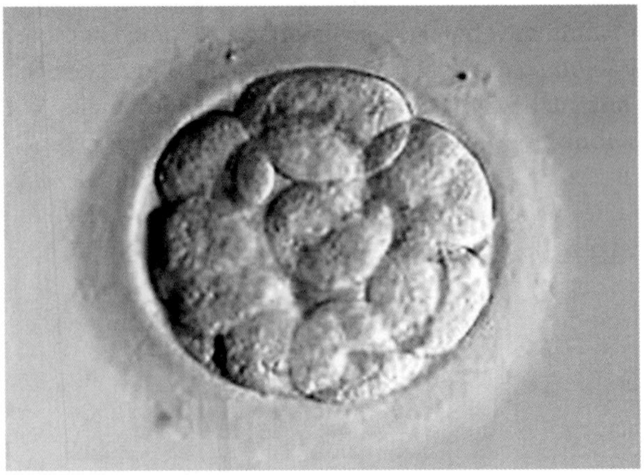

**Fig. 34:** Day 4: Grade I morula

## Day 5

At 106–108 hours postinsemination, a healthy embryo turns into a blastocyst **(Fig. 36)**. However, not all blastocysts are

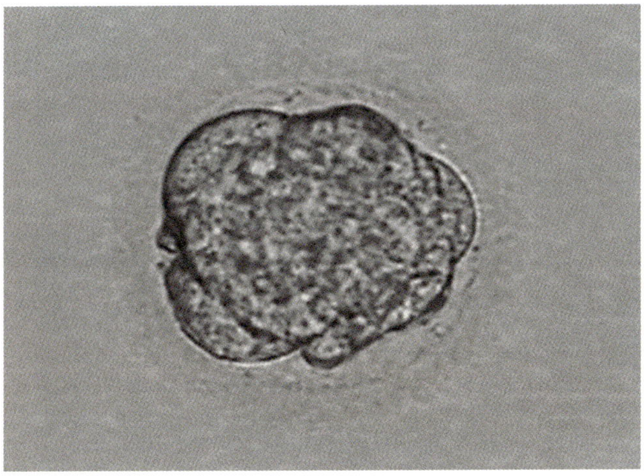

**Fig. 35:** Day 4: Compacting stage.

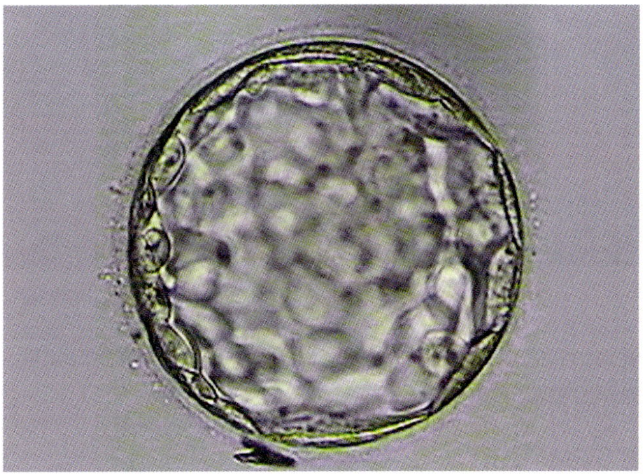

**Fig. 37:** An expanded blastocyst without inner cell mass.

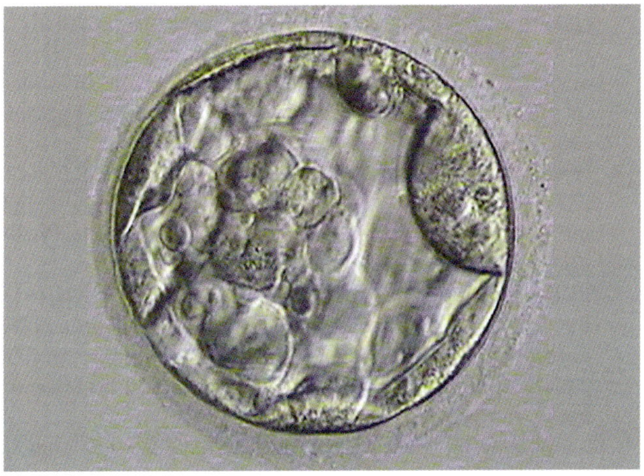

**Fig. 36:** Day 5: Grade I blastocyst.

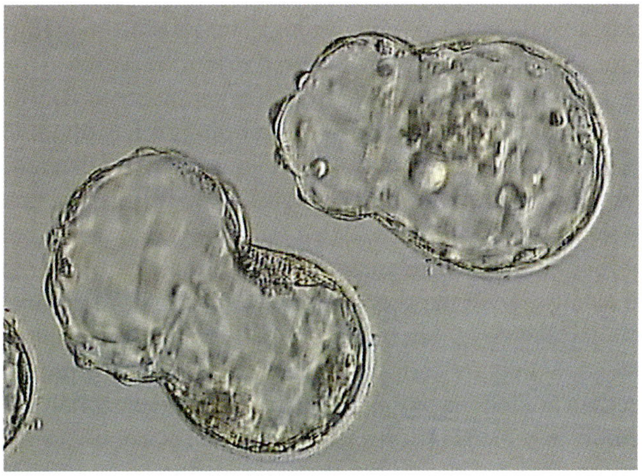

**Fig. 38:** Hatching blastocysts.

capable of implantation. Timing of blastocyst formation and its morphology is crucial for its viable status. An expanded blastocyst with thin zona, blastocoel filling almost entire area, clear sickle-shaped trophectoderm, and tightly packed inner cell mass (ICM) comprising about 25% of blastocoel are obvious markers to certify a blastocyst as grade I. Whereas, an expanded blastocyst with poorly developed or absent ICM is nonviable **(Fig. 37)** and, if transferred and gets implanted, may result in blighted ovum.

One can even observe a hatching blastocyst on day 5 or day 6 **(Fig. 38)**. It indicates healthy morphological status of the growing embryo.

## MORPHOLOGICAL ASSESSMENT USING MORPHOKINETICS

With the advanced scientific developments, dynamic growth of growing embryo can be monitored using techniques like time-lapse monitoring where embryo's images are taken at intermittent intervals throughout development without disturbing microenvironment **(Figs. 39A to E)**.

Using "time-lapse" imaging system, morphological competency can be checked in more predictive manner, where embryo can be assessed as:

- Those remained healthy throughout development stages
- Those which were healthy during early stages, but became unhealthy at later stages
- Those which were unhealthy initially, became healthy later
- Those showing unhealthy pattern throughout development.

These systems tell us which embryos display ideal growth pattern. However, they cannot tell with certainty that other embryos can never initiate a pregnancy. Question is—should we discard them or cryopreserve them and ultimately transfer in subsequent cycles, because there are pregnancies reported from grade II or even grade III embryos.

Though these devices do not have confidence in declaring noncompetency of poorly developed embryos, they help us in selecting "most probable" embryo that can result in live birth if transferred in a competent and receptive endometrium.[33] This presumably shortens number of efforts

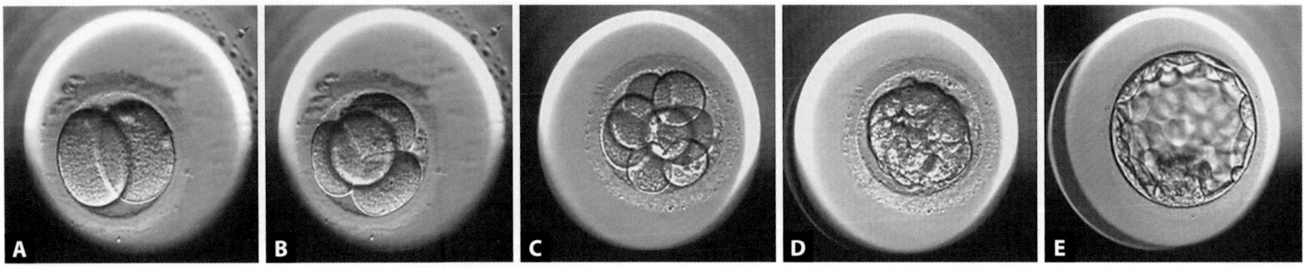


**Figs. 39A to E:** Time lapse images of growing embryo.

in terms of embryo transfers and hence duration for patient to become pregnant.

## SUMMARY

Selecting optimum embryo for transfer through morphological assessment under inverted microscope is most widely used criteria in IVF centers. Though, it is possible to predict probability of pregnancy to some extent, research is on to correlate genomics and proteomics involved during embryogenesis along with morphology of individual embryo to further enhance selection criteria. While using morphological assessment, it is important to note that embryo should not be selected only at the end point, but throughout its development. For example, an embryo showing grade I blastocyst after 20% fragments in embryo on day 2 or day 3 can be less optimum than one retaining its grade I status from day 2 through day 5. This imposes certain limitations on embryo culture like "group culture" of embryos, which is known to be beneficial. Secondly, detail evaluation of each embryo at each stage requires extended exposure during observation unless time-lapse imaging systems are used. This demands quick assessment with minimum fluctuations in culture system.

A combination of evaluation protocol involving morphology and biochemistry with practical and economical feasibility to select a single viable embryo for transfer is need of the time to improve take-home baby rates while reducing multiple gestations.

## REFERENCES

1. Mangoli V, Mangoli R. Gamete and embryo assessment in IVF. In: Desai S, Parihar M, Allahabadia G (Eds). Update on Infertility. New delhi: BI Publications Pvt. Ltd; 2004. pp. 124-9.
2. Kitasaka H, Yoshimi K, Mikiko T, Fukunaga N, Asada Y. Oocyte cytoplasmic diameter of >130 μm can be used to determine human giant oocytes. F S Sci. 2021;3(1):10-7.
3. Balaban B, Urman B, Sertac A, Alatas C, Aksoy S, Mercan R. Oocyte morphology does not affect fertilization rate, embryo quality and implantation rate after intracytoplasmic sperm injection. Hum Reprod. 1998;13:2431-3.
4. Maro B, Verlac M. Polar body formation: new rules for asymmetric divisions. Nat Cell Biol. 2002;4:281-3.
5. Kawakami M, Okimura T, Uchiyama K, Yabuuchi A, Kobayashi T, Kato K et al. The effect of zona pellucida thickness variation on fertilization and subsequent embryonic development: a large single center cohort study. Fertil Steril. 2019;112(3):e128-9.
6. Kahramam S, Yakin K, Donmez E, Samli H, Bahçe M, Cengiz G, et al. Relationship between granular cytoplasm of oocytes and pregnancy out- come following intracytoplasmic sperm injection. Hum Reprod. 2000;15:2390-3.
7. Hassan-Ali H, Hisham-Saleh A, El-Gezeiry D, Baghdady I, Ismaeil I, Mandelbaum J. Perivitelline space granularity: a sign of human menopausal gonadotropin overdose in intracytoplasmic sperm injection. Hum Reprod. 1998;13:3425-30.
8. Mandelbaum J, Junca AM, Balaisch-Allert J, Salat-Baroux J, Plachot M, Antoine JM, et al. Oocyte maturation and intracytoplasmic sperm injection. Contracept Fertil Sex. 1996; 24(7-8):534-8.
9. Eichenlaub-Ritter U, Schmiady H, Kentenich H, Soewarto D. Recurrent failure in polar body formation and premature chromosome condensation in oocytes from a human patient: indicator of asynchrony in nuclear and cytoplasmic maturation. Hum Reprod. 1995;10:2343-9.
10. Van Wissen B, Eisenberg C, Debey P, Pennehouat G, Auger J, Bomsel-Helmreich O. In vitro DNA fluorescence after in vitro fertilization (IVF) failure. J Assist Reprod Genet. 1992;9:564-71.
11. Ebner T, Moser M, Sommergruber M, Tews G. Selection based on morphological assessment of oocytes and embryos at different stages of preimplantation development: a review. Hum Reprod Update. 2003;9:251-62.
12. Massarotti C, Stigliani S, Ramone A, Bovis F, Sozzi F, Remorgida V, et al. Occurrence of smooth endoplasmic reticulum aggregates in metaphase II oocytes: relationship with stimulation protocols and outcome of ICSI and IVF cycles. Hum Reprod. 2021;18;36:907-17.
13. Ebner T, Moser M, Shebl O, Sommerguber M, Tews G. Prognosis of oocytes showing aggregation of smooth endoplasmic reticulum. Reprod Biomed Online. 2008;16:113-8.
14. Keef DL. Oocyte and zona imaging. In: Gardner D, RMB Rizk B, Falcone T. (Eds). Human Assisted Reproductive Technology: Future Trends in Laboratory and Clinical Practice. Cambridge: Cambridge University Press; pp. 205.
15. Tesarik J, Greco E. The probability of abnormal preimplantation development can be predicted by a single static observation on pronuclear stage morphology. Hum Reprod. 1999;14:1318-23.
16. Scott L, Alvero R, Leondires M, Miller B. The morphology of human pronuclear embryos is positively related to blastocyst development and implantation. Hum Reprod. 2000;15:2394-403.

17. Otsuki J, Iwasaki T, Enatsu N, Katada Y, Furuhashi K, Shiotani M. Noninvasive embryo selection: kinetic analysis of female pronuclear development to predict embryo quality and potential to produce live birth. Fertil Steril. 2019;112(5): 874-81.
18. Balaban B, Urman B, Isiklar A, Alatas C, Aksoy S, Mercan R, et al. The effect of pronuclear morphology on embryo quality parameters and blastocyst transfer outcome. Hum Reprod. 2001;16:2357-61.
19. Sadowy S, Tomkin G, Munné S, Ferrara-Congedo T, Cohen J. Impaired development of zygotes with uneven pronuclear size. Zygote. 1998;6:137-41.
20. Gianaroli L, Magli MC, Farraretti AP, Fortini D, Grieco N. Pronuclear morphology and chromosomal abnormalities as scoring criteria for embryo selection. Fertil Steril. 2003;80:341-9.
21. Salumets A, Hydén-Granskog C, Suikkari AM, Tiitinen A, Tuuri T. The predictive value of pronuclear morphology of zygotes in the assessment of human embryo quality. Hum Reprod. 2001;16:2177-81.
22. Weitzman VN, Schnee-Riesz J, Benadiva C, Nulsen J, Siano L, Maier D. Predictive value of embryo grading for embryos with known outcomes. Fertil Steril. 2010;93:658-62.
23. Terada Y, Hasegawa H, Takahashi A, Ugajin T, Yaegashi N, Okamura K. Successful pregnancy after oocyte activation by a calcium ionophore for a patient with recurrent intracytoplasmic sperm injection failure, with an assessment of oocyte activation and sperm centrosomal function using bovine eggs. Fertil Steril. 2009;91(3):935.
24. Hardarson T, Selleskog U, Reismer E, Wigander A, Wennerström S, Westin C, et al. Zygotes cleaving directly into more than two cells after 25-27 h in culture are predominantly chromosomally abnormal. Hum Reprod. 2006;21:i102.
25. Hardarson T, Hanson C, Sjögren A, Lundin K. Human embryos with unevenly sized blastomeres have lower pregnancy and implantation rates: indications for aneuploidy and multinucleation. Hum Reprod. 2001;16:313-8.
26. Van Royen E, Mangelschots K, De Neubourg D, Laureys I, Ryckaert G, Gerris J. Calculating the implantation potential of day 3 embryos in women younger than 38 years of age: a new model. Hum Reprod. 2001;16:326-32.
27. Antczak M, Van Blerkom J. Oocyte influence on early development: the regulatory proteins leptin and STAT 3 are polarized in mouse and human oocytes and differentially distributed within the cells of the preimplantation stage embryo. Mol Hum Reprod. 1997;3:1067-86.
28. Antczak M, Van Blerkom J. Temporal and spatial aspects of fragmentation in early human embryos: possible effects on developmental competence and association with the differential elimination of regulatory proteins from polarized domains. Hum Reprod. 1999;14:429-47.
29. Edwards RG, Beard HK. Oocyte polarity and cell determination in early mammalian embryos. Mol Hum Reprod. 1997;3:863-905.
30. Gulyas BJ. A reexamination of cleavage patterns in eutherian mammalian eggs: rotation of blastomere pairs during second cleavage of the rabbit. J Exp Zool. 1975;193:235-48.
31. Edwards RG, Hansis C. Initial differentiation of blastomeres in 4-cell human embryos and its significance for early embryogenesis and implantation. Reprod Biomed Online. 2005;11(2):206-18.
32. Prados FJ1, Debrock S, Lemmen JG, Agerholm I. The cleavage stage embryo. Hum Reprod. 2012;27 (Suppl 1):i50-71.
33. Racowsky C, Martins WP. Effectiveness and safety of time-lapse imaging for embryo culture and selection: it is still too early for any conclusion? Fertil Steril. 2017;108(3):450-2.

CHAPTER 108

# Blastocyst Culture and Transfer

*Rajvi H Mehta, Mohammed Ashraf C, Mir Jaffar*

## INTRODUCTION

The birth of a single, healthy baby is the desired outcome of any assisted reproductive technology (ART). But not all couples who undergo treatment for their infertile condition with ART manage to achieve this goal. Most embryos fail to implant when transferred into the uterus at the four- to eight-cell stage.

It has become a common practice to transfer multiple embryos into the uterus to improve the chances of a pregnancy. When more than one embryo was transferred, it was not possible to predict with certainty which of the embryos would implant and which would not. Transfer of multiple embryos did improve the chances of pregnancy, but along with it, there was an increase in the incidence of multiple pregnancies as well as the obstetric complications that go along with multiple gestations. It has been reported that the incidence of twinning has doubled, while that of triplets has increased sevenfold in the last few decades in the United States[1] and this has been attributed to some form of fertility treatment. Thus, an ideal situation would be to transfer only one embryo that has the highest potential of implantation, wherein the risk of multiple pregnancies is reduced without compromising on the chance of pregnancy itself. The crucial question that arises is what is the optimal stage at which the embryo should be transferred into the uterus.

## WHY CULTURE EMBRYOS TO THE BLASTOCYST STAGE IN VITRO?

In an in vivo situation, early embryonic development occurs in the fallopian tube, and it enters the uterus at the stage of a blastocyst. However, following conventional in vitro fertilization (IVF), embryos are only at the four- to eight-cell stage when they are transferred to the uterus either on day 2 or day 3. Are the embryos being transferred into the uterus too early?

Second, embryos from many mammalian species are known to undergo a "metabolic block" when cultured in vitro, i.e., a stage where the metabolism in the embryos switches from the control of the maternal genome to the embryonic genome. This embryonic gene expression occurs in humans at the four- to eight-cell stage.[2] Therefore, when embryos are transferred into the uterus at this stage, one is unsure whether the embryo is capable of further development after the activation of the embryonic genome. In fact, it is not even possible to determine whether the embryo is viable at the time of transfer.

The best option to overcome both of these limitations seems to be to culture the embryos in vitro till the blastocyst stage. Transfer of blastocysts into the uterus would be closer to the in vivo situation. Secondly, culturing embryos for an extended period will select the developing embryos from those that have undergone developmental arrest. Buster et al. reported high pregnancy rates following transfer of blastocysts obtained after uterine flushing from donors.[3] Thus, it only seemed logical to transfer blastocysts into the uterus after extended culture of embryos obtained after IVF.

### Culturing Blastocysts In Vitro

Attempts to extend the culture of embryos in vitro till they reached the blastocyst stage using conventional media remained unsuccessful. About 40% of oocytes fertilized in vitro, developed to blastocysts, but only 10% led to pregnancy after transfer on day 5 post insemination.[4] This was primarily because the metabolic requirements of early human embryonic development were unknown.

### Coculturing Embryos with Somatic Cell Lines

Coculture of human embryos with autologous or heterologous somatic cell lines offered a means of successfully culturing human blastocysts in vitro. In the early 1990s, Menezo's group in France and Bongso in Singapore cocultured human embryos with Vero cells and tubal ampullary cells, respectively.[5,6] Vero cells were selected over the others since the kidney cells have the same origin as the reproductive tract. Ampullary cells were the closest to the in vivo environment. Nearly 60% of the embryos did develop to the blastocyst stage in these studies.

What led to the improvement in the blastocyst formation rate following coculture remained unknown. It could be specific factors produced by the cocultured cells that promoted embryonic development or it could be the detoxification effect brought about by the cell line and the improved buffering systems. But neither of these could be characterized. The process of coculturing embryos with cell lines was cumbersome, and there was also the potential risk of using cell lines from animal species. Thus, this methodology did not become popular or attain routine application.

### *Blastocyst Culture using Sequential Media*

Another approach to culture blastocyst that has gained popularity is the culture of embryos in defined, serum-free, sequential culture media.[7,8] The principle behind the formulation of such media is to reflect the changing environment in the maternal reproductive tract. The requirements of early human embryos are minimal and do not require glucose as an energy source. Development of cleavage-stage embryos to morula and then blastocyst requires more nutrients. Hence, two or more media are used sequentially for the culture of blastocyst in vitro, which takes into consideration the changes in the metabolic requirements and the different stages of development. On an average, nearly 50% of the embryos developed to a blastocyst stage when cultured in sequential media, of which about 50% were viable. Many commercial brands of media are currently available for blastocyst culture, and several studies have compared the quality of the different commercial media for culturing cleavage-stage embryos and blastocysts.[9-11]

### *Extended Culture in a Single Defined Medium*

Biggers and Racowsky have reported a one-step protocol for culturing human embryos in the same medium till the blastocyst stage.[12] They report that a single-step protocol using potassium simplex optimized media (KSOM) is as efficacious as sequential culture for developing blastocysts. Five babies were born from transfer of nine blastocysts.

## MORPHOLOGICAL EVALUATION OF BLASTOCYSTS

Extended culture of human embryos till the blastocyst stage helps in improving the implantation rate by improving the selection of embryos. A further improved selection of blastocysts can help in further improving the implantation rates. The evaluation of blastocysts is primarily based on the morphological assessment of the embryos. Morphological assessment is limited by its subjectivity, but the development of grading and scoring makes the data on blastocyst quality comparable.

Normal blastocyst development required blastulation, a visible inner-cell mass, trophectoderm cells covering 60% of the inner zona surface and thinning of the zona.[13]

Gardner et al. developed a system to score the developmental potential of blastocysts based on their ability to implant following transfer of single or two blastocysts.[14] They observed that in 21% of the patients, one top-quality blastocyst was available for transfer, and the implantation and pregnancy rates in this group were as high as 50 and 70%, respectively. However, when a low-scoring blastocyst was available for transfer, the implantation and pregnancy rates were 28 and 44%, respectively.

Kovacic et al. classified 1,396 blastocysts and morula into eight morphological categories.[15] The optimal blastocysts were called B1. The other categories were characterized by different deviations from optimal blastocysts: Cytoplasmic fragments and necrosis in trophectoderm (B2), unexpanded blastocoele (B3), noncompact or small inner cell mass (ICM) (B4), fragments in trophectoderm and ICM (B5), up to 20% excluded blastomeres (B6), necrotic trophectoderm and ICM (B7), and >20% excluded cells from blastocysts (B8). The live birth rate was calculated from blastocysts with known outcomes after transfer. The birth rate declined from B1 to B8 in the same order and was 45.2, 32.8, 26.9, 23, 17.7, 16.7, 7.7, and 1.2%, respectively. Normal ICM was recognized as the most important parameter for implantation. They concluded that such a grading system is helpful in selecting the best of all available day 5 embryos for transfer.

### Morphological Characteristics of Blastocyst with Impact on Implantation

Embryoblast is considered to be optimal if the ICM shows a tight package of numerous cells. In contrast with a well-expanded cavity and a cohesive trophectoderm, ICM size was significantly related to implantation. Blastocysts showing an ICM of <3,800 $\mu m^2$ showed lower implantation rates (18%) compared to blastocysts with a larger ICM of 4,500 $\mu m^2$ (45%). An optimal human blastocyst at day 5 of development should exceed 60 cells and at least double its cell number on day 6.[16]

### Blastocyst Evaluation by Inner Cell Mass Morphometry

#### *Roundness Index*

The roundness index (RI) is an important scoring parameter with regard to clinical outcome. It can be defined as the length-to-width proportion of the ICM.

It is categorized into three shapes:
1. Round
2. Oval
3. Slightly oval

When the RI is <1.04 (almost round) and >1.20 (oval), it showed lower implantation rates of 7 and 33%, respectively, in comparison with an implantation rate of 58% for RI between 1.04 and 1.20 (slightly oval). However, high implantation rates of 71% were observed with optimal ICM size and shape.[16]

A mislead in the apoptotic process and a disproportionately oversized ICM increase the distance for diffusion of nutrients and oxygen. This leads to unhealthy central cells increasing the risks of large offspring syndrome.[17]

### Trophectoderm

The presence of numerous sickle-shaped cells forming a cohesive epithelium (grade A) in the outer layer of the trophectoderm is considered to be optimal **(Fig. 1)**.[18]

Lower implantation rates were prevalent in blastocysts with an impaired trophoblast (e.g., extremely flattened cells, no sickle-shaped cells, no junctions between trophectoderm cells, cells with granulation, pigmentation, and/or vacuolization).

## MORPHOLOGY OF POOR-QUALITY BLASTOCYSTS

These groups of blastocysts exhibit low cell numbers and higher degree of chromosomal aberrations.[19]

Poor-quality blastocysts consist of various morphological subtypes, namely blastocysts with excessive fragmentation, vacuoles, necrotic cells, and trophoblast vesicles.

### Trophoblast Vesicle

Trophoblast vesicles are characterized by the absence of the ICM[20,21] and a rather rudimentary trophectoderm. Thus, it is more or less a trophoblastic vesicle with a dominant blastocyst cavity. The cavity can also be a large vacuole **(Fig. 2)**.

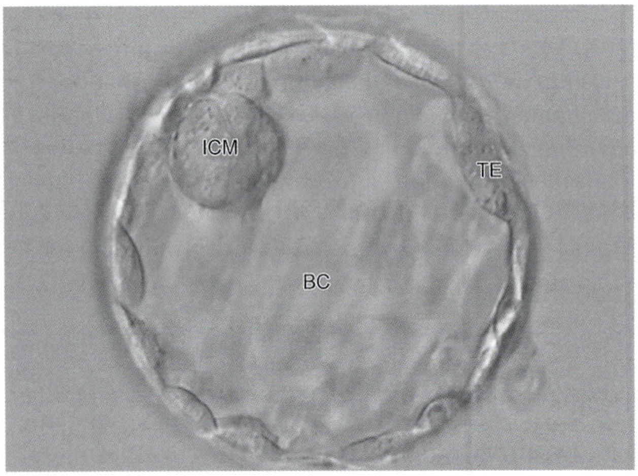


**Fig. 1:** Hatching blastocyst of optimal quality with the hatching site being at the 4 o'clock position.
(BC: blastocyst cavity; ICM: inner cell mass; TE: trophectoderm)

### Necrotic Foci

Necrosis is the irreversible damage to cells, where the cells get distended and rupture their membrane, ultimately leading to cell death.

The assessment of the degenerative areas revealed that implantation rates were lower when ICM was affected (23% live births) and slightly higher when only the trophectoderm was affected (32.8% live births). Therefore, the compactness and the multicellularity of the ICM were more essential for implantation than the cohesiveness of the trophectoderm **(Fig. 3)**.[15]

### Vacuoles

Vacuoles found within the blastocyst **(Figs. 4A and B)** tend to appear more in the trophectoderm than in the ICM. Vacuoles present in close proximity to ICM tend to have a more detrimental effect on the outcome. However, the restriction of these vacuoles to the trophectoderm yields better results.

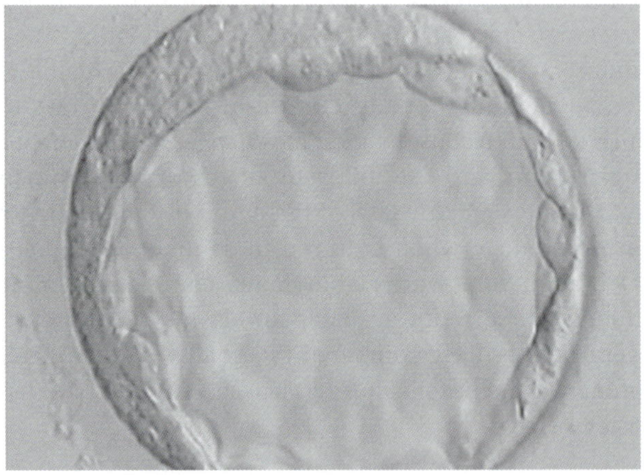

**Fig. 2:** Blastocyst with no visible inner cell mass (comparable to trophoblast vesicle).

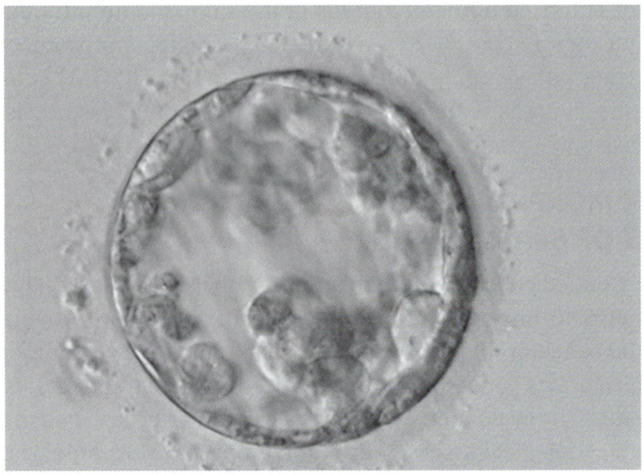

**Fig. 3:** Early blastocyst showing dark, degenerative changes.

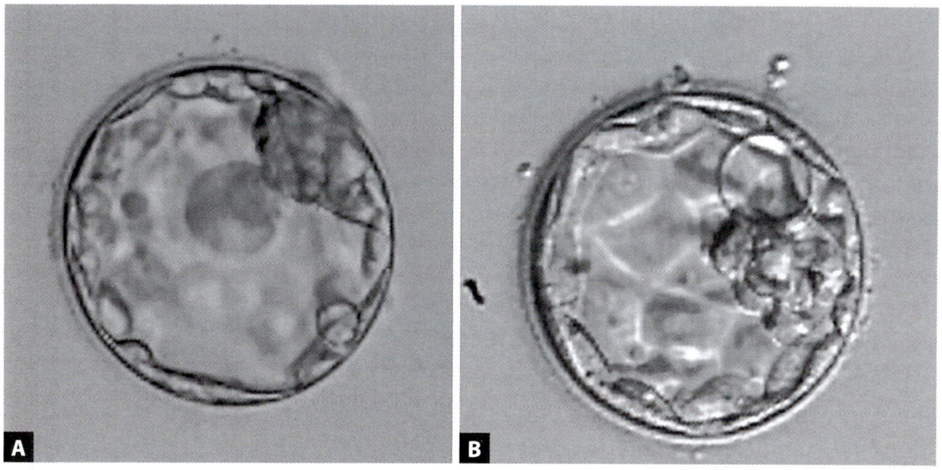

**Figs. 4A and B:** Blastocysts showing vacuole.

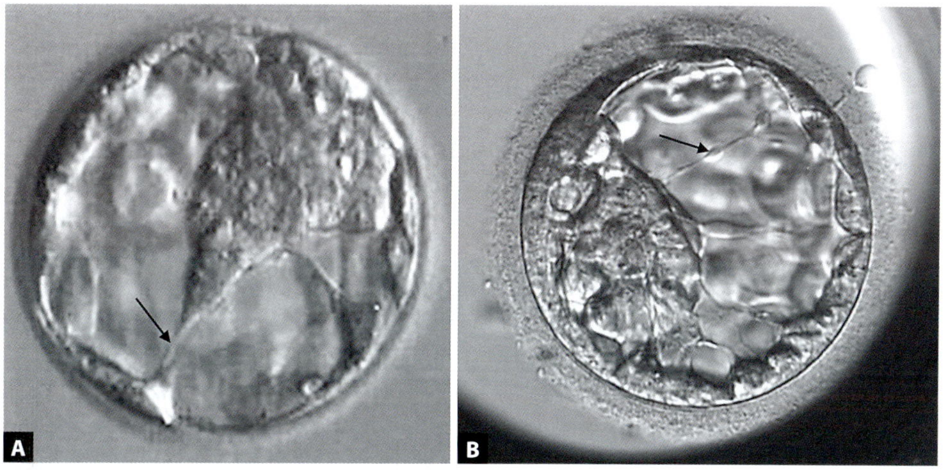

**Figs. 5A and B:** Blastocysts showing cytoplasmic strings (arrows).

## Cytoplasmic Strings

Cytoplasmic strings are specialized projections that connect the cells of ICM and trophectoderm. The implantation behavior is affected by the presence of these cytoplasmic extensions that bridge the blastocyst cavity at the expansion stage or the later stages **(Figs. 5A and B)**.

They are commonly observed in nearly half of the junctional trophectoderm cells across the boundary between the polar and mural regions of trophectoderm and are directed at the blastocoelic surface of the ICM.[22] As these cytoplasmic extensions are linked to the polarized flow of cells from the polar to the mural trophectoderm, they tend to withdraw as the cells reach their destination. Strings vary in both shape (from broad triangles to string-like projections) and length (some fail to reach the ICM surface). Since early blastocysts are characterized by cytoplasmic extensions that cover the surface of the ICM, majority of the surface remains unaffected in the later stages of the blastocyst. Cytoplasmic strings were more likely to be found in fair and good quality blastocysts, and blastocysts with more cytoplasmic strings (>4) were associated with increased clinical pregnancies and live birth rates. However, when the cytoplasmic strings persist even in the expanded phase, they mark the developmental lability of the blastocysts, which possibly indicate polarization breakdown leading to diminished embryo quality and lower implantation rates.

# EVALUATION OF ZYGOTES AND EMBRYOS AND THEIR POTENTIAL TO DEVELOP INTO BLASTOCYSTS

The improved implantation rate following blastocyst culture was not attributed to improvement in embryo quality by extended culture but to the selection process. Therefore, attempts were also made to develop grading systems whereby it may be possible to predict which of the zygotes and cleavage-stage embryos are capable of developing into blastocysts. Such systems would give the advantages of blastocyst culture without actually attempting it.

Zygotes were scored according to distribution and size of nucleoli within each nucleus. Zygotes displaying equality between the nuclei had 49.5% blastocyst formation, and those with unequal sizes, numbers, or distribution of nucleoli had 28% blastocyst formation.[23]

Fisch et al. attempted to culture 983 embryos up to the blastocyst stage.[24] When ranked by cell number and morphology alone, 34% of embryos with more than or equal to seven cells and <20% fragmentation formed good-quality blastocysts. This is corroborated by other investigators.[25] Stone et al. also analyzed the rate of blastocyst formation against the type of fragmentation 72 hours after insemination.[13] Embryos exhibiting no fragmentation or type I fragmentation had significantly higher blastocyst development rates (27.9 and 19.9%) than embryos with type 2 or 3 fragmentation. Vidaeff et al. reported that blastocysts developed when the embryos were at least eight cells on day 3.[1]

A reduction in the cytoplasmic volume of an embryo leads to a significant loss of cells in the blastocyst stage. This reduction in cytoplasmic volume is mainly caused due to cryoinjury or fragmentation. The embryos when subjected to cryopreservation drastically lowered the blastocyst cell numbers on day 6 in comparison to blastocysts obtained from fully intact cleavage-stage embryos post thawing. Fragmentation also had the same effect in lowering the cell number.[17] However, when the fragmentation was at minimal or moderate levels, ICM cell numbers remained the same, with reduced cell numbers limited to the trophectoderm.

## FACTORS INFLUENCING BLASTOCYST DEVELOPMENT

The factors that influence the development of blastocyst in vitro are the age of the woman, number of oocytes retrieved, intrinsic factors, and culture conditions.[26] For example, Bedaiwy et al. analyzed the levels of reactive oxygen species (ROS) in the culture media and found that media associated with a low blastocyst rate had high levels of ROS in the media.[27]

- *Age of the woman:* The blastocyst developmental rate does get compromised in women over 40 years. It is just 22.2% in contrast to nearly 40% in younger women, and so pregnancy and implantation rates decrease in older women.[28]

  Shapiro et al. further analyzed the relationship between the age of the women and the blastocyst development and pregnancy rate.[29] The proportion of cycles with expandable blastocysts decreased with age although there was no difference with reference to fertilization rates. Pregnancy rates per stimulation cycle decreased, but the pregnancy rate per transfer was not related to age.
- *Embryonic development rate:* Jones et al. observed a significant positive correlation between the number of blastocysts formed and the number of oocytes, pronuclear zygotes, and eight-cell embryos formed on day 3.[30] There was a negative correlation with male factor infertility.
- *Culture conditions:* The culture conditions with reference to the volume of culture medium or the culturing of embryos in groups or individually did not influence the blastocyst formation rate.[31]

## HATCHING PHENOMENON IN A BLASTOCYST

In vitro, the hatching process is supported by the increasing internal pressure due to the gradual accumulation of blastocoel fluid and cellular proliferation mainly originating from the trophectoderm. In vitro, the hatching process begins with the protrusion of small vesicles through the zona pellucida (ZP). However, this blebbing is not an indicator of the exact location of the subsequent hatching.[32] With the creation of this small opening, the herniation of the trophectoderm begins and creates a larger opening due to the mechanical forces governed by the trophectodermal projections.[33] Under the electron microscope, specialized cells known as "zona-breaker cells" lining both sides of the trophectoderm were observed at the hatching sites. Superficial microvilli and bundles of contractile tonofilaments allow these cells to interact with the ZP, somewhat acting like a sphincter.

The occurrence of blastocyst "breathing" provides an additional mechanical assistance by a series of rapid collapses and slow reexpansions to allow for its final extrusion from the ruptured ZP. The presence of secretory vesicles such as lysosomes indicates the involvement of biochemical processes, in addition to the mechanical forces. Hatching in close proximity to the ICM has the tendency to accelerate the contact among the trophectodermal cells that draw the blastocyst to the uterine wall and the endometrium. The presence of hernia opposite to the ICM may delay the interaction between the blastocyst and the uterus.

## CRYOPRESERVATION OF BLASTOCYSTS

The improvement in implantation rates following blastocyst transfer results in supernumerary embryos requiring cryopreservation. Slow freezing as well as vitrification protocols have been successfully used to freeze blastocysts.

Stehlik et al. compared blastocyst freezing by slow freezing and vitrification.[34] 83% of the blastocysts survived thawing after slow freezing, while all the blastocysts survived thawing following vitrification. The pregnancy rate was only 16.7% following transfer of thawed embryos frozen slowly, in contrast to a pregnancy rate of 50%, i.e., 10 out of the 20 following transfer of thawed vitrified embryos.

The relatively poor pregnancy rates following frozen-thawed cleavage-stage embryos are due to two factors—the metabolic block of embryonic development in vitro due to maternal, paternal and the embryonic genomes as well as the culture conditions. The metabolic block is overcome in the blastocyst-stage embryos, so the number of embryos available for freezing may be lower, but the pregnancy rates following the transfer of thawed blastocysts are better.[35]

### Optimal Time for Freezing Blastocysts

What is the right time to freeze blastocysts? Should they be frozen as soon as the cavity is formed or as advanced-stage blastocysts? Van den Abbeel froze blastocysts either at an early stage or at an advanced stage or hatching blastocysts.[36] Morphological survival post thawing was better for early blastocysts, while developmental potential of advanced-stage blastocysts was better.

### Optimal Time for Transferring Thawed Blastocysts

Not all blastocysts that are frozen survive on thawing. Therefore, it becomes crucial to select the "right" thawed blastocyst for transfer. Most protocols incubate blastocysts for a few hours before transferring as that not only helps the selection process but also gives the blastocyst time to hydrate and adapt to environment. Guerif et al. compared the implantation rate after transferring blastocysts incubated for 4 or 20 hours after thawing and found that the implantation rates were better after a longer duration of incubation prior to transfer.[37]

## ADVANTAGES AND APPLICATIONS OF BLASTOCYST CULTURE

### Improved Pregnancy and Implantation Rates

Several studies suggest that embryo transfer at the blastocyst stage results in higher implantation rates compared to early cleavage-stage replacement on day 3.[38-40] In a retrospective analysis of 4,165 transfers, Pantos et al. also found improved pregnancy and implantation rates in blastocyst transfer as compared with day 2 transfer.[41] In a prospective, randomized trial of patients who responded well to ovulation induction, the implantation rate following blastocyst transfer was significantly higher (50.5%) than embryo replacement on day 3 (30.1%), although it should be noted that different culture systems were used for the two treatment groups.[38]

Barrenetexea et al. reported a 46% blastocyst formation rate and 23% implantation rate in patients in whom at least three previous cleavage-stage embryo transfers had failed to lead to a pregnancy, clearly suggesting that blastocyst transfer did have an advantage over cleavage-stage embryos in a certain group of patients.[42] Blastocyst transfer was found to be beneficial and led to pregnancies in patients in whom two previous cycles with day 2 or 3 transfer had failed.[43]

A recent Cochrane review of 12 randomized controlled trials that reported live birth following cleavage or blastocyst transfer was evidence of a significant difference in live birth rate per couple favoring blastocyst culture (days 2–3: 31%; days 5–6: 38.8%). This means that for clinics that use early cleavage-stage cycles, the rate of live births would increase from 32 to 42% if clinics used blastocyst transfer.[44]

### Blastocyst Transfer—Decreased Risk of Multiple Gestations

As mentioned earlier, multiple pregnancies have become a serious concern following ART with reference to the obstetric complication and the health of the children born. The high implantation rates of blastocyst transfer, accompanied by the methods used for selecting the best embryo for transfer, make it possible to achieve a respectable ongoing pregnancy rate after the transfer of a single embryo with no dizygotic twinning.[45,46]

### Preimplantation Genetic Diagnosis

The implantation rates and clinical pregnancy can be improved by the application of techniques like embryo biopsy and preimplantation genetic screening (PGS). These techniques can analyse the complete chromosomal status of the embryo. During a biopsy, a single cell at the cleavage stage or several trophectoderm cells are retrieved. However, PGS has limited applications due to technical issues and its effect on the long-term health of the off springs. Recently, the introduction of techniques like noninvasive methods of PGT (niPGT) can analyse the genomic DNA from embryo culture medium or blastocyst cavity fluid provides a less invasive alternative to embryo biopsy.[47]

#### *Derivation of Human Embryonic Stem Cells*

One of the most vital applications of blastocyst culture is the derivation of human embryonic stem (hES) cell lines from the ICM of the blastocyst. The potential benefits of hES cells are beyond the scope of this chapter as they may offer treatment of some chronic, untreatable diseases facing mankind.[48]

## LIMITATIONS OF BLASTOCYST TRANSFER

Although blastocyst culture and transfer has many advantages, it has still not become a routine application in ART laboratories because of certain justifiable concerns. Blastocyst culture also imposes additional requirements in terms of personnel, equipment, and cost.

### Poor Rate of Blastocyst Development In Vitro and Cancellation of Transfer

One of the major limitations of blastocyst transfer is that not all cleavage-stage embryos develop into blastocysts. Some patients may not have any blastocysts available for transfer on day 5 despite having cleavage-stage embryos on day 3[38] leading to cancellation of transfer. The question that would then remain unanswered is whether that woman would have conceived with a day 3 transfer? A meta-analysis of 29 trials showed a significant number of cancellations of transfer when transfer was scheduled on day 5 because no blastocysts were formed.[49]

## Monozygotic Twinning

Many studies have reported a higher incidence of monozygotic twinning following blastocyst transfer as compared to cleavage-stage transfer.[50,51] Peramo et al. were the first to report that the incidence of monozygotic twinning increased after blastocyst transfer.[52]

da Costa et al. reported that 3% of the pregnancies following blastocyst transfer were complicated by monozygotic twinning as compared with 0.7% after four- to eight-cell stage embryo transfer,[53] while 0.42% of natural pregnancies result in monozygotic twinning (Bulmer, 1970). The obstetric outcome of these pregnancies was poor.[54] It was thought that this incidence is higher in embryos developed after intracytoplasmic sperm injection (ICSI) or assisted hatching possibly because the drilling may have caused premature herniation of the blastocyst. But Sills et al. did not find a difference in monozygotic twinning rate between manipulated embryos such as those with ICSI or assisted hatching as compared with those obtained after conventional IVF.[55] The increased incidence of monozygotic twinning is clearly a result of blastocyst culture and transfer and has been corroborated by many more studies. Milki et al. showed that the incidence of monozygotic twinning was 5.6% with day 5 (blastocyst) transfer as compared with 2% with day 3 (cleavage-stage embryo) transfer.[56] The incidence was identical in ICSI and non-ICSI groups. A recent retrospective analysis of 14,956 clinical pregnancies from single blastocyst transfer indicated a 1% monozygotic twinning with an odds ratio (OR) of 2.0 irrespective of zona drilling, ICSI, or type of stimulation used.[57]

While monozygotic twinning need not be considered as a major disadvantage of blastocyst culture, it is important to take this phenomenon into account while deciding on the number of blastocysts to be transferred as well as appropriately counsel the patients. As of now, the mechanism by which the incidence of monozygotic twinning increases following blastocyst transfer is unclear.

## Failure of Blastocyst Development and No Embryos Available for Transfer

There are several reasons that prevent an embryo from developing into a blastocyst like reduced metabolic activity. This results in the slow embryo development which eventually leads to its degeneration. Embryo development can be affected at any stage of its development. The failure in the process of embryo development is multifactorial which includes chromosomal errors, cell division errors and mitochondrial function.

Molecular failures can occur which can increase the chances of the onset of imprinting disorders in the offspring like large offspring syndrome.[58]

### *Large Offspring Syndrome*

In vitro culture of embryos for 5–7 days in vitro has been associated with large offspring syndrome in certain animal species. This has been attributed to the suboptimal embryo culture conditions. This syndrome manifests as abnormal growth and development at fetal, neonatal, and later stages of life.[59] It has been shown that extended culture of embryos to the blastocyst stage can compromise many aspects of development including metabolism,[60] differentiation,[61] gene expression,[62] imprinting,[63] and subsequent fetal development after embryo transfer[64] in several mammalian species.

Menezo et al. did not find any difference in the birth weights of babies born after spontaneous conception and blastocyst transfer.[65] Although several healthy babies have been born following the transfer of blastocysts, there has been a concern that the birth of healthy babies does not preclude the possibility of long-term effects. Continued research and follow-up of the children conceived after transfer of blastocysts cultured in vitro is recommended.

## Obstetric and Perinatal Outcomes

Fernando et al. studied the obstetric and perinatal outcomes in women who underwent day 2 or 3 and day 5 or 6 transfer. Multivariate analysis found no statistically significant difference between transfers on days 5 and 6 and days 2 and 4 for all maternal and perinatal outcomes.[66] However, Kalra et al. studied 69,039 live births following either cleavage-stage transfer or blastocyst transfer. Singleton IVF births conceived after blastocyst transfer, as compared with cleavage-stage transfer, were at an increased risk for preterm delivery (18.6% compared with 14.4%, respectively; adjusted OR 1.39, $p < 0.001$) and very preterm delivery (2.8% compared with 2.2%, respectively; adjusted OR 1.35, $p < 0.001$) but not low birth weight.[67]

## KEY POINTS

- Blastocyst culture, although a little time consuming and has inherent limitations, is an important step ahead in the field of ARTs. However, before it can be routinely applied in an ART laboratory, it is essential that the laboratory first has the requisite infrastructure, maintenance, and skills.

- Although the pregnancy rate per blastocyst transfer is higher than pregnancy rates following cleavage-stage transfer, if one were to look at the cumulative pregnancy rate per cycle started or per patient, then the results are not that dramatic. The number of embryos that grow to blastocysts and are available for transfer or cryopreservation is much lesser. Till the concerns about the potential epigenetic changes that extended culture could lead to,[68] one should use extended culture to blastocyst only when there are multiple cleavage-stage embryos available for transfer so that those that do not develop to the blastocyst get deselected. As of now, its routine application for ART in all cases does not seem justified.
- Further studies are still required to have an optimal understanding of the metabolism of embryos and nutritional requirements. In the luminal secretions, the embryo is exposed to a variety of growth factors and cytokines[69] that are not routinely added to culture media. Growth factors are known to have pleiotropic effects on embryo development including blastocyst formation and hatching,[70] and it needs to be seen whether the addition of these would further improve the development of *blastocysts* in vitro.

## REFERENCES


1. Vidaeff AC, Racowsky C, Rayburn WF. Blastocyst transfer in human in vitro fertilization. A solution to the multiple pregnancy epidemic. J Reprod Med. 2000;45:529-39.
2. Braude P, Bolton V, Moore S. Human gene expression first occurs between the four- and eight-cell stages of preimplantation development. Nature. 1988;332:459-61.
3. Buster JE, Bustillo M, Rodi IA, Cohen SW, Hamilton M, Simon JA, et al. Biologic and morphologic development of donated human ova recovered by nonsurgical uterine lavage. Am J Obstet Gynecol. 1985;153:211-7.
4. Bolton V, Wren ME, Parsons JH. Pregnancies after in vitro fertilization and transfer of human blastocysts. Fertil Steril. 1991;55:830-2.
5. Bongso A, Ng SC, Fong CY, Ratnam S. Cocultures: a new lead in embryo quality improvement for assisted reproduction. Fertil Steril. 1991;56:179-91.
6. Menezo YJ, Guerin JF, Czyba JC. Improvement of human early embryo development in vitro by coculture on monolayers of Vero cells. Biol Reprod. 1990;42:301-6.
7. Behr B, Pool TB, Milki AA, Moore D, Gebhardt J, Dasig D. Preliminary clinical experience with human blastocyst development in vitro without co-culture. Hum Reprod. 1999;14:454-7.
8. Gardner DK, Lane M. Culture and selection of viable blastocysts: a feasible proposition for human IVF? Hum Reprod Update. 1997;3:367-82.
9. Balaban B, Urman B. Comparison of two sequential media for culturing cleavage-stage embryos and blastocysts: embryo characteristics and clinical outcome. Reprod Biomed Online. 2005;10:485-91.
10. Artini PG, Valentino V, Cela V, Cristello F, Vitè A, Genazzani AR. A randomized control comparison study of culture media (HTF versus P1) for human in vitro fertilization. Eur J Obstet Gynecol Reprod Biol. 2004;116:196-200.
11. Utsunomiya T, Naitou T, Nagaki M. A prospective trial of blastocyst culture and transfer. Hum Reprod. 2002;17:1846-51.
12. Biggers JD, Racowsky C. The development of fertilized human ova to the blastocyst stage in KSOM(AA) medium: is a two- step protocol necessary? Reprod Biomed Online. 2002;5:133-40.
13. Stone BA, Greene J, Vargyas JM, Ringler GE, Marrs RP. Embryo fragmentation as a determinant of blastocyst development in vitro and pregnancy outcomes following embryo transfer. Am J Obstet Gynecol. 2005;192:2014-9.
14. Gardner DK, Lane M, Stevens J, Schlenker T, Schoolcraft WB. Blastocyst score affects implantation and pregnancy outcome: towards a single blastocyst transfer. Fertil Steril. 2000;73:1155-8.
15. Kovacic B, Vlaisavljevic V, Reljic M, Cizek-Sajko M. Developmental capacity of different morphological types of day 5 human morulae and blastocysts. Reprod Biomed Online. 2004;8:687-94.
16. Richter KS, Harris DC, Daneshmand ST, Shapiro BS. Quantitative grading of human blastocyst: optimal inner cell mass size and shape. Fertil Steril. 2001;76:1157-67.
17. Hardy K, Stark J, Winston RML. Maintenance of the inner cell mass in human blastocysts from fragmented embryos. Biol Reprod. 2003;68:1165-9.
18. Gardner DK, Schoolcraft WB. In vitro culture of human blastocysts. In: Jansen R, Mortimer D (Eds). Towards Reproductive Certainty: Infertility and Genetics Beyond. Carnforth, UK: Parthenon Press; 1999. pp. 378-88.
19. Hardarson T, Caisander G, Sjögren A, Hanson C, Hamberger L, Lundin K. A morphological and chromosomal study of blastocysts developing from morphologically suboptimal human pre-embryos compared with control blastocysts. Hum Reprod. 2003;18:399-407.
20. Ménézo YJR, Kaufmann R, Veiga A, Servy EJ. A mini-atlas of the human blastocyst in vitro. Zygote. 1999;7:61-5.
21. Sathananthan H, Menezes J, Gunasheela S. Mechanisms of human blastocyst hatching in vitro. Reprod Biomed Online. 2003;7:228-34.
22. Ma BX, Yang L, Tian Y, Jin L, Huang B. Cytoplasmic strings between ICM and mTE are a positive predictor of clinical pregnancy and live birth outcomes: A time-lapse study. Front Med. 2022;9.
23. Scott L, Alvero R, Leondires M, Miller B. The morphology of human pronuclear embryos is positively related to blastocyst development and implantation. Hum Reprod. 2000;15:2394-403.
24. Fisch JD, Rodriguez H, Ross R, Overby G, Sher G. The Graduated Embryo Score (GES) predicts blastocyst formation and pregnancy rate from cleavage-stage embryos. Hum Reprod. 2001;16:1970-5.
25. Boostanfar R, Jain JK, Slater CC, Tourgeman DE, Francis MM, Paulson RJ. The prognostic significance of day 3 embryo cleavage stage on subsequent blastocyst development in a sequential culture system. J Assist Reprod Genet. 2001;18:548-50.

26. Smith AL. Blastocyst culture in human IVF: the final destination or a stop along the way? Theriogenology. 2002;57:97-107.
27. Bedaiwy MA, Falcone T, Mohamed MS, Aleem AAN, Sharma RK, Worley SE, et al. Differential growth of human embryos in vitro: role of reactive oxygen species. Fertil Steril. 2004;82:593-600.
28. Pantos K, Athanasiou V, Stefanidis K, Stavrou D, Vaxevanoglou T, Chronopoulou M. Influence of advanced age on the blastocyst development rate and pregnancy rate in assisted reproductive technology. Fertil Steril. 1999;71:1144-6.
29. Shapiro BS, Richter KS, Harris DC, Daneshmand ST. Influence of patient age on the growth and transfer of blastocyst-stage embryos. Fertil Steril. 2002;77:700-5.
30. Jones GM, Trounson AO, Lolatgis N, Wood C. Factors affecting the success of human blastocyst development and pregnancy following in vitro fertilization and embryo transfer. Fertil Steril. 1998;70:1022-9.
31. Rijnders PM, Jansen CA. The predictive value of day 3 embryo morphology regarding blastocyst formation, pregnancy and implantation rate after day 5 transfer following in-vitro fertilization or intracytoplasmic sperm injection. Hum Reprod. 1998;13:2869-73.
32. Veeck LL, Zaninovic N. Human blastocysts in vitro. In: Veeck L, Zaninovic N (Eds). An Atlas of Human Blastocysts. Boca Raton, FL: Parthenon Publishing; 2003. pp. 99-137.
33. Schiewe MC, Araujo Jr E, Asch RH, Balmaceda JP. Enzymatic characterization of zona pellucida hardening in human eggs and embryos. J Assist Reprod Genet. 1995;12:2-7.
34. Stehlik E, Stehlik J, Katayama KP, Kuwayama M, Jambor V, Brohammer R, et al. Vitrification demonstrates significant improvement versus slow freezing of human blastocysts. Reprod Biomed Online. 2005:11:53-7.
35. Menezo Y. Cryopreservation of IVF embryos: which stage? Eur J Obstet Gynecol Reprod Biol. 2004;113(Suppl 1): S28-32.
36. Van den Abbeel E, Camus M, Verheyen G, Van Waesberghe L, Devroey P, Van Steirteghem A. Slow controlled-rate freezing of sequentially cultured human blastocysts: an evaluation of two freezing strategies. Hum Reprod. 2005:20:2939-45.
37. Guerif F, Cadoret V, Poindron J, Lansac J, Royere D. Overnight incubation improves selection of frozen–thawed blastocysts for transfer: preliminary study using supernumerary embryos. Theriogenology. 2003;60:1457-66.
38. Gardner DK, Vella P, Lane M, Wagley L, Schlenker T, Schoolcraft WB. Culture and transfer of human blastocysts increases implantation rates and reduces the need for multiple embryo transfers. Fertil Steril. 1998;69:84-8.
39. Marek D, Langley M, Gardner DK, Confer N, Doody KM, Doody KJ. Introduction of blastocyst culture and transfer for all patients in an in vitro fertilization program. Fertil Steril. 1999;72:1035-40.
40. Milki AA, Hinckley MD, Fisch JD, Dasig D, Behr B. Comparison of blastocyst transfer with day 3 embryo transfer in similar patient populations. Fertil Steril. 2000;73:126-9.
41. Pantos K, Makrakis E, Karantzis P, Stavrou D, Grammatis M, Chronopoulos K. Blastocyst versus early cleavage embryo transfer: a retrospective analysis of 4,165 transfers. Clin Exp Obstet Gynecol. 2004;31:42-4.
42. Barrenetexea G, Lopez de Larruzea A, Ganzabal T, Jiménez R, Carbonero K, Mandiola M. Blastocyst culture after repeated failure of cleavage-stage embryo transfers: a comparison of day 5 and day 6 transfers. Fertil Steril. 2005;83:49-53.
43. Guerif F, Bidault R, Gasnier O, Couet ML, Gervereau O, Lansac J, et al. Efficacy of blastocyst transfer after implantation failure. Reprod Biomed Online. 2004;9:630-6.
44. Glujovsky D, Blake D, Farquhar C, Bardach A. Cleavage stage versus blastocyst stage embryo transfer in assisted reproductive technology. Cochrane Database Syst Rev. 2012;(7): CD002118.
45. Gerris JMR. Single embryo transfer and IVF/ICSI outcome: a balanced appraisal. Hum Reprod Update. 2005;11:105-21.
46. Van Royen E, Mangelschots K, De Neubourg D, Valkenburg M, Van de Meerssche M, Ryckaert G, et al. Characterization of a top quality embryo, a step towards single embryo transfer. Hum Reprod. 1999;14:2345-9.
47. Fang R, Yang W, Zhao X, Xiong F, Guo C, Xiao J, et al. Chromosome screening using culture medium of embryos fertilised in vitro: a pilot clinical study. J Transl Med. 2019;17:73.
48. Trounson AO. The derivation and potential use of human embryonic stem cells. Reprod Fertil Dev. 2001;13:523-32.
49. Blake D, Proctor M, Johnson N, Olive D. Cleavage stage versus blastocyst stage embryo transfer in assisted conception. Cochrane Database Syst Rev. 2002;(2):CD002118.
50. Behr B, Fisch JD, Racowsky C, Miller K, Pool TB, Milki AA. Blastocyst-ET and monozygotic twinning. J Assist Reprod Genet. 2000;17:349- 51.
51. Jain JK, Boostanfar R, Slater CC, Francis MM, Paulson RJ. Monozygotic twins and triplets in association with blastocyst transfer. J Assist Reprod Genet. 2004;21:103-7.
52. Peramo B, Ricciarelli E, Cuadros-Fernandez JM, Huguet E, Hernandez ER. Blastocyst transfer and monozygotic twinning. Fertil Steril. 1999;72:1116-7.
53. da Costa ALE, Abdelmassih S, de Oliveira FG, Abdelmassih V, Abdelmassih R, Nagy ZP, et al. Monozygotic twins and transfer at the blastocyst stage after ICSI. Hum Reprod. 2001;16:333-6.
54. Bulmer MG. The Biology of Twinning in Man. Oxford: Clarendon Press; 1970.
55. Sills ES, Tucker MJ, Palermo GD. Assisted reproductive technologies and monozygous twins: implications for future study and clinical practice. Twin Res. 2000;3:217-23.
56. Milki AA, Jun SH, Hinckley MD, Behr B, Giudice LC, Westphal LM. Incidence of mono- zygotic twinning with blastocyst transfer compared to cleavage-stage transfer. Fertil Steril. 2003;79:503-6.
57. Kawachiya S, Bodri D, Shimada N, Kato K, Takehara Y, Kato O. Blastocyst culture is associated with an elevated incidence of monozygotic twinning after single embryo transfer. Fertil Steril. 2011;95:2140-2.
58. Paonessa M, Borini A, Coticchio G. Genetic causes of preimplantation embryo developmental failure. Mol Reprod Dev. 2021;88:338-48.
59. McEvoy TG, Sinclair KD, Young LE, Wilmut I, Robinson JJ. Large offspring syndrome and other consequences of ruminant embryo culture in vitro: relevance to blastocyst culture in human ART. Hum Fertil (Camb). 2000;3:238-46.
60. Martin KL, Leese HJ. Role of glucose in mouse preimplantation embryo development. Mol Reprod Dev. 1995;40:436-43.

61. Hardy K, Handyside AH, Winston RM. The human blastocyst: cell number, death and allocation during late preimplantation development in vitro. Development. 1989;107:597-604.
62. Khosla S, Dean W, Reik W, Feil R. Culture of preimplantation embryos and its long-term effects on gene expression and phenotype. Hum Reprod Update. 2001;7:419-27.
63. Doherty AS, Mann MR, Tremblay KD, Bartolomei MS, Schultz RM. Differential effects of culture on imprinted H19 expression in the preimplantation mouse embryo. Biol Reprod. 2000;62:1526-35.
64. Sinclair KD, Young LE, Wilmut I, McEvoy TG. In-utero overgrowth in ruminants following embryo culture: lessons from mice and a warning to men. Hum Reprod. 2000;(Suppl. 5):68-86.
65. Menezo YJ, Chouteau J, Torello J, Girard A, Veiga A. Birth weight and sex ratio after transfer at the blastocyst stage in humans. Fertil Steril. 1999;72:221-4.
66. Fernando D, Halliday JL, Breheny S, Healy DL. Outcomes of singleton births after blastocyst versus nonblastocyst transfer in assisted reproductive technology. Fertil Steril. 2012;97:579-84.
67. Kalra SK, Ratcliffe SJ, Barnhart KT, Coutifaris C. Extended embryo culture and an increased risk of preterm delivery. Obstet Gynecol. 2012;120:69-75.
68. Chason RJ, Csokmay J, Segars JH, DeCherney AH, Randall Armant D. Environmental and epigenetic effects upon preimplantation embryo metabolism and development. Trends Endocrinol Metab. 2011;22:412-20.
69. Smotrich DB, Stillman RJ, Widra EA, Gindoff PR, Kaplan P, Graubert M, et al. Immunocytochemical localization of growth factors and their receptors in human pre-embryos and Fallopian tubes. Hum Reprod. 1996;11:184-90.
70. Martin KL, Barlow DH, Sargent IL. Heparin-binding epidermal growth factor significantly improves human blastocyst development and hatching in serum-free medium. Hum Reprod. 1998;13:1645-52.

CHAPTER 109

# Cryopreservation of Oocytes

Goral Gandhi

## INTRODUCTION

Cryopreservation of human cells is an integral part of assisted reproductive technology (ART). Unlike the human sperms and preimplantation embryos, it has been extremely difficult to cryopreserve the metaphase II (MII) oocyte. Even though the ability to store oocytes successfully at –196°C has numerous practical and financial advantages, together with ethical considerations, surprisingly, there was not much interest in cryopreserving oocytes. Chen reported the first human birth using cryopreserved oocytes as early as in 1986.[1] However, the failure to reproduce this early success became a major setback. The possibility of oocyte cryopreservation becoming a routine technique seemed unlikely for many years.

For a long time, oocyte cryopreservation was considered as an experimental procedure at best. A significant resurgence of interest in the human egg freezing came about in recent times owing to its perceived potential to preserve fertility. Vitrification was applied to oocyte cryopreservation techniques, which produced more consistent and reproducible results. Kuleshova et al. reported the first birth from vitrified human oocytes.[2] Various studies followed, which showed the superiority of vitrification over slow freezing in the postthaw survival of vitrified oocytes.[3,4] Vitrification was proposed as an alternative to conventional slow freezing methods. Recent advances in cryobiology have led to a newer option or protocols available for the oocyte cryopreservation in terms of technique used, media composition, and various storage devices used for vitrification. This has resulted in an improved survival of cryopreserved oocytes.

In fact, the results after oocyte vitrification have been extremely promising. As a result, a 2011 guideline from the Practice Committees of the American Society for Reproductive Medicine (ASRM) and the Society for Assisted Reproductive Technology (SART) indicated that mature oocyte vitrification and warming should no longer be considered as an experimental procedure[5] because this technology is recommended in cases of gonadotoxic therapies when there is a lack of alternative options for fertility preservation.

These guidelines have resulted in the vitrification of oocytes being offered as an option for women who wish to preserve their fertility to allow them to have a possibility of having their own genetic offspring in the future. Cancer patients as well as patients with other diseases who need to undergo potentially gonadotoxic treatments benefit from this. Another population to benefit from oocyte freezing is women who wish to postpone childbearing for a variety of "nonmedical" reasons. This form of egg freezing is popularly known as "social egg freezing."

## INDICATIONS FOR OOCYTE FREEZING

- Loss of reproductive function due to chemotherapy, radiation, and/or surgery for cancer
- Premature menopause and ovarian failure
- Overcoming ethical and legal issues involved in embryo freezing
- Oocytes cryobanking for facilitation of egg donation program
- To prevent age-related infertility and options for delaying motherhood
- Prevention of ovarian hyperstimulation syndrome
- Male factor infertility or inadequate seminal samples
- Poor egg quality due to endometriosis
- Immunological disorders

## HURDLES ASSOCIATED WITH OOCYTE CRYOPRESERVATION

In spite of so many reasons to freeze oocytes, it took scientists many years to successfully preserve oocytes. The reason was the extreme cryosensitive nature of the human oocyte. Oocyte cryopreservation is technically more challenging than embryo cryopreservation. Differences in membrane permeability and in physiology are two main reasons why successful oocyte cryopreservation had remained elusive and also explain why it has taken so long to introduce oocyte cryopreservation even though the first embryo was cryopreserved as early as 1978.

## FACTORS AFFECTING OOCYTE SURVIVAL

- *Spherical shape and surface area:* Oocytes are extremely difficult to cryopreserve because of their low surface area to volume ratio and high susceptibility to intracellular ice formation. Perfect sphere of the oocyte slows down permeation and equal distribution of cryoprotectant in the oocyte. This continuous concentration gradient results in a longer exposure of the oocyte to cryoprotectants, which may lead to toxic damage in one part of the oocyte offering less than optimal protection in other.[6]
- *Size:* Size is a very important parameter in cryobiology. Larger the cell, more difficult to cryopreserve it. Oocytes are the largest cell of the human body. Size of the oocyte widely affects crystal formation and the slow dilution or accumulation of toxic cryoprotectants, thus increasing the challenge of survival.
- *Monocellular nature:* Since oocyte is a single-cell structure, there is no backup to regenerate from serious injuries as compared to multicellular embryo, which can survive up to 50% loss of its cells.[6]
- *Physiology of the membrane:* It is very difficult to predict the membrane permeability characteristics of human oocytes along with other biophysical parameters.[7] Studies have also revealed the negative effects of cryopreservation on the stability of microtubules and microfilaments in mammalian oocytes, which are vital for normal chromosomal segregation.[8]
- *Cryoinjuries*: The oocyte is highly susceptible to the cryoinjuries to the cytoplasmic content and the nuclear spindle.[9] Chilling injury occurs at high temperature and induces irreversible damage to the cytosolic content, membrane, and zona pellucida. Hardening of the zona due to premature cortical granule release may result in the decreased fertilization rate. Therefore, a very careful approach has to be applied for oocyte freezing. There is an increase in the intracellular calcium concentration following cryopreservation. This can cause cortical granule release, zona pellucida hardening, and parthenogenic activation of the oocyte.[10-12]

Due to these varied difficulties associated with oocyte vitrification, for many years, oocyte vitrification was considered experimental, and therefore, embryo cryopreservation was the only established option for fertility preservation in female cancer patients.[13]

However, with the advent of vitrification, everything changed. The optimization and widespread use of vitrification methods for human oocytes in laboratories worldwide have been one of the major advancements in the field of ART. The traditional slow freezing methods of cryopreservation also underwent improvements in the last decade, but the real game-changer in the field of cryopreservation has been vitrification.

## VITRIFICATION

*Vitrification* is a process of cryopreservation which involves exposure of oocyte to high concentration of cryoprotectants and ultra-rapid cooling to solidify the cell into glass-like state without the formation of ice crystals. There are five principal steps in vitrification:

1. Add cryoprotectants.
2. Cool the cells to –196°C.
3. Store at –196°C.
4. Warm the cells.
5. Remove cryoprotectants.

There are many factors that impact successful vitrification during these five steps.

### Cryoprotectants

Vitrification dramatically increased the survival rates of the oocytes. However, one of the major concerns surrounding vitrification is the high concentration of cryoprotectants that are used in vitrification solutions.

There are mainly two types of cryoprotectants. The penetrating cryoprotectants, as the name suggests, penetrate the cell membrane. They protect the cells and tissues by replacing some of the water they contain, thus increasing the viscosity in the cells, preventing the formation of ice crystals, and making the vitrification process easier by inducing the transition to the glass state. The commonly used penetrating cryoprotectants are ethylene glycol (EG), dimethyl sulfoxide (DMSO), and propylene glycol [1,2-propanediol (PrOH)]. The nonpenetrating cryoprotectants protect the cells from the outside. They guard against osmotic damage, especially during the warming procedures. During the warming process, the transfer of the oocytes from a solution containing a high concentration of cryoprotectant to an isotonic solution can lead to a reverse osmotic shock and swelling of the oocyte. This may be dangerous for the oocyte. Use of a hypertonic solution containing nonpenetrating cryoprotectants can prevent this osmotic shock by slowing down the movement of water across the membrane.[14] The typically used nonpenetrating cryoprotectants are sucrose and trehalose. Protein in the vitrification solution helps due to its surfactant characteristics.

During the first phase of research and development of vitrification, efforts were focused on decreasing the toxic and osmotic effects of cryoprotectants. The double or triple amount of cryoprotectants required for vitrification compared to traditional freezing was a big concern.

To decrease the specific toxicity, mixtures of two or three cryoprotectants were applied. At least one of these compounds was permeable. With two cryoprotectants, the concentration of each can be lower than that needed when either is used separately, thereby making the solution less toxic.

## Freezing Rate

A high freezing rate is crucial to achieving proper vitrification and survival. This can be achieved via direct contact between the sample and liquid nitrogen or indirect contact if the sample is contained in a closed carrier.

Decreasing the temperature of the liquid nitrogen can also increase the freezing rate. This way, the freezing rate can increase in two ways. More rapid heat transfer is achieved by a wider temperature difference and it may also minimize the chances of the formation of gas bubbles that can insulate the heat transfer.

The liquid nitrogen temperature can be decreased in two ways: (1) By applying a vacuum over the liquid nitrogen, or (2) By the use of liquid nitrogen slush.[14-16]

In order to achieve the maximal freezing rates, current vitrification loading devices hold a minimal volume of solution, such as the EM grid, CryoLoop™, CryoTip™, CryoTec, CryoTeb, CryoTop, and Cryoleaf™ high security straws. Currently, the most acceptable target in designing vitrification loading devices for oocytes or embryos is to use a small volume (<1 μL) of high-concentration cryoprotectant (approximately 30%) and very rapid freezing rates of 15,000–30,000°C/min.[17]

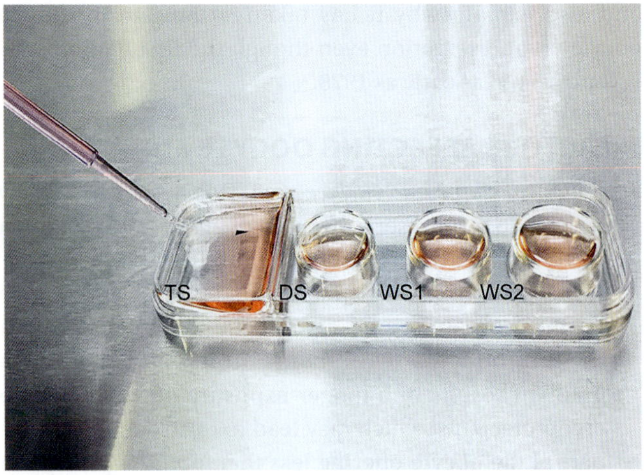


**Fig. 1:** Warming plate by Cryotech Japan which has a warm well included in the plate to facilitate rapid warming rates. (DS: diluent solution; TS: thawing solution; WS: washing solution)

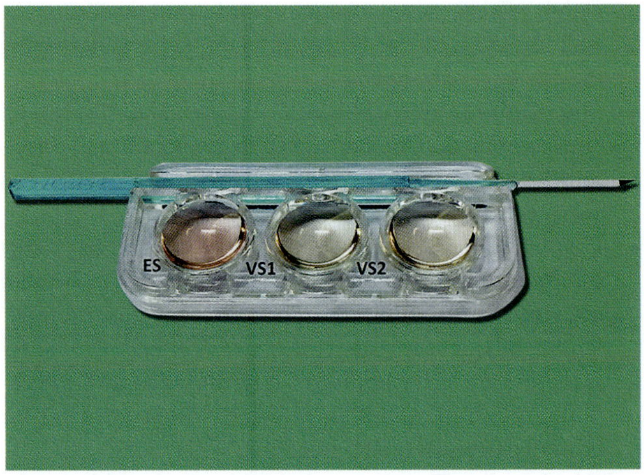


**Fig. 2:** Vitriplate by Cryotech Japan with a holder for the Cryotech. Loading becomes very efficient due to the special plates. (ES: equilibration solution; VS: vitrification solution)

## Warming Rate

The cells are more sensitive to the warming rate compared to the cooling rate during vitrification. It has been suggested that slow warming is lethal for the cells since it allows the growth of tiny ice crystals by recrystallization.

To achieve high-warming rates, it is essential that minimum volumes are used during vitrification. Mixing the cells in pre-warmed media will aid in achieving high-warming rates.

In open system vitrification, very high-warming rates can be achieved by mixing the sample in the thawing solution that is warmed to 37°C **(Fig. 1)**.

### *Loading of the Carrier*

Choose a carrier that facilitates rapid heat transfer. Choose a system that is easy for the embryologist. This will ensure reproducibility of consistently high survival rates **(Fig. 2)**.

## Open versus Closed System Vitrification

There are two types of vitrification methods. In one method, the cells come into direct contact with liquid nitrogen. This is called "open system vitrification." There has been much concern about the risk of disease transmission through the use of this method. As a result, another method was developed, where the cells do not come in direct contact with liquid nitrogen. The carrier is closed before plunging into liquid nitrogen. This is known as "closed system vitrification." The cooling rate achieved with the closed system is, however, reported to be much lower than those achieved with open system.

### *Effectiveness of Open and Closed Systems*

A review of the literature shows that the best survival rates reported for oocytes using closed system vitrification are between 70 and 85%[18] whereas a survival rate of 98–100% for oocytes is reported by many workers using the open system.[19] Hence, clearly for oocytes, open system vitrification seems to be working much more effectively than closed system vitrification.

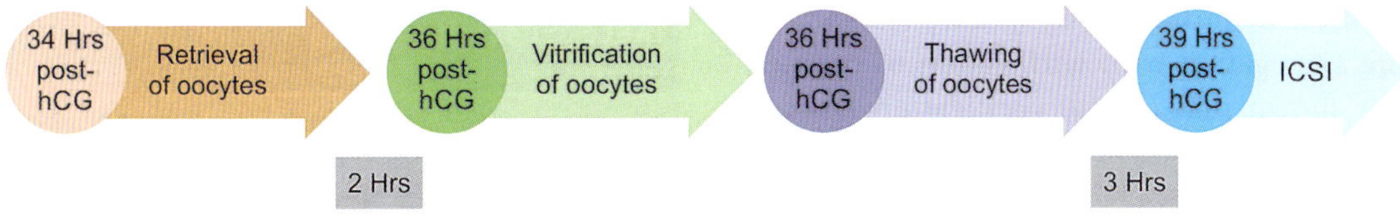


**Fig. 3:** Time schedule to be observed for oocyte vitrification and warming.
(hCG: human chorionic gonadotropin; ICSI: intracytoplasmic sperm injection)

### *Risk of Disease Transmission*

The main concern against the use of open systems is the risk of disease transmission. However, no such disease transfer has yet been reported, although estimated 600,000–1,000,000 vitrified embryos or embryos derived from vitrified oocytes by using open systems have been transferred. So, is this risk applicable to real-life situations?[20]

Vajta et al. have compared the open and closed systems of vitrification and have noted that overwhelming evidence shows that open systems are efficient for both blastocyst and oocyte vitrification; relevant data on closed systems, however, are sporadic, especially in the case of human oocytes, and far from convincing. The authors recommended that a pragmatic approach in legislation and scientific evaluation should be used. They advised to consider the facts instead of theories and acknowledge the value of methods that are used in a huge number of cases.

There are ways of preventing contamination during storage that can be adopted:

- Proper sealing of carriers containing oocytes is an effective measure against contamination during storage.
- An alternative preventive step is filtration of liquid nitrogen and the application of accessory protective storage containers.
- Cross contamination may be prevented by storing oocytes/embryos from patients with known infections in separate liquid nitrogen tanks.

## DYNAMICS OF MEIOTIC SPINDLES OF FROZEN-THAWED OOCYTES

The spindle is very sensitive to cryoprotectants and low temperature. Oocytes analyzed immediately after thawing displayed severe disorganization or disappearance of spindles. This disappearance of the meiotic spindle is one of the most significant changes caused by oocyte cryopreservation. The meiotic spindles are crucial for the events following fertilization at completion of meiosis, the second polar body (PB) formation, and migration of the pronuclei. Incubation for 1–3 hours resulted in recovery of spindles.[21-23] Even though spindle abnormalities in cryopreserved oocytes were originally of concern, the incidence of chromosomal abnormalities in human embryos derived from cryopreserved oocytes is not statistically different from that of control embryos.[8,24]

## TIME SCHEDULE FOR VITRIFICATION OF OOCYTES AND FERTILIZATION

The optimum time for intracytoplasmic sperm injection (ICSI) for human oocytes is between 37 and 41 hours posthuman chorionic gonadotropin (hCG).

We know that inseminating oocytes soon after thawing, when there is serious spindle disorganization, adversely affects fertilization outcome.[1]

Choosing the optimum time interval between oocyte thawing and ICSI is crucial for normal fertilization and subsequent development.

Oocyte recovery can be performed at 34 hours post-hCG, vitrification of oocytes being performed at 2 hours after oocyte recovery, and ICSI being performed at 3 hours postthaw (post-hCG 39 hours) **(Fig. 3)**.

## SAFETY OF VITRIFICATION

There have been many concerns regarding the safety of vitrification and the metabolomics, proteomics, and epigenetic risks involved with vitrification.

A study on the metabolomics profile of embryos developed from fresh and vitrified oocytes has suggested that the embryonic metabolomics profile is not disturbed by oocyte vitrification.[25] The influence of vitrification on the oocyte proteome of in vitro grown germinal vesicle (GV) as well as MII oocytes was assessed in a study on mouse oocytes. Transient changes in mitochondrial activity by vitrification occur at the preantral stage, but proteome of in vitro grown and matured oocyte is not affected.[26] Oocyte proteome and developmental potential may get affected[27] because of changes in cellular integrity and protein alterations with the use of high concentration of cryoprotectant in an animal model.[28,29]

In a study where messenger ribonucleic acid (mRNA) contents in MII oocytes after slow freezing/rapid thawing and vitrification/warming protocols were compared with the fresh MII oocytes, it was found that mRNA abundance may decrease in both types of cryopreservation methods which may result in molecular injury. However, the mRNA content level in vitrified oocyte remains sufficient to sustain biological function.[30]

Recovery of the meiotic spindle occurs after cryopreservation in both conventional and vitrification technology.[31-33] Thus, it is suggested that there are no increased risks of disturbances in spindle formation or chromosome segregation with vitrification of oocytes.[34] Studies have shown that oocyte vitrification does not increase the rate of aneuploidy or diminish the implantation potential of viable blastocysts.[35]

In a study conducted to check the neonatal outcomes of babies born using vitrified oocytes, a total of 58 reports were reviewed from 1996 to 2008. Of the total 936 newborn, 1.3% had birth anomalies. No difference was noted in the birth defect rates when compared with naturally conceived babies.[36] A similar study has revealed no difference in birth weight or congenital anomalies among those born from vitrified oocytes as compared to children conceived after fresh in vitro fertilization (IVF).[35,37] A successful live birth has been reported from vitrified oocytes after 5 years of cryopreservation.[38] These findings suggest that there are no reported increase in miscarriages, chromosome abnormalities, and birth defect in the infants born from vitrified oocytes. With many recent studies now reporting similar findings, vitrification procedures have certainly become mainstream and led to an increase in our confidence in oocyte vitrification.

**TABLE 1:** Comparative data showing survival, fertilization, and cleavage rates between fresh and frozen–thawed human oocytes.

| | *Fresh oocytes* | *Frozen-thawed oocytes* | *p-value* |
|---|---|---|---|
| Number of oocytes | 792 | 884 | |
| Survival rate (%) | NA | 98.8 | |
| Fertilization rate (%) | 85.0 | 83.8 | NS |
| Cleavage rate (%) | 98.2 | 98.6 | NS |

(NA: not applicable; NS: not significant)

**TABLE 2:** Clinical outcomes of fresh and frozen-thawed human oocytes.

| | *Fresh oocytes* | *Frozen-thawed oocytes* | *p-value* |
|---|---|---|---|
| Number of cycles | 99 | 110 | NS |
| Pregnancy rate | 76 (76.76%) | 84 (76.36%) | NS |
| Biochemical pregnancy rate | 5 (5.05%) | 6 (5.45%) | NS |
| Missed abortion rate | 6 (6.06%) | 7 (6.36%) | NS |
| Live birth rate | 64 (64.65%) | 71 (64.55%) | NS |

(NS: not significant)

## OUR RESULTS WITH OOCYTE VITRIFICATION

The oocytes were subjected to vitrification by using the Cryotech vitrification method (Repro-Support Medical Research Centre, Co. Ltd., 2-5-5-8F Shinjuku, Tokyo, Japan).

A retrospective analysis was done to study the outcome of oocyte vitrification using the Cryotech method. We compared the outcome of fresh versus frozen oocytes in the oocyte donation program. The data was evaluated over a period from January 2015 to December 2016. A total of 2,095 oocytes were obtained from 174 oocyte donors. The study included 1,676 mature oocytes. From this, 792 eggs were used in fresh cycles and 884 oocytes were vitrified using the Cryotech method. The oocytes were later warmed using the Cryotech warming solutions, fertilized by ICSI, and the embryos thus created were transferred into the recipients. A total of 171 embryo transfer cycles were performed on day 3 of embryo development. The parameters which were assessed and compared between the two groups included survival rate, fertilization rate, cleavage rate, embryo development, and the clinical pregnancy rates.

## OUR EXPERIENCE WITH OOCYTE VITRIFICATION

A comparative study to evaluate the outcome of oocyte vitrification using the Cryotech method, observed in an egg donation program with fresh versus frozen oocyte, was done. The data was evaluated over a period from January 2011 to December 2011. A total of 1,210 oocytes were obtained from 112 oocyte donors. The analysis included a total of 1,029 mature oocytes, 485 oocytes were used in fresh cycle, and the remaining 544 oocytes were vitrified using the Cryotech method. The vitrified oocytes were subsequently warmed using the Cryotech warming method. The warmed oocytes were fertilized by ICSI and the embryos thus created were transferred into the recipients. A total of 209 embryo transfers were performed on day 3 of the embryo development. The laboratory and clinical parameters of both the groups were compared **(Tables 1 and 2)**.

Our results with oocyte vitrification are extremely encouraging. It has proved that the current vitrification protocols are extremely efficient and effective in cryopreserving oocytes. Excellent clinical outcome indicates that this technology can be applied successfully for cryopreserving oocytes for various indications including preserving fertility for cancer patients, building donor oocyte banks, and preserving female fertility for age-related reasons.

## IMMATURE OOCYTES

Oocyte cryopreservation is associated with many factors, such as different human oocyte sources including in vivo mature, in vitro mature, and immature oocytes. There are reports about babies born using vitrified oocytes of the three types.

However, studies have shown that in vivo and in vitro mature human oocytes are more suitable to vitrification than immature human oocytes.[39]

## POOR MORPHOLOGY OOCYTES

It is well known that the majority of the oocytes retrieved from stimulated cycles (60–70%) exhibit one or more abnormal morphological characteristics.[40]

The presence of large PB, large perivitelline space (PVS), refractile bodies, or vacuoles is associated with decreased oocyte fertilization. It is generally hypothesized that morphologically abnormal oocytes could be more affected by the vitrification procedure than normal oocytes. Embryologists tend to expect a negative influence of oocyte morphological abnormalities on survival rates postvitrification and ICSI outcomes. However, studies have shown that oocyte morphology, observed prior to vitrification, does not predict postwarming survival.[41,42] The noninvasive identification of predictive markers for oocyte survival potential remains a difficult task. Hence, it would not be wise to omit poor morphology oocytes from vitrification, especially for autologous cases of oocyte cryopreservation.

## KEY POINTS

- Very efficient protocols for oocyte vitrification are now available. It is our duty as reproductive scientists to use these protocols efficiently and preserve precious human life till the patient's dream of becoming parents comes true.
- Vitrification is highly skill dependent, and close adherence to the prescribed protocol is absolutely essential for excellent results.
- As per the current technology available, open system vitrification is more efficient for oocyte vitrification than close system vitrification.
- It is advised to vitrify the oocytes within 2 hours of retrieval and to wait for 3 hours after warming before fertilizing them. This will take care of meiotic spindle recovery as well as avoid oocyte aging.
- Oocyte vitrification does not increase the rate of aneuploidy or decrease the implantation potential of the embryos. This makes oocyte vitrification a very valuable tool for young women wanting to preserve their fertility for either medical or age-related reasons.

## REFERENCES


1. Chen C. Pregnancy after human oocyte cryopreservation. Lancet. 1986;1:884-6.
2. Kuleshova L, Gianaroli L, Magli C, Ferraretti A, Trounson A. Birth following vitrification of a small number of human oocytes: case report. Hum Reprod. 1999;14:3077-9.
3. Oktay K, Cil AP, Bang H. Efficiency of oocyte cryopreservation: a meta-analysis. Fertil Steril. 2006;86:70-80.
4. Smith GD, Serafini PC, Fioravanti J, Yadid I, Coslovsky M, Hassun P, et al. Prospective randomized comparison of human oocyte cryopreservation with slow-rate freezing or vitrification. Fertil Steril. 2010;94:2088-95.
5. Practice Committees of American Society for Reproductive Medicine, Society for Assisted Reproductive Technology. Mature oocyte cryopreservation: a guideline. Fertil Steril. 2013;99:37-43.
6. Kuwayama M, Cobo A, Vajta G. Vitrification of oocytes—general considerations and the use of the Cryotop method. In: Tucker MJ, Liebermann J (Eds). Vitrification in Assisted Reproduction. Oxon: Informa Healthcare; 2007. pp. 119-28.
7. Fuller BJ, Hunter JE, Bernard AG, Mcgrath JJ, Curtis P, Jackson A. The permeability of unfertilised oocytes to 1,2-propanediol: a comparison of mouse and human-cells. Cryo Lett. 1992;13:287-92.
8. Pickering SJ, Johnson MH. The influence of cooling on the organization of the meiotic spindle of the mouse oocyte. Hum Reprod. 1987;2:207-16.
9. Vincent C, Johnson MI. Cooling, cryoprotectants and the cytoskeleton of the mammalian oocyte. Oxf Rev Reprod Biol. 1992;14:73-100.
10. Gook DA. History of oocyte cryopreservation. Reprod Biomed Online. 2011;23:281-9.
11. Kim TJ, Hong SW, Chung HM, Lee SH, Cha KY. Pregnancy and delivery after vitrification of human oocytes. Fertil Steril. 2005;83:S13.
12. Kim T, Hong S, Cha K. Pregnancies from cryopreserved oocytes using vitrification protocol. Fertil Steril. 2005;84: S174.
13. Ethics Committee of the American Society for Reproductive Medicine. Fertility Preservation and Reproduction in Cancer Patients. Fertil Steril. 2005;83:1622-8.
14. Fuller BJ, Bernard A. Successful in vitro fertilization of mouse oocytes after cryopreservation using glycerol. Cryo Lett. 1984;5:307-12.
15. Nakagata N. High survival rate of unfertilized mouse oocytes after vitrification. J Reprod Fertil. 1989;87:479-83.
16. Martino A, Songsasen N, Leibo SP. Development into blastocysts of bovine oocytes cryopreserved by ultra-rapid cooling. Biol Reprod. 1996;54:1059-69.
17. Vajta G, Holm P, Kuwayama M, Booth PJ, Jacobsen H, Greve T, et al. Open pulled straw (OPS) vitrification: a new way to reduce cryoinjuries of bovine ova and embryos. Mol Reprod Dev. 1998;51:53-8.
18. Pensis M, Loumaye E, Psalti I. Screening of conditions for rapid freezing of human oocytes: preliminary study toward their cryopreservation. Fertil Steril. 1989;52:787-94.
19. Seki S, Mazur P. Effect of warming rate on the survival of vitrified mouse oocytes and on the recrystallization of intracellular ice. Biol Reprod. 2008;79:727-37.
20. Kuwayama M, Vajta G, Kato O, Leibo SP. Highly efficient vitrification method for cryopreservation of human oocyte. Reprod Biomed Online. 2005;11:300-8.
21. Bielanski A, Vajta G. Risk of contamination of germplasm during cryopreservation and cryobanking in IVF units. Hum Reprod. 2009;24:2457-67.
22. Eroglu A, Toth TL, Toner M. Alterations of the cytoskeleton and polyploidy induced by cryopreservation of metaphase II mouse oocytes. Fertil Steril. 1998;69:944-57.
23. Rienzi L, Martinez F, Ubaldi F, Minasi MG, Iacobelli M, Tesarik J, et al. Polscope analysis of meiotic spindle changes in living

metaphase II human oocytes during the freezing and thawing procedures. Hum Reprod. 2004;19:655-9.

24. Sathananthan AH, Ng Sc, Trounson AO, Bongso A, Ratnam SS, Ho J, et al. The effect of ultrarapid freezing on meiotic and mitotic spindle of mouse oocytes and embryos. Mol Reprod Dev. 1988;21:385-401.
25. Dominguez F, Castello D, Remohí J, Simón C, Cobo A. Effect of vitrification on human oocytes: a metabolic profiling study. Fertil Steril. 2013;99:565-72.
26. Demant M, Trapphoff T, Fröhlich T, Arnold GJ, Eichenlaub-Ritter U. Vitrification at the pre-antral stage transiently alters inner mitochondrial membrane potential but proteome of in vitro grown and matured mouse oocytes appears unaffected. Hum Reprod. 2012;27:1096-111.
27. Aye M, Di Giorgio C, De Mo M, Botta A, Perrin J, Courbiere B. Assessment of the genotoxicity of three cryoprotectants used for human oocyte vitrification: dimethyl sulfoxide, ethylene glycol and propylene glycol. Food Chem Toxicol. 2010;48:1905-12.
28. Fahy GM. Cryoprotectant toxicity neutralization. Cryobiology. 2010;60:S45-53.
29. Fahy GM, Lilley TH, Linsdell H, Douglas MS, Meryman HT. Cryoprotectant toxicity and cryoprotectant toxicity reduction: in search of molecular mechanisms. Cryobiology. 1990;27:247-68.
30. Chamayou S, Bonaventura G, Alecci C, Tibullo D, Di Raimondo F, Guglielmino A, et al. Consequences of metaphase II oocyte cryopreservation on mRNA content. Cryobiology. 2011;62:130-4.
31. Chen CK, Wang CW, Tsai WJ, Hsieh LL, Wang HS, Soong YK. Evaluation of meiotic spindles in thawed oocytes after vitrification using polarized light microscopy. Fertil Steril. 2004;82:666-72.
32. Bianchi V, Coticchio G, Fava L, Flamigni C, Borini A. Meiotic spindle imaging in human oocytes frozen with a slow freezing procedure involving high sucrose concentration. Hum Reprod. 2005;20:1078-83.
33. Larman MG, Minasi MG, Rienzi L, Gardner DK. Maintenance of the meiotic spindle during vitrification in human and mouse oocytes. Reprod Biomed Online. 2007;15:692-700.
34. Trapphoff T, El Hajj N, Zechner U, Haaf T, Eichenlaub-Ritter U. DNA integrity, growth pattern, spindle formation, chromosomal constitution and imprinting patterns of mouse oocytes from vitrified pre-antral follicles. Hum Reprod. 2010;25:3025-42.
35. Forman EJ, Li X, Ferry KM, Scott K, Treff NR, Scott Jr RT. Oocyte vitrification does not increase the risk of embryonic aneuploidy or diminish the implantation potential of blastocysts created after intracytoplasmic sperm injection: a novel, paired randomized controlled trial using DNA fingerprinting. Fertil Steril. 2012;98:644-9.
36. Noyes N, Porcu E, Borini A. Over 900 oocyte cryopreservation babies born with no apparent increase in congenital anomalies. Reprod Biomed Online. 2009;18:769-76.
37. Chian RC, Huang JY, Tan SL, Lucena E, Saa A, Rojas A, et al. Obstetric and perinatal outcome in 200 infants conceived from vitrified oocytes. Reprod Biomed Online. 2008;16:608-10.
38. Kim TJ, Hong SW. Successful live birth from vitrified oocytes after 5 years of cryopreservation. J Assist Reprod Genet. 2011;28:73-6.
39. Song WY, Peng ZF, Chen XM, Jin HX, Yao GD, Shi SL, et al. Effects of vitrification on outcomes of in vivo-mature, in vitro-mature and immature human oocytes. Cell Physiol Biochem. 2016;38:2053-62.
40. Fabbri R, Porcu E, Marsella T, Rocchetta G, Venturoli S, Flamigni C. Human oocyte cryopreservation: new perspectives regarding oocyte survival. Hum Reprod. 2001;16:411-6.
41. Maldonaldo I, Bermudez A, Varghese A, Gaytan J, Sharma R, Agarwal A. Oocyte dysmorphism is not a limiting factor for post-thaw survival following vitrification by Cryotop method. Fertil Steril. 2008;90:S283.
42. Rienzi L, Vajta G, Ubaldi F. Predictive value of oocyte morphology in human IVF: a systematic review of the literature. Hum Reprod Update. 2010;17:34-45.

CHAPTER 110

# Embryo Cryopreservation

Nitin Laxmikant Lad, Mir Jaffar

## INTRODUCTION

The history of cryopreservation dates back to as long as 2000 BCE where the Mesopotamians used ice houses to store food. The magical use of "cold" temperatures soon became a "hot" topic of interest for many. Reproductive biologists too, left no opportunity to explore the use of ultra-cool temperatures for storage of gametes and embryos. Since its inception in the 1980s, embryo cryopreservation has thereafter seen a profound expansion in its routine clinical use. A report from the US Center for Disease Control and Prevention has stated that the proportion of frozen embryo transfers has risen from 20% in 2005 to almost 50% in 2014.[1,2] Initially, embryo freezing was restricted to patients with medical indications, because back then in vitro fertilization (IVF) was carried out in natural menstrual cycles. So, only one oocyte used to be available, the embryo of which, would immediately be transferred in the same cycle. Advancements in ovarian stimulation, tailored treatments and efficient cryopreservation have expanded the demand for embryo freezing. Some nonelective and elective reasons for embryo freezing include: (1) *Fertility preservation:* embryo freezing allows cancer patients to freeze healthy embryos in order to negate the ill effects of radiation or chemotherapy; (2) *OHSS:* embryo freezing allows time for ovarian recovery in patients prone to OHSS and its related complications; (3) *Elevated progesterone:* high levels of progesterone have a detrimental effect on the implantation rates, thus, embryo freezing allows the privilege to transfer at a suitable time; (4) *Preimplantation genetic testing (PGT) screening:* embryo freezing allows time for patients to select a suitable euploid embryo to be identified for transfer; (5) *Patients or physicians choice:* freezing allows a chance to reduce the risk of multiple pregnancies and need for repeated stimulation cycles; (6) *Personal reasons:* embryo freezing allows couple to conceive at their time-of-choice without compromising on age-related side effects.[2-6] Although cryotechnology has come a long way and made substantial advancements there is still scope for improvement. Great scientific efforts are being made to discover more logical, ethical and economical procedures in order to ensure utmost success without compromising on the safety of these cryoprocedures.

Mammals, being homoeothermic, are not capable of surviving cold temperatures or tolerating freeze injuries unlike some poikilothermic animals that can easily tolerate freezing temperatures. Cryoinjury is the root cause of cell death at low temperatures. When temperatures go below 0°C, the aqueous fluids of the cell supercool to form ice crystals. Ice crystals pose a threat as they mechanically tear into the organelles or at times also rupture the entire cell. Secondly, low temperatures send the cell into an osmotic stress thereby creating a concentrated environment within the cell, eventually leading to cell death. To survive low temperatures, the cell first needs to be sufficiently dehydrated in order to minimize the formation of ice crystals. This can be easily achieved with the use of cryoprotective agents (CPAS).

## CRYOPROTECTIVE AGENTS

Spermatozoa were the most popular cells used by cryobiologists to test the protective ability of different compounds. Since sperms are motile cells, their motility gave direct indications of their viability. All this could be observed simply using a light microscope without having to use any fancy apparatus. Such was the advantage of using sperm cells. This came as a natural advantage to reproductive biologists since most of the cryoresearchers used spermatozoa as their study model. In the 1940s, it became clear that certain sugar solutions give more cellular protection at low temperatures than others. Glycerol is one of the most commonly used cryoprotectants; but how it was discovered, is a story of serendipity. Cryobiologist, Sir Alan Parkes and his student Chris Polge were testing the efficiency of fructose solutions in protecting spermatozoa. They were testing different concentrations of fructose solutions, but to their nightmare after every warming cycle they saw non-motile, dead spermatozoa. One fine day, surprisingly, they saw almost all the thawed spermatozoa were happily motile. This accidental success was because two of the stock bottles in the refrigerator had lost their labels and they had mistakenly used glycerol instead of fructose. From there on began the quest for finding a good CPA.

Cryoprotective agents cause lowering of freezing point of solution, displace water from the intracellular to extracellular environment and alter the solute concentration in the liquid phase. Extracellular CPA increases the extracellular osmolarity, thereby generating an osmotic gradient across the cell. This facilitates dehydration of the cell. During warming, CPA also prevents the rapid entry of water into the cell during the process of rehydration.[6-9] Thus a good CPA must be of a small size with low molecular weight, should easily penetrate cell membrane at high concentrations, should be highly water soluble and should "ideally" be non-toxic.[10] Based upon the nature of the CPA, they are divided into two groups—(1) permeating CPAs and (2) non-permeating CPAs.

## Permeating Cryoprotective Agents

As the name suggests, permeating CPAs are small molecules that readily permeate into the cell membrane. They form hydrogen bonds with water molecules to prevent ice crystallization.[9] To create a higher osmotic gradient, highly concentrated solution of CPAs needs to be used. Since these CPAs enter the cell, higher the concentration of CPA, higher will be the risk of cytotoxicity. In order to minimize the risk of cytotoxicity, scientists came up with the idea of combining two CPAs. For example, ethylene glycol has a low molecular weight and high permeability, therefore it is widely used. But when used by itself, it needs to be used in a very high concentration of about ≥5.5 M. So, it is usually combined with dimethyl sulfoxide (DMSO) in 1:1 ratio, thereby reducing the concentration of either of them by half, without compromising on the effective CPA working concentration. Some commonly used permeating CPAs are:

- Glycerol
- Ethylene glycol (EG)
- Dimethyl sulfoxide (DMSO)
- 1,2-propanediol (PrOH).

## Non-permeating Cryoprotective Agents

In contrast to permeating CPAs, non-permeating CPAs work extracellularly. They draw out intracellular water by creating an osmotic imbalance. They are usually used in combination with permeating CPAs, so that the dual action of extra- and intracellular CPAs dehydrates the cell more efficiently during freezing. Non-permeating CPAs also play a crucial role in the process of warming. During warming, the intracellular ice melts quickly thereby increasing the risk of osmotic swelling of the cell. It is very necessary that the intracellular cryoprotectants (used during freezing) are diffused out of the cell quickly to avoid swelling and rupture of the cell. Nonpermeating CPAs, during warming, prevent excessive influx of free water and draw out permeating CPAs quickly.

Some commonly used non-permeating CPAs are:

- Sugars such as sucrose, trehalose, galactose, mannose
- Polymers such as polyvinylpyrrolidone (PVP), polyethylene glycol (PEG), polyvinyl alcohol (PVA), ficoll and dextran
- Hydroxypropyl cellulose (HPC), human serum albumin (HSA), serum substitute supplement (SSS), dextran serum substitute (DSS).

## Safety and Cytotoxicity of Cryoprotective Agents

Even though most of the permeating CPAs are natural metabolites, they are used in super-physiological concentrations. Thus, the fact that there certainly will be some cytotoxic effects is inevitable. However, the mechanism and the extent to which CPAs negatively affect embryo preservation remains a topic of interest. Studies have shown that temperature fluctuations and exposure to CPAs independently lead to disruption/disorientation of the cytoskeleton such as the microfilaments or the meiotic microtubule assembly, therefore potentially creating a risk of chromosomal abnormalities.[11-13] In fact, higher incidences of chromosomal abnormalities were reported after oocyte cryopreservation. CPA toxicity studies done in thawed oocytes revealed that there is an increased likelihood of oocytes to undergo parthenogenetic activation as a result of various physical and chemical stimuli used during the process.[14-16] Certain studies indicated CPA toxicity to be related to the hydrophobic interactions between CPAs and proteins and the extent of hydrogen binding between CPA molecules and water. It has also been shown that CPAs change the intracellular pH, cause intracellular $Ca^{2+}$ release and formaldehyde formation in the cryopreservation medium.[17-19] Scientists are also trying to figure out whether the toxicity of CPA arises from the wide changes in osmolarity induced due to CPAs or the actual exposure of cells to chemical CPAs. Nonetheless, valuable efforts are being made to mitigate the cytotoxic effects of CPAs.

## Tips for Minimizing the Toxicity of Cryoprotective Agents

While it is impossible to entirely eliminate the toxicity and osmotic injuries posed by CPAs on the embryos, the following can minimize its negative effects.

- Use highly permeable CPAs at lowest required concentrations.
- Keep exposure time of CPAs to bare minimum
- Permeation of CPAs is a temperature dependent process. High temperature accelerates the rate of permeation

and thereby increases the risk of cytotoxicity. Thus it is essential to maintain optimum temperatures of the solutions.

- Combine a balanced concentration of a strong glass former such as DMSO and a weak glass former such as EG or acetamide.
- Increasing the viscosity of vitrification solution (VS) is used as one of the strategies to assist dehydration and reduce cytotoxicity.

## FREEZING OR SLOW FREEZING

Slow freezing or equilibrium freezing is a technique where cryopreservation of cell occurs at a sufficiently slow rate to allow adequate cellular dehydration while minimizing intracellular ice formation. The first successful pregnancy of frozen embryo used a cooling rate of about 1°C/min to -70°C. The principle behind this process is that when cells are loaded with CPAs, they transiently shrink by osmosis since their membranes are more permeable to water than to the solute. When ice nucleates in the extracellular space, the overall concentration of the solutes rises, causing a secondary and lasting dehydration of the cell.[10]

The process involves two main steps: (1) *Equilibration* and (2) *Freezing*. An overview of the process is discussed here. In the first step, embryos are transferred from an isotonic culture medium to a hyperosmotic medium containing one or more permeating CPAs. The embryo is allowed a brief period to take up the CPA. During this period due to difference in the intracellular and extracellular osmotic pressure, the embryos undergo a transient shrinkage. Water and CPAs gradually reenter the cells to maintain the intracellular osmotic equilibrium. Once equilibrium is achieved between the efflux of water and influx of CPA, the shrinkage stops. This is the equilibration state. Equilibration is complete when no further osmotic and chemical gradients between CPA and water exist. At this point, embryos are loaded onto plastic straws and cooled at the rate of 0.5–2°C/min from room temperature to a temperature slightly below the melting point of the solution, which is approximately -5°C to -7°C. Manual seeding is performed at this temperature by manually touching the cryo-container with prechilled forceps, to initiate extracellular ice formation and avoid supercooling. The embryos are further allowed to equilibrate for another 5–10 minutes. After this step, the temperatures are lowered at the rate of 0.3–0.5°C/min until below -30°C. During this period, increasing extracellular ice crystal formation drives intra cellular water out of the cells, leading to a gradual increase in the intracellular ice crystals. The cooling process continues until the intracellular CPA concentration is high enough to allow the solidification of intracellular water without ice crystal formation. At this point in time, the embryos are plunged into liquid nitrogen. The process of warming involves retrieval from liquid nitrogen, warming to 37°C and gradual rehydration to remove CPAs from the embryo.

Slow freezing has its own advantages and drawbacks. The most crucial advantage is the use of less-concentrated CPAs. This serves the critical purpose of achieving dehydration without exerting cytotoxic effects on the embryo. The major limitation of slow freezing is that it is a very lengthy and time-consuming process. Secondly, there are chances of mechanically damaging the embryo in the process. Over time, vitrification has proved to be more efficient than slow freezing. Nonetheless, the journey of embryo freezing began with the concept of slow freezing, after which vitrification took its shape and became renowned.

## VITRIFICATION

Vitrification is a term applied to refer the physical phenomenon where the solidification of water or water-based solutions into a glass-like amorphous liquid state (called vitreous state), due to extreme elevation in viscosity during cooling, without the formation of ice crystals.[20,21] Successful vitrification depends on two factors are following:

1. A very high concentration of CPA to inhibit the crystallization water into ice.
2. Extremely high cooling and warming rates (up to 20,000°C/min) to rapidly pass through the dangerous temperature zone between +15°C and –5°C to avoid cryoinjuries.

Since most CPAs are toxic under high concentrations, it is imperative to reduce its exposure time to embryo. If the exposure is too brief, its permeation to the embryo may be inadequate and intracellular ice will form even in the absence of extracellular ice. Vitrification procedure circumvents' two major limiting factors for exceeding optimal cryopreservation: (1) cryoinjury; (2) ice formation. The common protocol for vitrification of embryo is to first equilibrate them in a solution (called equilibration solution or ES) containing a lower concentration of one or more permeable CPA and then transferring it into a final solution, called vitrification solution (VS) containing a full-strength permeable CPA and a nonpermeable CPA.

Vitrification of embryos are generally carried out with carrier systems such as electron microscopy (EM) grid, open pulled straw (OPS), Cryotop, Cryoleaf, and Cryotip, successfully. However, in human assisted reproductive techniques, Cryotop and its derivatives such as Hemi-Straw System (HSS), Cryolock, Cryoleaf, Cryoloop, EM grid and OPS are more widely used.

### Laboratory Procedure for Vitrification

Commercial kits are quite similar in their composition with certain modifications in their protocol. While performing the procedures kindly follow the protocol as per the manufacturers' instructions.

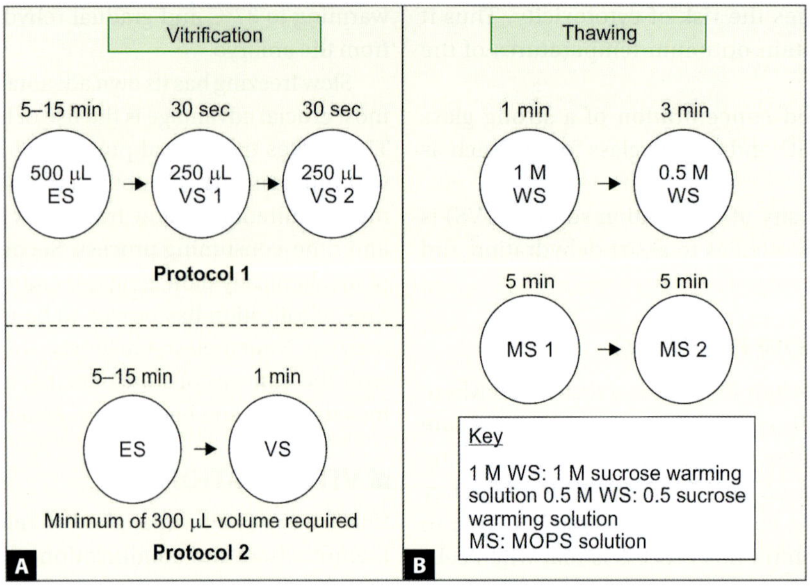


**Figs. 1A and B:** (A) Two commonly used protocols of vitrification; (B) Protocol commonly followed for thawing.

Vitrification is a two-step procedure which involves moving embryos first to the equilibration solution (ES) and then to the vitrification media. In general, two protocols are most commonly used for embryo vitrification **(Figs. 1 A and B)**. The main differences between the commercial protocols includes the number of vitrification drops (varies between one drop to four drops) and the recommended volume of use (varies between 0.1 and 1 mL). To enhance uniformity in procedures, scientists are now developing universal protocols for vitrification and warming. Parmegiani and team have tested the efficacy of a universal warming protocol for embryos frozen using different commercial kits. The experiments have shown promising results with a single universal protocol that is based on sequential use of 1 M and 0.5 M concentration of extracellular cryoprotectant (ECCP).[22]

## *Vitrification Protocol*

- Prepare all the materials prior to starting the process of vitrification. Keep all things handy, since time is very crucial during the process of vitrification. Prewarming of media, dishes, pipettes and tips, labeling of cryo-devices, keeping marker, stop watch etc., are some things to be prepared beforehand.
- Carry out all procedures at room temperature (22–27°C).
- Gently shake all vials before use (do not homogenize the solution by pipetting). Dispense 0.1–1 mL of equilibration solution (ES) into well/dish (SAGE, Origio, Denmark).
- Dispense 0.1–1 mL of vitrification solution (VS) into the second well/dish (SAGE, Origio, Denmark).
- Transfer the embryo(s) to the first well (ES) and let it equilibrate for 5–15 min. The equilibration time depends on the stage of embryo. Broadly, cleavage stage need 5–7 min, collapsed blastocysts need 5 min and expanded blastocysts need 12–15 min.
- While the embryos are equilibrating, prepare the cryo-devices under sterile conditions. Label under appropriate witnessing.
- At the end of equilibration time, transfer the embryos to the second well containing VS. Incubate it for 1 min.
- At the end of incubation, load the embryos onto the cryo-device in minimum volumes. Remove excess medium.
- Place the device in liquid nitrogen and stir gently.
- Cap the device, whilst under liquid nitrogen and store until further use.
- Perform all procedures under a microscope. Adjust the focus well, since embryos tend to float in the medium.

## *Warming Protocol*

- Prepare all the materials prior to starting the process of warming. Keep all things handy, since time is very crucial during the process of warming. Media, dishes, pipettes and tips should be pre-warmed at 37°C.
- Note that all the warming procedures should be carried out 37°C.
- First start by preparing the dishes. Gently shake and dispense 500 μL of 1 M warming solution (WS) (SAGE, Origio, Denmark) into a dish. The frozen embryos will be removed into this dish first.
- In a well dispense 500 μL of 0.5 M WS.
- In well number two and three, dispense 250 μL of MOPS solution (MS).
- Now it is time to remove the cryo-device. Remove the correctly labeled cryo-device from liquid nitrogen under appropriate witnessing.

- Quickly open the cryo-device and place the tip in dish containing 500 μL of 1 M WS. Incubate for 1 min.
- Transfer the embryo(s) to 500 μL of 0.5 M W for 3 min.
- Now transfer the embryo(s) to the first drop of MS for 5 min.
- Transfer the embryo(s) to the second drop of MS for 5 min.
- Transfer the embryo(s) to your preferred culture medium and place them in the incubator.

### *Tips for Optimizing Vitrification Success*

- Maintain and follow Standard Operating Procedures (SOPs) in the clinic and take all small considerations into account. All operators, regardless of their experience should follow this SOP. This maximizes success rate by reducing interperson variability. Back tracing of problems is also easier if a SOP is maintained in the clinic.
- Try to use good quality embryo(s). Embryos of questionable quality can be vitrified, but they limit the success of survival. Hence try to vitrify top quality embryos.
- Be particular with the control of timing, temperature, osmolarity and pipetting.
- Do not exceed the maximum number of embryos recommended for the cryo-device.
- Load the embryos in minimal volumes to support an appropriate cooling rate.
- Carry all procedures under a microscope. Ensure that the lens is properly focused since embryos tend to float in the medium.

## "FREEZE-ALL" STRATEGY

The last decade or so has seen a substantial rise in the concept of "freeze-all' strategy wherein all the embryos following IVF are first frozen, thawed and then transferred in subsequent cycles. The rationale behind this strategy is that the transfer of embryos in a non-IVF cycle would provide a more "physiologically natural" environment which would result not only in higher pregnancy rates but also reduce the risks of maternal and perinatal morbidity as compared to fresh cycle transfer.[23] Some occasional reports have shown increased reproductive outcomes using this strategy whereas some groups suggest that this strategy is more beneficial for certain subgroups of patients and detrimental to others. An interesting SWOT (strengths, weakness, opportunities, and threats) analysis of "freeze-all" strategy was done by Blockeel and group.[24] They suggest the following SWOT's of the "freeze-all" strategy—

*Strengths:*

- Increased maternal safety, OHSS-free clinic
- Improved pregnancy rates
- Lower ectopic pregnancies
- Better obstetric and perinatal outcomes

*Weakness:*

- Evidences of three RCTs only
- Less evidences providing promising results in all groups

*Opportunities:*

- Stimulation can be started at any time of the cycle
- Scheduling possibilities
- Patient friendliness

*Threats:*

- Cost increment.

Thus, all in all it seems to be on the physicians acumen to decide whether to use "freeze-all" strategy for "all" patients or a certain subgroup of them. Subgroup of patients being poor ovarian responders or those prone to OHSS. Promising results have been shown in these subgroups.[24]

## SAFETY OF REPRODUCTIVE CRYOPRESERVATION

Higher birth-weight associated with FET has been observed in large epidemiological populations in the UK. However, it is a matter of debate whether the actual process of FET contributes to higher birth-weight or are there any other factors. An increased risk of placental problems (placenta accreta), pregnancy-induced hypertension and preeclampsia have been observed following FET.[25] One of the reasons for preeclampsia has been attributed to the use of estrogens in endometrial priming protocols during FET cycles.[26-28] Also, the epigenetic effect of cryopreservation remains a question of study in FET babies. According to the Developmental Origins of Health and Diseases, it is hypothesized that cryopreservation of gametes and embryos may alter the epigenetic make-up of the DNA, which could result in altered developments of the fetus.[29-32]

Although scientists have seen the abovementioned outcomes in FET groups, these outcomes still remain a question of debate. In all of the mentioned outcomes there are contradicting evidences that show no differences between frozen and fresh embryo transfer cycles.[2,28,29]

## CONCLUSION

Cryopreservation has seen a pragmatic boom in the field of ART since its advent in the 1980s. Scientific advancements have led to higher success rates of survival post cryopreservation, making cryopreservation accessible to clinicians and patients alike. It is undoubtedly a boon for many. However, it is necessary to explore the fine physiological effects of cryopreservation. It is imperative that there is a need for larger studies, long-term evaluation of FET born babies and thorough evaluation of toxicity-related studies to determine the safety of reproductive cryopreservation.

## REFERENCES


1. US Centers for Disease Control and Prevention. Available from: https://www.cdc.gov/art/artdata/index.html.
2. Ernesto B, De Vos M, Peter H. The future of cryopreservation in Assisted Reproductive Technologies. Front Endocrinol. 2020:11:67.
3. Coates A, Kung A, Mounts E, Hesla J, Bankowski B, Barbieri E, et al. Optimal euploid embryo transfer strategy, fresh versus frozen, after preimplantation genetic screening with next generation sequencing: a randomized control trial. Fertil Steril. 2017;107(3):723-30.
4. Argyle C, Harper JC, Davies MC. Oocyte cryopreservation: where are we now? Hum Reprod Update. 2016;22:440-9.
5. Santos S, Polyzos NP, Haentjens P, Smitz J, Smitz J, Camus M, Tournaye H, et al. Live birth rates after IVF are reduced by low and high progesterone levels on the day of human chorionic gonadotrophic administration. Hum Reprod. 2014;29(8):1698-705.
6. Bosch E, Labarta E, Crespo J, Simón C, Remohí J, Jenkins J, et al. Circulating progesterone levels and ongoing pregnancy rates in controlled ovarian stimulation cycles for in vitro fertilization: analysis of over 4000 cycles. Hum Reprod. 2010;25(8):2092-100.
7. Lieberman J. Potential importance of vitrification in reproductive medicine. Biol Reprod. 2002;67:1671-80.
8. Lieberman J, Tucker MJ. Effect of carrier system on the yield of human oocytes and embryos as assessed by survival and development potential after vitrification. Reproduction. 2002;124:483-9.
9. Principles of freezing and thawing of cells: basic cryobiology. Embryol Begin. 2021;14:234-45.
10. Roger G. General principles of cryopreservation. Hum Fertil. 2014;11:261-8.
11. Pickering SJ, Johnson MH. The influence of cooling on the organization of the meiotic spindle of the mouse oocyte. Hum Reprod. 1987;2: 207-16.
12. Aman RR, Parks JE. (1994) Effects of cooling and rewarming on the meiotic spindle and chromosomes of in vitro-matured bovine oocytes. Biol Reprod. 1994;50:103-10.
13. Vincent C, Garnier V, Heyman Y, Renard JP. Solvent effects on cytoskeletal organization and in-vivo survival after freezing of rabbit oocytes. J Reprod Fertil. 1989;87:809-20.
14. Cuthbertson KS. Parthenogenetic activation of mouse oocytes in vitro with ethanol and benzyl alcohol. J Exp Zool. 1983;226:311-4.
15. Steinhardt RA, Epel D, Carroll EJ Jr, Yanagimachi R. Is calcium ionophore a universal activator for unfertilised eggs? Nature. 1974;252: 41-3.
16. Kaufman MH. Early mammalian development: parthenogenetic studies. Cambridge: Cambridge University Press; 1983.
17. Arakawa T, Carpenter JF, Kita YA, Crowe JH. The basis for toxicity of certain cryoprotectants: a hypothesis. Cryobiology. 1990;27:401-15.
18. Damien M, Luciano AA, Peluso JJ. Propanediol alters intracellular pH and developmental potential of mouse zygotes independently of volume change. Hum Reprod 1990;5:212-6.
19. Gardner DK, Sheehan CB, Rienzi L, Katz-Jaffe M, Larman MG. Analysis of oocyte physiology to improve cryopreservation procedures. Theriogenology. 2007;67: 64-72.
20. Whittingham DG, Leibo SP, Mazur P. Survival of mouse embryos frozen to -196 degrees and -269 degrees celsius. Science. 1972:178.
21. Fahy GM, MacFarlane DR, Angell CA, Meryman HT. Vitrification as an approach to cryopreservation. Cryobiology. 1984;21:407-26.
22. Parmegiani L, Beilby KH, Arnone A, Bernardi S, Maccarini AM, Nardi E, et al. Testing the efficacy and efficiency of a single universal warming protocol for vitrified human embryos: prospective randomized controlled trial and retrospective longitudinal cohort study. J Assist Reprod Genet. 2018;35:1887-95.
23. Evans J, Hannan NJ, Edgell TA, Vollenhoven BJ, Lutjen PJ, Osianlis T, et al. Fresh vs. frozen embryo transfer: backing clinical decisions with scientific and clinical evidences. Hum Reprod Update. 2014;20:808-21.
24. Blockeel C, Drakopoulos P, Santos-Ribeiro S, Polyzos NP, Tournaye H. A fresh look at the 'freeze-all' protocol: a SWOT analysis. 2016;31:491-97.
25. Ishihara O, Araki R, Kuwahara A, Itakura A, Saito H, Adamson GD. Impact of frozen-thawed single-blastocyst transfer on maternal and neonatal outcome: an analysis of 277,042 single-embryo transfer cycles from 2008 to 2010 in Japan. Fertil Steril. 2014;101:128-33.
26. Roque M, Haahr T, Geber S, Esteves SC, Humaidan P. Fresh versus elective frozen embryo transfer in IVF/ICSI cycles: a systematic review and meta-analysis of reproductive outcomes. Hum Reprod Update. 2019;25:2-14.
27. Pinborg A, Henningsen AA, Loft A, Malchau SS, Forman J, Andersen AN. Large baby syndrome in singletons born after frozen embryo transfer (FET): is it due to maternal factors or the cryotechnique? Hum Reprod. 2014;29:618-27.
28. Shi Y, Sun Y, Hao C, Zhang H, Wei D, Zhang Y, et al. Transfer of fresh versus frozen embryos in ovulatory women. N Engl J Med. 2018;378:126-36.
29. Belva F, Bonduelle M, Roelants M, Verheyen G, Van Landuyt L. Neonatal health including congenital malformation risk of 1072 children born after vitrified embryo transfer. Hum Reprod. 2016;31:1610-20.
30. Fleming TP, Watkins AJ, Velazquez MA, Mathers JC, Prentice AM, Stephenson J, et al. Origins of lifetime health around the time of conception: causes and consequences. Lancet. 2018;391:1842-52.
31. Hanson MA, Gluckman PD. Early developmental conditioning of later health and disease: physiology or pathophysiology? Physiol Rev. 2014:94:1027-76.
32. Xue Y, Tong X, Zhu H, Li K, Zhang S. Freeze-all embryo strategy in poor ovarian responders undergoing ovarian stimulation for in vitro fertilization. Gynaecol Endocrinol. 2018;34(8):680-3.

CHAPTER 111

# Viral Contamination Risk to Gametes and Embryos in Cryostorage during COVID-19

*Prathima Tholeti, Satish Kumar Adiga*

## INTRODUCTION

Cryopreservation is an essential component of a successful assisted reproduction technology (ART) program that involves freezing of gametes and embryos of infertile couples at ultralow temperatures, thereby providing flexibility of time for effective management.[1] This technique also forms the crux in fertility preservation programs recommended by the American Society of Clinical Oncology to young and adult cancer patients,[2,3] as well as in non-oncological medical conditions,[4] thereby helping them preserve their reproductive cells such as spermatozoa, oocytes, testicular, or ovarian tissues for a fertile future.

The success of cryopreservation has led to an increased number of in vitro fertilization (IVF) clinics across the globe routinely freezing their patients' samples for future use, highlighting the need to ensure safe and reliable storage, both short- and long term.[5] One of the major concerns with cryostorage is the contamination of liquid nitrogen (LN2), a commonly used cryogenic medium, by viral pathogens, especially leading to transmission of infectious diseases between samples[6,7] or transmission to the patient itself during fertility restoration. Severe acute respiratory syndrome coronavirus 2 (SARS-CoV-2), which is responsible for the recent coronavirus disease 2019 (COVID-19) pandemic, is one such viral pathogen that has shown to infect reproductive cells and can therefore pose a relevant risk in cryostorage and potential disease transmission.[7]

## SARS-COV-2 AND ITS IMPACT ON REPRODUCTIVE CELLS

SARS-CoV-2 virus is a single-strand ribonucleic acid (RNA) virus belonging to the coronavirus family and shares 82% genome similarity with SARS-CoV. SARS-CoV-2 facilitates its entry by binding to angiotensin-converting enzyme 2 (ACE2) receptor of the host cell, after which the viral spike glycoprotein priming occurs through transmembrane serine protease 2 (TMPRSS2).[8] This allows for the fusion of viral and host cell membranes enabling successful entry and invasion of the host cell. Most of the tissues of the human reproductive system, gametes, or embryos express ACE2 receptors and are therefore highly susceptible to a SARS-CoV-2 infection. However, the effect of COVID-19 infection on these cells and its impact on reproductive outcomes are not completely known.[9] Alternate binding receptors such as BSG (basigin/CD147) have also been reported; however, their direct role in enabling viral invasion is yet to be established.[10]

### Effect of SARS-CoV-2 in Male Reproductive Cells

SARS-CoV-2 infection appears to affect male fertility in various ways such as a direct impact on the sperm parameters or testicular function, on male steroidogenesis, or indirectly through an immune response mounted by the virus causing damage to the male reproductive cells.[11] The testis is a potential target for SARS-CoV-2 infection as ACE2 receptors have been shown to be expressed in spermatogonia and Leydig and Sertoli cells.[12] Some of the patients infected with COVID-19 have shown symptoms similar to those of Sertoli cell-only syndrome suggesting that SARS-CoV-2 infection could cause viral orchitis resulting in impaired spermatogenesis.[13] A few other reports have suggested autoimmune orchitis due to COVID-19 infection leading to disruption of the blood–testis barrier.[14,15]

The presence of SARS-CoV-2 in human semen remains controversial due to insufficient literature. While some studies have reported the presence of SARS-CoV-2 in the semen of patients during the acute phase of infection,[14] others have failed to detect the virus through reverse transcription polymerase chain reaction (RT-PCR) in the semen of COVID-19 patients or in a postmortem testicular sample of a patient diagnosed with COVID-19.[16-18] However, impaired sperm parameters have been reported in patients with moderate COVID-19 infection though the presence of virus was not detected in the semen; hence, it is unclear whether the infection or treatment itself is causing the impairment.[19] Overall, there is no conclusive evidence to draw a firm conclusion on the effect of SARS-CoV-2 on spermatozoa, the severity of infection at the time of semen sampling, and the possibility of SARS-CoV-2 presence in the semen of the asymptomatic COVID-19 patients which cannot be completely ruled out.[20]

### Effect of SARS-CoV-2 in Female Reproductive Cells

The female reproductive tract appears to be less impacted by SARS-CoV-2 than the males,[21] although ACE2 is widely expressed in the ovary,[22] uterus, and vagina.[23] While the presence of ACE2 is indicative of the female reproductive organs being potential targets for SARS-CoV-2 infection, no evidence so far has been convincing of infection or sexual transmission.[24] However, it has been observed that the hormonal profile and ovarian reserve in SARS-CoV-2 infected patients reveal lower anti-Müllerian hormone (AMH), increased follicle-stimulating hormone (FSH), and higher testosterone and prolactin levels compared to the age-matched control group, thereby suggesting an impact of COVID-19 infection on the ovarian function.[25] The presence of SARS-CoV-2 in follicular fluid of infected patients has also been reported, but it appears to have no significant effect on oocyte yield and fertilization rate;[26,27] however, top-quality embryos on days 3 and 5 were significantly lower.[28,29]

The American Society for Reproductive Medicine (ASRM) recommends following standard universal precautions while handling gametes from patients with other viral illnesses, such as human immunodeficiency virus (HIV) and hepatitis, to reduce vertical transmission to noninfected partner and cross-contamination of reproductive tissue within the ART laboratory.[30] However, whether these special precautions are to be recommended even for SARS-CoV-2, given the lack of insufficient evidence for transmission through blood or sexual contact, is still not clear.[24,31]

## FERTILITY PRESERVATION

Oncofertility is an upcoming area of science,[2] and with the American Society of Clinical Oncology recommending guidelines to offer fertility preservation services to oncological patients,[3] many young and adult cancer patients preserve their spermatozoa, testicular tissues, ovarian tissues, oocytes, or embryos for a fertile future. Various cryopreservation protocols have been developed for each of the reproductive material to ensure efficient long-term storage and recovery while also sustaining the fertility potential.[1] These samples are usually cryopreserved in either open or closed cryodevices, which are then plunged in LN2 that maintains an ultralow temperature of –196°C,[32] facilitating prolonged cryostorage of reproductive material. However, one of the main concerns of fertility preservation in patients with a virus infection, including SARS-CoV-2, is the risk of cross-contamination through the storage devices or LN2 and reintroduction of the virus when patients need fertility restoration, which could even be decades later in the case of prepubertal patients.[7]

## CROSS-CONTAMINATION OF VIRUSES IN LIQUID NITROGEN CRYOTANKS

Several concerns exist pertaining to contamination of LN2, which could result in transmission of infectious diseases either between the stored samples[6,7] or transmission of infection to the patient itself years later during fertility restoration.

While there have been no reports of transmission of viral pathogens in cryotanks of fertility centers,[33] other reports of cross-contamination of hepatitis virus from cryopreserved bone marrow transplant to other frozen samples in the same LN2 tank[34] have been reported. Viruses such as HIV, hepatitis, influenza, and papillomavirus seem to retain their infectivity even after cryopreservation, thereby highlighting the biohazard that LN2 can pose when exposed to the virus, hence leading to cross-contamination.[34-38] The use of cryoprotectants in protecting reproductive cells during freeze–thawing also seems to confer protection to the enveloped viruses, thereby making them cryoresistant and thus leading to transmission of the pathogen between stored biomaterials.[5,39-41] An experimental contamination of LN2 with bovine viral diarrhea virus (BVDV) and bovine herpesvirus-1 (BHV-1) has shown that while there was no transmission from infected semen samples to noninfected samples stored in the same LN2 tanks, cross-contamination of the same viruses to frozen embryos was seen during this experiment.[41]

It is reassuring that upon screening LN2 used for gamete or embryo cryopreservation in chronic HIV, hepatitis C virus (HCV), hepatitis B virus (HBV) seropositive patients undergoing ART treatment, RNA or deoxyribonucleic acid (DNA) sequences could not be detected.[42] Also, since no studies have demonstrated the SARS-CoV-2 virus binding to the zona pellucida (ZP) of human oocytes, other studies reporting the penetration of ZP by other viruses such as BHV-1 and bovine herpesvirus 5 should be taken into consideration.[43,44] However, breaching of ZP during manipulation such as intracytoplasmic sperm injection (ICSI), laser-assisted hatching, or embryo biopsy could facilitate SARS-CoV-2 entry.[45] Nevertheless, ASRM has recommended repeated washings of gametes or embryos to effectively eliminate the viral pathogens.[46]

As a precautionary measure for safe cryostorage and to assure patients that their gametes or embryos would not be infected by SARS-CoV-2 or other viral pathogens, viral testing can be made mandatory for all patients cryopreserving their reproductive samples.[47]

Additionally, there is a risk of iatrogenic transmission of pathogens from either laboratory personnel or LN2 operators to the frozen samples. As stated earlier, the particles of SARS-CoV-2 or other viruses are cryotolerant, and therefore, could survive the freeze–thaw process.[46] Hence, there is a need for standard guidelines for safe handling and cryopreservation of reproductive samples during fertility preservation.

## RISK MITIGATION STRATEGIES AND SAFETY DURING CRYOSTORAGE

Due to the various concerns associated with SARS-CoV-2, international reproductive societies and clinical groups have provided guidelines for the smooth conducting of ART cycles in lieu of the global pandemic. The same guidelines can also be applied to infertile patients with other viral infections. The risk prevention strategies that can be incorporated at IVF clinics are as follows:

- Viral testing including SARS-CoV-2 for infertile patients before starting the ART cycle and also in oncofertility patients recruited for fertility preservation.[46-49]
- Ensuring implementation of disinfection protocols in semen collection rooms and procedure rooms.[50]
- Handling or culture of gametes/embryos/reproductive tissue of suspected or infected patients in class II biological safety laminar hoods and incubators, thereby reducing the risk of contamination, keeping in mind aerosol generation.[51]
- Oocyte retrieval of patients who are suspected or infected can be performed only in IVF clinics with expertise in managing infectious specimens and should also be equipped to offer better protection to healthcare providers.[52]

Strategies for risk mitigation in cryostorage include proper selection of carrier devices, sterilization of LN2 tanks, and appropriate washing steps during gamete/embryo handling[7] as detailed below.

## CRYOSYSTEMS AND CARRIER DEVICES

Depending on whether open or closed cryopreservation systems are used, the carrier devices can vary. Closed devices, such as sealed straws, help ensure that the reproductive samples are not directly exposed to LN2, therefore reducing the hazard of cross-contamination.[53] Other closed carrier systems for cryopreservation include microvolume air cooling (MVAC) device,[54] high-security vitrification straw (HSV), or Cryotip, which have been used for human embryo vitrification in order to hermetically isolate the reproductive samples.[55-57] Hence, for patients with COVID-19 or other viral infections, the use of high-security straws and vapor-phase storage for cryopreservation of reproductive samples can be recommended.[48] However, most laboratories use screw-capped plastic vials that can lead to contact with surrounding LN2 by generation of vacuum in the vial through atmospheric condensation at such low temperatures, thereby drawing in LN2.[58] In such cases, it may be safe to use a secondary enclosure for such cryodevices or to store samples of patients who are suspected/infected in separate LN2 cryotanks, thereby avoiding the risk of disease transmission through contaminated LN2.[39] While using the open carrier system during vitrification, in order to avoid contamination, other alternatives to LN2 can be used such as a bench-top device that produces cooled clean liquid air (CLAir) with similar temperature to that of LN2.[59] It is also advisable not to share LN2 between patient samples during cryopreservation.[60] Vapor phase nitrogen can also be used as a safer alternative,[56] although the risk cannot be completely negated.[61] This can be a more practical option, especially in cases of storing unwashed semen samples or for those awaiting viral test results.[62]

## LIQUID NITROGEN STERILIZATION

Liquid nitrogen is an efficient cryogenic medium but considering the risk of cross-contamination, it would be advisable to ensure the sterility of LN2,[39,46,63] either by using certain devices (http://www.freepatentsonline.com/5737926.html) or by filtering LN2 using 0.2 μm pore size disposable filters[64,65] and also by exposure to ultraviolet (UV) radiation in a temperature-controlled manner in a short interval for effective sterilization.[66] However, the efficacy of such methods on eliminating the different viruses including SARS-CoV-2 remains to be seen. Other methods to sterilize LN2 include periodic disinfection of the cryotanks as well as the tools used during cryopreservation, by UV exposure or chemical disinfectants.[39,63] Irradiation with ultraviolet C (UVC) rays of 254 nm for >15 minutes has shown to be effective in deactivating the SARS-CoV-virus, but whether the same exposure would be sufficient for use in LN2 remains to be seen.[67] It is worth noting that care should be taken to avoid putting the stored reproductive samples at risk during removal from cryotanks while cleaning.[68]

## WASHING PROCEDURES TO ELIMINATE PATHOGENS

To minimize the risk of contamination, a safe three-step washing procedure of carrier devices with sterile LN2 has been reported to eliminate bacterial and fungal pathogens from human cryopreserved specimens.[69] It may be advisable to implement a similar strategy for viral pathogens as gentle repeated washes of gametes and embryos before cryopreservation and after thawing can minimize the infectivity by high dilution of viral particles.[39,46] It has been shown that such washing-dilution procedures can dilute the infective agents to a probability of <0.0002% even with open vitrification systems, far below the threshold level required for causing clinical infection.[70] Established sperm-washing procedures such as double density gradient followed by swim-up have been known to effectively separate motile sperm free of viral particles in males infected with HIV or HCV; therefore, such sperm-wash procedures could also be used for other viral infections[30] such as SARS-CoV-2.

## SAFETY ISSUES

While the above precautionary strategies offer protection to the cryosamples, it is equally important to implement standard precautions for the safety of the laboratory personnel while handling LN2,[71] to prevent any health hazards. One of the risks during cryohandling, especially with contaminated LN2, is the generation of aerosol mist particles of 1–5 µm sizes which are generated near the LN2 surface, even up to a distance of 10–20 cm, resulting from evaporation and floating of particles.[72] This, in turn, could pose a risk to the personnel while handling contaminated LN2 containers. Hence, it is advisable for the laboratory personnel to use safety cryoaccessories such as goggles or face visors and protective clothing while working with LN2, thereby ensuring safety and efficiency.[7,71]

## CONCLUSION

It is essential for healthcare providers to be aware not only of the effect of viral infections, such as SARS-CoV-2, on male and female reproductive cells but also of the risk of cross-contamination and transmission through cryobanking services. Recent literature is controversial on the presence of SARS-CoV-2 and its impact on sperm parameters as well as on the ovarian reserve. However, as the human gonadal tissues are abundant in ACE2 receptors, they are potential targets for SARS-CoV-2 infection which can, in turn, lead to the transmission of infections to other samples in cryostorage due to cross-contamination. Hence new strategies must be adopted when offering fertility services, especially pertaining to cryopreservation, to combat viral infections including COVID-19.

Cryostorage commonly uses LN2 for long-term cryopreservation, however, it carries the risk of cross-contamination by viral pathogens that can lead to disease transmission among cryosamples or to the patient itself later when they come for fertility restoration. Hence, it is important to identify and mitigate such risks involved in cryostorage through safety and precautionary measures. Some of the strategies include viral testing, including COVID-19 testing of both partners before initiating ART cycle, utility of closed-carrier cryodevices, and sanitary cryostorage protocols followed by efficient washing of gametes or embryos during cryopreservation, all of which would minimize the risk of disease transmission. However, each IVF laboratory, especially in developing countries, will have to decide on the feasibility of adopting these strategies depending on their setting and available resources without compromising on patient and laboratory personnel safety.

## KEY POINTS

- SARS-Cov-2 virus can pose as a relevant risk during cryostorage of fertility preservation biomaterials.
- Important to identify and employ risk mitigation measures in cryo-facilities to ensure safety of patient as well as laboratory personnel
- Depending on the available resources, each IVF laboratory can adopt feasible strategies to minimize risk of disease transmission during cryostorage.

## REFERENCES


1. Rodriguez-Walberg KA, Waterstone M, Anastácio A. Ice age: cryopreservation in assisted reproduction—an update. Reprod Biol. 2019;19:119-26.
2. Woodruff TK. Oncofertility: a grand collaboration between reproductive medicine and oncology. Reproduction. 2015; 150(3):S1-10.
3. Oktay K, Harvey BE, Partridge AH, Quinn GP, Reinecke J, Taylor HS, et al. Fertility preservation in patients with cancer: ASCO Clinical Practice Guideline update. J Clin Oncol. 2018;36:1994-2001.
4. Gidoni Y, Holzer H, Tulandi T, Tan SL. Fertility preservation in patients with non-oncological conditions. Reprod Biomed Online. 2008;16(6):792-800.
5. Alikani M. Cryostorage of human gametes and embryos: a reckoning. Reprod Biomed Online. 2018;37:1-3.
6. Tomlinson M. Managing risk associated with cryopreservation. Hum Reprod. 2005;20:1751-6.
7. Adiga SK, Tholeti P, Uppangala S, Kalthur G, Gualtieri R, Talevi R. Fertility preservation during the COVID-19 pandemic: mitigating the viral contamination risk to reproductive cells in cryostorage. Reprod Biomed Online. 2020;41(6):991-7.
8. Hoffmann M, Kleine-Weber H, Schroeder S, Krüger N, Herrler T, Erichsen S, et al. SARS-CoV-2 cell entry depends on ACE2 and TMPRSS2 and is blocked by a clinically proven protease inhibitor. Cell. 2020;181:271-80.e8.
9. Delamuta LC, Monteleone PAA, Ferreira-Filho ES, Heinrich-Oliveira V, Soares-Júnior JM, Baracat EC, et al. Coronavirus disease 2019 and human reproduction: a changing perspective. Clinics (Sao Paulo). 2021;76:e3032.
10. Shilts J, Crozier TWM, Greenwood EJD, Lehner PJ, Wright GJ. No evidence for basigin/CD147 as a direct SARS-CoV-2 spike binding receptor. Sci Rep. 2021;11(1):413.
11. He Y, Wang J, Ren J, Zhao Y, Chen J, Chen X. Effect of COVID-19 on male reproductive system—a systematic review. Front Endocrinol (Lausanne). 2021;12:677701.
12. Wang W, Xu Y, Gao R, Lu R, Han K, Wu G, et al. Detection of SARS-CoV-2 in different types of clinical specimens. JAMA. 2020;323:1843-4.
13. Ma X, Guan C, Chen R, Wang Y, Feng S, Wang R, et al. Pathological and molecular examinations of postmortem testis biopsies reveal SARS-CoV-2 infection in the testis and

spermatogenesis damage in COVID-19 patients. Cell Mol Immunol. 2021;18(2):487-9.

14. Li D, Jin M, Bao P, Zhao W, Zhang S. Clinical characteristics and results of semen tests among men with coronavirus disease 2019. JAMA Netw Open. 2020;3:e208292.
15. Peirouvi T, Aliaghaei A, Eslami Farsani B, Ziaeipour S, Ebrahimi V, Forozesh M, et al. COVID-19 disrupts the blood-testis barrier through the induction of inflammatory cytokines and disruption of junctional proteins. Inflamm Res. 2021;70(10-12):1165-75.
16. Pan F, Xiao X, Guo J, Song Y, Li H, Patel DP, et al. No evidence of severe acute respiratory syndrome-coronavirus 2 in semen of males recovering from coronavirus disease 2019. Fertil Steril. 2020;113:1135-39.
17. Song C, Wang Y, Li W, Hu B, Chen G, Xia P, et al. Detection of 2019 novel coronavirus in semen and testicular biopsy specimen of COVID-19 patients. medRxiv. 2020.
18. Guo L, Zhao S, Li W, Wang Y, Li L, Jiang S, et al. Absence of SARS-CoV-2 in semen of a COVID-19 patient cohort. Andrology. 2021;9(1):42-7.
19. Holtmann N, Edimiris P, Andree M, Doehmen C, Baston-Buest D, Adams O, et al. Assessment of SARS-CoV-2 in human semen—a cohort study. Fertil Steril. 2020;114(2):233-8.
20. Kashi AH. COVID-19 and semen: an unanswered area of research. Urol J. 2020;17:328.
21. Segars J, Katler Q, McQueen DB, Kotlyar A, Glenn T, Knight Z, et al. Prior and novel coronaviruses, coronavirus disease 2019 (COVID-19), and human reproduction: what is known? Fertil Steril. 2020;113(6):1140-9.
22. Jing Y, Run-Qian L, Hao-Ran W, Hao-Ran C, Ya-Bin L, Yang G, et al. Potential influence of COVID-19/ACE2 on the female reproductive system. Mol Hum Reprod. 2020;26:367-73.
23. Vaz-Silva J, Carneiro MM, Ferreira MC, Pinheiro SVB, Silva DA, Silva-Filho AL, et al. The vasoactive peptide angiotensin-(1-7), its receptor Mas and the angiotensin-converting enzyme type 2 are expressed in the human endometrium. Reprod Sci. 2009;16(3):247-56.
24. Cui P, Chen Z, Wang T, Dai J, Zhang J, Ding T, et al. Clinical features and sexual transmission potential of SARS-CoV-2 infected female patients: a descriptive study in Wuhan, China. medRxiv. 2020.
25. Ding Y, He L, Zhang Q, Huang Z, Che X, Hou J, et al. Organ distribution of severe acute respiratory syndrome (SARS) associated coronavirus (SARS-CoV) in SARS patients: implications for pathogenesis and virus transmission pathways. J Pathol. 2004;203(2):622-30.
26. Herrero Y, Pascuali N, Velázquez C, Oubiña G, Hauk V, de Zúñiga I, et al. SARS-CoV-2 infection negatively affects ovarian function in ART patients. Biochim Biophys Acta Mol Basis Dis. 2022;1868(1):166295.
27. Bentov Y, Beharier O, Moav-Zafrir A, Kabessa M, Godin M, Greenfield CS, et al. Ovarian follicular function is not altered by SARS-CoV-2 infection or BNT162b2 mRNA COVID-19 vaccination. Hum Reprod. 2021;36(9):2506-13.
28. Wang M, Yang Q, Rena X, Hu J, Li Z, Long R, et al. Investigating the impact of asymptomatic or mild SARS-CoV-2 infection on female fertility and in vitro fertilization outcomes: a retrospective cohort study. EClinicalMedicine. 2021;38:101013.
29. Orvieto R, Segev-Zahav A, Aizer A. Does COVID-19 infection influence patients' performance during IVF-ET cycle? An observational study. Gynecol Endocrinol. 2021;37:895-7.
30. Practice Committee of American Society for Reproductive Medicine. Recommendations for reducing the risk of viral transmission during fertility treatment with the use of autologous gametes: a committee opinion. Fertil Steril. 2013;99:340-6
31. Chang L, Yan Y, Wang L. Coronavirus disease 2019: coronaviruses and blood safety. Transfus Med Rev. 2020;34:75-80.
32. Joaquim DC, Borges ED, Viana IGR, Navarro PA, Vireque AA. Risk of contamination of gametes and embryos during cryopreservation and measures to prevent cross-contamination. Biomed Res Int. 2017;2017:1840417.
33. Yakass MB, Woodward B. COVID-19: should we continue to cryopreserve sperm during the pandemic? Reprod Biomed Online. 2020;40:905.
34. Tedder RS, Zuckerman MA, Goldstone AH, Hawkins AE, Fielding A, Briggs EM, et al. Hepatitis B transmission from contaminated cryopreservation tank. Lancet. 1995; 346(8968):137-40.
35. Merrill DR, Wade CD, Fahnestock P, Baker RO. (2018). Long-term and short-term stability of viruses depend on storage temperature and preservation method. bei RESOURCES Poster. [online] Available from: https://www.beiresources.org/Portals/2/PDFS/Long-Term%20and%20Short-Term%20Stability%20of%20Viruses.pdf. [Last accessed December, 2022].
36. Bielanski A. A review of the risk of contamination of semen and embryos during cryopreservation and measures to limit cross-contamination during banking to prevent disease transmission in ET practices. Theriogenology. 2012;77:467-82.
37. Byers KB. Risks associated with liquid nitrogen cryogenic storage systems. J Am Biol Saf Assoc. 1999;3:143-6.
38. Schaffer TW, Everett J, Silver GH, Came PE. Biohazard potential: recovery of infectious virus from the liquid nitrogen of a virus repository. Health Lab Sci. 1976;13:23-4.
39. Bielanski A, Vajta G. Risk of contamination of germplasm during cryopreservation and cryobanking in IVF units. Hum Reprod. 2009;24:2457-67.
40. Hubálek Z. Protectants used in the cryopreservation of microorganisms. Cryobiology. 2003;46:205-29.
41. Bielanski A, Nadin-Davis S, Sapp T, Lutze-Wallace C. Viral contamination of embryos cryopreserved in liquid nitrogen. Cryobiology. 2000;40:110-6.
42. Cobo A, Bellver J, de los Santos MJ, Remohí J. Viral screening of spent culture media and liquid nitrogen samples of oocytes and embryos from hepatitis B, hepatitis C, and human immunodeficiency virus chronically infected women undergoing in vitro fertilization cycles. Fertil Steril. 2012;97:74-8.
43. Silva-Frade C, Martins Jr A, Borsanelli AC, Cardoso TC. Effects of bovine herpesvirus type 5 on development of in vitro-produced bovine embryos. Theriogenology. 2010;73:324-31.
44. Queiroz-Castro VLD, da Costa EP, Alves SVP, Machado-Neves M, Guimarães JD, Gomes LL, et al. Correction: bovine herpesvirus 1 can cross the intact zona pellucida of bovine oocytes after artificial infection. PLoS One. 2019;14(9):e0222645.

45. Yan L, Yang M, Guo H, Yang L, Wu J, Li R, et al. Single-cell RNA-Seq profiling of human preimplantation embryos and embryonic stem cells. Nat Struct Mol Biol. 2013;20(9):1131-9.
46. American Society of Reproductive Medicine (2020). Patient management and clinical recommendations during coronavirus (COVID-19) pandemic. Second update published 13th April 2020. [online] Available from: https://www.asrm.org/globalassets/asrm/asrm-content/news-and-publications/covid-19/covidtaskforceupdate2.pdf.
47. Dellino M, Minoia C, Paradiso AV, De Palo R, Silvestris E. Fertility preservation in cancer patients during the coronavirus (COVID-19) pandemic. Front Oncol. 2020;10:1009.
48. European Society of Human Reproduction and Embryology. (2020). News and statements. Assisted reproduction and COVID-19: an updated statement from ESHRE 23rd April 2020. Available from: https://www.eshre.eu/Guidelines-and-Legal/Position-statements/COVID19.
49. Esteves SC, Lombardo F, Garrido N, Alvarez J, Zini A, Colpi GM, et al. SARS-CoV-2 pandemic and repercussions for male infertility patients: a proposal for the individualized provision of andrological services. Andrology. 2021;9(1):10-8.
50. Society for Assisted Reproductive Technology. (2020). Laboratory guidance for commencing or continuing ART operations during the ongoing COVID-19 pandemic. [online] Available from: https://www.asrm.org/globalassets/__sart/covid-19/laboratory-guidance-for-covid.pdf [Last accessed December, 2022].
51. Huyser C. Prevention of infections in an ART laboratory: a reflection on simplistic methods. Facts Views Vis Obgyn. 2014;6(4):231-4.
52. Vaiarelli A, Bulletti C, Cimadomo D, Borini A, Alviggi C, Ajossa S, et al. COVID-19 and ART: the view of the Italian Society of Fertility and Sterility and Reproductive Medicine. Reprod Biomed Online. 2020;40(6):755-9.
53. Shapiro H, Zaman L, Kennedy VL, Dean N, Yudin MH, Loutfy M. Managing and preventing blood-borne viral infection transmission in assisted reproduction: a Canadian Fertility and Andrology Society clinical practice guideline. Reprod Biomed Online. 2020;41(2):203-16.
54. Punyawai K, Anakkul N, Srirattana K, Aikawa Y, Sangsritavong S, Nagai T, et al. Comparison of Cryotop and micro volume air cooling methods for cryopreservation of bovine matured oocytes and blastocysts. J Reprod Dev. 2015;61(5):431-7.
55. Arav A. A recommendation for IVF lab practice in light of the current COVID-19 pandemic. J Assist Reprod Genet. 2020;37:1543.
56. AbdelHafez F, Xu J, Goldberg J, Desai N. Vitrification in open and closed carriers at different cell stages: assessment of embryo survival, development, DNA integrity and stability during vapor phase storage for transport. BMC Biotechnol. 2011;11:29.
57. Kuwayama M, Vajta G, Ieda S, Kato O. Comparison of open and closed methods for vitrification of human embryos and the elimination of potential contamination. Reprod Biomed Online. 2005;11:608-14.
58. Woods EJ, Thirumala S. Packaging considerations for biopreservation. Transfus Med Hemother. 2011;38:149-56.
59. Arav A, Natan Y, Levi-Setti PE, Menduni F, Patrizio P. New methods for cooling and storing oocytes and embryos in a clean environment of –196°C. Reprod Biomed Online. 2016;33(1):71-8.
60. Pomeroy KO, Schiewe MC. Cryopreservation and IVF in the time of Covid-19: what is the best good tissue practice (GTP)? J Assist Reprod Genet. 2020;37(10):2393-8.
61. Grout BWW, Morris GJ. Contaminated liquid nitrogen vapour as a risk factor in pathogen transfer. Theriogenology. 2009;71:1079-82.
62. Schiewe MC, Freeman M, Whitney JB, VerMilyea MD, Jones A, Aguirre M, et al. Comprehensive assessment of cryogenic storage risk and quality management concerns: best practice guidelines for ART labs. J Assist Reprod Genet. 2019;36(1):5-14.
63. Larman MG, Hashimoto S, Morimoto Y, Gardner DK. Cryopreservation in ART and concerns with contamination during cryobanking. Reprod Med Biol. 2014;13:107-17.
64. McBurnie LD, Bardo B. Validation of sterile filtration of liquid nitrogen. Pharm Technol North Am. 2002;26:74-82.
65. Vajta G, Lewis IM, Kuwayama M, Greve T, Callesen H. Sterile application of the Open Pulled Straw (OPS) vitrification method. Cryo Lett. 1998;19:389-92.
66. Parmegiani L, Cognigni GE, Filicori M. Ultra-violet sterilization of liquid nitrogen prior to vitrification. Hum Reprod. 2009;24:2969.
67. Darnell MER, Subbarao K, Feinstone SM, Taylor DR. Inactivation of the coronavirus that induces severe acute respiratory syndrome, SARS-CoV. J Virol Methods. 2004;121(1):85-91.
68. Tao Y, Sanger E, Saewu A, Leveille MC. Human sperm vitrification: the state of the art. Reprod Biol Endocrinol. 2020;18:17.
69. Parmegiani L, Accorsi A, Bernardi S, Arnone A, Cognigni GE, Filicori M. A reliable procedure for decontamination before thawing of human specimens cryostored in liquid nitrogen: three washes with sterile liquid nitrogen (SLN2). Fertil Steril. 2012;98(4):870-5.
70. Vajta G, Rienzi L, Ubaldi FM. Open versus closed systems for vitrification of human oocytes and embryos. Reprod Biomed Online. 2015;30:325-33.
71. Vajta G, Reichart A, Ubaldi FM, Rienzi L. From a backup technology to a strategy-outlining approach: the success story of cryopreservation. Expert Rev Obst Gynecol. 2014;8:181-90.
72. Lee BU. Cryogenic aerosol generation: airborne mist particles surrounding liquid nitrogen. Int J Environ Res Public Health. 2020;17:1071.

SECTION

# 16 Advances in Assisted Reproductive Technologies

CHAPTER 112

# Assisted Hatching in Assisted Reproductive Technology

*Gaurav Majumdar*

## INTRODUCTION

Over the last decade, many attempts have been made to improve embryo implantation in in vitro fertilization (IVF). A high incidence of chromosomal anomalies has been observed in embryos generated from IVF. However, genetic factors alone cannot explain the low implantation rate of morphologically normal embryos, indicating that a number of other factors could be involved. One of these factors is possibly the inability of the embryo to hatch out successfully from within its outer covering, i.e., the zona pellucida (ZP). It has been reported that 25–30% of embryos fail to hatch in optimal culture conditions in vitro.[1-3] If the rate of hatching is similar in vivo, it may explain in part the low implantation rates after IVF. An embryo must hatch out completely before it can implant into the uterine endometrium.

The impaired hatching may be due to the extended time in culture, in an artificial environment, causing hardening of the ZP. Hence, the strategy of assisted hatching, which involves artificial thinning or breaching of the ZP to facilitate embryo hatching, has been proposed to improve implantation rates in selected patients.[4,5] Several approaches have been adopted since then for assisted hatching, such as mechanical incision of the zona, chemical zona drilling with acidic medium, and laser-assisted drilling or thinning of the zona. Assisted hatching can be performed on both cleavage-stage embryos and blastocysts. Assisted hatching may be associated with certain adverse effects, such as damage to individual blastomeres resulting in reduced embryo viability; therefore, the procedure did not gain access as a routinely used adjunct treatment to all cases undergoing assisted reproductive technology (ART). In addition, there have been very few reports to support the efficacy of assisted hatching after the initial randomized controlled trials (RCTs) published by Cohen et al.[6] in 1992. This chapter shall, therefore, focus on identifying the patient groups that would benefit most from assisted hatching to maximize pregnancy rates.

## CAUSES FOR IMPAIRED HATCHING

Embryo hatching involves a spontaneous breach in the zona, thus allowing the expanding blastocyst to "hatch out" of the ZP and gain access to the endometrium for further implantation to occur. During the normal course of embryonic development in vitro, as a blastocyst undergoes expansion, it results in thinning of the zona to a point where finally the zona spontaneously ruptures. Subsequently, either the expanding blastocyst herniates out of the breached ZP or the embryo undergoes repeated cycles of contraction and expansion, which ultimately enables the blastocyst to break out of the zona. In addition to mechanical factors, lysins of embryonic and uterine origin are also involved in ZP thinning and hatching. The normal process of hatching may be impaired due to one of the following conditions:

- *Zona hardening:* This can occur either spontaneously or following gonadotropin therapy, cryopreservation, or after extended culture in vitro.
- *Increased zona thickness:* A thick zona is defined as having a mean ZP >18 µm. This measurement is dependent on the duration of follicular stimulation and maternal age.[7]
- *Reduction in zona lysins*: Lysins are compounds that are produced by the embryo and/or the endometrium that dissolve the ZP, thereby reducing its thickness. The blastocyst expands and contracts repeatedly before hatching, leading to further thinning and eventual rupture of the zona. Therefore, a reduction in these lysins may impair the normal process of hatching.
- *Embryos with extensive fragmentation or cell death:* After freezing and thawing, these embryos may also encounter hatching difficulties.

## ASSISTED HATCHING: PLAUSIBLE MECHANISMS

Primarily, a breach in the zona may help the embryo to hatch by overcoming the mechanical barrier of a hard or thick zona. Cellular energy requirement for hatching might be insufficient in patients with poor prognosis. Therefore, assisted hatching may also decrease this energy requirement of the embryo to commence hatching. Artificially rupturing the zona promotes early hatching[8] and may therefore increase chances of implantation by optimizing the implantation window. Normally, hatching occurs 5 days postfertilization in a nonstimulated cycle, after which an embryo has 48 hours more to implant as judged by the presence of endometrial pinopods (120–168 hours post insemination). However, in a gonadotropin-stimulated cycle, the phenomenon of endometrial advancement may lead to a premature shift of the implantation window to between 72 and 120 hours postfertilization. Thus, if hatching occurs at 120 hours, then endometrial advancement may result in limiting the opportunity for implantation to occur. Assisted hatching seems to allow earlier hatching and therefore offers higher chances of implantation, obviating the closing of the implantation window in stimulated patients.

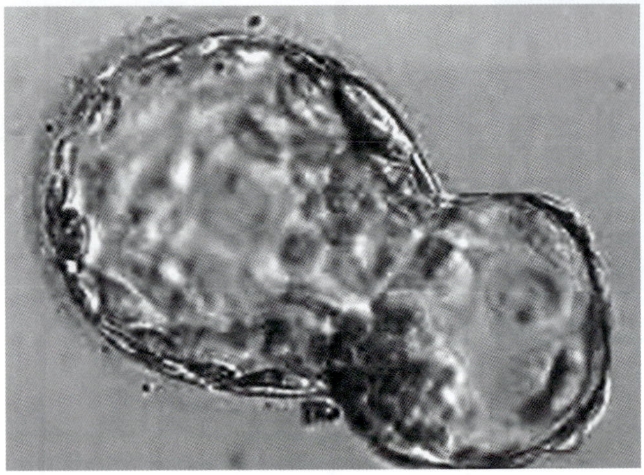

**Fig. 1:** A day 5 blastocyst seen hatching from its outer covering zona pellucida. Part of the embryo has herniated out of a breach in zona pellucida at 4'o clock position with the remainder of the embryo still inside the zona.

## Overview of Techniques

It has been observed that although human blastocysts expand readily in vitro, about 20% of such blastocysts have hatching problems. Therefore, it was proposed that such embryos could be rescued by disrupting the zona physically on day 2 or day 3, thereby promoting the natural process of hatching. The reason for delaying the procedure until the third day is that intercellular connections start to form at this stage, thereby preventing loss of blastomeres following opening of the ZP **(Fig. 1)**. Thereafter, various approaches have been adopted, some of which have been shown to be useful. The different techniques that have been tried are given in the following text.

### *Mechanical: Partial Zona Dissection on Day 2*

Originally, the technique of partial zona dissection (PZD) had been used to assist or enhance fertilization in vitro, mainly in cases of male factor infertility, where patients could not be helped by conventional IVF. This technique was subsequently given up because of poor fertilization rates. However, in 1993, Cohen et al. demonstrated that the same technique could be used on day 2 embryos to assist hatching and improve implantation rates of these embryos, which otherwise may have failed to implant.

In this technique **(Fig. 2)**, (1) the embryo is held firmly in place by a holding micropipette; (2) a sharp dissection micropipette is inserted through the ZP, at the other end, in the perivitelline space between two adjacent blastomeres; and (3) a slit in the ZP is created by gently rubbing the holding pipette over the small part of the zona trapped against the micropipette until the embryo is released. This technique is preferably performed on day 2 embryos since the embryo does not have more than four blastomeres, and therefore, there is enough perivitelline space between adjacent blastomeres to assist the procedure of PZD.

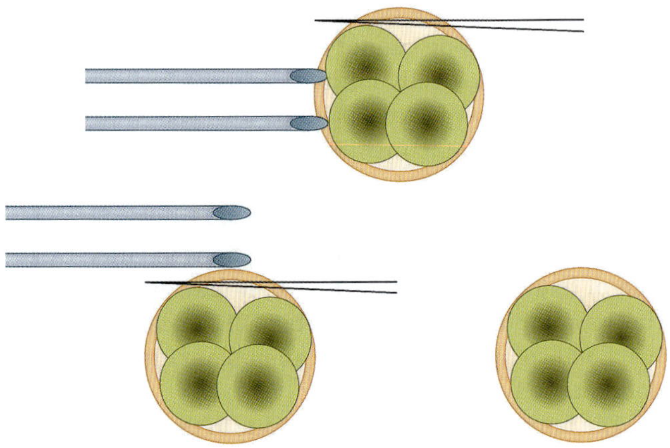

**Fig. 2:** Partial zona dissection.

### *Chemically Assisted Hatching: Zona Drilling with Acid Tyrode's Solution (pH 2.5)*

Zona drilling involves creating an opening in the zona measuring 15–20 μm on the inside and 30–50 μm on the outside, by spraying acid Tyrode's solution on the zona **(Fig. 3)**. This is generally done on day 3 embryos. Initially, it was shown that zona drilling significantly improved the implantation rates in patients whose embryos had thick zona. The best results were achieved for patients with elevated basal follicle-stimulating hormone (FSH) levels or for those older than 38 years. Nonetheless, both these techniques of mechanical and chemical manipulation did not turn out to be very popular since there were a lot of practical problems associated with the procedures, some of which were simply the result of technical drawbacks and/or lack of standardized protocols. For instance, it was observed that embryos with a thin zona (<13 μm) appeared to get damaged following the

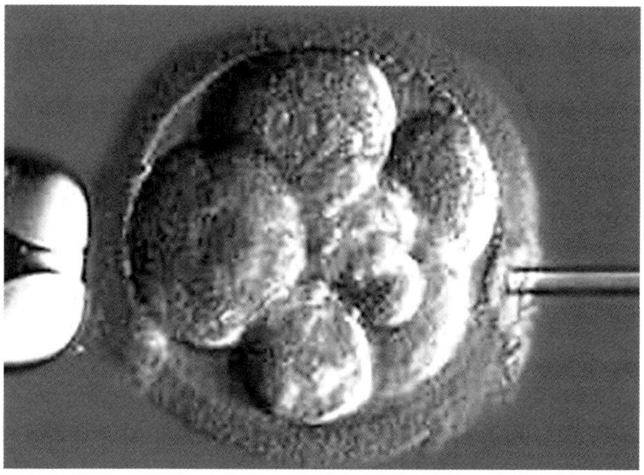

**Fig. 3:** Opening in the zona by drilling with the help of acid Tyrode's solution.

zona drilling procedure.[9] Some of the common problems with respect to PZD and zona drilling are as follows:

- Formation of holes <10 µm, which may lead to trapping of embryos during hatching or cell separation
- Formation of holes >25 µm, which may lead to cell loss during a traumatic embryo transfer
- Excessive exposure to acid Tyrode's solution, which could damage the adjacent cells in the embryo.

Several recent studies evaluating the impact of chemically assisted hatching with zona thinning have been inconclusive with respect to any improvement in outcomes. Interestingly, majority of these studies were focused on fresh embryos. However, data emerging from retrospective analysis as well as from prospective randomized studies evaluating the effect of assisted hatching on frozen/thawed cycles have shown an improvement in implantation rates but no improvement in pregnancy rates.[9]

### *Enzymatic: Zona Softening or Complete Removal with Pronase*

Enzymatic treatment of the ZP to either soften or remove the zona totally before blastocyst transfer has resulted in high implantation rates.[10] The zona is usually completely dissolved after 1.5 minutes of exposure to 10 IU pronase at 37°C. The increase in implantation rates may be due to better cell-to-cell anchorage between the trophectoderm (TE) and endometrium as a result of complete zona removal.[11] In the method described by Fong et al., day 5 blastocysts were transferred to 10 IU/mL pronase for 1 minute.[11] Embryos were quickly checked (on a heated stage) for zona stretching, zona becoming faint, and subsequent increase in perivitelline space. Thereafter, the embryos were washed in culture medium and incubated until transfer. All the embryos that were transferred either had a faint zona or were zona free. Complete zona removal should not be done before compaction due to lack of junctional complexes between adjacent blastomeres.

### *Laser-assisted Drilling*

Laser technology has found widespread use in medicine. It is especially appreciated for its precise and atraumatic mode of action. This fact encouraged the application of lasers for micromanipulation, especially to perform assisted hatching. This easy and precise procedure offers a gentle way to create an opening in the zona using only a few laser pulses within seconds. However, keeping in mind the delicate nature of micromanipulation techniques, it is recommended that the following four criteria be taken into account before selecting a suitable laser system for your embryology laboratory:

1. Absolute avoidance of thermal effects causing coagulation or vaporization, thereby causing irreversible denaturation of proteins
2. Prevention of genetic damage by a wavelength well above the absorption maximum of deoxyribonucleic acid (DNA) (268 nm)
3. Low ablation threshold to ensure precision and to minimize mechanical vibration
4. Easy handling using existing micromanipulation equipment.

There are two types of laser systems:

1. Contact laser in which the laser beam is guided through a glass/optical fiber. The fiber is fitted to the micromanipulator by a pipette holder and is brought in direct contact with the zona, but the tip is not forced further into it before application of the laser beam. This prevents any contact of the fiber with the surface of the ooplasm or blastomere once it penetrates the zona. The laser fiber should be either disposable or sterilizable before being used on other patients' embryos.
2. Noncontact laser systems[12] are more popular since they are very easy to use. In this system, the laser beam is guided through an optical lens and focused on the specimen. None of the equipment comes in contact with the embryo or culture media; therefore, this system ensures complete sterility, high precision, and selectivity avoiding all problems of cross-contamination. The simplicity of the procedure does not require skilled laboratory technicians or a great deal of training.

Lasers can be used in thinning[13] of the ZP, creating a complete breach,[12] through the zona. Thinning of the zona has been preferred because a complete breach may impair the natural process of blastocyst expansion and zona thinning. The opening results in releasing any pressure exerted by the expanding embryo on the zona and consequently the zona remain relatively thick. Furthermore, a larger than normal opening may lead to loss of blastomeres or loss of the whole embryo during contractions of the reproductive tract.[14] Nevertheless, in either case, the use of laser for assisted hatching has proven to be much more advantageous than that with PZD or acid Tyrode's since laser allows making holes of standardized sizes, avoiding both the escape of blastomeres or embryo trapping. Also, compared to mechanical or chemical methods, the use of lasers greatly reduces the risk of damaging the embryo because of its high precision and ease of handling.

A number of laser systems have now been reported, and there is continuing evaluation to determine the most effective and the least hazardous of these systems. In the "contact mode," different lasers have been used to drill holes: Argon fluoride at 193 nm[15] and the neodymium-doped yttrium aluminum garnet (Nd:YAG) at 1,064 nm.[16] Strohmer and Feichtinger made use of an erbium YAG (infrared) laser at a wavelength of 2.94 μm along with a glass fiber with a 20 μm tip diameter.[17] In 1994, Obruca et al. reported the use of the same laser system obtaining an improvement in implantation and pregnancy rates.[18] Antinori et al. again used the same erbium YAG system for zona thinning.[13]

A PALM UV laser at 337 nm operating in a "noncontact mode" was used to assist hatching in embryos by making complete holes in the zona.[12] The other laser systems that have been used in the noncontact mode are the xenon chloride excite laser at 248 nm,[19] the krypton fluoride laser at 248 nm,[20] and the diode laser at 1.48 μm.[21]

The use of laser technology for ZP thinning has been shown to be of benefit in some studies. The results were obtained in favor of the partial zona thinning as compared to the complete breaching of the ZP in studies comparing different laser-based techniques.[9]

### *Piezo-assisted Drilling*

In 1999, Nakayama et al.[22] demonstrated that assisted hatching, using a piezo-micromanipulator, improved the pregnancy and implantation rates in infertile patients with a poor prognosis with good-quality embryos for transfer. Piezo-assisted drilling of holes in the ZP has been achieved in animal models. The technique entails the use of electromagnetic pulses wherein the zona is corked off without any bending.[23] Piezo-assisted drilling is very fast and extremely easy with no potential detrimental effects on the embryo. The procedure has been used to perform nuclear transfers (in all animal species except the cow) and might, in future, be considered as the method of choice for clinical application in humans.

## PITFALLS OF ASSISTED HATCHING

In some instances, the creation of a hole or thinning of ZP may not be enough to improve the chances of the embryo to adequately hatch. Current research shows that the benefits of assisted hatching are limited to selected cases and there is no evidence of benefit for the overall patient population. Some of the common problems identified with assisted hatching are as follows:

- It deprives the embryo of its protective coat, which otherwise shields it from detrimental factors such as bacteria and viruses in the female reproductive tract.[24]

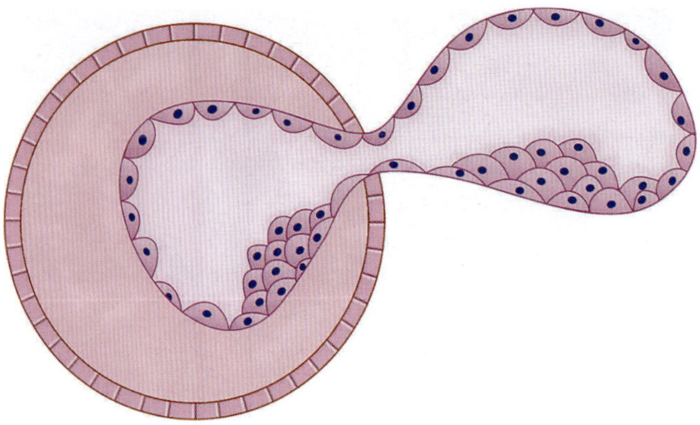

**Fig. 4:** Figure-of-eight configuration of the embryo.

- The absence of an intact ZP may lead the embryo to be immunocompromised. This may fail to support the implantation of ZP-dissected human embryos.[24]
- There is possibility of an increased loss of blastomeres or whole embryos during contractions of the female reproductive tract.[14]
- The natural expansion of blastocysts with breached ZP may fail to occur.
- A higher incidence of monozygotic twinning as a result of smaller hole size in ZP has been reported.[25]

### Monozygotic Twinning

The size of the hole in the ZP has a major impact on the hatching embryo. A blastocyst with narrow artificial holes may lose trophoblastic vesicles as they expand and attempt to hatch through the narrow gap. Most importantly, a very small hole may lead to a figure-of-eight configuration of the embryo **(Fig. 4)** at the time of hatching, while multiple gaps of the same dimension promote multiple herniations. Any of these situations may also lead to splitting of the inner cell mass (ICM), forming dichorionic or diamniotic twins. If this takes place after the differentiation of the trophoblast, then a monochorionic or diamniotic twin pregnancy may result.[26]

It is important to note that monozygotic twin formation may be viewed as an adverse effect of assisted hatching, as it creates a complex obstetric situation by potentially increasing morbidity and mortality rates of the fetus before and after birth. Monoamniotic twin pregnancies may lead to an increased risk of intrauterine fetal death, due to fetal entanglement, umbilical cord accidents, or formation of conjoint twins.

Currently, the available evidence is insufficient to conclude that assisted hatching increases the rate of monozygotic twinning since the outcome is rare and conflicting results have been obtained from different studies.[27] A meta-analysis, evaluating the risk factors for monozygotic twinning after IVF, which included 16 studies that compared IVF with and without assisted hatching, demonstrated a statistically significant association between monozygotic twinning and assisted hatching [odds ratio (OR) 1.17; 95% confidence interval (CI) 1.09–1.27; $p < 0.0001$]. However, this association could not be confirmed when the analysis was limited to only high-quality cohort and case-control studies.[28] A study analyzing the results from the Society for Assisted Reproductive Technology (SART) database between 2004 and 2010 demonstrated that although monozygotic twinning was more likely with day 5 or day 6 embryos, addition of assisted hatching had no significant effect, whereas assisted hatching had a substantial effect on day 2 or day 3 embryos (OR 2.05–2.48).[29]

There are a similar number of studies showing no increase in monozygotic twinning rates with assisted hatching; however, majority of studies are underpowered or inconsistent in the number of embryos transferred or the method of assisted hatching used.[30]

## PATIENT SELECTION FOR ASSISTED HATCHING

The criterion for selecting individual embryos for assisted hatching is dependent on many variables. It is believed that a thick or hard zona may act as a mechanical barrier for a hatching embryo. Zona hardening may occur as a natural consequence of in vitro embryo culture and cryopreservation. Similarly, zona thickness, which correlates negatively with implantation rates, may be influenced by factors such as maternal age and elevated basal FSH. Therefore, assisted hatching may be considered in the following cases.

### Indications

- Women aged >38 years
- Elevated basal FSH levels
- Zona thickness >18 μm
- Repeatedly failed IVF or intracytoplasmic sperm injection (ICSI) cycles after transfer of multiple good-quality embryos
- Embryos generated from in vitro matured oocytes
- Embryos generated from cryopreserved oocytes
- Frozen–thawed embryos in cryopreservation cycles.

### Contraindications of Assisted Hatching

- If a traumatic embryo transfer is anticipated, assisted hatching should not be attempted.
- Assisted hatching may not be performed if the blastomeres do not appear to be in interphase; for example, a dividing four-cell embryo might be more sensitive to external influences as compared to an embryo with cells at the interphase stage.

A Cochrane review assessing the impact of assisted hatching, including 39 RCTs with 2,486 clinical pregnancies, reported a slight increase in clinical pregnancy rate (OR 1.20; 95% CI 1.09–1.33) as well as multiple pregnancy rate (OR 1.38; 95% CI 1.13–1.68); however, the quality of evidence was poor. They reported no beneficial impact of assisted hatching on the live birth rate (OR 1.09; 95% CI 0.92–1.29). Miscarriage rates were also similar in both the groups. On accounting for the heterogeneity in the studies included, there may also be little to no difference in clinical pregnancy rates.[31]

## MEDICAL MANAGEMENT

The ZP is the protective covering for the embryo and its blastomeres during its passage through the female reproductive tract. Breach in the zona, while the embryo is still lying in the uterine cavity, waiting to hatch and to be implanted, exposes it to microorganism and immune factors, including antigens. Therefore, use of antibiotics and immunosuppressive drugs has been proposed for patients, whose embryos undergo assisted hatching, as prophylactic therapy, to possibly protect the embryo from local insults. The most preferred therapy is methylprednisolone (16 mg four times a day) and tetracycline (250 mg four times a day) started from the day of oocyte retrieval. However, the utility of these drugs is still not established and should be regarded as empirical for the time being.

## CONCLUSION

The latest guidelines published by the American Society for Reproductive Medicine (ASRM) and SART (2022) (investigating the role of assisted hatching in IVF) state that there is moderate evidence that assisted hatching does not significantly improve live birth rates in fresh IVF cycles. In patients with poor prognosis (such as those of advanced maternal age or with recurrent implantation failure) or undergoing frozen embryo transfer cycles,[30] the available data are insufficient to demonstrate any benefit of laser-assisted hatching. Hence, ASRM in its recommendations states that currently, laser-assisted hatching should not be incorporated in to routine clinical practice for all patients undergoing IVF.[27]

## KEY POINTS

- Assisted hatching has been applied during IVF treatment in an attempt to improve pregnancy rates. However, the application of assisted hatching as a technique has still not gained widespread acceptance, even though some publications report improved implantation rates with its use.
- The laser system has been better appreciated for its precise and atraumatic mode of action when compared to PZD or zona drilling with acid solution, and therefore might be very important in future as an adjunct to IVF treatment.
- Use of prophylactic steroid and antibiotic treatment is controversial and may not be recommended for routine use after embryo transfer.
- Further research is needed, utilizing more recent and standardized techniques, with properly conducted prospective RCTs in a well-defined subgroup of patients to allow better appraisal of results.

## REFERENCES

1. Fehilly CB, Cohen J, Simons RF, Fishel SB, Edwards RG. Cryopreservation of cleaving embryos and expanded blastocysts in the human: a comparative study. Fertil Steril. 1985;44:638-44.
2. Lindenberg C, Hyttel P, Sjogren A, Greve T. A comparative study of attachment of human, bovine and mouse blastocysts to uterine epithelial monolayer. Hum Reprod. 1989;4:446-56.
3. Dokras A, Sargent H, Ross C, Gardner RL, Barlow DH. The human blastocyst: morphology and human chorionic gonadotropin secretion in vitro. Hum Reprod. 1991;6:1143-51.
4. Cohen J, Elsner C, Kort H, Malter H, Massey J, Mayer MP, et al. Impairment of the hatching process following IVF in the human improvement of implantation by assisted hatching using micromanipulation. Hum Reprod. 1990;5:7-13.
5. Tucker MJ, Cohen J, Massey JB, Mayer MP, Wiker SR, Wright G. Partial dissection of the zona pellucida of frozen-thawed human embryos may enhance blastocyst hatching, implantation, and pregnancy rates. Am J Obstet Gynecol. 1991;165:341-4; discussion 344-5.
6. Cohen J, Alikani M, Trowbridge J, Rosenwaks Z. Implantation enhancement by selective assisted hatching using zona drilling of human embryos with poor prognosis. Hum Reprod. 1992;7:685-91.
7. Cohen J, Willadsen S, Schimmel T. Micromanipulation as a clinical tool. In: Trounson AO, Gardner DK (Eds). Handbook of In Vitro Fertilization. Boca Raton, FL: CRC Press; 2000. p. 265.
8. Liu HC, Cohen J, Alikani M, Noyes N, Rosenwaks Z. Assisted hatching facilitates earlier implantation. Fertil Steril. 1993;60:871-5.
9. Alteri A, Viganò P, Maizar AA, Jovine L, Giacomini E, Rubino P. Revisiting embryo assisted hatching approaches: a systematic review of the current protocols. J Assist Reprod Genet. 2018;35(3):367-91.
10. Fong CY, Bongso A, Ng SC, Kumar J, Trounson A, Ratnam S. Blastocyst transfer after enzymatic treatment of the zona pellucida: improving in-vitro fertilization and understanding implantation. Hum Reprod. 1998;13(10):2926-32.
11. Fong CY, Bongso A, Sathananthan H, Ho J, Ng SC. Ultrastructural observations of enzymatically treated human blastocysts: zona-free blastocyst transfer and rescue of blastocysts with hatching difficulties. Hum Reprod. 2001;16:540-6.
12. Antinori S, Selman HA, Caffa B, Panci C, Dani GL, Versaci C. Zona opening of human embryos using a non-contact UV laser for assisted hatching in patients with poor prognosis of pregnancy. Hum Reprod. 1996;11(11):2488-92.
13. Antinori S, Panci C, Selman HA, Caffa B, Dani G, Versaci C. Zona thinning with the use of laser: a new approach to assisted hatching in humans. Hum Reprod. 1996;11:590-4.
14. Nicholas J, Gardner RL. Effect of damage to zona pellucida on development of preimplantation embryos in the mouse. Hum Reprod. 1989;4:180-7.
15. Palanker D, Ohad S, Lewis A, Simon A, Shenkar J, Penchas S, et al. Technique for cellular microsurgery using the 193-nm excimer laser. Laser Surg Med. 1991;11:580-6.
16. Coddington CC, Veek LL, Swanson RJ, Kaufmann RA, Lin J, Simonetti S, et al. The YAG laser used in micromanipulation to transect the zona pellucida of hamster oocytes. J Assist Reprod Genet. 1992;9:557-63.
17. Strohmer H, Feichtinger W. Successful clinical application of laser for micromanipulation in an in vitro fertilization program. Fertil Steril. 1992;58:212-4.
18. Obruca A, Strohmer H, Sakkas D, Menezo Y, Kogosowski A, Barak Y, et al. Use of lasers in assisted fertilization and hatching. Hum Reprod. 1994;9:1723-6.
19. Neev J, Tadir Y, Ho PD, Berns MW, Asch RH, Ord T. Microscope-delivered ultraviolet laser zona dissection: principles and practices. J Assist Reprod Genet. 1992;9:513-23.
20. Blanchet GB, Russel JB, Fincher Jr CR, Portmann M. Laser micromanipulation in the mouse embryo: a novel approach to zona drilling. Fertil Steril. 1992;57:1337-41.
21. Germond M, Nocera D, Senn A, Rink K, Delacrétaz G, Fakan S. Microdissection of mouse and human zona pellucida using a 1.48-microns diode laser beam: efficacy and safety of the procedure. Fertil Steril. 1995;64:604-11.
22. Nakayama T, Fujiwara H, Yamada S, Tastumi K, Honda T, Fujii S. Clinical application of a new assisted hatching method using a piezo-micromanipulator for morphologically low-quality embryos in poor-prognosis infertile patients. Fertil Steril. 1999;71(6):1014-8.
23. Nakayama T, Fujiwara H, Tastumi K, Fujita K, Higuchi T, Mori T. A new assisted hatching technique using a piezo-micromanipulator. Fertil Steril. 1998;69:784-8.
24. Cohen J, Malter H, Elsner C, Kort H, Massey J, Mayer MP. Immunosuppression supports implantation of zona pellucida dissected human embryos. Fertil Steril. 1990;53:662-5.
25. Schieve L, Meikle S, Peterson H, Jeng G, Burnett NM, Wilcox LS. Does assisted hatching pose a risk for monozygotic twinning in pregnancies conceived through in vitro fertilization? Fertil Steril. 2000;74:288-94.
26. Hershlag A, Paine T, Cooper G, Scholl GM, Rawlinson K, Kvapil G. Monozygotic twinning associated with mechanical assisted hatching. Fertil Steril. 1999;71:144-6.
27. Practice Committee of the American Society for Reproductive Medicine. The role of assisted hatching in in vitro fertilization: a guideline. Fertil Steril. 2022;117(6):1177-82.
28. Busnelli A, Dallagiovanna C, Reschini M, Paffoni A, Fedele L, Somigliana E. Risk factors for monozygotic twinning after in vitro fertilization: a systematic review and meta-analysis. Fertil Steril. 2019;111(2):302-17.
29. Luke B, Brown MB, Wantman E, Stern JE. Factors associated with monozygosity in assisted reproductive technology pregnancies and the risk of recurrence using linked cycles. Fertil Steril. 2014;101(3):683-9.
30. Nakasuji T, Saito H, Araki R, Nakaza A, Nakashima A, Kuwahara A, et al. The incidence of monozygotic twinning in assisted reproductive technology: analysis based on results from the 2010 Japanese ART national registry. J Assist Reprod Genet. 2014;31(7):803-7.
31. Lacey L, Hassan S, Franik S, Seif MW, Akhtar MA. Assisted hatching on assisted conception (in vitro fertilisation (IVF) and intracytoplasmic sperm injection (ICSI)). Cochrane Database Syst Rev. 2021;3(3):CD001894.

CHAPTER 113

# Preimplantation Genetic Screening and Diagnosis: Laboratory Aspects

*Krishna Chaitanya M, Durga G Rao, Sushma Baxi, Abhishek Shah*

## INTRODUCTION

Assisted reproductive technologies (ARTs) are currently focused on introducing advanced technologies to improve live birth rate (LBR), which includes extending embryo culture till the blastocyst stage, along with algorithms and annotations including the time-lapse technology to select the single embryo for transfer that has the best implantation potential. Above criteria help in the ultimate goal of safe mother and a healthy child. Preimplantation genetic testing (PGT) is one of the advanced ART methods which has been introduced to enhance the reproductive outcomes further. Since its first report in 1990,[1,2] till date, there has been a lot of developments with PGT, in both clinical application and laboratory aspects for embryo biopsy and genetic screening; currently, the updated version in practice is 3.0 as suggested by the European Society of Human Reproduction and Embryology (ESHRE) special interest group. This chapter, in particular, will deal with the laboratory aspects of PGT. A prerequisite for successful implantation of PGT program is the laboratory setup, which will be dealt with in detail in this chapter. Ideal embryo stages for biopsy, ideal platform for chromosomal screening, and ways to handle the limitations of PGT have been extensively researched in the past few years. Despite advancing technology and successful implementation of PGT, controversy still exists about the application of PGT routinely to all infertile couples seeking ART.

## TERMINOLOGY

In the past few years, the terminologies of preimplantation genetic screening (PGS) and preimplantation genetic diagnosis (PGD) have changed and are currently referred to as preimplantation genetic testing.

Preimplantation genetic testing is divided into three subtypes as mentioned below:

1. *PGT-A (aneuploidy):* PGT-A determines whether the correct numbers of chromosomes are present in the embryo. It was previously known as PGS (pregenetic screening). It is indicated in cases such as advanced maternal age (AMA), recurrent implantation failures (RIF), recurrent pregnancy loss (RPL), and severe male factor (SMF) couples. PGT-A deals with aneuploidy in embryos alone.
2. *PGT-SR (structural rearrangement):* PGT-SR screens for chromosomal translocations, inversions, and deletions. This also identifies the embryos with the correct amount of genetic material (balanced/normal) and embryos that have extra or missing genetic material. PGT-SR deals with screens for structural rearrangements such as translocations, inversions, and deletions in an embryo.
3. *PGT-M (monogenic):* PGT-M screens for deoxyribonucleic acid (DNA) pathogenic variant(s) causing single-gene disorders, also called monogenic disorders.[3] It was previously known as PGD (pregenetic diagnosis). It is indicated in cystic fibrosis, cancer (autosomal dominant disorders), Huntington's disease, thalassemia, sickle cell anemia, hemophilia, fragile X syndrome, etc.

*Human leukocyte antigens (HLA) typing:* HLA-matched embryo selection via PGT is the best option in couples who already have an affected child with malignancy, genetic disorder, or an acquired disorder where the affected child can be treated with stem cell therapy from an HLA-matched sibling.[3]

This change in terminology to PGT along with the usage of comprehensive chromosomal screening (CCS) methods such as next-generation sequencing (NGS) has been termed PGT 3.0 version by the Preimplantation Genetic Diagnosis International Society (PGDIS).

## SETTING UP A STATE OF ASSISTED REPRODUCTIVE TECHNOLOGY LABORATORY AND AN EFFICIENT PROGRAM FOR PREIMPLANTATION GENETIC SCREENING/ PREIMPLANTATION GENETIC DIAGNOSIS

A PGT program involves several units. Ensuring optimal communication between these units has to be clear and informative with the implementation of strict quality control.[4]

Informed consent from all patients entering the PGT program regarding the expected results, details of the PGT cycle from start to end, and the limitations of the technique should be undertaken. Treatment consent forms should be discussed with the patients in detail, in the language they understand, and a written consent to be obtained prior to starting the procedures.

Every couple seeking PGT needs detailed evaluation of reproductive history and adequate genetic counseling as a part of the preliminary workup, particularly for couples at high genetic risk due to chromosome structural abnormalities or monogenic diseases.

It is advisable to set up the embryology laboratory as per the guidelines for good practice in an in vitro fertilization (IVF) laboratory prepared by the ESHRE Embryology Special Interest Group.[4] Standard operating procedures (SOPs) should be collected in a manual that is kept updated by the laboratory director; the current version should be accessible to every member of the staff. This ensures strict uniformity of treatment. The procedures for single-embryo culture, cell biopsy, tubing of the tissue, transportation of the tissue post biopsy, details of the genetic laboratory, and later transfer of the selected embryos on the basis of the genetic results are additional aspects expressly related to the PGT program, which should be clearly explained in the SOPs.

Considering the risk of contamination and the risk of embryo toxicity with the extensive use of cleaning solutions, it is recommended to have a separate designated area exclusively for embryo biopsy and cell tubing.

Standard operating procedures should also have a detailed checklist for carrying out the embryo biopsy in the IVF laboratory.

Following are few of the aspects the checklist should have:

- Details of validation and calibration of various laboratory equipment
- Adequate stock of consumables, disposables, and culture media required for the biopsy
- Proper planning of IVF cycles and other procedures in the IVF laboratory to ensure balance between ongoing cycles, manpower, and the load acceptability of the laboratory
- Availability of the adequate laboratory staff is mandatory.
- Ensuring optimal cleaning of IVF laboratory pre- and post-biopsy.
- Intimation to the genetic laboratory through a test requisition form about the indication for PGT, expected oocyte retrieval date, number of embryos, stage of biopsy, tentative plan for embryo transfer fresh or frozen cycle, and organizing the transportation of samples post biopsy.

### Equipment and Disposables for Embryo Biopsy

- Class 100 vertical laminar air flow (LAF) with a stereo zoom microscope
- Micromanipulator with an inverted microscope, heated stage, and a diode laser
- Benchtop incubator to temporarily store embryos during the biopsy process
- -20°C freezer to store the biopsied tissue till it is transported to the genetic laboratory.
- Inverted microscope equipped with:
  - Micropipettes:
    - Holding pipettes
    - Biopsy aspiration pipettes.

### Reagents

- 2.1 media for biopsy
- $Ca^{2+}$ and $Mg^{2+}$ free buffer
- Human serum albumin (HSA)
- Mineral oil.

All of these above-mentioned reagents have to be new, unopened bottles.

## PATIENT MANAGEMENT

An important prerequisite for PGT is patient counseling and informed consent.

The need for PGT is to be discussed in detail. Especially in couples undergoing PGT, feasibility of the genetic laboratory to handle the underlying gene defect and the process has to be elaborated. For PGT cycles, pre-PGT workup for designing the probes for the particular single gene has to be planned beforehand. This might involve transportation of blood samples of the couple, parents of the couple, and sometimes the affected child. The genetics laboratory will design the necessary probe and use this at the time of PGT and arrive at a final report of normal embryos, carrier embryos, and affected embryos. Pre-PGT workup might take 2–6 weeks; therefore, keeping the patient informed about the timelines is very important. However, karyomapping is a new technique that is evolving which is a universal probe and the pre-PGT step can be skipped, which ensures a quicker process time for PGT couples. Further data for routine usage is yet to be established.

Reproductive counseling would involve an in-depth evaluation of reports and formulation of a plan. Counseling should also address the success rates, financial logistics, and limitations of PGT.

## HISTORY, COUNSELING, CONSENTING, AND DOCUMENTATION

Before starting a clinical cycle, extensive genetic and reproductive counseling is provided to the prospective parent(s). Psychological support may be offered as well.

Detailed couple history and family history are of upmost importance before offering genetic analysis options and starting clinical treatment.

- Complete medical history of the couple and child/children if applicable.
- Complete medical and genetic history of the family of the couple with direct blood relation.
- Possible karyotype of the couple and child/children if applicable.
- Complete counseling of the stimulation cycle, oocyte retrieval and risk of medical complications, embryo formation rate and biopsy stage, risks associated, and survival of embryo biopsy and cryopreservation.
- Counseling of embryo transfer policy of the organization and local regulations.
- Minimal risk of no conclusive results, misdiagnosis rate, limitations of the testing methods, and possibility of epigenetic disorders can arise with the continuation of pregnancy, etc., which are to be explained in detail.
- Percentage of conception with PGT embryos and miscarriage rates to be counseled.
- Cost factor for the entire process and timeline required for it should be estimated to the couple.
- In embryos having genetic abnormalities and not selected for transfer, the option of donation for research or training should be selected as per the country's regulations and guidelines.
- Entire counseling, all risk factors, and possibilities to be counseled by the treating physician and genetic counselor, and written consents are to be taken, framed by local regulations and organization.
- Entire counseling and consenting (preferably) is to be done in the couple's local or known language.

## IN VITRO FERTILIZATION STIMULATION PROTOCOLS

Preimplantation genetic diagnosis/preimplantation genetic testing is an expensive and laborious process. There is no probability as to how many embryos will have a normal genetic status after screening. Hence, it is always desired to have a good ovarian response to hormonal stimulation.

Poor responders should be counseled regarding their reduced success rates, and also a balance needs to be maintained between feasibility for PGT, cost, success, and alternative approaches to optimize reproductive outcomes in this group of patients.

Stimulation protocols should be devised to increase the optimal number of retrieved oocytes but a calculated approach to avoid ovarian hyperstimulation syndrome (OHSS).

## CHOICE OF ASSISTED REPRODUCTIVE TECHNOLOGY FOR PREIMPLANTATION GENETIC SCREENING/PREIMPLANTATION GENETIC DIAGNOSIS

In cases where fluorescence in situ hybridization (FISH) is used for screening, there are no restrictions on the technique of insemination. However, for carriers of single-gene disorders where polymerase chain reaction (PCR) will be applied or for molecular [comparative genomic hybridization (CGH) and DNA microarrays] assessment of chromosome status, intracytoplasmic sperm injection (ICSI) is recommended in order to avoid sperm contamination.[5] For the same reason, the removal of corona cells should be especially meticulously performed. Additionally, to ensure an optimal tracking of embryo post biopsy, keeping them in individual culture drops prior to cryopreservation is mandatory. Therefore, necessary culture plates with provision for single droplet culture depending on the number of embryos for biopsy are to be planned. A recent guideline by the American Society for Reproductive Medicine (ASRM) recommends the usage of ICSI for PGT in the absence of male factor infertility, which should be restricted to situations where contamination of extraneous sperm could affect the accuracy of test results.

## IDEAL STAGE FOR EMBRYO BIOPSY

Scientists have attempted embryo biopsy for genetic screening at various stages. This segment will address the pros and cons of each stage and discuss the ideal stage for biopsy in the current scenario. Considering that the traditional biopsy techniques are invasive, the current focus has been to introduce noninvasive techniques to perform genetic screening, but further validation and efficiency of traditional biopsy techniques are yet to be proven.

## POLAR BODY BIOPSY

Polar body (PB) is extruded after completion of the first meiotic division in a mature metaphase II (MII) oocyte and after completion of the second meiotic division in a zygote. PBs are a haploid set of chromosomes in an MII oocyte, and in zygote, it is the extra set of chromosomes.

PB biopsy is considered to mirror the genetic status of the oocyte or zygote. PB biopsy is relatively less invasive when compared to the blastomere or trophectoderm (TE) biopsy. In countries where regulations do not permit blastomere or TE biopsy, PB biopsy is the preferred stage. As per ESHRE, PGT consortium use of PB biopsy for genetic screening is still debatable. Several studies have highlighted technical, economical, biological, and clinical deficiencies underlying this approach. Capalbo et al.[6] inferred that PB biopsy gives high false-positive and -negative error rates when compared against other stages. There is an operative concern and lack of consensus on whether to biopsy the first PB of mature metaphase oocyte in one sitting and the second PB in a separate sitting or should it be biopsied simultaneously at the zygote stage. There is no consensus on the timing of PB biopsy, although 8–14 hours post fertilization seems to be optimal. There is a risk of enucleation due to spindle remnants if biopsy is performed too early or a risk of degeneration if biopsy is delayed.[7]

In the current scenario, the application of PB biopsy is gradually reducing in favor of TE biopsy due to lack of supporting data in terms of its efficacy and diagnostic accuracy.[8]

## CLEAVAGE STAGE BIOPSY—BLASTOMERE BIOPSY

Cleavage stage biopsy is normally performed on day 3 embryos post insemination with at least six blastomeres.

Cleavage stage embryos are briefly exposed to calcium/magnesium (Ca/Mg) free medium to loosen up the gap junction and compaction between the blastomeres making the process of biopsy easier. Scientists have posed a concern with the inappropriate use of Ca/Mg free medium, which would adversely affect the blastulation process.[9] Mice models have shown this exposure to be detrimental.[10,11] A final conclusion is still elusive. As per ESHRE, PGT consortium cleavage stage biopsy still remains to be the most commonly followed method for PGT than TE biopsy.[12]

After exposure to Ca/Mg-free medium, the next step is assisted hatching. Assisted hatching of zona pellucida to facilitate biopsy can be done by laser-assisted hatching (LAH)[13] or Tyrode drilling[14] or mechanically by use of pipettes.[15] Randomized controlled trials (RCTs) on sibling embryos have shown all three methods to be safe and show no detrimental effects on clinical outcomes.[16,17]

## PROTOCOL FOR EMBRYO BIOPSY AND TUBING

### General Rules to Prevent Contamination

Always use gloves for the manipulation of all the material and samples. All disposables, consumables, and gloved hands have to be wiped with 70% ethanol to avoid contamination.

## PROTOCOL—BLASTOMERE BIOPSY

- Warm buffer supplemented with 5% HSA at 37°C for 20 minutes before starting (to make this buffer, take 1.8 mL of Ca/Mg free buffer and add 200 µL of HSA in a 5 mL tube and leave in the gassed incubator with a tightly closed cap).
- Place the culture plates in the laminar flow hood over the heated area.
- Check day 3 embryo morphology. Use the following criteria to choose embryos to biopsy:
  - *Cell number:* More than six cells
    - *Fragmentation:* <20%
    - *Multinucleate:* <50%
    - *Nucleus:* Present
- Place the aspiration (right hand) and holding (left hand) pipettes at the microinjectors and focus them.
- Prepare a biopsy plate with drops of biopsy media covered by mineral oil. For each embryo: Prepare one drop to wash the embryo (50 µL), one drop to wash the pipette (35 µL), and one drop to place the embryo (35 µL). There should not be more than two embryos per plate. See **Figure 1** for an example of two embryos.
- Turn on the laser.
- Label the plate with the patient's name at the top and the embryo number in the base, close to the corresponding drop.
- Place the embryos into the biopsy plate (one per drop).
- Wash the aspiration pipette in the washing buffer drop.
- Focus the embryo and hold it with the holding pipette. Rotate the embryo to select a blastomere for removal (choose one with only one nucleus).
- Make a hole of approximately 30 µm diameter in the zona pellucida using as few laser pulses as possible.
- Gently insert a biopsy pipette through the hole while holding the embryo with the holding pipette.
- Wash the aspiration pipette after the first embryo is biopsied. Use a new pipette if there is remaining cytoplasm from the previous cell.

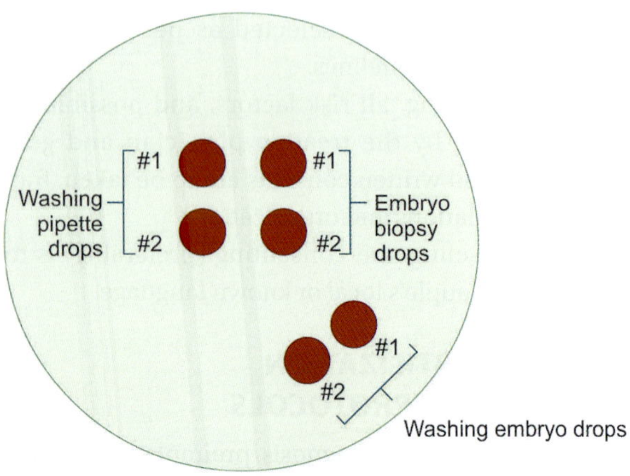


**Fig. 1:** Preparation of biopsy plate with drops of biopsy media covered by mineral oil: No more than two embryos per plate.

- Apply a gentle suction to grasp one blastomere and gently pull out the biopsy pipette while maintaining the suction. *Caution:* If the blastomere is still attached, extreme care should be taken at this point to avoid breaking the plasma membrane. Any sudden aspiration or movement should be avoided.
- Remove the blastomere with the pipette completely out of the embryo and gently expel the blastomere in the medium.
- Remove the embryos from the biopsy plate and wash them in drops of cell culture medium (CCM) to remove traces of buffer. Place embryos in their prolonged culture drops/wells.
- The blastomeres should remain on the biopsy plate until further processing based on the subsequent analysis type [FISH, array comparative genomic hybridization (aCGH), and PCR].

## ADVANTAGES OF CLEAVAGE STAGE BIOPSY

- Biopsy at this stage is less operator dependent.
- More reproducible.
- Embryos in the cleavage stage are more synchronous and are similar in terms of morphology, and biopsy can be attempted in one sitting.
- It is easier and convenient to biopsy a second blastomere immediately at the cleavage stage for any reason. Contrary to this, when a TE biopsy is done, a second biopsy immediately might be difficult due to the collapse of the blastocoel cavity.
- Embryo biopsy at the cleavage stage and fresh embryo transfer at the blastocyst stage are possible in the same cycle. On the other hand, a fresh transfer after TE biopsy is difficult unless there is an in-house genetic laboratory.

## LIMITATIONS OF CLEAVAGE STAGE BIOPSY

- Breaching of zona for biopsy at cleavage stage would impact blastocyst formation rates.[18]
- Removal of a few blastomeres would adversely affect clinical outcomes.[19]
- Kirkegaard et al.[20] did a comparative study of cleavage stage biopsied embryos and nonbiopsied embryos using time-lapse technology. Their findings showed that there was delayed compaction and blastocoel expansion in biopsied embryos at cleavage stage.
- Blastomere biopsy is associated with a high rate of amplification failure.[21]
- Chromosomal mosaicism is highest at the cleavage stage, and this might lead to errors in clinical management. In order to avoid this, two blastomere biopsies were suggested, but this would negatively impact the embryonic cell mass and the clinical outcomes further.[22]
- In 2013, Scott et al. did an RCT of transferring one biopsied (cleavage stage biopsied embryo) and one nonbiopsied good-quality embryo from the same cohort. A dramatic 39% relative reduction in implantation rate was reported when cleavage stage biopsy was conducted with respect to control.[23]
- Considering the fact that embryos at cleavage stage are relatively fragile since embryonic genome activation and cell differentiation processes are not completed, removal of a cell at this stage would compromise further developmental events and clinical outcomes.[24-26]

Though at this point TE biopsy seems to be a preferable option over cleavage stage biopsy, owing to the ease of cleavage biopsy, there are a lot of RCTs ongoing to further evaluate its efficacy with newer CCS methods as most of the studies have been done with FISH in the past.

## MORULA STAGE BIOPSY

Morula stage biopsy is not a common practice; however, some groups have shown morula biopsy to be beneficial owing to the more number of blastomeres available for biopsy.[27] Technically, the biopsy process is similar to cleavage stage biopsy, and similar limitations are applicable. The risk of mosaicism still remains a concern at the morula stage in comparison with TE biopsy. Hence, morula stage biopsy is not widely practiced.

## BLASTOCYST STAGE BIOPSY

In the year 2004, de Boer et al. reported successful biopsy and PGT of TE tissue,[28] and later in 2005, live births were reported by McArthur et al. and Kokkali et al.[29,30] TE biopsy of blastocysts was a major breakthrough in the field of PGT.

## PROTOCOL FOR TROPHECTODERM BIOPSY

- On day 3 of embryo development or day 5, make a small hole (approximately 20 µm) in the zona pellucida using the laser or acid Tyrode's in each embryo.
- On day 5 of embryo development, pretemper and precalibrate the biopsy medium for at least 4 hours.
- Place the culture plates in the laminar flow hood over the heated area.
- Check day 5 embryo morphology. Hatching TE is the ideal situation. In case the embryo is not hatching, locate the hole created on day 3 and attempt to reach the TE through the hole. Try to avoid the use of laser near the inner cell mass (ICM).
- In the case of vitrified embryos without assisted hatching, you can force the hatching of a cavitated blastocyst by making a small hole at the zona pellucida with a laser. The blastocyst will likely collapse, and then you have to wait for re-expansion before performing the biopsy.
- Prepare a biopsy plate with drops of biopsy media covered by mineral oil. For each embryo, prepare one drop to wash the embryo (50 µL), one drop to wash the pipette (35 µL), and one drop to place the embryo (35 µL). Only one embryo per plate should be used. See **Figure 2**.

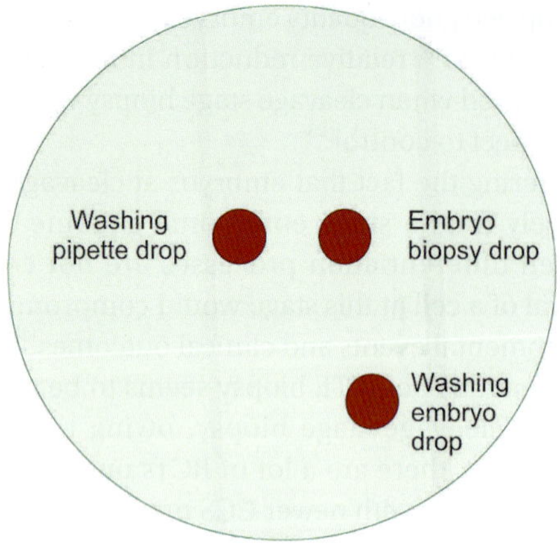


**Fig. 2:** Preparation of biopsy plate with drops of biopsy media covered by mineral oil: Only one embryo per plate.

- Label the plate with the patient's name at the top and the embryo number in the base, close to the corresponding drop.
- Place the plates in the dry incubator at 37°C.
- Place the aspiration (right hand) and holding (left hand) pipettes on the microinjectors and focus them.
- Place the blastocyst into the biopsy plate (one per drop).
- Turn on the laser.
- Hold the blastocyst so that hole created on day 3 is at 3 o'clock. If possible, the ICM should be at 6 or 12 o'clock. If this placement is not possible, try to avoid aspirating near the ICM.
- Change to the laser objective.
- Place the aspiration area on the target.
- Slowly bring the biopsy pipette close to the blastocyst.
- Apply gentle suction to grasp several cells and use four to six laser pulses to cut the TE. Caution: If the TE is still attached, release the blastocyst and squeeze the aspiration pipette to the holding pipette and make a quick movement down to separate the group of cells. Gently expel the TE in the medium.
- Remove the blastocyst from the biopsy plate and wash it in drops of CCM. Place blastocyst in its prolonged culture drops/wells.
- The TE remains on the biopsy plate until further processing according to the subsequent analysis type (FISH, aCGH, and PCR).
- Wash the aspiration pipette before the biopsy of each embryo. If there is any remaining debris from the previous embryo, use a new pipette to avoid cross contamination.

## TUBING PROTOCOL: ARRAY AND SINGLE-GENE DISORDERS (BLASTOMERE OR TROPHECTODERM)

### Materials Required

#### *Equipment*

- Stereomicroscope for cell manipulation from plate to PCR tube
- Automatic pipette 2–20 μL. Use exclusively for this purpose and always with gloves
- Sterile tips, with filter and DNA/ribonucleic acid (RNA) free
- Microcapillaries of a diameter between 100 and 130 μm
- Petri dishes (6 cm dishes from BD Falcon 3002)
- Sterile 0.2 mL PCR tubes with 2 μL of phosphate-buffered saline (PBS) solution—provided by genetic laboratory (stored at -20°C)
- Sterile safelock 1.5 mL tubes with 1 mL of cell washing media [1% PBS-polyvinylpyrrolidone (PVP)]—(stored at 4°C)
- Laminar flow hood with ultraviolet (UV) lamp
- PCR cooler rack
- Minicentrifuge for 0.2 mL PCR tubes.

### Methodology

#### *General Rules to Prevent Contamination*

- Always use gloves cleaned with alcohol for manipulation of all the material and samples of this procedure.
- Switch off the heated stage of LAF. Tubing to be performed at room temperature (RT).
- The embryologist should wear a disposable operating room gown and cap.
- Before starting the procedure, turn on the UV lamp and the laminar flow for at least 15 minutes. Clean with alcohol the surface of the cabinet and the external surface of all the material that will be used for tubing (tip boxes, automatic pipettes, capillaries boxes, etc.). The placement of the cell within the PCR tube must be performed inside the laminar flow hood and under the stereo microscope.
- Things to be kept in the LAF for tubing:
  - 3 mL transfer pipettes (BD Falcon 7575)—two of them
  - Oil in 14 mL tubes at RT for making the dishes for washing the biopsied material
  - 2–20 μL micropipette tip from Gilson2
  - Micropipette—2–20 μL volume
  - 6 cm dishes from BD Falcon 3002—two dishes for every four embryos
  - Glass denuding pipettes—one per embryo
  - Two sterile semen collection containers
  - PBS + PVP tube—stored at 4°C
  - PCR tubes with the rack—this is stored at -20°C
  - Mouth pipette/stripper handle with glass stripper
  - Marker pens
- An isolated room is recommended for single-cell manipulation, if possible a room separate from the IVF laboratory. Avoid manipulating DNA in this room and in the freezer and fridge where the solutions are stored.

### Protocol

- Every step should be performed using gloves, and all the material (not the embryos) should be exposed to UV light before starting the procedure.

- Use one new capillary for each individual cell (day 3 biopsy) or TE biopsy
- Place the mini spin inside the hood and spin the PCR tubes with 2 μL of PBS before starting. Check that there are no bubbles inside the PCR tubes and confirm that liquid is at the bottom of the tube. Manually, we can just shake the tubes to bring the PBS solution to the bottom of the tube.
- Prepare a Petri dish with one row with three droplets of 5 μL of cell washing media (1% PBS–PVP) for each embryo (include six rows maximum in one plate) and cover with mineral oil. Each blastomere/TE sample should be rinsed in these droplets.
- Place the blastomere/TE sample inside the PCR tube under the stereoscope. The embryologist should observe the release of the cell(s) inside the tube. This step is a key point of the procedure, and the cell(s) should be released inside the tube with a minimal volume of washing media (maximum 0.5 μL).
- For genetic disease testing only, submit one blank for each embryo sample. A blank is not needed for array testing.
- *Creating a blank*: After releasing each cell into the collection tube, release the remaining fluid in the capillary into a new collection tube to create a blank. If there is not enough solution left in the capillary, aspirate a small amount of the last washing drop used for this embryo with the same capillary and release into a new collection tube.
- For arrays and genetic disease testing also, include two PCR tubes with the solution but without cells which will be used as positive and negative control during the analysis.
- Close the PCR tubes and place them inside the cooler rack.
- Once every cell has been processed, cover the cool rack with parafilm. Place the cool rack inside the shipping box with at least two freezer packs/negative accumulators securely so the cooler does not move inside the box during shipping.

## ADVANTAGES OF TROPHECTODERM BIOPSY

*Following are the advantages of TE biopsy:*

- TE biopsy has an advantage of higher technical and biological robustness.
- There is a lesser incidence of procedural errors and a lower impact of mosaicism on molecular analysis.[8]
- In general, as per the last Cochrane review, blastocyst stage embryos have higher LBR per embryo transfer than cleavage stage. Additionally, cleavage stage embryos have shown to impact embryo implantation and developmental kinematics compared to a blastocysts stage TE biopsy, inferring TE biopsy beneficial over other stages.[31]
- Considering the current trend of freeze-all policy and an elective single-embryo transfer (eSET) in a frozen embryo replacement cycle has helped to control the incidence of OHSS and multiple pregnancies. Doing a TE biopsy and picking a genetically normal embryo for eSET would give the best results.[23-25]
- At blastocyst biopsy, more TE cells can be obtained and this prevents the risk of nonamplification due to inadequate tissue, which can be a common occurrence in cleavage stage biopsy.
- Not all cleavage stage embryos make it to the blastocyst stage; hence on day 5 we will have a lesser number but competent embryos, which will be subjected to biopsy.

## LIMITATIONS OF TROPHECTODERM BIOPSY

- The major limitation is the extended embryo culture system, which requires higher laboratory standards and technical expertise.
- TE biopsy is found to be beneficial only for good prognosis patients. In poor responders and couples with poor embryo quality, the proportion of blastocysts formed and the possibility of TE biopsy are limited.
- Considering the heterogeneous nature of herniation of TE tissue post-LAH for embryo biopsy, there might be a need for multiple sittings for biopsy. On the other hand, in cleavage stage biopsy with six to eight cells, we can do the biopsy in one sitting.
- Possibility for a re-biopsy for technical reasons can be done immediately in a cleavage stage biopsy but might be challenging in a blastocyst due to collapse of the blastocoel cavity.
- Blastocyst formation after extended embryo culture is again heterogeneous and might happen on day 5 or day 6, and in some instances, day 7 also. This calls for multiple sittings of biopsy, which increases not only the operational challenges but also the cost, which could be a major limitation.
- TE tissue is very sticky compared to a blastomere of a cleavage stage embryo. Hence, handling of TE tissue needs a lot of skill and care.
- Care needs to be extended to avoid manipulations with the ICM, which eventually forms the fetus properly.
- TE biopsy does not totally eliminate the risk of mosaicism,[32] but the incidence is lesser than cleavage stage biopsy.

## NONINVASIVE METHODS FOR EMBRYO BIOPSY

The earlier embryo biopsy methods, though have been the most common practice, are still considered invasive.

There has been a constant effort to come up with methods which are noninvasive and have similar reproducibility to the traditional methods. A few of the noninvasive methods for genetic screening are as follows.

### Blastocoel Fluid Sampling

Palini et al. showed for the first time that blastocoel fluid (BF) has presence of genomic DNA and can be used to screen for single-gene disorders.[33] Magli et al. used array CGH screening technique to evaluate the efficacy of BF biopsies for ploidy prediction in comparison with the conventional biopsy methods, i.e., blastocyst, blastomere, and PB biopsy, and inferred that BF biopsy was comparable to conventional biopsy materials for chromosomal analysis.[34] Nevertheless, embryo quality did show discordance of ploidy prediction between BF and blastocyst biopsy, suggesting that more experiments and clinical trials should be performed before BF sampling is ready for PGT.[34]

### Assay of Cell-free Nucleic Acid in Culture Medium

Using cell-free nucleic acids released from embryos in the culture medium, DNA is extracted and screened for chromosomal analysis. This showed higher diagnosis efficacy than blastomere biopsy. However, this method still needs to be further validated by eliminating potential contamination and providing more robust evidence in PGT.[35,36]

### Time-lapse Technology for Assessment of Embryo Quality

Continuous time-bound assessment of cellular morphology and morphokinetics is another noninvasive recent technology that is researched extensively. Studies have tried to correlate the timing of morphokinetics with embryo aneuploidy. Meanwhile, different assessment assays and statistical models were applied to refine the morphokinetic variables and increase the chance of predicting a top-quality blastocyst.[37] However, considering the potential technical and statistical error in time-lapse imaging, one should be cautious in over-interpreting the results.[38,39]

Current consensus about the best stage for embryo biopsy for PGT is yet to arrive. PB biopsy has become obsolete. Cleavage and morula stage biopsies have shown to bring about adverse clinical outcomes. TE biopsy seems to be encouraging and optimizing clinical outcomes, but its efficacy in terms of the delivery rate per intention to treat is yet to be proven.

## CRYOPRESERVATION OF EMBRYOS

An efficient embryo-freezing program with maximum survival rates is another essential element for PGT program. Improved extended embryo culture systems, TE biopsies of blastocysts, freeze-all embryo policy, and policy of an eSET of a genetically normal embryo in a frozen embryo replacement cycle are all dependent on an efficient embryo cryopreservation program. Over the years, vitrification and warming protocols of oocytes and embryos have dramatically improved and enabled improved reproductive outcomes worldwide. Embryos need to be vitrified single on each cryo device after embryo biopsy. Proper witnessing system to track the identity of embryos from biopsy till cryopreservation is essential. Vitrification at 1.5–3 hours post biopsy in blastocyst is recommended.[40]

Comparative studies on post-thaw survival of biopsied embryos have shown similar survival rates with nonbiopsied embryos, in both cleavage and blastocyst stages.[41,42] Intactness of blastomeres and blastulation process post thaw has shown to be good in cleavage stage embryos after freeze and thaw post biopsy.

## IDEAL PLATFORM FOR GENETIC SCREENING

After embryo biopsy, the tissue is tubed in small PCR tubes or it is fixed if the plan is FISH and sent to the genetic laboratory for further evaluation and screening. PGT can be performed at either the chromosomal level or at DNA level. FISH, PCR-based methods, and single-cell genomic methods are few of the techniques applied for PGT. For identifying single-gene mutations, PCR was the first technique introduced for PGT. On the other hand, FISH was introduced to screen for aneuploidies and translocation.

## FLUORESCENCE IN SITU HYBRIDIZATION

Fluorescence in situ hybridization is a traditional method practiced for a very long time, for both PGT and prenatal diagnostic tests. Owing to its limitations, FISH is now becoming obsolete. The incidence of false positive and negatives has been shown to be high due to incapability of detecting de novo genetic mutations, contamination, and sensitivity issues.[43] A review and meta-analysis of all RCTs was done in 2011 and compared aneuploidy testing with FISH versus standard IVF without PGT.[44] As per this meta-analysis, aneuploidy screening with FISH showed no beneficial effect on LBRs. On the other hand, AMA patients had even lesser chance to attain live birth. The author's explanation for such results was that it could be due to technical drawbacks and proposed the need for novel screening methods. Technically, FISH screens limited chromosomes and not the entire 24 chromosomes, which is one of the major limitations. FISH is considered to be a low-resolution technique in comparison to newer CCS methods. The combination of these two limitations led to high technical variability, overestimation of mosaicism, and false positives and negative rates as high as 10%.[41]

## Application of Single-cell Genomics in Preimplantation Genetic Diagnosis/ Preimplantation Genetic Screening

Single-cell genomics with high resolution has led to a major makeshift in the field of PGT, which enables screening with limited sample size. Whole genome amplification (WGA) and high throughput are the two major basic steps in single-cell genomics. WGA amplifies DNA from a single cell and generates sufficient templates for either microarray or next-generation sequencing (NGS) assays.

New diagnosis methods, such as aCGH, single nucleotide polymorphism (SNP) microarray, multiplex quantitative polymerase chain reaction (qPCR), karyomapping, and NGS, are developed to improve clinical efficiency and outcomes.

### Microarrays

Single nucleotide polymorphism and CGH arrays are the two commonly used genetic tests for PGT. The TE cells are lyzed and amplified for WGA for both the microarray platforms.

#### *Single Nucleotide Polymorphism Microarrays*

Single nucleotide polymorphisms are pairs of single nucleotides (A, T, C, or G) in genomic DNA. SNPs microarray for PGT evaluates nonexon coding segments of the genome, and approximately 300,000 SNPs are spaced throughout the genome.[45,46] Using this platform, we can identify whole chromosome aneuploidy and it can also detect approximately 250 common structural chromosome aberrations throughout the genome. If enough TE cells are provided, these arrays can identify mosaicism. SNP arrays can generate genotype; hence they can identify uniparental disomy, which other microarray methods cannot. Limitations of SNP arrays are failure to identify aneuploidies in couples with consanguinity, limited ability to identify triploidy, and abnormalities below the resolution of 300,000 that can be significantly missed.

#### *Comparative Genomic Hybridization Microarrays*

Comparative genomic hybridization microarrays are less dense than SNP microarrays. These aCGH chips approximately have 4,000 markers spaced throughout the genome. The principle of aCGH is ratio labeling, where the clinical sample is compared to normal 46,XY and 46,XX DNA samples.[47,48] The major advantage of CGH arrays is their time frame to complete the entire analysis in 12–15 hours, whereas it takes around 30–40 hours with SNP arrays. aCGH cannot identify uniparental disomy. It can only identify the whole chromosome aneuploidies but cannot identify structural chromosomal aberrations. Though aCGH can identify mosaicism, there are some studies which have shown that aCGH has an approximate error rate of 15–30%.[49] A comparative study of 400 TE samples with aCGH and NGS has shown similar results and 99% concordance,[50] which encourages its application in the ART industry for PGT.

### Quantitative Polymerase Chain Reaction or Real-time Polymerase Chain Reaction

Quantitative polymerase chain reaction or real-time polymerase chain reaction (RT-PCR) is a PCR assay which identifies whole chromosome aneuploidy by detecting the copy number of each chromosome analyzed.[51,52] This assay identifies aneuploidies of all 23 chromosomes in a very shorter time frame but is very labor intensive.[51,52] Even this assay cannot identify structural chromosomal aberrations and uniparental disomy.[49]

### Next-generation Sequencing

Next-generation sequencing is a newer CCS method based on ultra-high throughput parallel DNA sequencing that achieves genome-scale sequencing faster. It has an advantage of detecting genetic mutations at a single nucleotide level and can detect aneuploidies such as triploidy and uniparental disomy. NGS is an efficient and robust technology and can be applied for both PGT and PGT.[53] Studies have reported successful live births with its application.[54,55] It has been validated with all stages of biopsy PB, blastomere, and TE.[56-58] There are few studies trying to combine newer noninvasive methods of sampling and NGS, and this would be bringing new excitement and revolutionize the clinical application of PGT.

However, the technical obstacle of nonlinear amplification limits these WGA methods. Single-cell genomics has been applied to comprehensively study the genome and transcriptome of individual cells to select an optimal embryo in IVF.

## ERRORS WITH PREIMPLANTATION GENETIC SCREENING TECHNIQUES

Errors could be biological and are termed mosaicism or technical errors.

### Mosaic Embryos and the Current Consensus

Mosaicism is defined as the presence of two or more cell populations with different genotypes. In other words, it is the presence of more than one chromosomally distinct cell line in a single sample originating from one individual.[59]

Fluorescence in situ hybridization of sex chromosomes demonstrated mosaicism at cleavage stage in preimplantation human embryos.[60] Occurrence of mosaicism is due to mitotic errors after fertilization during cleavage of embryos.[61] Mosaic embryos can be classified into two categories based on the extent of blastomere involvement: (1) Aneuploid mosaic, where two different aneuploid genotypes exist and 100% of the cells within the embryo are abnormal, and

(2) diploid—aneuploid mosaic, where one population of the cell is euploid and the other is aneuploid.[61]

At fertilization, the human embryo is genomically inactive, and this makes the embryo prone to meiotic errors. After fertilization, the first three cell divisions are dependent on oocyte cytoplasmic transcriptome. Anaphase lag, mitotic nondisjunction, inadvertent chromosome demolition, and premature cell division before DNA duplication[62,63] are few of the reasons explained in the literature for the occurrence of mosaicism. All these reasons support the higher incidence of mosaicism in cleavage stage embryos. In 50% of cases, there is an autocorrection of mosaic cleavage stage embryos to euploid blastocysts. Few theories which explain the autocorrection of aneuploidy are increased apoptosis of aneuploid cells, decreased division of aneuploid cells in relation to euploid cells, or preferential development of euploid cells within the ICM.[64] Trisomic cell populations may self-correct by losing the extra chromosome via anaphase lag or nondisjunction.[65]

New CCS techniques for PGT, such as NGS, have led to increased reporting of mosaicism.[66] The interpretation of mosaicism is complicated, and there is a dilemma whether to transfer such an embryo or not. Literature reports live births from the transfer of mosaic embryos in the past and hence the controversy.[67,68] On the other hand, the transfer of mosaic embryos leads to decreased implantation and decreased pregnancy potential as well as increased risk of genetic abnormalities and adverse pregnancy outcomes.[69] It is preferable to transfer genetically normal embryos over mosaic embryos. However, if there is a need to transfer, this should be done with proper genetic counseling. There are certain mosaic trisomies such as 2, 7, 13, 14, 15, 16, 18, and 21, which have potential risks to the pregnancy outcome and should be avoided in all circumstances. One of the recent studies suggested encouraging the couples to undergo another cycle to obtain euploid embryos, when possible, rather than transferring a mosaic embryo.[69] There is no consensus about transferring a mosaic embryo after PGT currently. However, discussion about the uncertain reproductive outcomes has to be put forward to the couple to make a conscious decision.

### Technical Source of Error

A newer technique or newer embryo selection parameter can only be introduced in clinical practice after a structured validation protocol. Any new technique needs assessment for accuracy of specificity and sensitivity. All the CCS methods adapted to or designed to perform PGT screening showed very high consistency in the detection of whole chromosome imbalances when compared to the blinded validation study performed by Capalbo et al. and published in 2015.[49] Till date, there is no consensus on which CCS method gives 100% accuracy; each method has its own benefits and drawbacks.

## EMBRYO TRANSFER

After the genetic screening of embryos, the next step is embryo transfer. For cleavage stage embryos, it is possible to consider a fresh embryo transfer. For TE biopsy, a fresh transfer might be challenging. Considering that the frozen embryo transfer (FET) cycle has better uterine implantation rates than a stimulated cycle, FET is preferred to have the best reproductive outcome. At embryo transfer, communication between clinical and embryology laboratory teams is essential to decide on which embryo to transfer. Embryos recommended for transfer should be clearly indicated. Discussing the PGT report with the patient and the intended plan is recommended. Couples where no normal embryos are obtained after PGT need an in-depth discussion about the report and the possible alternatives as the next step.

It is advisable to counsel the couples toward eSET. Forman et al., in their study, showed that eSET after PGT equals double untested embryo transfer in the general population in terms of LBR. This study further emphasizes the need for eSET for PGT patients.

Especially in PGT cases, where a confirmatory prenatal amniocentesis or chorionic villi sampling is advisable to ensure that the fetus is normal, a singleton pregnancy is preferable. Considering the error rates after single cell analysis is not negligible, prenatal diagnostic tests are still recommended. Hence, eSET should be encouraged to couples post PGT.

Embryo transfer catheter, transfer technique, and culture media remain similar to the routine practice of your individual clinics.

Double witnessing of patient ID at embryo thawing and embryo transfer is mandatory.

## FOLLOW-UP OF PREGNANCIES

Follow-up of pregnancies is important to evaluate the efficacy of screening methods. Follow-up should be till live birth to ensure and document any adverse outcomes.

Follow-up of infants for identification of major and minor malformations will help determine the effects related to the embryo biopsy procedures and error rates of the screening methods. An extended follow-up would be especially valuable for the evaluation of long-term effects possibly derived from the invasiveness of the technique.

## QUALITY CONTROL AND QUALITY ASSURANCE: OUTCOME MEASURES

Considering PGT being multidisciplinary work, the results should be monitored on a systematic basis from each individual center.[4] Outcome measures include the following:

- Proportion of cells overtly damaged during embryo biopsy
- Proportion of cells for which a diagnosis was not obtained
- Misdiagnosis rate per embryo and per pregnancy calculated in vitro

- Misdiagnosis rate calculated in vivo. Implantation rate and clinical pregnancy loss rate
- Take-home baby rate. Multiple pregnancy rate (monozygotic versus dizygotic)
- Minimum number of preclinical assays to be performed in a given laboratory before clinical application
- Criteria to assess the competence of the staff involved in the different steps of PGT.

## EFFECTIVENESS AND EFFICACY OF PREIMPLANTATION GENETIC SCREENING IN THE FIELD OF ASSISTED REPRODUCTIVE TECHNOLOGY

In a review published in 2015,[70] Lee et al. summarized all the RCTs, observational and prospective studies that approached CCS-based PGT in comparison to standard care. They were able to show that in both young and AMA patient populations, PGT results in a higher delivery rate per embryo transferred. An eSET after PGT screening is shown to have better clinical outcomes compared to a double embryo transfer in unscreened population. Dahdouh et al. and Chen et al. in 2015 published meta-analyses,[19,20,71,72] which showed that embryo transfer with PGT-screened embryos results in a higher sustained implantation rate per transfer as well as a lower miscarriage rate with respect to the control. These studies also prove the efficacy of advanced embryology techniques introduced to optimize the reproductive outcomes such as extended culture to blastocyst stage, TE biopsy, and CCS, and by adopting a freeze-all and eSET strategy. Ubaldi et al. in 2015 conducted a retrospective study in AMA patient population across the years through all of the above-mentioned advanced embryology techniques and demonstrated similar cumulative LBR per cycle, while the miscarriage, and especially the multiple pregnancy rates, significantly decreased in comparison with non-PGT cycles.[73] Application of PGT in the field of ART is encouraging but needs further data on identifying groups of patients in whom it is beneficial. Multicenter RCTs comparing PGT cycles to standard care, where primary outcome should be the delivery rate per intention to treat, are still eagerly needed. Finally, there is an urgent need for cost-effectiveness analysis for PGT cycles. Majority of the studies published in the literature are on the good prognosis of patient and role of PGT in poor responders and RPL in women is debated, and financial logistics is one of the reasons for concern in poor responders and additionally time to pregnancy in RPL women.[74] Hence, there is a need for cost analysis with a specification to each subgroup.

## KEY POINTS

- For successful implementation of PGT program, laboratory setup has to be state of ART and as per the guidelines of ESHRE special interest group.
- Both laboratory and laboratory teams should be geared up to handle extended embryo culture till blastocyst stage.
- ICSI is the preferred ART technique for PGT cases.
- Blastocyst stage seems to be a beneficial stage for embryo biopsy and PGT.
- FISH for genetic screening is obsolete.
- Single genomic techniques such as aCGH and NGS seem to address the technical issues of the traditional screening methods.
- eSET of genetically normal embryos after PGT seems to offer better reproductive outcomes than double-embryo transfers.
- Follow-up of pregnancies till live birth is an essential aspect of the quality management system of the PGT program.

## REFERENCES


1. Munné S, Lee A, Rosenwaks Z, Grifo J, Cohen J. Diagnosis of major chromosome aneuploidies in human preimplantation embryos. Hum Reprod. 1993;8(12):2185-91.
2. Handyside AH, Kontogianni EH, Hardy K, Winston RM. Pregnancies from biopsied human preimplantation embryos sexed by Y-specific DNA amplification. Nature. 1990;344(6268):768-70.
3. ESHRE PGT Consortium Steering Committee, Carvalho F, Coonen E, Goossens V, Kokkali G, Rubio C, et al. ESHRE PGT Consortium good practice recommendations for the organisation of PGT. Hum Reprod Open. 2020;2020:hoaa021.
4. Magli MC, Van den Abbeel E, Lundin K, Royere D, Van der Elst J, Gianaroli L, et al. Revised guidelines for good practice in IVF laboratories. Hum Reprod. 2008;23(6):1253-62.
5. Preimplantation Genetic Diagnosis International Society (PGDIS). Guidelines for good practice in PGD: programme requirements and laboratory quality assurance. Reprod Biomed Online. 2008;16(1):134-47.
6. Capalbo A, Bono S, Spizzichino L, Biricik A, Baldi M, Colamaria S, et al. Sequential comprehensive chromosome analysis on polar bodies, blastomeres and trophoblast: insights into female meiotic errors and chromosomal segregation in the preimplantation window of embryo development. Hum Reprod. 2013;28(2):509-18.
7. Montag M, Köster M, Strowitzki T, Toth B. Polar body biopsy. Fertil Steril. 2013;100(3):603-7.
8. Cimadomo D, Capalbo A, Ubaldi FM, Scarica C, Palagiano A, Canipari R, et al. The impact of biopsy on human embryo developmental potential during preimplantation genetic diagnosis. Biomed Res Int. 2016;2016:7193075.
9. Dumoulin JC, Bras M, Coonen E, Dreesen J, Geraedts JP, Evers JL. Effect of $Ca^{2+}/Mg^{2+}$-free medium on the biopsy procedure for preimplantation genetic diagnosis and further development of human embryos. Hum Reprod. 1998;13(10):2880-3.
10. Pratt HP, Ziomek CA, Reeve WJ, Johnson MH. Compaction of the mouse embryo: an analysis of its components. J Embryol Exp Morphol. 1982;70:113-32.
11. Pey R, Vial C, Schatten G, Hafner M. Increase of intracellular $Ca^{2+}$ and relocation of E-cadherin during experimental decompaction of mouse embryos. Proc Natl Acad Sci USA. 1998;95(22):12977-82.

12. Moutou C, Goossens V, Coonen E, De Rycke M, Kokkali G, Renwick P, et al. ESHRE PGD Consortium data collection XII: cycles from January to December 2009 with pregnancy follow-up to October 2010. Hum Reprod. 2014;29(5):880-903.
13. Feichtinger W, Strohmer H, Fuhrberg P, Radivojevic K, Antinori S, Pepe G, et al. Photoablation of oocyte zona pellucida by erbium-YAG laser for in-vitro fertilisation in severe male infertility. Lancet. 1992;339(8796):811.
14. Cohen J. Assisted hatching of human embryos. J In Vitro Fert Embryo Transf. 1991;8(4):179-90.
15. Cohen J, Malter H, Elsner C, Kort H, Massey J, Mayer MP. Immunosuppression supports implantation of zona pellucida dissected human embryos. Fertil Steril. 1990;53(4):662-5.
16. Eldar-Geva T, Srebnik N, Altarescu G, Varshaver I, Brooks B, Levy-Lahad E, et al. Neonatal outcome after preimplantation genetic diagnosis. Fertil Steril. 2014;102(4):1016-21.
17. Jones AE, Wright G, Kort HI, Straub RJ, Nagy ZP. Comparison of laser-assisted hatching and acidified Tyrode's hatching by evaluation of blastocyst development rates in sibling embryos: a prospective randomized trial. Fertil Steril. 2006;85(2):487-91.
18. Schmoll F, Schneider H, Montag M, Wimmers K, Rink K, Schellander K. Effects of different laser-drilled openings in the zona pellucida on hatching of in vitro-produced cattle blastocysts. Fertil Steril. 2003;80(Suppl. 2):714-9.
19. Duncan FE, Stein P, Williams CJ, Schultz RM. The effect of blastomere biopsy on preimplantation mouse embryo development and global gene expression. Fertil Steril. 2009;91(4 Suppl.):1462-5.
20. Kirkegaard K, Hindkjaer JJ, Ingerslev HJ. Human embryonic development after blastomere removal: a time-lapse analysis. Hum Reprod. 2012;27(1):97-105.
21. Brodie D, Beyer CE, Osborne E, Kralevski V, Rasi S, Osianlis T. Preimplantation genetic diagnosis for chromosome rearrangements—one blastomere biopsy versus two blastomere biopsy. J Assist Reprod Genet. 2012;29(8):821-7.
22. Bielanska M, Tan SL, Ao A. Chromosomal mosaicism throughout human preimplantation development in vitro: incidence, type, and relevance to embryo outcome. Hum Reprod. 2002;17(2):413-9.
23. Scott Jr RT, Upham KM, Forman EJ, Zhao T, Treff NR. Cleavage-stage biopsy significantly impairs human embryonic implantation potential while blastocyst biopsy does not: a randomized and paired clinical trial. Fertil Steril. 2013;100(3):624-30.
24. Staessen C, Verpoest W, Donoso P, Haentjens P, Van der Elst J, Liebaers I, et al. Preimplantation genetic screening does not improve delivery rate in women under the age of 36 following single-embryo transfer. Hum Reprod. 2008;23(12):2818-25.
25. Debrock S, Melotte C, Spiessens C, Peeraer K, Vanneste E, Meeuwis L, et al. Preimplantation genetic screening for aneuploidy of embryos after in vitro fertilization in women aged at least 35 years: a prospective randomized trial. Fertil Steril. 2010;93(2):364-73.
26. Hardarson T, Hanson C, Lundin K, Hillensjö T, Nilsson L, Stevic J, et al. Preimplantation genetic screening in women of advanced maternal age caused a decrease in clinical pregnancy rate: a randomized controlled trial. Hum Reprod. 2008;23(12):2806-12.
27. Zakharova EE, Zaletova VV, Krivokharchenko AS. Biopsy of human morula-stage embryos: outcome of 215 IVF/ICSI cycles with PGS. PLoS One. 2014;9(9):e106433.
28. de Boer KA, Catt JW, Jansen RP, Leigh D, McArthur S. Moving to blastocyst biopsy for preimplantation genetic diagnosis and single embryo transfer at Sydney IVF. Fertil Steril. 2004;82(2):295-8.
29. Kokkali G, Vrettou C, Traeger-Synodinos J, Jones GM, Cram DS, Stavrou D, et al. Birth of a healthy infant following trophectoderm biopsy from blastocysts for PGD of beta-thalassaemia major. Hum Reprod. 2005;20(7):1855-9.
30. McArthur SJ, Leigh D, Marshall JT, de Boer KA, Jansen RP. Pregnancies and live births after trophectoderm biopsy and preimplantation genetic testing of human blastocysts. Fertil Steril. 2005;84(6):1628-36.
31. Glujovsky D, Blake D, Farquhar C, Bardach A. Cleavage stage versus blastocyst stage embryo transfer in assisted reproductive technology. Cochrane Database Syst Rev. 2012;(7):CD002118.
32. Munné S, Blazek J, Large M, Martinez-Ortiz PA, Nisson H, Liu E, et al. Detailed investigation into the cytogenetic constitution and pregnancy outcome of replacing mosaic blastocysts detected with the use of high-resolution next-generation sequencing. Fertil Steril. 2017;108(1):62-71.e8.
33. Palini S, Galluzzi L, DeStefani S, Bianchi M, Wells D, Magnani M, et al. Genomic DNA in human blastocoele fluid. Reprod Biomed Online. 2013;26(6):603-10.
34. Magli MC, Pomante A, Cafueri G, Valerio M, Crippa A, Ferraretti AP, et al. Preimplantation genetic testing: polar bodies, blastomeres, trophectoderm cells, or blastocoelic fluid? Fertil Steril. 2016;105(3):676-83.e5.
35. Assou S, Aït-Ahmed O, El Messaoudi S, Thierry AR, Hamamah S. Non-invasive pre-implantation genetic diagnosis of X-linked disorders. Med Hypotheses. 2014;83(4):506-8.
36. Wu H, Ding C, Shen X, Wang J, Li R, Cai B, et al. Medium-based noninvasive preimplantation genetic diagnosis for human α-thalassemias-SEA. Medicine (Baltimore). 2015;94(12):e669.
37. Storr A, Venetis CA, Cooke S, Susetio D, Kilani S, Ledger W. Morphokinetic parameters using time-lapse technology and day 5 embryo quality: a prospective cohort study. J Assist Reprod Genet. 2015;32(7):1151-60.
38. Rienzi L, Capalbo A, Stoppa M, Romano S, Maggiulli R, Albricci L, et al. No evidence of association between blastocyst aneuploidy and morphokinetic assessment in a selected population of poor-prognosis patients: a longitudinal cohort study. Reprod Biomed Online. 2015;30(1):57-66.
39. Swain JE. Could time-lapse embryo imaging reduce the need for biopsy and PGS? J Assist Reprod Genet. 2013;30(8):1081-90.
40. Maggiulli R, Giancani A, Cimadomo D, Ubaldi FM, Rienzi L. Human blastocyst biopsy and vitrification. J Vis Exp. 2019;(149).
41. Zheng WT, Zhuang GL, Zhou CQ, Fang C, Ou JP, Li T, et al. Comparison of the survival of human biopsied embryos after cryopreservation with four different methods using non-transferable embryos. Hum Reprod. 2005;20(6):1615-8.
42. Chang LJ, Huang CC, Tsai YY, Hung CC, Fang MY, Lin YC, et al. Blastocyst biopsy and vitrification are effective for preimplantation genetic diagnosis of monogenic diseases. Hum Reprod. 2013;28(5):1435-44.
43. Lu L, Lv B, Huang K, Xue Z, Zhu X, Fan G. Recent advances in preimplantation genetic diagnosis and screening. J Assist Reprod Genet. 2016;33(9):1129-34.
44. Mastenbroek S, Twisk M, van der Veen F, Repping S. Preimplantation genetic screening: a systematic review and meta-analysis of RCTs. Hum Reprod Update. 2011;17(4):454-66.

45. Treff NR, Levy B, Su J, Northrop LE, Tao X, Scott Jr RT. SNP microarray-based 24 chromosome aneuploidy screening is significantly more consistent than FISH. Mol Hum Reprod. 2010;16(8):583-9.
46. Handyside AH. PGD and aneuploidy screening for 24 chromosomes by genome-wide SNP analysis: seeing the wood and the trees. Reprod Biomed Online. 2011;23(6):686-91.
47. Wells D, Alfarawati S, Fragouli E. Use of comprehensive chromosomal screening for embryo assessment: microarrays and CGH. Mol Hum Reprod. 2008;14(12):703-10.
48. Fiegler H, Geigl JB, Langer S, Rigler D, Porter K, Unger K, et al. High resolution array-CGH analysis of single cells. Nucleic Acids Res. 2007;35(3):e15.
49. Capalbo A, Treff NR, Cimadomo D, Tao X, Upham K, Ubaldi FM, et al. Comparison of array comparative genomic hybridization and quantitative real-time PCR-based aneuploidy screening of blastocyst biopsies. Eur J Hum Genet. 2015;23(7):901-6.
50. Brezina PR, Anchan R, Kearns WG. Preimplantation genetic testing for aneuploidy: what technology should you use and what are the differences? J Assist Reprod Genet. 2016;33(7):823-32.
51. Treff NR, Tao X, Ferry KM, Su J, Taylor D, Scott Jr RT. Development and validation of an accurate quantitative real-time polymerase chain reaction-based assay for human blastocyst comprehensive chromosomal aneuploidy screening. Fertil Steril. 2012;97(4):819-24.
52. Treff NR, Scott Jr RT. Four-hour quantitative real-time polymerase chain reaction-based comprehensive chromosome screening and accumulating evidence of accuracy, safety, predictive value, and clinical efficacy. Fertil Steril. 2013;99(4):1049-53.
53. Zheng H, Jin H, Liu L, Liu J, Wang WH. Application of next-generation sequencing for 24-chromosome aneuploidy screening of human preimplantation embryos. Mol Cytogenet. 2015;8:38.
54. Fiorentino F, Biricik A, Bono S, Spizzichino L, Cotroneo E, Cottone G, et al. Development and validation of a next-generation sequencing-based protocol for 24-chromosome aneuploidy screening of embryos. Fertil Steril. 2014;101(5):1375-82.
55. Tan Y, Yin X, Zhang S, Jiang H, Tan K, Li J, et al. Clinical outcome of preimplantation genetic diagnosis and screening using next generation sequencing. Gigascience. 2014;3(1):30.
56. Lukaszuk K, Pukszta S, Ochman K, Cybulska C, Liss J, Pastuszek E, et al. Healthy baby born to a Robertsonian translocation carrier following next-generation sequencing-based preimplantation genetic diagnosis: a case report. AJP Rep. 2015;5(2):e172-5.
57. Fishel S, Gordon A, Lynch C, Dowell K, Ndukwe G, Kelada E, et al. Live birth after polar body array comparative genomic hybridization prediction of embryo ploidy-the future of IVF? Fertil Steril. 2010;93(3):1006.e7-10.
58. Łukaszuk K, Pukszta S, Wells D, Cybulska C, Liss J, Płóciennik Ł, et al. Routine use of next-generation sequencing for preimplantation genetic diagnosis of blastomeres obtained from embryos on day 3 in fresh in vitro fertilization cycles. Fertil Steril. 2015;103(4):1031-6.
59. Practice Committee and Genetic Counseling Professional Group (GCPG) of the American Society for Reproductive Medicine. Clinical management of mosaic results from preimplantation genetic testing for aneuploidy (PGT-A) of blastocysts: a committee opinion. Fertil Steril. 2020;114:246.
60. Delhanty JD, Griffin DK, Handyside AH, Harper J, Atkinson GH, Pieters MH, et al. Detection of aneuploidy and chromosomal mosaicism in human embryos during preimplantation sex determination by fluorescent in situ hybridisation, (FISH). Hum Mol Genet. 1993;2(8):1183-5.
61. Munné S, Weier HU, Grifo J, Cohen J. Chromosome mosaicism in human embryos. Biol Reprod. 1994;51(3):373-9.
62. Mantzouratou A, Delhanty JD. Aneuploidy in the human cleavage stage embryo. Cytogenet Genome Res. 2011; 133(2-4):141-8.
63. Mantikou E, Wong KM, Repping S, Mastenbroek S. Molecular origin of mitotic aneuploidies in preimplantation embryos. Biochim Biophys Acta. 2012;1822(12):1921-30.
64. Delhanty JD. The origins of genetic variation between individual human oocytes and embryos: implications for infertility. Hum Fertil (Camb). 2013;16(4):241-5.
65. Bazrgar M, Gourabi H, Valojerdi MR, Yazdi PE, Baharvand H. Self-correction of chromosomal abnormalities in human preimplantation embryos and embryonic stem cells. Stem Cells Dev. 2013;22(17):2449-56.
66. Fiorentino F, Bono S, Biricik A, Nuccitelli A, Cotroneo E, Cottone G, et al. Application of next-generation sequencing technology for comprehensive aneuploidy screening of blastocysts in clinical preimplantation genetic screening cycles. Hum Reprod. 2014;29(12):2802-13.
67. Greco E, Minasi MG, Fiorentino F. Healthy babies after intrauterine transfer of mosaic aneuploid blastocysts. N Engl J Med. 2015;373(21):2089-90.
68. Maxwell SM, Colls P, Hodes-Wertz B, McCulloh DH, McCaffrey C, Wells D, et al. Why do euploid embryos miscarry? A case-control study comparing the rate of aneuploidy within presumed euploid embryos that resulted in miscarriage or live birth using next-generation sequencing. Fertil Steril. 2016;106(6):1414-9.e5.
69. Sachdev NM, Maxwell SM, Besser AG, Grifo JA. Diagnosis and clinical management of embryonic mosaicism. Fertil Steril. 2017;107(1):6-11.
70. Lee E, Illingworth P, Wilton L, Chambers GM. The clinical effectiveness of preimplantation genetic diagnosis for aneuploidy in all 24 chromosomes (PGD-A): systematic review. Hum Reprod. 2015;30(2):473-83.
71. Dahdouh EM, Balayla J, García-Velasco JA. Preimplantation genetic screening using comprehensive chromosome screening: evidence and remaining challenges. Hum Reprod. 2015;30(6):1515-6.
72. Chen M, Wei S, Hu J, Quan S. Can comprehensive chromosome screening technology improve IVF/ICSI outcomes? a meta-analysis. PLoS One. 2015;10(10):e0140779.
73. Ubaldi FM, Capalbo A, Colamaria S, Ferrero S, Maggiulli R, Vajta G, et al. Reduction of multiple pregnancies in the advanced maternal age population after implementation of an elective single embryo transfer policy coupled with enhanced embryo selection: pre- and post-intervention study. Hum Reprod. 2015;30(9):2097-106.
74. Munné S, Grifo J, Wells D. Mosaicism: "survival of the fittest" versus "no embryo left behind". Fertil Steril. 2016;105:1146-9.

CHAPTER

# 114 In Vitro Maturation of Oocytes: A Practical Approach

*Varsha Samson Roy*

## INTRODUCTION

In vitro fertilization (IVF) is now a well-accepted and standard technique. Since the first report on the successful live birth in human IVF, this technique has been used to treat millions of infertile couples worldwide. Replacing natural cycle IVF with controlled ovarian hyperstimulation (COH) gave the added advantage of increasing the oocyte yield and the number of embryos for transfer. However, COH does carry a higher risk of ovarian hyperstimulation syndrome (OHSS), which can be potentially a life-threatening iatrogenic complication. In vitro maturation (IVM) was first used successfully in humans in 1991.[1] This technique has been practiced for 25 years with the intention to reduce the risk of OHSS, especially in patients with polycystic ovary syndrome (PCOS). Moreover, the procedure costs were less due to reduced requirement or at times there was no requirement of exogenous gonadotropins. However, the recent developments in COH, such as the use of gonadotropin-releasing hormone (GnRH) antagonist to prevent premature luteinization or the use of GnRH agonist for trigger, and the improved embryo survival rates by vitrification seem to have changed the primary indication of IVM. The fact that IVM oocytes show a lower developmental potential as compared to the in vivo matured IVF oocytes has contributed in its limited use. Recently, IVM has found a new indication in patients undergoing cancer treatment as a means of fertility preservation.[2] A paper published by Pincus and Enzmann[3] in 1935 raised a possibility that mammalian eggs can undergo normal development in vitro; this of course was based on their experience on rabbit oocytes. Later in 1969, Edwards[4] mentioned that human immature oocytes left in culture can undergo maturation in vitro. The first birth after IVM of immature oocytes was reported by Cha[5] in 1991. These oocytes were collected during gynecological surgeries for oocyte donation. It was Trounson et al.[6] who in 1994 reported the first birth through IVM with a patient's own oocytes. The categories of patients selected were the polycystic ovary (PCO) or PCOS group. They also advocated IVM by transvaginal aspiration under ultrasound guidance, thus making IVM seem more "possible and realistic" and paved way in making it more popular and acceptable. Introduction of IVM in regularly cycling women with normal gonadotropin sensitivity was reported by Mikkelsen[7] in 2004. Today, approximately 400 babies have been born through the procedure of IVM.[8]

## OOCYTE MATURATION IN VIVO

At birth, there are about a million primordial follicles (female germ cells) in the ovaries. Each primordial follicle is enclosed by a basement membrane which is covered by a single layer of flattened pregranulosa cells. From this pool, a large number of them will grow but only a few are destined to be selected, mature, and will ovulate. At puberty, these follicles will respond to the growing levels of gonadotropins. During each menstrual cycle, a few will respond to the rising follicle-stimulating hormone (FSH) levels to grow, mature, and ovulate. Majority of them will undergo apoptosis and atresia at the early antral stage. During a woman's reproductive life span, she ovulates approximately 400 oocytes with the potential to fertilize and develop further.

During the process of haploidization, the oocytes get arrested at prophase I of meiosis during fetal development (first meiotic arrest). Following puberty, these oocytes undergo extensive growth and completion of the first meiotic division. This is an asymmetric cytokinesis resulting in a secondary oocyte and first polar body formation. These oocytes now undergo the second meiotic arrest at metaphase of meiosis II. The penetration of the sperm during the process of fertilization initiates the resumption of meiosis producing the haploid chromosomal complement within the oocyte. The oocyte is now ready to combine with the haploid chromosomal complement brought in by the sperm resulting in fertilization.

Oocyte maturation is defined as the process by which the oocyte attains the competence to undergo fertilization and embryogenesis. It involves both the nuclear and the cytoplasmic maturation. Nuclear maturation is identified by the resumption of meiosis, and the extrusion of the first polar body. The events required in preparing the cytoplasm for fertilization and embryogenesis constitute cytoplasmic maturation. This, however, has no visual parameter unlike the nuclear counterpart and involves complex pathways required for protein synthesis and phosphorylation, reorganization of the cytoplasmic organelles (e.g., exocytosis of the cytoplasmic granules, formation and localization of the microfilaments), and activation of particular metabolic pathways to assist in the process. The human oocyte has a size-dependent ability to resume meiosis and complete the maturation in vitro, and this increases significantly as the size of the oocyte increases to 90–120 μm in diameter.[9,10]

For optimum outcome, both the nuclear and the cytoplasmic maturation should be well programmed and synchronous. As both can proceed independent of each other, oocytes can acquire competence to undergo cytoplasmic maturation independent of competence to complete nuclear maturation.[11] This asynchrony between the nuclear and cytoplasmic maturation seems to be one of the major hurdles in the process of successful IVM culture.

Granulosa cells seem to play a vital role in the process of oocyte development and maturation. By retaining the granulosa cell viability and function and the primary elements of follicular culture, Staigmiller and Moor[12] were able to maintain maturation and developmental competence of oocyte–cumulus complexes (OCCs) in the mouse when removed from their follicular environment. Oocyte growth is proportional to the granulosa cells. They increase the surface area of the oocyte and hence increase the maturation regulatory and nutritional molecules entering the egg. They are essential for the metabolic needs of the oocyte and also improve the competence of the oocyte to undergo nuclear maturation.

## ADVANTAGES AND INDICATIONS FOR IN VITRO MATURATION

Historically, patients with PCOS were the selected group for IVM. Of recent, patients with different causes of infertility—tubal, endometriosis, and male factor—and those with a history of poor response to gonadotropin stimulation seem to be considered for IVM.[13]

The advantages provided by IVM include reducing or curtailing the risk of OHSS by reducing the requirement of gonadotropins and hence making the procedure cost-effective. Reduction in the monitoring aspect by scan and blood tests makes it more patient friendly. IVM seems a safer option in terms of the long-term theoretical risks of exogenous gonadotropins, which is yet to be determined.[14] In patients undergoing chemotherapy or radiotherapy which is gonadotoxic, fertility preservation becomes an important aspect because of the better survival rates of these patients post treatment. Cryopreservation of their immature oocytes followed by IVM years later has become a very important practical advantage of IVM.

About 15–20% of the oocytes retrieved during the standard IVF cycles are immature; IVM of these oocytes can put them to good use. These could be a compromised group of follicles.[15] However, immature oocytes obtained from conventional stimulation cannot be compared to those obtained from small antral follicles during IVM, as they exhibit poor developmental potential. One of the reasons for this could be poor perfusion of these follicles and poor response to gonadotropin stimulation.

The field of oncology has seen marked changes in the diagnosis and treatment options which reflect in the increased cancer survival rates. However, the impact of these treatment options on lowering the fertility remains to be a concern. The options for fertility preservation in women are embryo, oocyte, and ovarian tissue cryopreservation. Though embryo cryopreservation is the most effective among them all, it is not suitable for women without a male partner. Ovarian tissue cryopreservation requires repeated operations and lack of standard reliable protocols for ovarian tissue freezing. Oocyte cryopreservation overcomes these shortcomings and is currently regarded the most promising option for female fertility preservation. IVM can be performed urgently irrespective of the phase of menstrual cycle and even without ovarian stimulation.

The potential indications for IVM include:
- PCOS- and PCO-like ovaries
- Hyper-responders and patients with a history of OHSS
- History of oocyte maturation abnormalities
- Emergency oocyte aspiration due to malignancy (estrogen-sensitive tumors)
- IVM for oocytes retrieved from ovarian tissue prior to its cryopreservation
- IVM for rescuing immature oocytes obtained during conventional IVF
- Resistant ovary syndrome.

## CLINICAL ASPECTS OF IN VITRO MATURATION

The technique of IVM is far from standardized. The patient selection, stimulation protocols, culture conditions, and stage of embryo transfer (ET) vary considerably between clinics. These reflect in the extremely variable pregnancy rates that are being reported. There also seems to be a substantial difference of opinion among the clinicians relating to IVM. PCO and PCOS patients seem to be the ideal candidates for IVM; not only are they at the risk of OHSS but also they possess a huge number of resting follicles as compared to the non-PCO group. There is a huge cohort of growing follicles within the cortex and failure of dominance of a particular follicle. It is not uncommon to find ≥20 small- to medium-sized antral follicles in this group.

It was suggested that oocytes from patients with PCOS would be suboptimal as they are in an abnormal endocrine environment with stasis of follicular growth.[16] It is interesting to note that most of the oocytes obtained from these follicles do not show atresia or reduced developmental competence.[17] It has been reported and has been our experience as well that oocytes recovered during the cesarean section can also mature in vitro and form embryos and blastocysts.[18,19]

In natural cycle IVM, the regular baseline scan is done on day 2 or day 3 of periods. Between day 6 and day 8, another scan is done to assess not only the follicular size but also the endometrial thickness. Follicular aspiration is timed when the dominant follicle reaches 12 mm but does not exceed 14 mm in size. This would usually be seen between day 8 and day 10 of the cycle. Human chorionic gonadotropin (hCG) trigger may or may not be given though there are obvious benefits of administering hCG. The endometrium at least needs to be 5–6 mm on the day of oocyte pickup (OPU).[17] Some investigators also believe that if the leading follicle is >10 mm, the blastocyst developmental potential is impaired.[20,21] The pregnancy rates can be low in cycles where dominant follicle was >13 mm.[22]

Controlled ovarian hyperstimulation for IVM cycles has involved the use of clomiphene citrate, letrozole, recombinant or urinary FSH, or human menopausal gonadotropin (hMG). COH protocol involving hMG or FSH priming and hCG trigger seems to have a better maturation rate and developmental competence.[23] Gonadotropin priming improves the maturation rate and adds to rapid progression of meiosis I and improves the first polar body extrusion rate.[1,24,25] However, not all studies were able to prove any beneficial effect of gonadotropin priming on maturation rate and fertilization rate on embryo development.[26]

In vitro maturation done with mild ovarian stimulation involves a baseline scan followed by 75 IU of gonadotropin for 4–6 days. This dose can be continued till the follicles reach 11–12 mm in size. On an average, a total dose of 300–450 IU may be required. Physiologically, FSH priming with or without insulin-sensitizing agents would be a better choice to overcome the androgenic intrafollicular environment that causes ovulatory dysfunction in patients with PCOS. hCG trigger is given at 11–12 mm follicle size and aspiration is done 35–36 hours post-hCG administration.

Endometrial preparation is considered mandatory as the follicular phase length is reduced due to reduced exposure to estradiol (E2) in the proliferative phase. Also, the nonexisting corpus luteum can lead to loss of hormonal support in the secretory phase of the endometrium. For endometrial preparation, patients receive E2 valerate daily (6–10 mg orally in divided doses) beginning on the day of oocyte retrieval. This is followed by progesterone support (600 mg/day of micronized progesterone per vaginally) beginning on day after retrieval. Starting E2 very early in the follicular phase may reduce the maturation and the cleavage rates.[27] Child et al.[28] found the endometrial thickness at the time of ET to be different in pregnancy cycles as 10.2 ± 2.0 mm versus that in nonpregnancy cycles (9.4 ± 2.1 mm).

If the endometrial buildup is not satisfactory, then the decision to freeze the embryos can be considered. All freeze cycles are being practiced in many centers and recommending it for IVM cycles seems appropriate.

### Triggering before Oocyte Pickup

Both hCG and gonadotropin-releasing hormone agonist (GnRHa) can be used for the final trigger, though most of the available data is related to hCG. The dose of hCG is 10,000 units and there seems to be no dose-dependent effect on the maturation rate between 10,000 and 20,000 IU.[29] But other embryo developmental parameters need to be studied. Controlled ovarian stimulation (COS) with FSH and an hCG trigger is considered as a "truncated IVF" cycle.

The number of oocytes retrieved with dispersed cumulus complex seemed higher (64.3%) when oocytes were exposed to hCG for 38 hours as compared to the 35-hour group (37.5%).[30] In this study, the number of oocytes matured in vivo and in vitro on day 1 of culture was higher in the 38-hour group and so was the clinical pregnancy rate. The authors concluded that the better pregnancy rate in the 38-hour group is attributed to an increase in the quantity of embryos produced from oocytes matured in vivo and matured faster in vitro.

The hypothesis is that hCG may promote initiation of oocyte maturation in vivo and hasten the rate of maturation in vitro. This may also improve the pregnancy rates. It loosens the cumulus contact with the follicular wall, hence making aspiration of the smaller follicles easier and thus increasing the oocyte retrieval rate. In studies comparing different protocols of IVM in PCOS, hCG priming which was not dose-dependent raised the maturation rate from 69 to 84%, fertilization rate from 45 to 80%, pregnancy rate from 31 to 38.5%, and live birth rate (LBR) to 33%.[31]

However, a recent Cochrane review found no conclusive evidence of the beneficial effect of hCG trigger on the clinical pregnancy rate and LBR.[32] In a randomized controlled trial (RCT) involving 172 cancer patients comparing no trigger, hCG trigger, and GnRH agonist trigger, the authors found no difference in the oocyte retrieval rate or the maturation rate between these three interventions.[33]

## IN VITRO MATURATION ASPIRATION

Specially designed 17-gauge single-lumen aspiration needles are used which may be single or double lumen. These needles are more rigid with a shorter bevel and of a lesser length as compared to the conventional needle. The shorter bevel prevents the needle from going through the small-diameter follicles aspirated in IVM. The shorter length of the needle helps to accumulate less aspirate volume. The aspiration pressure is reduced to 50–80 mm Hg. Higher aspiration pressure poses the risk of disrupting the immature oocyte of the granulosa cells. Flushing follicles may lead to reduced retrieval rate due to loss of these oocytes. It is not uncommon to have a blood-stained aspirate, and frequent flushing and rinsing of the needle may be needed to avoid blocking. Unlike in conventional IVF, the visual collapse of aspirated follicles is not readily seen in IVM retrievals and one needs to apply multiple passes of the needle in a back-and-forth motion while also simultaneously rotating the bevel of the needle.

## OOCYTE IDENTIFICATION

The follicular aspirates are collected in tubes containing HEPES-buffered media with heparin (2–5 IU/mL). As follicles of smaller diameter are aspirated for IVM, it is not unusual to find most of the aspirates to be smaller in volume with greater proportion of blood products. The blood products are due to the ovarian trauma during aspiration. Hence, addition of heparin to the media is extremely important to prevent the formation of blood clots. Secondly, unlike in conventional IVF aspiration, multiple needle punctures may be needed in IVM, again predisposing the aspirates to be extremely blood stained **(Figs. 1A and B)**.

Once the tubes containing the follicular aspirates are passed on to the laboratory, identification of the OCC forms the next important step. This can be the most frustrating part of IVM. These OCCs do not have the typical mucoid and "sun ray" appearance. Identification of these IVM OCCs needs to be done meticulously and patiently.

There are two ways of doing this. First, the follicular aspirates are directly poured into the Petri dish and examined under the microscope; they are most likely to sink to the bottom of the dish or tube. Hence, pouring the aspirates into Petri dishes and waiting for the OCCs to sink to the bottom will help in identification. These dishes with the follicular aspirate can be kept in the incubator for a few minutes prior to observing them under the microscope. The disadvantage of this method, however, is the time factor and the longer interaction of the OCCs with the blood clots which may be detrimental.

The second method is by using a cell strainer device made of nylon mesh, the pore size being 70 μm.[17,34] The follicular aspirates are filtered through this strainer. These collected aspirates can be washed to remove the red blood cells (RBCs) and small cells and then screened under the microscope to identify the OCCs.

Each laboratory will have its own protocol; some might utilize both methods. In protocols involving hCG priming, identification by the first method is possible as the cumulus is dispersed. However, in non-hCG-primed cycles, the cumulus will be more compact and their identification by the cell filter method is a better and faster option.

Special attention should be given to temperature and pH settings during multiple manipulations done during IVM as this can affect the protein synthesis and spindle morphology.

## IN VITRO MATURATION CULTURE

There is very little data available on the composition of culture media for human IVM. Experience gained from IVM on mammalian species is what forms the basis for the composition of media used for human IVM. Historically simple salt solutions were used. Complex culture media such as tissue culture media 199 (TCM-199), Ham's F-10, P-1, Chang's medium, and Eagle's minimum essential media (EMEM) have been widely used. These media are supplemented with serum. Owing to potential sources of infectious agents, it was preferred to use patient's own serum. Human serum albumin (HSA) or synthetic serum has also been used as substitute for protein supplementation. Significantly higher maturation pregnancy and implantation rates were obtained in media supplemented with serum as compared to HSA. This could indicate that factors other

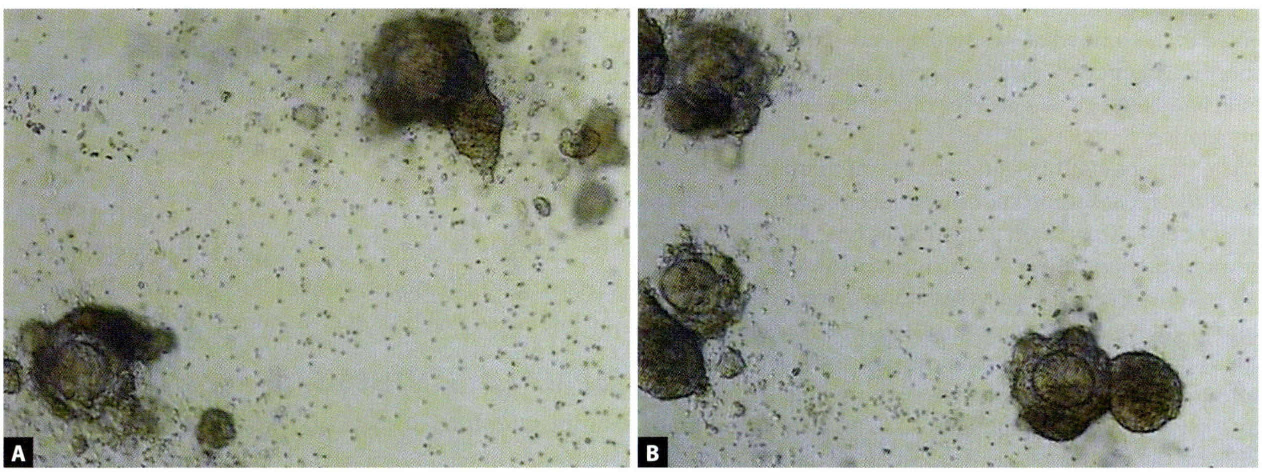

**Figs. 1A and B:** Immature oocytes obtained during in vitro maturation aspiration.

than albumin in the maternal serum may play a role in the maturation and embryo development.[35] Several other factors such as epidermal growth factor (EGF), activin, and inhibin may also be present in the serum which may play a role in the maturation process.[36] Hence, the addition of EGF could be a useful supplementation in the IVM media. Some IVM protocols also suggest supplementation of media with FSH and/or luteinizing hormone (LH); their effects on embryonic development, however, are still controversial. Media supplemented with FSH and LH in the ratio of 1:10 resulted in significantly higher developmental competent embryos with increased development to blastocyst stage in vitro as compared with FSH alone or no gonadotropins.[37] Addition of hCG in the culture media seems to have no effect on the maturation rate and further embryonic development.[21] Further studies are indicated to clarify the role of gonadotropins and other supplements used in the culture media for IVM. Of late, commercially made IVM media are available.

## ASSESSMENT OF OOCYTE MATURITY

Assessment of the oocyte maturity immediately after retrieval is required to separate the metaphase II (MII) from the immature oocytes. It is not uncommon to obtain MII eggs in hCG-primed cycles, especially if the trigger is given at >12 mm follicle diameter. The tight cumulus makes the identification of maturity a difficult task. However, this can be identified by sliding method or spreading method.[21,38]

The sliding method involves allowing the OCCs to slide from one end to the other at the bottom of the Petri dish; tilting of the dish can make identification easier. The spreading method allows for spreading of the cumulus complex with Pasteur pipette with minimal media or follicular aspirate retained in the Petri dish. This will allow easy spreading of the cumulus, so as to allow observation of the oocyte cytoplasm under the dissecting microscope. Different radiate appearances can be observed in oocytes collected from different sizes of follicles and the maturity of these oocytes can still be at MII stage. Hence, it is very important to identify the in vivo matured oocytes in hCG-primed cycles immediately after retrieval. If this check is not done, the MII oocytes would be aged at the next check which would be 24 hours later and affect the further developmental competence.[35]

The hours of culture required for maturation could be one of the most important criteria deciding the outcome of that oocyte. Most of the IVM studies have shown 40–60% maturation rates after 24–30 hours of culture.[21,39] It is important to assess the oocyte maturity after 1-day culture. There might be some oocytes arrested at MII stage for more than 24 hours before insemination and this could reflect in poor fertilization rates. This was seen in earlier studies in which oocytes were inseminated at 48 or 56 hours without assessing the oocyte maturity between 24 and 30 hours of culture.[6,40]

## FERTILIZATION OF IN VITRO MATURATION OOCYTES

Most of the studies prefer intracytoplasmic sperm injection (ICSI) even in the absence of male factor, due to the concerns regarding zona hardening as an effect of prolonged hours of culture. Denuding of the oocytes for ICSI also helps to identify the maturation status of the oocyte. Fertilization rates seem to be higher with ICSI as compared to IVF.[41]

Irrespective of the method of insemination, the developmental potential of the fertilized oocyte did not show any significant difference. Söderström-Anttila et al.[42] reported a higher fertilization rate with ICSI compared to IVF, but a higher pregnancy and implantation rate with IVF as compared to ICSI. Hence, it is not clear as to which is the best form of inseminating the IVM oocytes in the absence of a male factor.

In vitro maturation oocytes obtained from COH cycles are sensitive to postmaturation aging, and delayed ICSI can result in abnormal fertilization, pronucleus size asynchrony, and cleavage failure.[43] Hence, determining the optimal interval between the first polar body extrusion and ICSI is important to obtain normal fertilization and embryo development.

Human oocytes matured in vitro needed at least 1 hour after the extrusion of the first polar body to complete nuclear maturation.[44] Spindle imaging system could be a useful device in deciding the timing of ICSI for IVM oocytes. Source of immature oocytes, primed or nonprimed cycles (FSH and/or hCG), patient categories, and the IVM culture systems could all affect the nuclear maturation and hence the timing of the first polar body extrusion.

## EMBRYO DEVELOPMENT

Most studies suggest ET being done on day 2 or day 3. This could be because of poor quality and quantity of embryos formed. IVM embryos may show a higher incidence of cleavage arrest as compared to the conventional IVF embryos. They also seem to show an increase in multinucleation owing to cell division arrest. Son et al.[38] in their studies obtained a good blastocyst formation (41.6%), clinical pregnancy (51.9%), and implantation (26.8%) in IVM patients who had more than seven zygotes and three or more good-quality embryos on day 3.

Use of assisted hatching can also be considered and frozen ETs using IVM oocytes have also been used successfully. The numbers with both these techniques are too low to accurately predict outcomes **(Table 1)**.

## PROTEIN SYNTHESIS

During the period of oocyte growth, a large number of genes are transcripted and translated. During oocyte maturation, the protein translation activity continues and these

**TABLE 1:** Clinical aspects of in vitro maturation.

| Author | No. of cycles | No. of immature oocytes | Maturation rate | Fertility rate | Cleavage rate | Pregnancies |
|---|---|---|---|---|---|---|
| Cha and Chian[1] | 72 | 832 | 60% | 80% (ICSI) | 90% | 1 twin 15 singleton |
| Cobo et al.[20] | 90 | 112 | 37–52% | 66–88% (ICSI) | 36–57% develop to blastocyst | NR |
| Mikkelsen[45] | 32 | 115 | 71–81% | 61–79% (ICSI) | 53–72% | 2—Singleton delivered<br>3—Ongoing<br>1—Singleton miscarriage |
| Chian et al.[46] | 11 | 81 | 69% | 84% | 96% | Three clinical |
| Le Du et al.[47] | 45 | 509 | 63% | 70.1% | 96.3 | 11—Biochemical<br>6—Ongoing<br>5 (+1)—Births |
| Child[48] | 107 | 1,102 | 75% | 78% | – | 28—Biochemical<br>23—Ongoing<br>17—Births |
| Cha[40] | 94 | 1,139 | 62 | 75 | – | 23—Biochemical<br>20—Births |

(ICSI: intracytoplasmic sperm injection; NR: not reported)

play an integral role in meiotic progression and embryo developmental competence.

Studies have revealed that in vitro matured MII human oocytes obtained from ovaries of untreated women have reduced protein content as compared to in vivo matured MII oocytes obtained from gonadotropin-treated patients.[6] Similar reduction in oocyte protein content has also been reported in bovine oocytes matured in vitro.[49] The role of these protein deficiencies and their impact on transcriptional inadequacies or translational defects is unknown. Further studies on the specific protein content and their role need to be assessed.

## PREGNANCY RATES WITH IN VITRO MATURATION

Pregnancy rates per transfer vary between 4 and 27% and implantation rates between 2 and 14%. The reasons for the lower pregnancy rates have not been a subject of randomized trial. Some of the reasons suggested are nuclear and cytoplasmic asynchrony wherein the nuclear maturation is achieved without the cytoplasm undergoing maturation, thus resulting in poor embryo quality and higher pregnancy loss. Other factors contributing could be inadequate culture conditions inherent or induced abnormalities, failure of the embryonic gene expression, suboptimal timing of insemination, and asynchronous endometrium.[50,51]

### Fresh or Freeze-only Embryo Transfer

Due to a shorter follicular phase, the endometrial exposure to estradiol is truncated in IVM cycles. This short proliferative phase and insufficient exposure to progesterone impact the endometrial receptivity by altering the expression pattern of the steroid receptors and deficient midluteal phase.[52] The LBR in frozen transfers was significantly higher compared to the fresh ET as reported by an RCT in non-hCG IVM cycles.[53] Thus, it appears that the endometrium in non-hCG cycles is suboptimal; hence, a freeze-all strategy should be considered.

## SAFETY OF IN VITRO MATURATION

It is estimated that approximately 400 babies have been born through the procedure of IVM. A report by Buckett et al.[8] in 2007 did not find any increased incidence of malformation or disturbed development in babies born through the procedure of IVM as compared to that following natural conception. There have been reports of increased chromosomal abnormalities in embryos derived from IVM.[54-56] Comparison of the aneuploidy rate in the IVF and IVM embryos in 2010 was reassuring as it concluded that it was similar in both the groups (58.7% IVM vs. 57.4% IVF).[57] Another point highlighted by the study was that based on the maturation time of the IVM oocytes, the oocyte that matured early (<24 hours) had lesser incidence of aneuploidy as compared to those matured late (>48 hours). These studies do have a few limitations; the number of probes used is limited and different studies use different methods for assessment of aneuploidy. The patient population and selection of patient vary in different studies.

Cha et al.[58] reported 20 singletons and four twin live births; three congenital anomalies (7.9%) were noted, including two major congenital anomalies (5.3%) detected by ultrasonography: hydrops fetalis ($n$ = 1), omphalocele ($n$ = 1), and cleft palate ($n$ = 1). Hydrops fetalis was associated with normal chromosomes. Mikkelsen[59] reported 47 births. No specific abnormalities were related to IVM procedure. One 46,XX with *CCNH* gene variation, inherited paternally (no clinical significance), one intrauterine death (IUD), induction failure, and asphyxia were reported. Söderström-Anttila et al.[60] reported 40 singletons and three sets of twins. At the age of 12 months, eight children (19%) expressed minor developmental problems and one girl was found to have optical glioma. At 2 years of age, neuropsychological development was within the normal range. Fadini et al.[61] in 2012 reported the birth of 200 IVM babies, none of them with any major congenital anomalies.

We need to be cautious as the numbers of babies born are low, and there is no standardization of protocols on both the clinical and embryology front. The information available on their long-term development is scanty. Prolonged culture may instill certain epigenetic alterations. However, the findings from a recent meta-analysis regarding neonatal outcomes, including preterm birth, iatrogenic or spontaneous, low or high birth rate, and large for gestational age, have been reassuring.[62]

### Recent Advances in In Vitro Maturation

A recent development has been the introduction of biphasic IVM. The prematuration step (24 hours) involves culture in presence of C-type natriuretic peptide (CNP) followed by maturation step (30 hours) in the presence of FSH and amphiregulin (AREG). The basic principle here is to maintain the oocyte meiotically arrested in the germinal vesicle (GV) stage in vitro while retaining their physical contact with the cumulus cells to facilitate an environment which allows the OCCs to acquire developmental competence followed by introducing an environment similar to post-LH surge, which will elicit maturation. A first prospective study by Sanchez et al.[63] involving sibling oocytes from 15 PCOS patients to study the impact of IVM culture on embryo yield in comparison to standard IVM protocol was followed by a second prospective study on 15 PCOS patients. The latter study involved evaluation of oocyte meiotic arrest, oocyte chromatin configuration, preservation of cumulus-oocyte transzonal projections, and cumulus cell apoptosis. Oocyte developmental assessment 24 and 46-hour prematuration culture (PMC) + IVM along with aneuploidy rate in 20 good blastocysts by next-generation sequencing (NGS) was analyzed.

This method showed a significant increase in maturation rate in comparison to standard IVM (70 vs. 49%; $p \geq 0.001$).

Also, the number of good-quality day 3 embryos and blastocysts was higher with no increase in aneuploidy rates.

## KEY POINTS

- The optimization of IVM is ongoing.
- Although it may be premature to offer IVM to all types of infertility patients at this time, it does offer huge promise in the field of oncofertility.
- The practice of IVM requires flexibility and adjustment in the routine IVF program in the clinic.
- IVM holds a great promise as another type of assisted reproductive technology when fully developed.
- Further research and understanding of the human oocyte within the follicular environment are crucial for the advancement of IVM.

## REFERENCES

1. Cha KY, Chian RC. Maturation in vitro of immature human oocytes for clinical use. Hum Reprod Update. 1998;4:103-20.
2. Oktay K, Buyuk E, Rodriguez-Wallberg KA, Sahin G. In vitro maturation improves oocyte or embryo cryopreservation outcome in breast cancer patients undergoing ovarian stimulation for fertility preservation. Reprod Biomed Online. 2010;20:634-8.
3. Pincus G, Enzmann EV. The comparative behavior of mammalian eggs in vivo and in vitro. The activation of ovarian eggs. J Exp Med. 1935;62:655.
4. Edwards RG. Maturation in vitro of mouse, sheep, cow, pig, rhesus monkey and human ovarian oocytes. Nature (London). 1965;208:349-51.
5. Cha KY, Koo JJ, Ko JJ, Choi DH, Han SY, Yoon TK. Pregnancy after in vitro fertilization of human follicular oocytes collected from nonstimulated cycles, their culture in vitro and their transfer in a donor oocyte program. Fertil Steril. 1991;55:109-13.
6. Trounson A, Wood C, Kausche A. In vitro maturation and the fertilization and developmental competence of oocytes recovered from untreated polycystic ovarian patients. Fertil Steril. 1994;62:353-62.
7. Mikkelsen AL. In vitro maturation of human ova. International Congress Series, Elsevier. 2004;1266:160-6.
8. Buckett WM, Chian RC, Holzer H, Dean N, Usher R, Lin Tan S. Congenital abnormalities and perinatal outcome in pregnancies following IVM, IVF, and ICSI delivered in a single center. Fertil Steril. 2006;85:11-2.
9. Durinzi KL, Wentz AC, Saniga EM, Johnson DE, Lanzendorf SE. Follicle stimulating hormone effects on immature human oocytes: in vitro maturation and hormone production. J Assist Reprod Genet. 1997;14:199-204.
10. Durinzi KL, Saniga EM, Lanzendorf SE. The relationship between size and maturation in vitro in the unstimulated human oocyte. Fertil Steril. 1995;63:404-6.
11. Eppig JJ, O'Brien MJ. Development in vitro of mouse oocytes from primordial follicles. Biol Reprod. 1996;54:197-207.
12. Staigmiller RB, Moor RM. Effect of follicle cells on the maturation and developmental competence of ovine oocytes matured outside the follicle. Gamete Res. 1984;9:221-9.
13. Russell JB. In vitro oocyte maturation-human aspects. Contemporary Endocrinology: Assisted Fertilization and Nuclear Transfer in Mammals. Clifton, New Jersey: Humana Press; 2001. pp. 67-79.
14. Lerner-Geva L, Geva E, Lessing JB, Chetrit A, Modan B, Amit A. The possible association between in vitro fertilization treatments and cancer development. Int J Gynecol Cancer. 2003;13:23-7.
15. Strassburger D, Komarovky D, Bern O. The outcome of intracytoplasmic sperm injection in immature (M1) oocytes

with or without in vitro maturation. Abstract of the 15th Annual Meeting of ESHRE, June 27–30, Tours, France. Hum Reprod. 1999;14:6.
16. Almahbobi G, Anderiesz C, Hutchinson P, McFarlane JR, Wood C, Trounson AO. Functional integrity of granulosa cells from the polycystic ovaries. Clin Endocrinol (Oxf). 1996;44:571-80.
17. Mikkelsen AL, Smith S, Lindenberg S. Possible factors affecting the development of oocytes in in-vitro maturation. Hum Reprod. 2000;15(Suppl. 5):11-7.
18. Barnes FL, Kausche A, Tiglias J, Wood C, Wilton L, Trounson A. Production of embryos from in vitro-matured primary human oocytes. Fertil Steril. 1996;65:1151-6.
19. Hwu YM, Lee RK, Chen CP, Su JT, Chen YW, Lin SP. Development of hatching blastocysts from immature human oocytes following in vitro maturation and fertilization using a co-culture system. Hum Reprod. 1998;13:1916-21.
20. Cobo AC, Requena A, Neuspiller F, Aragons M, Mercader A, Navarro J, et al. Maturation in vitro of human oocytes from unstimulated cycles: selection of the optimal day for ovum retrieval based on follicular size. Hum Reprod. 1999;14:1864-8.
21. Ge HS, Huang XF, Zhang W, Zhao JZ, Lin JJ, Zhou W. Exposure to human chorionic gonadotropin during in vitro maturation does not improve the maturation rate and developmental potential of immature oocytes from patients with polycystic ovary syndrome. Fertil Steril. 2008;89:98-103.
22. Fadini R, Dal Canto MB, Renzini MM, Brambillasca F, Comi R, Fumagalli D, et al. Predictive factors in in vitro maturation in unstimulated women with normal ovaries. Reprod Biomed Online. 2009;18:251-61.
23. Trounson A, Anderiesz C, Jones G. Maturation of human oocytes in vitro and their developmental competence. Reproduction. 2001;121:51-75.
24. Gomez E, Tarin JJ, Pellicer A. Oocyte maturation in humans: the role of gonadotropins and growth factors. Fertil Steril. 1993;60:40-6.
25. Wynn P, Picton HM, Krapez JA, Rutherford AJ, Balen AH, Gosden RG. Pretreatment with follicle stimulating hormone promotes the numbers of human oocytes reaching metaphase II by in vitro maturation. Hum Reprod. 1998;13:3132-8.
26. Mikkelson AL, Lindenberg S. Benefit of FSH priming of women with PCOS to the in vitro maturation procedure and the outcome: a randomized prospective study. Reproduction. 2001;122:587-92.
27. Russell JB, Knezevich KM, Fabian KF, Dickson JA. Unstimulated immature oocyte retrieval: early versus midfollicular endometrial priming. Fertil Steril. 1997;67:616-20.
28. Child TJ, Gulekli B, Sylvestre C, Tan SL. Ultrasonographic assessment of endometrial receptivity at embryo transfer in an in vitro maturation of oocyte program. Fertil Steril. 2003;79:656-8.
29. Gulekli B, Buckett W, Chian RC, Child TJ, Abdul-Jalil AK, Tan SL. Randomized, controlled trial of priming with 10,000 IU versus 20,000 IU of human chorionic gonadotropin in women with polycystic ovary syndrome who are undergoing in vitro maturation. Fertil Steril. 2004;82:1458-9.
30. Son WY, Chung JT, Chian RC, Herrero B, Demirtas E, Elizur S, et al. A 38-hour interval between hCG priming and oocyte retrieval increases in vivo and in vitro oocyte maturation rate in programmed IVM cycles. Hum Reprod. 2008;23:2010-6.
31. Siristatidis CS, Vrachnis N, Creatsa M, Maheshwari A, Bhattacharya S. In vitro maturation in subfertile women with polycystic ovarian syndrome undergoing assisted reproduction. Cochrane Database Syst Rev. 2013;10: CD006606.
32. Reavey J, Vincent K, Child T, Granne IE. Human chorionic gonadotrophin priming for fertility treatment with in vitro maturation. Cochrane Database Syst Rev. 2016;11:CD008720.
33. Sonigo C, Le Conte G, Boubaya M, Ohanyan H, Presse M, El Hachem H, et al. Priming before in vitro maturation cycles in cancer patients undergoing urgent fertility preservation: a randomized controlled study. Reprod Sci. 2020;27:2247-56.
34. Son WY, Yoon SH, Park SJ, Yoon HJ, Lee WD, Lim JH. Ongoing twin pregnancy after vitrification of blastocysts produced by in-vitro matured oocytes retrieved from a woman with polycystic ovary syndrome: case report. Hum Reprod. 2002;17:2963-6.
35. Miao YL, Kikuchi K, Sun QY, Schatten H. Oocyte aging: cellular and molecular changes, developmental potential and reversal possibility. Hum Reprod Update. 2009;15:573-85.
36. Son WY, Han SY, Son JO, Park EH, Lee KA, Ko JJ, et al. Direct positive effect of EGF on nuclear maturation of human oocytes. Hum Reprod. 1997;12:39.
37. Anderiesz C, Ferraretti AP, Magli C, Fiorentino A, Fortini D, Gianaroli L, et al. Effect of recombinant human gonadotropins on human, bovine and murine oocyte meiosis, fertilization and embryonic development in vitro. Hum Reprod. 2000; 15:1140-8.
38. Son WY, Lee SY, Yoon SH, Lim JH. Pregnancies and deliveries after transfer of human blastocysts derived from in vitro matured oocytes in in vitro maturation oocytes. Fertil Steril. 2007;87:1491-3.
39. Son WY, Yoon SH, Lim JH. Effect of gonadotropin priming on in-vitro maturation of oocytes collected from women at risk of OHSS. Reprod Biomed Online. 2006;13:340-8.
40. Cha KY, Han SY, Chung HM, Choi DH, Lim JM, Lee WS, et al. Pregnancy and deliveries after in vitro maturation culture followed by in vitro fertilization and embryo transfer without stimulation in women with polycystic ovary syndrome. Fertil Steril. 2000;73:978-83.
41. Hwang JL, Lin YH, Tsai YL. In vitro maturation and fertilization of immature oocytes: a comprehensive study of fertilization techniques. J Assist Reprod Genet. 2000;17:39-43.
42. Söderström-Anttila V, Mäkinen S, Tuuri T, Suikkari AM. Favourable pregnancy results with insemination of in vitro matured oocytes from unstimulated patients. Hum Reprod. 2005;20:1534-40.
43. Goud P, Goud A, Van Oostveldt P, Van der Elst J, Dhont M. Fertilization abnormalities and pronucleus size asynchrony after intracytoplasmic sperm injection are related to oocyte postmaturity. Fertil Steril. 1999;72:245-52.
44. Hyun CS, Cha JH, Son WY, Yoon SH, Kim KA, Lim JH. Optimal ICSI timing after the first polar body extrusion in in vitro matured human oocytes. Hum Reprod. 2007;22:1991-5.
45. Mikkelsen AL, Smith SD, Lindenberg S. In-vitro maturation of human oocytes from regularly menstruating women may be successful without follicle stimulating hormone priming. Hum Reprod. 1999;14:1847-51.
46. Chian RC, Buckett WM, Tulandi T, Tan SL. Prospective randomized study of human chorionic gonadotrophin

priming before immature oocyte retrieval from unstimulated women with polycystic ovarian syndrome. Hum Reprod. 2000;15:165-70.
47. Le Du A, Kadoch IJ, Bourcigaux N, Doumerc S, Bourrier MC, Chevalier N, et al. In vitro oocyte maturation for the treatment of infertility associated with polycystic ovarian syndrome: the French experience. Hum Reprod. 2005;20:420-4.
48. Child T, Phillips S, Abdul-Jalil A, Gulekli B, Tan SL. A comparison of in vitro maturation and in vitro fertilization for women with polycystic ovaries. Obstet Gynecol. 2002;100:665-70.
49. Kastrop PM, Bevers MM, Destree OH, Kruip TA. Protein synthesis and phosphorylation patterns of bovine oocytes maturing in vivo. Mol Reprod Dev. 1991;29:271-5.
50. Buckett WM, Chian RC, Dean NL, Sylvestre C, Holzer HEG, Tan SL. Pregnancy loss in pregnancies conceived after in vitro oocyte maturation, conventional in vitro fertilization, and intracytoplasmic sperm injection. Fertil Steril. 2008;90:546-50.
51. Nagy ZP, Cecile J, Liu J, Loccufier A, Devroey P, Van Steirteghem A. Pregnancy and birth after intracytoplasmic sperm injection of in vitro matured germinal-vesicle stage oocytes: case report. Fertil Steril. 1996;65:1047-50.
52. Ortega-Hrepich C, Drakopoulos P, Bourgain C, Van Vaerenbergh I, Guzman L, Tournaye H, et al. Aberrant endometrial steroid receptor expression in in-vitro maturation cycles despite hormonal luteal support: a pilot study. Reprod Biol. 2019;19:210-7.
53. Walls ML, Hunter T, Ryan JP, Keelan JA, Nathan E, Hart RJ. In vitro maturation as an alternative to standard in vitro fertilization for patients diagnosed with polycystic ovaries: a comparative analysis of fresh, frozen and cumulative cycle outcomes. Hum Reprod. 2015;30:88-96.
54. Buckett WM, Chian RC, Barrington K, Dean N, Abdul-Jalil K, Tan SL. Obstetric, neonatal and infant outcome in babies conceived by in vitro maturation (IVM): initial five-year results 1998–2003. Fertil Steril. 2004;82:S133.
55. Buckett WM, Chian RC, Holzer H, Dean N, Usher R, Tan SL. Obstetric outcomes and congenital abnormalities after in vitro maturation, in vitro fertilization, and intracytoplasmic sperm injection. Obstet Gynecol. 2007;110:885-91.
56. Requena A, Bronet F, Guillen A, Agudo D, Bou C, García-Velasco JA. The impact of in-vitro maturation of oocytes on aneuploidy rate. Reprod Biomed Online. 2009;18:777-83.
57. Zhang XY, Ata B, Son WY, Buckett WM, Tan SL, Ao A. Chromosome abnormality rates in human embryos obtained from in-vitro maturation and IVF treatment cycles. Reprod Biomed Online. 2010;21(4):552-9.
58. Cha KY, Chung HM, Lee DR, Kwon H, Chung MK, Park LS, et al. Obstetric outcome of patients with polycystic ovary syndrome treated by in vitro maturation and in vitro fertilization-embryo transfer. Fertil Steril. 2005;83:1461-5.
59. Mikkelsen AL. Strategies in human in-vitro maturation and their clinical outcome. Reprod Biomed Online. 2005;10:593-9.
60. Söderström-Anttila V, Salokorpi T, Pihlaja M, Serenius-Sirve S, Suikkari AM. Obstetric and perinatal outcome and preliminary results of development of children born after in vitro maturation of oocytes. Hum Reprod. 2006;21:1508-13.
61. Fadini R, Renzini MM, Guarnieri T, Dal Canto M, De Ponti E, Sutcliffe A, et al. Comparison of the obstetric and perinatal outcomes of children conceived from in vitro or in vivo matured oocytes in in vitro maturation treatments with births from conventional ICSI cycles. Hum Reprod. 2012;27:3601-8.
62. Strowitzki T, Bruckner T, Roesner S. Maternal and neonatal outcome and children's development after medically assisted reproduction with in-vitro matured oocytes—a systematic review and meta-analysis. Hum Reprod Update. 2021;27:460-73.
63. Sanchez F, Lolicato F, Romero S, De Vos M, Van Ranst H, Verheyen G, et al. An improved IVM method for cumulus-oocyte complexes from small follicles in polycystic ovary syndrome patients enhances oocyte competence and embryo yield. Hum Reprod. 2017;32:2056-68.

CHAPTER

# 115 Ovarian Tissue Cryopreservation and its Eventual Transplantation: Is it Proficient Fertility Preservation Program?

*Pankaj Talwar, Pooja Awasthi*

## INTRODUCTION

Cryopreservation has proven as a boon for all the panoramas of reproductive medicine. A well-established program, tagged with proven medical laboratory protocol is required as an alternative to assist cases of women and adolescent girls facing urgent prerequisite for treatment of cancer and simultaneous management of their fertility preservation (FP). This section of the reproductive age group woman and adolescent girls suffering from various types of cancer may experience impaired fertility or hormone production as a result of their exposure to gonadotoxic chemoradiotherapy prior to or during the course of combating cancer.[1-3]

In current scenario, *ovarian tissue cryopreservation (OTC),* also known as ovarian cortex freezing, is considered as one of the best suited options that has gained substantial recognition as experimental tag has been removed from it recently in the year 2019. OTC is the only FP option that is readily available now in cases of cancer patients in whom traditional management such as oocyte and or embryo cryopreservation cannot be cogitated due to socio-psycho-medico issues. The main objective is the maintenance of the ovarian structure, physiology and endocrinology, benefiting multiple target patients facing different treatment and medical management situations.

Moreover, OTC is the only fertility preservation alternative for prepubertal patients, since in these cases, as neither the ovarian stimulation protocols nor oocyte collection can be applied.[4] Patients with benign conditions such as recurrent ovarian cysts, ovarian torsion, endocrine disorders, and autoimmune diseases may also benefit from this promising technique. Sometimes, individuals who wish to undergo gender affirmation surgery may also ask for preserving their ovarian cortex or whole ovary to be dissected into small pieces and cryopreserved.[5,6] However, some cases of women for whom surgery that requires removal of ovaries for medical condition or disease, e.g., prophylactic oophorectomy in BRCA patients and also for the patients who underwent previous treatment for cancer still has ovarian function is acceptable for choosing OTC. As the best suited option of their FP. OTC can also be indicated for postponing menopause.[7,8]

The main objective of OTC is to reimplant a few thawed cortical strips into the patient (i.e., auto transplantation) once the patient has completed cancer treatment, is disease free, and desires pregnancy. Pieces of ovarian cortex can be grafted to orthotopic (pelvis) or heterotopic (subcutaneous) sites, each having distinguished advantages and disadvantages. Very first pregnancy after orthotopic transplantation of OTC and live birth was reported in 2004 and according to the more recent literature, the number of live births after ovarian tissue cryopreservation exceeded 200 in 2020,[9] while the pregnancy and live birth rates reached 50 and 41%, respectively.[10] Though live births have also been reported by heterotopic transplantation,[11,12] the exact numbers are still unclear.

After eventual autotransplantation, success rates are high regarding the re-establishment of ovarian activity (63.9%) and natural live births (57.5%), according to a meta-analysis performed in 2017.[13] OTC requires a multidisciplinary approach to preserve the fertility in cases of females where necessity of husband or partner or donor sperms can be eradicated completely.[14] Concerted multidisciplinary discussions between hematologists, assisted reproductive technology (ART) teams and surgeons are required to improve the quality of patient information[15] in terms of procedures and measures for achieving OTC successfully. Radiosensitivity of the human ovary that leads to the loss of 50% of primordial follicles (LD50) is estimated to be 2 Gy.[16-18] The possibility of ovarian failure is also determined by the regimen and type of chemotherapy where block of DNA replication, double stranded (ds) DNA breaks, and induction of apoptosis primarily in the stroma and the granulosa cells of growing follicles occur.[19,20]

Ovarian tissue is collected surgically (laparoscopy or laparotomy) prior or during exposure of the young women to chemoradiotherapy. Afterwards, these strips are cryopreserved. Follicular viability and integrity of tissue compartments and cell-to-cell contacts must be ensured by the cryopreservation procedures.[21] Thus, studies investigating the most favorable cooling rates and dehydration times have been conducted. It is now well-established that for obtaining satisfactory results, adequate penetration of cryoprotectant through the stroma and granulosa cells to the oocytes is required.[22] Slow freezing[23-25] and vitrification techniques[26,27] are two proven methods applied. However, when compared to vitrification, very few reports of successful births were reported in comparison to implementing the slow freezing method for OTC based FP. Although OTC is expected to bridge an important gap in FP in the field of oncofertility in cases where it is impossible to create embryos for cryopreservation, especially in pediatric oncology mostly among young girls prior to adolescence.[27,28]

Ovarian tissue cryopreservation comes with four key components that involve: (1) ovarian surgical procurement, (2) ovarian tissue processing, (3) tissue cryopreservation, and (4) Storage followed by ovarian tissue transplantation (OTT). Ethically, providing inadequate information about OTC/OTT including surgeries, procedures and probabilities of success, should be obstructed and informed consent form should be taken from the patients. In cases of adolescent girls, written and signed informed consent form should be taken from both patient and her parents/guardian stating all uncertainty specially related to the long-term complications and benefits of the procedures. A unique feature of OTC is that in future, the patient can choose to reimplant the ovarian cortical tissue orthotopically or heterotrophically for fertility purposes or to restore ovarian endocrine function. We as an expert are not only suggesting and recommending OTC as FP method that is being applied to benefit cancer patients, but also the women who want to postpone their fertility and menopause can opt OTC.[29]

In 1999, the first successful autotransplantation of frozen-thawed ovarian cortical tissue was performed, but it was not until 2006 when Meirow et al. reported the first live birth obtained from OTC.[30] However, claims of the first live human birth coming from ovarian tissue which was cryopreserved using the slow freeze technique and then transplanted was described by Donnez et al.[31] Orthotopic transplantation is more frequently used approach but reports of live births from heterotopic autotransplantation methodology has also been started to serve the society.[32-35] Since orthotopic transplantation can allow both live birth and the recovery of endocrine function more efficiently but the reimplantation of malignant cells is always a major risk and should always be considered in serious manner. It was suggested that the histological analysis, immunohistochemical studies and molecular methods, are needed in order to improve the search for malignant cells before transplantation of ovarian tissue. OTC/OTT appears to be a method with specific benefits, indications and risks which can be an important tool in terms of preserving fertility in younger women and adolescent girls.[36-38]

OTC in turner syndrome is under investigation but there is no published report showing any success in such cases.[39] The medical, surgical and laboratory techniques/methodology are required to be improved further to advance the technology for intensification of the reach of OTC for different groups of needy women where no other options are relatable, to offer OTC as FP in an efficient manner.[40]

Though, the cryopreservation and reimplantation of whole ovaries are areas where extensive research needs to be performed prior to offering such high-end medical service to the necessitous, in future.

A well-focused effort in terms of research work also needs to be conducted where more attention needs to be given to clarify criteria and establishment of guidelines for accurate selection of the patients to offer OTC. From technical point of view, it is advisable to optimize the protocol of OTC (slow freezing or rapid vitrification) to achieve higher follicular survival. Ultimately, the surgical technique for revascularization of thawed/warmed ovarian tissue and whole ovary are required to be sharpened. The present stance of OTC is hopeful for young cancer sufferer females and future perspective of OTC/OTT seems to be promising enough, to help the society specially cancer victims. However, OTC along with its subsequent thawing/warming and eventual transplantation techniques are relatively new. The long term associated and unseen risks of metastasis in young female patients with malignancies who had ovarian cortex reimplanted is still a matter of research and concern and needs to be explored.

## REFERENCES


1. DeSantis CE, Lin CC, Mariotto AB, Siegel RL, Stein KD, Kramer JL, et al. Cancer treatment and survivorship statistics, 2014. CA: Cancer J Clin. 2014;64(4):252-71.
2. International Agency for Research on Cancer. Lyon: Cancer Today; 2018.
3. Gosden RG, Baird DT, Wade JC, Webb R. Restoration of fertility to oophorectomized sheep by ovarian autografts stored at –196 degrees C. Hum Reprod. 1994; 9(4):597-603.
4. Donnez J. Fertility preservation in women, focusing on cancer, benign diseases and social reasons. Minerva Ginecol. 2018;70(4):385-6.
5. Gellert SE, Pors SE, Kristensen SG, Bay-Bjørn AM, Ernst E, Yding Andersen C. Transplantation of frozen-thawed ovarian tissue: an update on worldwide activity published in peer-reviewed papers and on the Danish cohort. J Assist Reprod Genet. 2018;35(4):561-70.
6. Donnez J, Dolmans MM. Fertility Preservation in Women. N Engl J Med. 2017;377(17):1657-65.
7. Amorim CA, Goncalves PB, Figueiredo JR. Cryopreservation of oocytes from pre-antral follicles. Hum Reprod Update. 2003;9(2):119-29.

8. Amorim CA, Leonel ECR, Afifi Y, Coomarasamy A, Fishel S. Cryostorage and retransplantation of ovarian tissue as an infertility treatment. Best Pract Res Clin Endocrinol Metab. 2019;33(1):89-102.
9. Dolmans MM, Falcone T, Patrizio, P. Importance of patient selection to analyze in vitro fertilization outcome with transplanted cryopreserved ovarian tissue. Fertil Steril. 2020;114:279-80.
10. Shapira M, Dolmans MM, Silber S, Meirow D. Evaluation of ovarian tissue transplantation: Results from three clinical centers. Fertil Steril. 2020;114:388-97.
11. Stern CJ, Gook D, Hale LG, Agresta F, Oldham J, Rozen G, et al. First reported clinical pregnancy following heterotopic grafting of cryopreserved ovarian tissue in a woman after a bilateral oophorectomy. Hum Reprod. 2009;24(7):1670-83.
12. Oktay K, Buyuk E, Veeck L, Zaninovic N, Xu K, Takeuchi T, et al. Embryo development after heterotopic transplantation of cryopreserved ovarian tissue. Lancet. 2004;363(9412):837-40.
13. Pacheco F, Oktay K. Current success and efficiency of autologous ovarian transplantation: a meta-analysis. Reprod Sci. 2017;2 4(8):1111-20.
14. Salle B, Demirci B, Frank M, Rudigoz RC, Guerin JF, Lornage J. Normal pregnancies and live births after autograft of frozen-thawed hemi-ovaries in ewes. Fertil Steril. 2002;77(2):403-8.
15. Mancini J, Rey D, Preau M. Infertility induced by cancer treatment: inappropriate or no information provided to majority of French survivors of cancer. Fertil Steril. 2008;90(5):1616-25.
16. Wallace WH, Thomson AB, Kelsey TW. The radio sensitivity of the human oocyte. Hum Reprod. 2003;18:117-21.
17. Wallace WH, Thomson AB, Saran F, Kelsey TW. Predicting age of ovarian failure after radiation to a field that includes the ovaries. Int J Radiat Oncol Biol Phys. 2005;62:738-44.
18. Meirow D, Biederman H, Anderson RA, Wallace WH. Toxicity of chemotherapy and radiation on female reproduction. Clin Obstet Gynecol. 2010;53:727-39.
19. Lopes F, Smith R, Anderson RA, Spears N. Docetaxel induces moderate ovarian toxicity in mice, primarily affecting granulosa cells of early growing follicles. Mol Hum Reprod. 2014;20:948-59.
20. Roti Roti EC, Leisman SK, Abbott DH, Salih SM. Acute doxorubicin insult in the mouse ovary is cell- and follicle-type dependent. PLoS One. 2012;7:e42293.
21. Fuller B, Paynter S. Fundamentals of cryobiology in reproductive medicine. Reprod Biomed Online. 2004;9:680-91.
22. Hovatta O. Methods of cryopreservation of human ovarian tissue. Reprod Biomed Online. 2005;10:729-34.
23. Suzuki N, Yoshioka N, Takae S, Sugishita Y, Tamura M, Hashimoto S, et al. Successful fertility preservation following ovarian tissue vitrification in patients with primary ovarian insufficiency. Hum Reprod. 2015;30(3):608-15.
24. Grave T, Clasen-Linde E, Andersen MT, Andersen MK, Sørensen SD, Rosendahl M, et al. Cryopreserved ovarian cortex from patient with leukemia in complete remission contains no apparent viable malignant cells. Blood. 2012;123-4311-6.
25. Diaz AA, Kubo H, Handa N, Hanna M, Laronda MM. A Systematic Review of Ovarian Tissue Transplantation Outcomes by Ovarian Tissue Processing Size for Cryopreservation. Front Endocrinol (Lausanne). 2022;13:918899.
26. Gandolfi F, Paffoni A, Papasso Brambilla E, Bonetti S, Brevini TA, Ragni G. Efficiency of equilibrium cooling and vitrification procedures for the cryopreservation of ovarian tissue: comparative analysis between human and animal models. Fertil Steril. 2006;85:1150-6.
27. Jadoul P, Dolmans MM, Donnez J. Fertility preservation in girls during childhood: it is feasible, efficient and safe and to whom should it be proposed. Hum Reprod Update. 2010;16: 617-630.
28. Practice Committee of American Society for Reproductive Medicine. Ovarian tissue cryopreservation: a committee opinion. Fertil Steril. 2014;101:1237-43.
29. Kim S, Lee Y, Lee S, Ravau J, De Vos M, Demeestere I, et al. Ovarian tissue cryopreservation and transplantation in patients with cancer. Obstetrics Gynecol Sciences. 2018;61(4):431.
30. Meirow D, Levron J, Eldar-Geva T, Hardan I, Fridman E, Zalel Y, et al. Pregnancy after transplantation of cryopreserved ovarian tissue in a patient with ovarian failure after chemotherapy. N Engl J Med. 2005;353(3):318-21.
31. Donnez J, Dolmans MM, Demylle D, Jadoul P, Pirard C, Squifflet J, et al. Livebirth after orthotopic transplantation of cryopreserved ovarian tissue. Lancet. 2004;364:1405-10.
32. Ruan X, Du J, Lu D, Duan W, Jin F, Kong W, et al. First live birth in China after cryopreserved ovarian tissue transplantation to prevent premature ovarian insufficiency. Climacteric. 2022;25(4):421-4.
33. Tammiste T, Kask K, Padrik P, Idla K, Rosenstein K, Jatsenko T, et al. A case report and follow-up of the first live birth after heterotopic transplantation of cryopreserved ovarian tissue in Eastern Europe. BMC Women Health. 2019;19(1):65.
34. Marin L, Bedoschi G, Kawahara T, Oktay KH. History, Evolution and Current State of Ovarian Tissue Auto-Transplantation with Cryopreserved Tissue: a Successful Translational Research Journey from 1999 to 2020. Reprod Sci. 2020; 27(4):955-62.
35. Kristensen GS, Macklon KT. Methods and Techniques of Ovarian Tissue Harvesting and Preparation before Cryopreservation. In: Principles and practice of Ovarian Tissue Cryopreservation and Transplantation. New York: Elsevier; 2022. pp. 49-59; 169-75.
36. Ruan X, Cheng J, Korell M, Du J, Kong W, Lu D, et al. Ovarian tissue cryopreservation and transplantation prevents iatrogenic premature ovarian insufficiency: first 10 cases in China. Climacteric. 2020;23(6):574-80.
37. Arapaki A, Christopoulos P, Kalampokas E, Triantafyllidou O, Matsas A, Vlahos NF. Ovarian Tissue Cryopreservation in Children and Adolescents. Children (Basel). 2022;9(8):1256.
38. Rivas Leonel EC, Lucci CM, Amorim CA. Cryopreservation of Human Ovarian Tissue: A Review. Transfus Med Hemother. 2019;46(3):173-181.
39. Ye M, Yeh J, Kosteria I, Li L. Progress in Fertility Preservation Strategies in Turner Syndrome. Front Med (Lausanne). 2020;7:3.
40. Lee S, Ozkavukcu S, Ku SY. Current and Future Perspectives for Improving Ovarian Tissue Cryopreservation and Transplantation Outcomes for Cancer Patients. Reprod Sci. 2021;28(6):1746-58.

CHAPTER 116

# Polarization Microscopy and its Clinical Applications

*Taswin Kaur, Mir Jaffar*

## INTRODUCTION

There is great importance in searching for parameters that can improve the assessment of the quality and the developmental potential of the human gametes and the embryos for a good implantation and a healthy viable pregnancy. Many microscope technologies are available to visualize the subcellular structures. One such revolutionary technology is the polarization microscopy.

Polarized light was used to investigate the structure and the development of skeletal and cellular components in animal cells by Schmidt about a century ago. Microtubule-dependent birefringence of the mitotic spindle has been visualized by polarized microscopy half a decade ago. Polarized light microscopy provides a unique window to view the internal structures of a cell.

## PRINCIPLE

The polarization microscopy works on a principle that when two orthogonally polarized light rays passes through orderly arranged filamentous structures; they exhibit birefringence.

Birefringence is known as double refraction. It is a property that is exhibited when a ray of light passes through an anisotropic material and gets split by polarization into two unequal waves (traveling at different velocities). This phenomenon was first described in 1669 by a Danish scientist, Rasmus Bartholin. Light entering an isotropic substance passes through the substance with a single velocity at a constant angle. On the other hand, anisotropic substances have a nonuniform spatial distribution of properties. When light enters these substances at a nonequivalent axis, it is reflected into two rays, each traveling at different velocities. This is exhibited either to a greater or to a lesser degree in all anisotropic substances **(Figs. 1 and 2)**.

Retardance is the relative measure of optical path difference. In other words, it is the measured path length between the two exciting beams of light as they pass through the birefringent structure. It is usually measured in nanometers and is the primary quantity measure by a polarizing microscope. The retardance measured is directly proportional to the density of the structures in the cell, i.e., greater the density of the microtubules in the oocyte, greater the retardance **(Figs. 3 and 4)**.

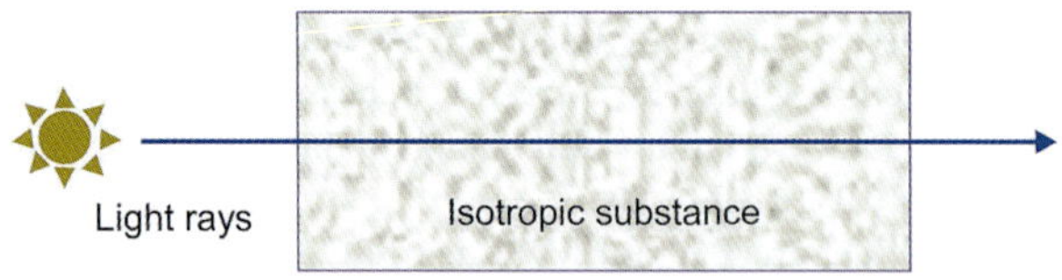


**Fig. 1:** Birefringence effect—when the light beam passes through an isotropic structure, no birefringence is seen. This is because light passes at a single velocity without being polarized.

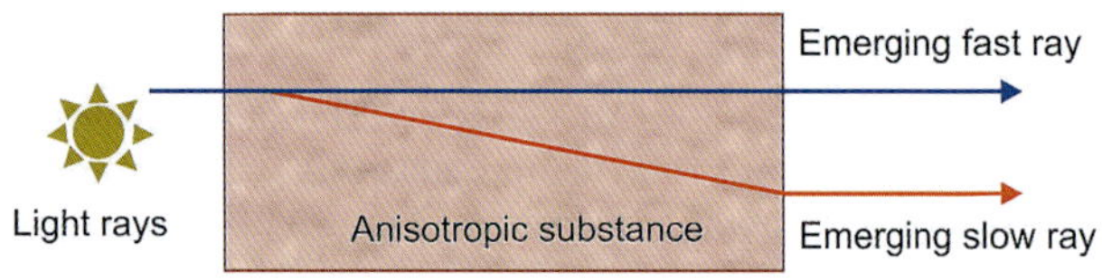


**Fig. 2:** Light rays passing through an anisotropic structure is split into two rays—an emerging fast and a slow ray.

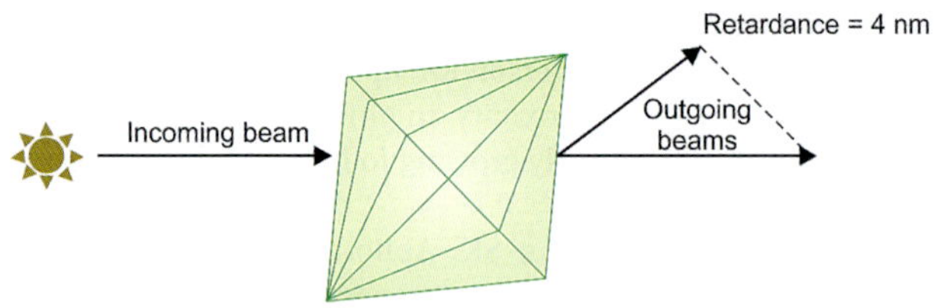


**Fig. 3:** Example of a spindle with a high birefringence. The spindle has a higher degree of molecular order.

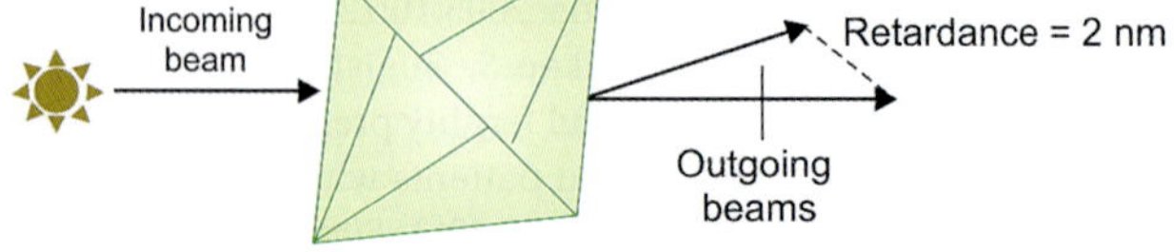


**Fig. 4:** Example of a spindle with low birefringence. These spindles have a lower degree of molecular order and are potentially less viable.

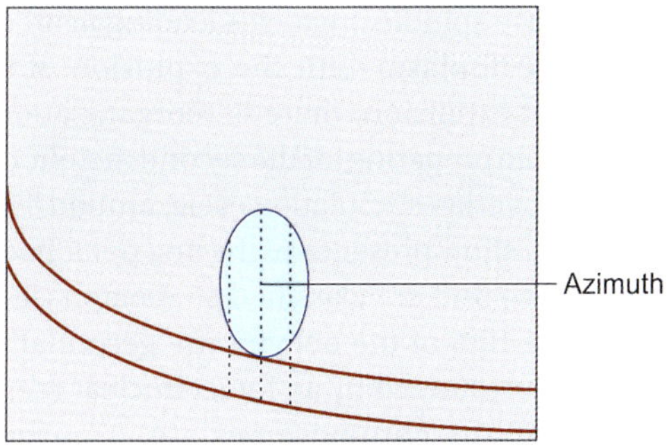


**Fig. 5:** Azimuth/orientation of a normal barrel-shaped spindle.

Azimuth is an angle, which refers to the orientation of the slow axis of a uniformly birefringent region. It is measured from the horizontal orientation with angles ranging from 0° to 180°. In case of the spindle apparatus, the azimuth follows the long axis of the spindle fibers. Therefore, normal and abnormal orientations can be identified **(Fig. 5)**.[1]

## DEVICE

A polarized microscope system has been designed to observe an optically anisotropic specimen. This specialized microscope has been developed as a variant adjustment of the standard light microscope equipped with a polarizer, motorized micromanipulator, and an analyzer **(Table 1)**.

Polarized light microscopy enhances the contrast between the cell and the background, which then helps to reveal specific important information about the structure and the composition of the substance. In the field of reproductive medicine, the oocyte appears translucent and appears to have little or no details when they are back illuminated by white light using a simple light microscope. However, when polarized light passes these same tissues (oocytes), there is splitting of the light beam and a shift in the plane of birefringence and retardance, causing the internal structures to become visible and therefore analyzed and seen on the computer screen as grayscale values. The polarizing microscope has a sensitivity of 0.1 nm of retardance **(Flowchart 1)**.[2]

In the market, both the traditional and the liquid crystal (LC) polarizing microscopes are available. The LC polarizing microscopes usually include an LC-based compensator, a circular polarizer, camera, and computer software for image rendering and processing **(Box 1)**.[3] The modifications done in a polarizing microscope from the traditional microscope are as follows:

- LC-based compensator is used instead of the traditional compensator.
- Specimen is illuminated with nearly circular polarized light.
- Magnitude and orientation of the birefringence are measured without mechanical movement of the specimen or the instrument.

**TABLE 1:** Components of polarization microscope and its functions.

| Components | Function |
|---|---|
| Eye piece | • Fitted with a cross wire reticule to mark the center of the field view<br>• "Bertrand" lens are used—specialized lens mounted within the observation tube |
| Compensator/ retardation plate | • Inserted between the cross polarizer<br>• Enhances the optical path difference in the specimen |
| Graduated circular rotating stage | • 360° rotating specimen stage<br>• Facilitates orientation with centralization of the objective and stage with the microscope's optical axis |
| Polarizer | Confines white light to vibrate in one plane when light passes through it |
| Analyzer | Image obtained is colorful |

**Flowchart 1:** Pathway of working system of a polarizing microscope.

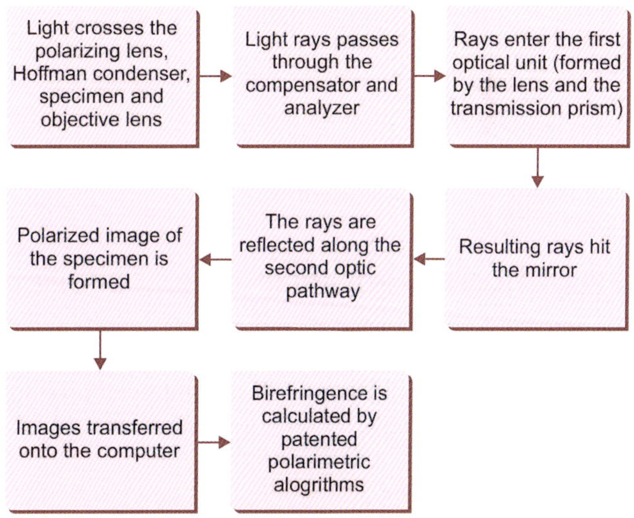


**TABLE 2:** Differences between the simple and polarizing microscopes.

| Parameters | Simple microscope | Polarizing microscope |
|---|---|---|
| Polarizer and analyzer | No | Yes |
| Working principle | Reflection and refraction | Interference |
| Specimen used | Any specimen | Optically anisotropic specimen |
| Image color | Not same as that of the specimen | Colorful image/grayscale image is obtained due to interference |
| Dishes used | Plastic/glass | Only glass dishes or slides |

Polarization microscopy is a new noninvasive tool to analyze the cell structures, mainly the meiotic spindle, zona pellucida, and the sperm acrosome **(Table 3)**.

**BOX 1:** Factors affecting the polarization microscope image.

- Orientation of the specimen
- Thickness of the specimen
- Orientation of the polarizer and analyzer with respect to each other
- Path difference between the two rays of light

**TABLE 3:** Advantages and disadvantages of the polarizing microscope.

| *Advantage* | *Disadvantage* |
|---|---|
| Noninvasive | The oocyte and the sperm have to be assessed separately and not as an embryo |
| No usage of exogenous dyes or labels | Can be only used with ICSI as the cumulus mass surrounding the oocyte has been stripped away |
| Allows spindle visualization in living oocytes | |
| Optimizes thermodynamic stability of the oocytes during ICSI | |
| Enables the dynamic architecture of the meiotic spindles | |

(ICSI: intracytoplasmic sperm injection)

## FUNCTIONS OF POLARIZING MICROSCOPE

The functions of a polarizing microscope are:

- Stage of meiosis
- Location of meiotic spindle during intracytoplasmic sperm injection (ICSI)
- Timing of ICSI
- Quality of the oocyte
- Laboratory conditions
- Sperm quality.

## APPLICATION OF POLARIZING MICROSCOPE

### Spindle Imaging

#### *Spindle Dynamics in the Meiotic Cycle*

Oocyte maturation is a complex process involving both the nuclear and the cytoplasm maturation. Oocytes are arrested at the prophase of the first meiotic division. Post puberty, under the stimuli of the luteinizing hormone (LH) surge, via its action on the granulosa cells, there is a decrease in the cyclic adenosine monophosphate (cAMP) concentration. This in turn leads to the resumption of meiosis I followed by the extrusion of the first polar body. Oocyte nuclear maturity begins when the meiosis resumes from the diplotene stage, and this is determined by the absence of a germinal vesicle and the expulsion of the first polar body present in the perivitelline space.

The metaphase spindle organizes leading to an unequal division of the cytoplasm with the expulsion of the first polar body. Post expulsion, there is reorganization of the metaphase spindle preparing for the second meiotic division. In any standard ovarian stimulation cycle, around 85% of the denuded oocytes show presence of the first polar body in the perivitelline space and are classified as metaphase II (MII) oocytes. Around 10% of the oocytes are germinal vesicles where they are surrounded by an intact nuclear membrane. In the MII stage, the chromosomes are arranged at the equatorial margin of the meiotic spindle.

#### *Determination of Stage of Meiosis*

The meiotic spindle is a highly dynamic structure, which changes during the transition from metaphase I (MI) to MII. It is made up of microtubules that are nucleated from the spindle polar bodies. Under the regular light microscope, the extrusion and the presence of the first polar body are synonymous with a mature MII oocyte. However, this scenario under a few circumstances may be false when these oocytes are viewed under a polarizing light. With the advent and examination of these oocytes under a PolScope, some of these oocytes were found to be in the early telophase I stage where the spindle forms a connecting strand between the ooplasm and the first polar body. For around 40–60 minutes, the spindle disappears in telophase I and then reappears followed by the formation of a MII oocyte.[4]

#### *Presence of the Meiotic Spindle*

It is known that without the help of the PolScope, it is almost impossible to identify the presence of the meiotic spindle and hence to clearly identify the oocytes undergoing the important maturational transition from MI to MII. With the advent of video cinematography, it is known that spindle disappearance in the cell cycle lasts for around an hour. Hence, it is important to reexamine the oocytes that did not have a spindle after 2–3 hours to avoid a misdiagnosis of an absent spindle as a result of this kinetic behavior. This is done to confirm the diagnosis of an absent spindle or that the oocyte was in the transition phase of late telophase I.

A study by Montag et al. showed that almost 50% of oocytes with an absent spindle initially displayed a meiotic spindle after an additional 2 hours of culture.[5] In ICSI procedures, studies have shown a positive correlation with the fertilization rate when the sperm injection was done in oocytes with a visible meiotic spindle.[6-8]

A meta-analysis by Petersen et al. evaluated the influence of the meiotic spindle visualization in human oocytes on the outcome of ICSI. The authors included 10 trials and concluded that the presence of the birefringent spindle was associated with a better fertilization rate and embryo development.[9] However, there was no benefit noted on the pregnancy or implantation rates.

A retrospective analysis done by Picinato et al. reported that there was an increased fertilization rate with the use of a polarization microscope, but a reduced cleavage rate and top-quality embryos were observed.[10]

### Location of the Meiotic Spindle

Majority of the spindles are located in the same equatorial plane as the first polar body, with the highest frequency of it being directly adjacent to the polar body, indicating that the position of the first polar body can be taken as a crude marker of spindle position. The vast availability of spindle imaging across in vitro fertilization (IVF) laboratories raised the question of the need of locating the position of the meiotic spindle during ICSI. The visualization of the spindle stamped that the location of the first polar body is not a reliable reference or predictor for the MII spindle location. The significance of the angle of meiotic spindle from the polar body position has been defined by various authors.[7,11] However, the association of the location of the meiotic spindle for the outcomes of ICSI has been investigated and debated in many publications with contradictory results in terms of fertilization rates, competent cleavage-stage embryos, blastocyst formation rates, and pregnancy or implantation rates.[3,12]

To avoid damaging the spindle during the ICSI procedure, the oocyte is usually rotated based on the position of the first polar body. However, we seldom realize that there may be possible movement of the polar body in the perivitelline space due to stress or physical displacement during oocyte denudation or the migration of the spindle in the oocyte. Hence, the relationship between these two structures is altered, leading to an impaired spindle if microinjection is done. Special care is usually taken not to damage the meiotic spindle when an isolated sperm is injected into the oocyte during ICSI.[13,14] Hence, the use of the PolScope is a useful tool in ICSI to allow the perfect orientation of the oocyte with the identification of the spindle, and not in relation to the polar body, thus, being as far as possible to the injection needle **(Fig. 6)**.

A recent study by Asa et al. reported that a close position of the meiotic spindle to the polar body was correlated with better fertilization and cleavage rates of the embryo.[15] This finding was consistent with the previous study by Rienzi et al., which demonstrated that oocytes with a spindle deviation of >90° from the polar body position had lower fertilization rates.[16] Kilani et al. demonstrated that spindle assessment was an early predictor of the pregnancy potential of that oocyte, especially in recurrent implantation failure patients.[17,18] However, on the other hand, in some researches, there was no significant correlation between spindle retardance and fertilization rates.[6,19]

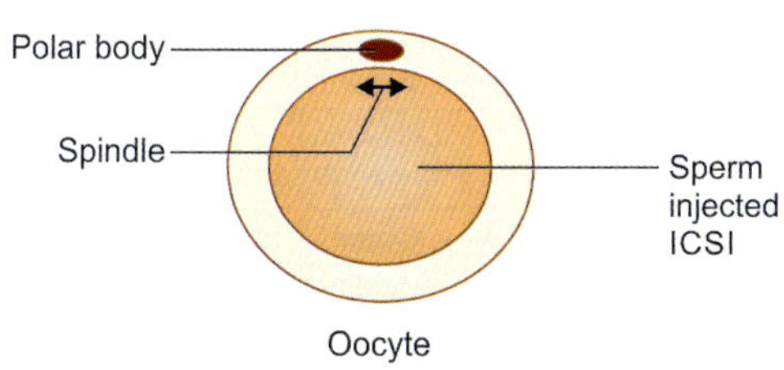


**Fig. 6:** Intracytoplasmic sperm injection (ICSI) injection site in relation to meiotic spindle and polar body.

### Quality of Oocytes

Spindle birefringence is contributed by the microtubules, and a positive correlation has been recorded between the spindle retardance and the microtubule density. Raju et al. observed that oocytes with a higher spindle retardance (>3 nm) and those with a longer spindle length (>12 nm) seemed to have a better-quality embryo and subsequently progressed to blastocyst.[20]

With an increasing age, there are changes in the spindle integrity leading to a decreased oocyte quality and ultimately a rise in aneuploidy rates.[21,22] Therefore, low retardance due to spindle abnormality is synonymous with an aged oocyte and thus an early predictor for a compromised oocyte quality and hence a deficient embryo.

In a recent study by Revelli et al., the increase of the meiotic spindle size has been found to be associated with an increased ovarian resistance to follicle-stimulating hormone (FSH), hence, translating to stimulation like a patient of increased reproductive age.[23]

### Prediction of Aneuploidy

The normal meiotic spindle is an important checkpoint in the cell cycle.[24] Its structure and function are crucial in mediating the mechanical alignment and segregation of chromosomes during MI and MII stages.

The noninvasive morphological assessment of these meiotic spindles by polarizing light microscopy identifies the oocytes with the greatest reproductive potential and least aneuploidy.[25] Five different types of oocyte spindle morphology—normal, dysmorphic, telophase, translucent, or no visible spindle—have been recently classified in a publication by Tilia et al. There were a higher percentage of aneuploid embryos with the presence of a translucent or absence of the meiotic spindle as compared to those with a dysmorphic spindle.[26] Hence, spindle visualization may be an important tool to predict better embryo outcomes.[27,28]

### Cryopreserved Oocytes

The meiotic spindle is the most obvious manifestation of the polarity of the mature oocyte. It is of central importance in the cell during chromatid segregation in the second meiotic division. Unfortunately, this cytoskeletal component is very sensitive, especially to temperature.[29]

Oocyte cryopreservation had not gained much limelight previously due to the poor survival rate of these frozen–thawed oocytes. With the introduction of slow cooling and recent vitrification protocols, there is a high recovery percentage of the thawed viable oocytes.[30]

Freezing of the MII oocyte to nonphysiological temperatures may result in depolymerization and damage to the oocyte. Repolymerization causes swelling of the cell back to the original state and is believed to be time dependent. The translucent structures of the oocyte can be viewed under a polarizing light post thawing and the time taken for the spindle to reform to its original length and birefringence has been studied.

In the first few initial studies when spindle-positive oocytes were subjected to the standard freeze–thaw cycles, around 50% of the oocytes repolymerized and spindles reappeared within 3–5 hours post warming.[31,32]

Along the years, multiple publications reported on the various slow-freezing methodologies, especially after increasing the sucrose content in the freeze–thaw solutions which has showed to improve the survival rates.[33,34] There is >80% spindle reformation of the frozen–thawed oocytes within 1 hour after warming in an efficient slow-freezing protocol.[35]

Vitrification is an alternative technique for cryopreservation of oocytes. Oocytes rewarmed post-vitrification were found to have the same fertilization and cleavage as a fresh gamete insemination.[36] Slow-freezing method has been found to be inferior to the vitrified human oocytes. Vitrification causes less damage to the spindle integrity and the chromosome alignment.[37,38]

A study by Chen et al. suggested that most of the spindle was visualized within an hour of vitrification and only in about 25% of cases the spindle of intact thawed oocytes was found to be undetected.[39]

### *In vitro Matured Oocytes*

Immature oocytes can be cultured in vitro to subsequent embryonic development, pregnancy, and a healthy live birth.[40] The timing of ICSI can be precisely determined by imaging the meiotic spindle under the polarizing microscope.[41] These in vitro matured oocytes show a varied time course compared to oocytes from stimulated cycles and develop faster.

### *Rescue Intracytoplasmic Sperm Injection*

Failed fertilization after ICSI can be emotionally disturbing to the couple. A rescue ICSI can be performed on these 1-day-old oocytes.[42] This procedure may reduce the cycle cancellation rate but has been reported to result in morphologically and genetically abnormal embryos. However, a few studies have reported a successful live birth after a rescue ICSI.[43] Polarization microscope allows the accurate visualization of the meiotic spindle.

### *Spindle Imaging as a Tool for Quality Assessment of Laboratory Parameters*

Microtubules are in the polymerized–depolymerized state. Oocyte meiotic spindle shows depolymerization to pH and temperature. The proper setting of laboratory parameters can be analyzed by these biochemical properties of the meiotic spindle.

Meiotic spindles start to disintegrate at the critical temperature of 33°C, and if the temperature falls below 25°C, repolymerization of the spindles is very unlikely.[44] Reassembly of the spindle depends on the minimum temperature and the duration that the microtubule was exposed to these harsh temperatures.[45,46] Hence, using this concept, the polarization microscope can be used to monitor the effects of cooling and rewarming not only in the oocytes but also in the laboratory. Therefore, the maintenance of the temperature at 37°C while oocyte manipulation is of utmost importance.

The meiotic spindle can also be disrupted by nonphysiological pH. Spindle disassembly can occur within 8–10 minutes of exposing the oocyte to an unbuffered culture.

If the meiotic spindles are consistently absent in most of the oocytes (>30%), it may be a wise decision to carefully monitor and troubleshoot the laboratory conditions.

## Zona Imaging

Visualizing under the conventional light microscopy, the zona pellucida appears as a uniform layer surrounding the oocyte. The same zona pellucida when visualized under a polarization microscope exhibits a multilaminar structure that can be distinguished by their birefringent properties **(Fig. 7)**.[47,48]

Oocytes with a higher zona birefringence reflect a better oocyte quality and are an indirect indication for a good follicular development.[49,50] There was a higher fertilization rate and higher conception cycles noted with oocytes, which had a higher birefringence in their inner zona layer.[51,52] According to a study by Cheng et al. and Safian et al., oocytes with a high birefringence were negatively correlated with the women's age.[53,54]

The potential of an embryo to progress and to develop into a blastocyst was higher when there was a retardance of >3 nm and a thickness between 10 and 12 nm in the zona inner layer.[20]

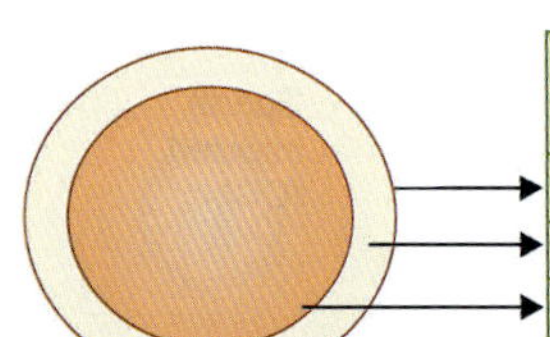

| *Layers in the zona* | *Filament arrangement* | *Birefringence* |
|---|---|---|
| Outer | Tangentially | Moderate |
| Middle | Random | Least |
| Inner | Radially | Maximum |

**Fig. 7:** Zona pellucida layers in an oocyte.

### Sperm Selection

Advanced sperm selection techniques are gaining importance in assisted reproductive technique cycles, especially cycles utilizing ICSI.[55] The use of polarization microscopy could assist the embryologist in selecting the most viable spermatozoa without an adverse effect on the sperm motility or membrane integrity.[56]

The polarization microscope is equipped with a 63× objective and the images obtained can be further enhanced by digital imaging on a screen. There is total magnification zoom of 2,500× and 5,500× and these specific birefringence characteristics can be visualized and measured in real time.

The anisotropic structure within the nuclear and the acrosome region of the sperm head exhibits birefringence. The protein filaments arranged longitudinally contribute to the acrosome birefringence.

Three types of birefringent patterns in the sperm head have been distinguished:[57]

1. Spermatozoa with totally birefringent head—represents sperms with an intact acrosome.
2. Spermatozoa with a partially birefringent head (localized at the postacrosomal region)—sperm cell that has undergone an acrosome reaction.
3. Sperm head with abnormal patterns of birefringence—due to presence of vacuoles, absence of birefringence, localized areas of birefringence in the acrosome or nuclear area.

A study by Vermey et al. reported that the optimum sperm retardance was between 0.56 and 0.91 nm. A low sperm birefringence is associated with better pregnancy outcomes.[58]

The selection of sperms with partial birefringence increases the probability of selecting a sperm with a lower deoxyribonucleic acid (DNA) fragmentation. Therefore, selecting a sperm with a higher birefringence prior to ICSI may result in poor fertilization and pregnancy outcomes.[59,60] Visualization of retardance of the spermatozoa prior to ICSI, especially in patients with severe male factor infertility, may yield a better embryo development, implantation, and pregnancy.[61,62] Hence, sperm birefringence can be a real-time robust indicator for a healthy sperm.

## CONCLUSION

The PolScope has been proven to be a boon for assessing the oocyte as well as the sperm. It is a real-time, noninvasive method that can be easily applied in an IVF-ICSI cycle. The use of this specialized microscope is a valuable add-on technique to identify the oocyte or the sperm that has the highest chance in developing a competent embryo, ultimately to reach the goal of a single healthy pregnancy.

## REFERENCES


1. Sato H, Ellis GW, Inoué S. Microtubular origin of mitotic spindle form birefringence. Demonstration of the applicability of Wiener's equation. J Cell Biol. 1975;67:501-17.
2. Oldenbourg R, Mei G. New polarized light microscope with precision universal compensator. J Microsc. 1995;180(2):140-7.
3. Koike-Tani M, Tani T, Mehta SB, Verma A, Oldenbourg R. Polarized light microscopy in reproductive and developmental biology. Mol Reprod Dev. 2015;82(7-8):548-62.
4. Rienzi L, Ubaldi F, Iacobelli M, Minasi MG, Romano S, Greco G. Meiotic spindle visualization in living human oocytes. Reprod Biomed Online. 2005;10:192-8.
5. Montag M, Schimming T, van der Ven H. Spindle imaging in human oocytes: the impact of the meiotic cell cycle. Reprod Biomed Online. 2006;12(4):442-6.
6. Moon JH, Hyun CS, Lee SW, Son WY, Yoon SH, Lim JH. Visualization of the metaphase II meiotic spindle in living human oocytes using the Polscope enables the prediction of embryonic developmental competence after ICSI. Hum Reprod. 2003;18(4):817-20.
7. Hatori A, Takahashi L, Nakano H. Examination of the relationship between the invisibility or location of visualized meiotic spindle in living human oocytes and embryonic development after ICSI. J Mamm Ova Res. 2011;28(4): 219-23.
8. Otsuki J, Iwasaki T, Tsuji Y, Shiotani M. The nuclear phase of human oocytes during ICSI and nuclear transfer procedures. J Mamm Ova Res. 2017;34(1):31-6.
9. Petersen CG, Oliveira JBA, Mauri AL, Massaro FC, Baruffi RLR, Pontes A, et al. Relationship between visualization of meiotic spindle in human oocytes and ICSI outcomes: a meta-analysis. Reprod Biomed Online. 2009;18(2):235-43.
10. Picinato MC, Martins WP, Giorgenon RC, Santos CKB, Ferriani RA, Navarro PAAS, et al. The impact of examining the meiotic spindle by polarization microscopy on assisted reproduction outcomes. Fertil Steril. 2014;101(2):379-84.e1.
11. Fang C, Miao B, Zhong Y, Zhou C, Zhuang G. Meiotic spindle location and embryo development of in vivo and in vitro matured human oocytes. Fertil Steril. 2008;90:S333.
12. Kim S, Eum J, Choi WY, Paek S, Kwon S, Kim J, et al. Spindle position and second polar body orientation enables the prediction of embryonic developmental potential after ICSI. Fertil Steril. 2016;106(3):e325.
13. Avery S, Blayney M. Effect of the position of the meiotic spindle on the outcome of intracytoplasmic sperm injection. Hum Fertil. 2003;6(1):19-22.
14. Mahfoudh AM, Moon JH, Henderson S, Garcia-Cerrudo E, Son WY, Dahan MH. Relationship between pre-ICSI meiotic spindle angle, ovarian reserve, gonadotropin stimulation, and pregnancy outcomes. J Assist Reprod Genet. 2017;34(5):609-15.
15. Asa E, Tabatabaee R, Farrokhi A, Nejatbakhsh R. Relationship between meiotic spindles visualization and intracytoplasmic sperm injection outcomes in human oocytes. Anat Cell Biol. 2017;50(1):26-32.
16. Rienzi L, Ubaldi F, Martinez F, Iacobelli M, Minasi MG, Ferrero S, et al. Relationship between meiotic spindle location with regard to the polar body position and oocyte developmental potential after ICSI. Hum Reprod. 2003;18(6):1289-93.

17. Kilani S, Cooke S, Tilia L, Chapman M. Does meiotic spindle normality predict improved blastocyst development, implantation and live birth rates? Fertil Steril. 2011;96(2):389-93.
18. Kilani S, Chapman MG. Meiotic spindle normality predicts live birth in patients with recurrent in vitro fertilization failure. Fertil Steril. 2014;101(2):403-6.e1.
19. Dib LA, Araújo MCPM, Giorgenon RC, Romão GS, Ferriani RA, Navarro PA. Noninvasive imaging of the meiotic spindle of in vivo matured oocytes from infertile women with endometriosis. Reprod Sci. 2013;20(4):456-62.
20. Raju G, Prakash GJ, Krishna KM, Madan K. Meiotic spindle and zona pellucida characteristics as predictors of embryonic development: a preliminary study using PolScope imaging. Reprod Biomed Online. 2007;14(2):166-74.
21. Shen Y, Stalf T, Mehnert C, De Santis L, Cino I, Tinneberg H, et al. Light retardance by human oocyte spindle is positively related to pronuclear score after ICSI. Reprod Biomed Online. 2006;12(6):737-51.
22. Tomari H, Honjou K, Kunitake K, Hidaka N, Nishimura K, Nagata Y. Relationship between the meiotic spindle size in human oocytes and embryo developmental potential after intracytoplasmic sperm injection. Fertil Steril. 2014;102(3):e341.
23. Revelli A, Canosa S, Bergandi L, Skorokhod OA, Biasoni V, Carosso A, et al. Oocyte polarized light microscopy, assay of specific follicular fluid metabolites, and gene expression in cumulus cells as different approaches to predict fertilization efficiency after ICSI. Reprod Biol Endocrinol. 2017;15(1):47.
24. Polanski Z. Spindle assembly checkpoint regulation of chromosome segregation in mammalian oocytes. Reprod Fertil Dev. 2013;25(3):472-83.
25. Shen Y, Betzendahl I, Tinneberg HR, Eichenlaub-Ritter U. Enhanced polarizing microscopy as a new tool in aneuploidy research in oocytes. Mutat Res. 2008;651(1-2):131-40.
26. Tilia L, Venetis C, Kilani S, Cooke S, Chapman M. Is oocyte meiotic spindle morphology associated with embryo ploidy? A prospective cohort study. Fertil Steril. 2016;105(4):1085-92.e7.
27. Madaschi C, de Souza Bonetti TC, de Almeida Ferreira Braga DP, Pasqualotto FF, Iaconelli Jr A, Borges Jr E. Spindle imaging: a marker for embryo development and implantation. Fertil Steril. 2008;90(1):194-8.
28. García-Oro S, Rey MI, Rodríguez M, Durán Á, Devesa R, Valverde D. Predictive value of spindle retardance in embryo implantation rate. J Assist Reprod Genet. 2017;34(5):617-25.
29. Gomes C, Merlini M, Konheim J, Serafini P, Motta ELA, Baracat EC, et al. Oocyte meiotic-stage-specific differences in spindle depolymerization in response to temperature changes monitored with polarized field microscopy and immunocytochemistry. Fertil Steril. 2012;97(3):714-9.
30. De Santis L, Cino I, Coticchio G, Fusi FM, Papaleo E, Rabellotti E, et al. Objective evaluation of the viability of cryopreserved oocytes. Reprod Biomed Online. 2007;15(3):338-45.
31. Bianchi V, Coticchio G, Fava L, Flamigni C, Borini A. Meiotic spindle imaging in human oocytes frozen with a slow freezing procedure involving high sucrose concentration. Hum Reprod. 2005;20(4):1078-83.
32. Rienzi L, Martinez F, Ubaldi F, Minasi MG, Iacobelli M, Tesarik J, et al. Polscope analysis of meiotic spindle changes in living metaphase II human oocytes during the freezing and thawing procedures. Hum Reprod. 2004;19:655-9.
33. De Santis L, Coticchio G, Paynter S, Albertini D, Hutt K, Cino I, et al. Permeability of human oocytes to ethylene glycol and their survival and spindle configurations after slow cooling cryopreservation. Hum Reprod. 2007;22:2776-83.
34. Coticchio G, De Santis L, Rossi G, Borini A, Albertini D, Scaravelli G, et al. Sucrose concentration influences the rate of human oocytes with normal spindle and chromosome configurations after slow-cooling cryopreservation. Hum Reprod. 2006;21:1771-6.
35. Sereni E, Sciajno R, Fava L, Coticchio G, Bonu MA, Borini A. A PolScope evaluation of meiotic spindle dynamics in frozen–thawed oocytes. Reprod Biomed Online. 2009;19(2):191-7.
36. Potdar N, Gelbaya TA, Nardo LG. Oocyte vitrification in the 21st century and post-warming fertility outcomes: a systematic review and meta-analysis. Reprod Biomed Online. 2014;29(2):159-76.
37. Cobo A, Diaz C. Clinical application of oocyte vitrification: a systematic review and meta-analysis of randomized controlled trials. Fertil Steril. 2011;96(2):277-85.
38. Doyle J, Richter KS, Lim J, Graham J, Tucker MJ. 128 autologous post-vitrification oocyte thaw cycles: warming, embryonic development, and pregnancy outcomes. Fertil Steril. 2015;104(3):e271.
39. Chen C, Wang C, Tsai W, Hsieh L, Wang H, Soong Y. Evaluation of meiotic spindles in thawed oocytes after vitrification using polarized light microscopy. Fertil Steril. 2004;82(3): 666-72.
40. Yang Z, Chian R. Development of in vitro maturation techniques for clinical applications. Fertil Steril. 2017; 108(4):577-84.
41. Faramarzi A, Khalili MA, Agha-Rahimi A, Omidi M. Is there any correlation between oocyte polarization microscopy findings with embryo time lapse monitoring in ICSI program? Arch Gynecol Obstet. 2017;295(6):1515-22.
42. Moon J, Son W, Henderson S, Mahfoudh A, Dahan M, Holzer H. Spindle examination in unfertilized eggs using the polarization microscope can assist rescue ICSI. Reprod Biomed Online. 2013;26(3):280-5.
43. Tanaka A, Nagayoshi M, Tanaka I, Miki T, Yamaguchi T. Faster and more accurate improved rescue ICSI by observing changing size and position of chromosome and spindle using polarization microscope and differential contrast microscope. Fertil Steril. 2016;106(3):e344.
44. Wang W, Meng L, Hackett RJ, Oldenbourg R, Keefe DL. Rigorous thermal control during intracytoplasmic sperm injection stabilizes the meiotic spindle and improves fertilization and pregnancy rates. Fertil Steril. 2002;77(6):1274-7.
45. Pickering SJ, Braude PR, Johnson MH, Cant A, Currie J. Transient cooling to room temperature can cause irreversible disruption of the meiotic spindle in the human oocyte. Fertil Steril. 1990;54(1):102-8.
46. Merlini M, Konheim J, Gomes C, Baracat EC, Serafini P, Smith GD. Oocyte meiotic-stage specific differences in spindle depolymerization in response to temperature changes. Fertil Steril. 2009;92(3):S216.
47. Canosa S, Adriaenssens T, Coucke W, Dalmasso P, Revelli A, Benedetto C, et al. Zona pellucida gene mRNA expression in human oocytes is related to oocyte maturity, zona inner layer retardance and fertilization competence. Mol Hum Reprod. 2017;23(5):292-303.

48. Keefe D, Tran P, Pellegrini C, Oldenbourg R. Polarized light microscopy and digital image processing identify a multilaminar structure of the hamster zona pellucida. Hum Reprod. 1997;12(6):1250-2.
49. Petersen CG, Vagnini LD, Mauri AL, Massaro FC, Silva LF, Cavagna M, et al. Evaluation of zona pellucida birefringence intensity during in vitro maturation of oocytes from stimulated cycles. Reprod Biol Endocrinol. 2011;9(1):53.
50. de Almeida Ferreira Braga DP, de Cássia Savio Figueira R, Queiroz P, Madaschi C, Iaconelli Jr A, Borges Jr E. Zona pellucida birefringence in in vivo and in vitro matured oocytes. Fertil Steril. 2010;94(6):2050-3.
51. Montag M, Schimming T, Köster M, Zhou C, Dorn C, Rösing B, et al. Oocyte zona birefringence intensity is associated with embryonic implantation potential in ICSI cycles. Reprod Biomed Online. 2008;16(2):239-44.
52. Madaschi C, Aoki T, de Almeida Ferreira Braga DP, de Cássia Sávio Figueira R, Francisco LS, Iaconelli Jr A, et al. Zona pellucida birefringence score and meiotic spindle visualization in relation to embryo development and ICSI outcomes. Reprod Biomed Online. 2009;18(5):681-6.
53. Cheng J, Huang L, He B, Lu F, Wang X, Wu Z, et al. Quantitative analysis of the intensity of zona pellucida birefringence of oocytes during IVF cycles. Reprod Fertil Dev. 2010;22(8):1167-74.
54. Safian F, Khalili M, Ashourzadeh S, Omidi M. Analysis of meiotic spindle and zona pellucida birefringence of IVM oocytes in PCOS patients. Turk J Med Sci. 2017;47:368-73.
55. McDowell S, Kroon B, Ford E, Hook Y, Glujovsky D, Yazdani A. Advanced sperm selection techniques for assisted reproduction. Cochrane Database Syst Rev. 2014(10):CD010461.
56. Collodel G, Serena C, Federico MG, Pascarelli NA, Geminiani M, Moretti E. Natural sperm birefringence can be used to estimate sperm viability and morphology. Syst Biol Reprod Med. 2010;56(6):465-72.
57. Gianaroli L, Magli MC, Collodel G, Moretti E, Ferraretti AP, Baccetti B. Sperm head's birefringence: a new criterion for sperm selection. Fertil Steril. 2008;90(1):104-12.
58. Vermey BG, Chapman MG, Cooke S, Kilani S. The relationship between sperm head retardance using polarized light microscopy and clinical outcomes. Reprod Biomed Online. 2015;30(1):67-73.
59. Magli MC, Crippa A, Muzii L, Boudjema E, Capoti A, Scaravelli G, et al. Head birefringence properties are associated with acrosome reaction, sperm motility and morphology. Reprod Biomed Online. 2012;24(3):352-9.
60. Petersen CG, Vagnini LD, Mauri AL, Massaro FC, Cavagna M, Baruffi RLR, et al. Relationship between DNA damage and sperm head birefringence. Reprod Biomed Online. 2011;22(6):583-9.
61. Gianaroli L, Magli MC, Ferraretti AP, Crippa A, Lappi M, Capitani S, et al. Birefringence characteristics in sperm heads allow for the selection of reacted spermatozoa for intracytoplasmic sperm injection. Fertil Steril. 2010;93(3): 807-13.
62. Garolla A, Cosci I, Menegazzo M, De Palo R, Ambrosini G, Sartini B, et al. Sperm selected by both birefringence and motile sperm organelle morphology examination have reduced deoxyribonucleic acid fragmentation. Fertil Steril. 2014;101(3):647-52.

CHAPTER 117

# OMICS in Assisted Reproductive Technology

*Syed Waseem Andrabi, Nivita Gugnani*

## INTRODUCTION

Approximately 15% of couples in the reproductive age are affected by infertility, which not only has significant medical and financial, but also many social implications. The number of couples opting for assisted reproductive technology (ART) is steadily increasing, to an extent, that, nearly four million babies have been born since the born of first in vitro fertilization (IVF) baby back in 1978. Although, ART does not overcome infertility completely, but it is like that light at the end of the tunnel for couples struggling to achieve their dream of parenthood.

The outcome of any ART procedure depends on multiple factors but, its ultimately the embryos, cultured inside the laboratory which are transferred into the female partner that play an important role in determining the overall outcome. Although, assessment of gametes and embryos can provide an idea about the overall outcome, however, even best of the best embryos with top grades, do not necessarily implant and vice-versa. Therefore, it is impossible to determine morphologically whether an embryo will result into a successful pregnancy or not.

The overall understanding of molecular physiology of endometrium, germ cells, embryo, and culture conditions is still very limited, but advancement in biotechnology over the last two decades has led to the emergence of new high-throughput techniques, generally grouped under the term "OMICS". Successful implantation of any embryo involves multiple events and is a consequence of regulated expression of embryonic and endometrial gene product. Diagnostic methods based on molecular interactions might be an encouraging tool for such assessments. So, owing to the simultaneous analysis of thousands of molecules in a single biological sample, OMICS approaches offer a global view of different biological processes, wherein particularly functional genomics is being used to determine information about the DNA sequence (Genomics), the mRNA (Transcriptomics), proteins encoded by mRNA (Proteomics) and the metabolic products (Metabolomics) **(Fig. 1)**. This, in

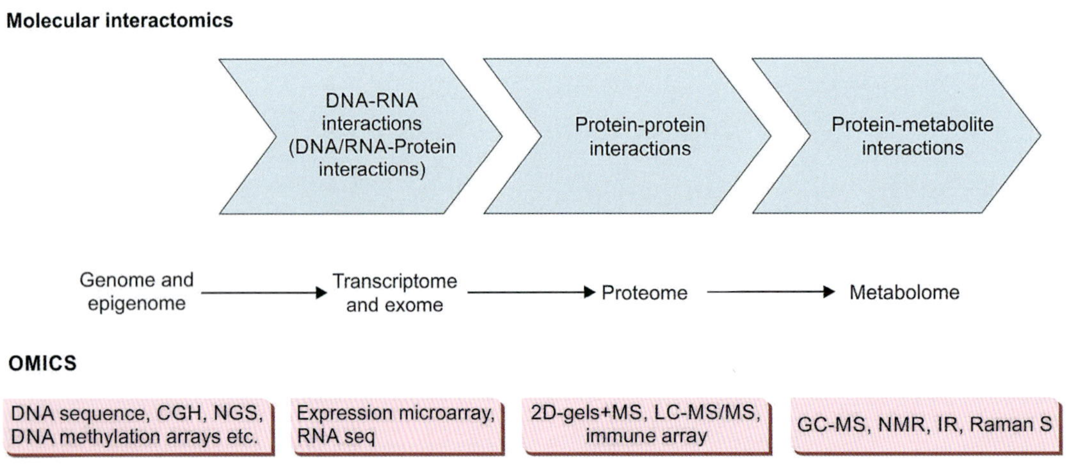


**Fig. 1:** Basic overview of OMICS.
(CGH: comparative genomic hybridization; GC: gas chromatography; IR: infrared spectroscopy; LC: liquid chromatography; MS: mass spectrometry; NGS: next generation sequencing; NMR: nuclear magnetic resonance)

turn is helping in decoding the complexity and behavior of biological systems.

The applications of OMICS in ART have become feasible due to the sensitivity, resolution and throughput of OMICS based assays, with the three most developed OMICS technologies being transcriptomics, proteomics and metabolomics. These technologies provide the platform to analyses all classes of biological molecules at different levels, that is, messenger RNA, proteins and metabolites using various techniques such as DNA sequencing for genomics; mass spectroscopy and protein microarray for proteomics; DNA microarray and real-time polymerase chain reaction (RTPCR) for transcriptomics; and Raman's infrared, proton nuclear magnetic resonance, near-infrared spectroscopy (NIR), and mass spectrometry (MS) technique for metabolites. Among these, metabolomic and proteomic approaches are emerging as promising noninvasive technologies for the evaluation of embryo viability.

The most important factor in any technology is the management of data, which in turn not only require proper planning but also great precision in order to produce reproducible data which can be easily translated into something biologically significant and OMICS fits this criterion through its expanding and more functional approaches. The example being exomics (analysis of exons), epigenomics (assessment of epigenetic modifications), secretomics (analysis of secreted products) and lipidomics (large-scale analysis of the whole lipid species).[1]

Studies of the interactome (entire network of molecular interactions in a system) and more integrative approaches, such as systems biology, are becoming increasingly significant in understanding the biological system and its activities as a whole, rather than a distinct component. OMICS and more broadly systems biology, are critical for the development of better diagnostic tools and treatments as they allow simultaneous investigation of numerous molecules. They are crucial not only in the determination of disease biomarkers, but they also provide information for a better knowledge of embryo implantation and pathological circumstances, with the goal of better patient care.[2]

## GENOMIC ANALYSIS

Analysis of embryonic DNA composition can provide insight into embryo viability by examining the number of chromosomes and their integrity. An abnormal chromosome in the form of aneuploidy in preimplantation embryos is believed to be the basic cause of implantation failure or embryo loss. Female age plays an important role in the outcome of any ART procedure, as advance age is directly linked to increase in incidence of aneuploidy in both oocytes and embryos.[3] Identifying and excluding aneuploid embryos can improve IVF results.

The three main methods for obtaining nuclear material for genetic analysis are polar body biopsy, the removal of one or two blastomeres from early embryos (cleavage stage biopsy) and biopsy of 5–10 cells from trophectoderm of an expanded day 5/6 blastocyst (trophectoderm biopsy). European Society for Human Reproduction and Embryology (ESHRE) labeled these techniques as preimplantation genetic testing (PGT).

### Fluorescent In-situ Hybridization

Previously, FISH, CGH, SNP-based arrays, and PCR SNP allele ratio analysis were methods used to study genomics. FISH was a frequently used method for chromosomal analysis, and the polymerase chain reaction (PCR) for the analysis of genes in cases of monogenic diseases. FISH was originally introduced in the clinic in 1992 using X and Y chromosome probes to treat families at risk of transmission of sex-linked disorders and to determine embryonic sex as an alternative to a PCR-based approach. In late 1993, the first FISH application for aneuploidy screening was run, and the number of chromosome copies of X, Y, 13, 18, and 21 chromosomes were evaluated as these chromosomal aneuploidies were mostly associated with birth defects. However, one limitation to this method was that the number of chromosomes that could be screened and the spectral resolution of the fluorescent dyes (red, yellow, green, light blue, blue). The chromosomes (16 and 22) most commonly associated with spontaneous abortion were then included with another set.[4] Irrespective of the stage of embryo biopsy, FISH technique has many drawbacks, one being that, FISH screens only up to 9–12 chromosomes and can detect only 60–80% of all aneuploid embryos. Given that aneuploidy does affect any chromosome, FISH cannot reliably detect a significant proportion of aneuploidy and segmental abnormalities present in the embryo. ESHRE and ASRM both stated that PGT with FISH was unjustified.

This problem was further solved by conventional comparative genomic hybridization array (CGH) where all 23 pairs of chromosomes were tested and copy number and entire chromosomal length details were analyzed. This comprehensive approach then provided a basis for array comparative genomic hybridization array (aCGH) technology and subsequently next-generation sequencing (NGS).

### Comparative Genomic Hybridization

Comparative genomic hybridization employs FISH principles by cohybridizing differentially labeled test and reference DNAs with normal metaphase chromosomes. But, in contrast to FISH, it allows for the assessment of chromosome copy number across the entire karyotype,[5] but with limited resolution.[6,7] This technique was first successfully applied to blastomeres in an IVF setting,[8] but was later described as tedious and time-consuming.[9] On the other hand, an aCGH (array CGH) involves whole genome amplification (WGA) and fluorescent labeling of samples where hybridization takes place on microarray (bacterial artificial chromosomes or synthetic oligonucleotides) instead of metaphase chromosomes and the results are further analyzed with specialized software such as Illumina. This method is not only fully automated and rapid but is also compatible with trophectoderm biopsy and subsequently allows fresh transfer. This has further been applied to polar body (PB) and cleavage stage biopsies as well (4).

### Next Generation Sequencing

Next generation sequencing (NGS) method is based on Omics technologies used to screen the entire embryonic genome with high accuracy, preventing the transfer of aneuploid (and possibly nonviable) embryos in poor-prognosis patients. NGS has slowly replaced CGH due to scalability and various other advantages such as assessment of aneuploidy, translocations, single-gene diseases, modest copy number variations, and low-level mosaicism (up to 25%) from the same biopsy sample while using the same platform technology. In this technique, WGA is followed by a barcoding step which allows embryo-specific sequences to be identified,[10] after which the amplified product is broken down into short sequence-ready fragments. For aneuploidy screening, these fragments are subsequently submitted to massively parallel sequencing with limited coverage. The number of reads per chromosome (binning) are then related to the number of copies on each chromosome, which is further used to determine aneuploidy. NGS allows a large number of samples to be evaluated at the same time, hence lowering costs and workload.[4]

Next generation sequencing has an advantage over aCGH in detecting mosaicism and triploidy and is an improved method with a positive impact on the clinical outcomes in terms of a decrease in the miscarriage rate.[11] In addition, it also collects both nuclear and mitochondrial DNA (mtDNA) in the same sequencing run.[12] Mitochondrial DNA has been proposed as a biomarker linked to implantation and embryo viability, as lower levels of mtDNA are being linked to higher embryo implantation rates.

### Epigenomics

Epigenetics, which is defined as changes in gene expression that occur without any changes in gene sequence can also be used in analysis of embryo viability biomarkers. With a major focus on long noncoding RNAs (lncRNAs) or microRNAs (miRNA), studies have analyzed some epigenetic modifications, wherein noncoding RNAs act as regulators of many target genes.[13] In a study of the expression profile of 12 miRNAs, it was found that aberrant miRNA in transferable blastocyst was linked to implantation failure associated with some specific infertility diagnosis. Data from a few studies also suggested that miRNAs might be an early indicator of the prognosis for human embryos of their development and that lncRNA has a regulatory role in embryo development and can be used as a marker of human embryo developmental potential.[14]

## TRANSCRIPTOMICS

Transcriptomics is the study of the level of mRNA expression in a specific cell population, which is commonly done using a high-throughput technique based on DNA microarray technology. Transcriptomics includes studying of almost fifty thousand known genes that are translated into RNA molecules. But, scarcity of human embryo material for research, particularly mRNA from a single biopsied cell has restricted transcriptomic research into the human embryos. Other probable reasons include plasticity of the embryonic transcriptome and the invasiveness of the process to obtain the biopsied sample.[15]

Microarray technology is a viable option and more recently, NGS has advanced the whole transcriptional analysis of an individual embryo. Exploiting these technologies, various studies have discovered distinct transcriptomes for each stage of preimplantation development in human embryos, with noteworthy changes before and after the maternal-to-zygote transition.[16-18]

While early maternal transcripts are primarily involved in the regulation of cellular processes necessary for the transition, those found in the blastocyst are mostly involved in cell proliferation and differentiation, as well as implantation pathways. In addition, a difference in transcriptomic analysis was observed between human aneuploid and euploid embryos.[19,20]

On the other hand, oocytes are delicate and examining gene expression profiles should be done in a way that does not harm them. Cumulus cells and granulosa cells, which are connected with the oocyte, can be investigated using a noninvasive oocyte mRNA microarray. Checking cumulus gene expression in oocytes serves as a marker and offers transcriptomics information about good quality oocytes, embryo potential, and successful pregnancy. BCL2L11, PCK1, and NFIB gene expression was discovered to be different in the cumulus of good morphology embryos that proceed into pregnancy, while VCAN, PTGS2, GREM1, and PFKP gene expression was linked to good quality oocytes, and oocyte quality can be predicted by the presence of cathepsins mRNA.[21]

Recently, several studies have also looked up at the transcriptome of SFC (somatic follicular cells) to see if there are any new biomarkers that can predict oocyte and embryo competency and/or pregnancy outcome.[22] This is one indirect but noninvasive approach suggesting that follicular environment, which is important for the maturation and acquisition of competence of a growing oocyte is influenced by bi-directional communication between the oocyte and its surrounding SFCs. These SFCs are exposed to the same environment as the oocytes they are linked with, which likely determines their transcriptome signature.[23]

## PROTEOMICS

Proteomics refers to the large-scale study of proteins, also defined as the "PROTEin complement of the genOME". Proteome is a complex and dynamic system that is always changing due to internal and external interactions and stimuli. It is made up of all the proteins that are translated from the transcriptome of a cell and are further responsible for the cellular activities. In order to attain a complete understanding of the cellular function and comprehend biological processes, it is important to investigate a cell's active proteome. Hence, various studies on changes in protein expression have revealed the underlying molecular mechanisms of physiological processes and disease states.[24] Because of the low protein concentration and huge number of proteins to be analyzed, embryonic proteome analyzation is extremely difficult. This, combined with a lack of sensitivity in proteomic platforms, has limited proteome investigations to the identification of specific proteins produced into the medium by the embryo.[25]

These problems have been addressed by some advances in MS as a result of which some sensitive, high-throughput methods have enabled the analysis of complete human embryonic proteome, detecting even the low molecular weight proteins. MS consists of an ion source that generates charged species in the gas phase and an analyzer that separates the ions based on their mass-to-charge (m/z) ratio. Electrospray ionization (ESI) and matrix assisted laser desorption/ionization (MALDI) are the two more commonly used ionization methods for MS analysis. The analyzer used in MS includes TOF, quadrupole, or ion trap. Ions that have been properly aligned by the mass analyzer are then detected and amplified, with the resulting data being processed through databases that predict the identity of the molecules based on their m/z ratio. Tandem mass spectrometry (MS/MS) provides more information about specific ions and is commonly used for protein sequencing.[24]

This technology is utilized as a proteomic platform to study the developing preimplantation embryo. Variation in protein profiles have been observed in early and expanded stage blastocysts as well as developing blastocysts and degenerate embryos.[25] In another study conducted on the protein profiles of human blastocyst lysates, it was discovered that degenerated embryos had a different proteome profile than growing blastocysts.[26]

### Microarray Analysis of the Proteomic Embryonic Secretome

In a study conducted by Dominguez and colleagues, to check the differential expression of protein in the secretome of implanted and the nonimplanted blastocysts using protein microarray, it was discovered that two proteins (CXCL-13, GM-CSF) were presumably consumed by implanted blastocyst.[27]

Subsequently, the same group conducted another study in which they proposed that, viable blastocysts consumed more IL-6 (Interleukin-6) than blastocysts that failed to implant, suggesting that IL-6 could be used as a potential predictor of good quality viable embryos.[28] Further, proteomic fingerprinting of individual human implanted embryos has also recently been combined with time-lapse morphokinetic analysis to create a superior embryo selection tool.[29]

### Targeted Protein-based Approach

When comparing ongoing blastocysts to arrested embryos, some proteins such as ubiquitin, apolipoprotein A1 and different hCG isoforms have been found to be differentially expressed in the secretome. However, the relationship between these proteins levels and implantation outcomes were not studied in these cases, so, additional validation studies are required before including their analysis in a noninvasive embryo viability assay.[2] A recent study also found that caspase-3 levels in the secretome could predict IVF outcome after transfer of day-2 cultured embryos. In future, it will be interesting to see if it can be a part of the decision-making process regarding which embryo to transfer for a positive pregnancy outcome. However, more research is needed to understand how these markers can be used in this context.[30]

## METABOLOMICS

The nutritional requirements and metabolic products of the preimplantation embryo at various stages of development have been studied, and their influence on the implantation process has been discovered. Therefore, human embryo metabolism has been extensively analyzed over the last three decades in order to help predict embryo potential. The majority of research has focused on the noninvasive quantification of a specific class of known metabolites used by the embryo, such as carbohydrates and amino acids. In the case of carbohydrate metabolism, while both pyruvate and glucose uptakes appear to correlate with blastocyst stage development, their relationship to implantation or pregnancy outcome is highly uncertain.[31,32] Hence, it was agreed that, carbohydrate metabolism cannot be considered as a suitable biomarker for embryo selection in clinical use.

Because of the differences in metabolic profile observed between embryos that grew into blastocysts and those that got arrested, specific quantification of amino acid turnover has also been proposed for selecting a competent embryo. Furthermore, some amino acids in culture media or the relative amino acid concentration are linked to the ploidy status of human embryos, as well as clinical pregnancy and live birth.[33,34] This correlation of metabolomic profile with the embryo viability has been validated in studies using media from embryos at different developmental stages after single or multiple embryo transfers. Fertilization rates and pregnancy outcomes were also linked to metabolic profiles of spent culture media from oocytes and follicular fluid.[2]

One of the most promising noninvasive methods for assessing embryo viability is based on measuring metabolite content in spent culture media as a clear reflection of its physiological or pathological status. Various platforms have been used to analyze the embryo metabolism. These include, gas or liquid chromatography (GC and LC, respectively) and/or MALDI coupled to MS, as well as nuclear magnetic resonance (NMR), Raman, or near infrared (NIR) spectroscopy. But due to the complex nature of embryo culture medium and low available sample volume, MS-based methods are considered ideal for this analysis. Vibrational spectroscopy is another technique for analyzing the metabolomic profile which is easily applicable for clinical use.[15] NMR is an efficient nondestructive analytical tool used for biomarker analysis, as it detects and quantifies specific metabolites within biological fluid or tissues. However, low sensitivity, high sample requirement and cost are some limitations associated with this technique.[32] Vibrational spectroscopy utilizes two approaches namely, Raman and IR, wherein scattering of electromagnetic radiation is measured by Raman spectroscopy while absorption of electromagnetic radiation results in an IR spectrum. Vibrational spectroscopy begins with exposing the sample to electromagnetic radiations which leads to the energy absorption by molecule's chemical bonds resulting in vibration to a large extent.[32]

### Follicular Fluid

Though NMR and tandem MS have been the methods of choice for the characterization of follicular fluid metabolome, but tandem MS has been found to be more sensitive and with the addition of different chromatographic methods, the number of metabolites that can be detected in the sample is increased. Studies have shown a significant correlation between low amino acid turnover in spent media of 4 to 8 cell embryos and development to blastocyst stage, while high turnover has been found to be an indicator of metabolic stress involved in the repair of damaged DNA, RNA and protein during development, further leading to embryo arrest. Furthermore, when individual amino acids were assessed, it was discovered that there is an abundance of glutamate metabolism in follicular fluid of oocytes that formed blastocyst. As glutamate is one of the main components of fluid in the fallopian tube, therefore it also promotes blastocyst formation.

Overall, the majority of the statistically significant metabolites have been observed to be downregulated in the follicular fluid of embryos that formed a blastocyst, hence supporting the "quiet embryo hypothesis" which states the importance of endogenous resources over nutrient supplementation in embryo survival.[35]

### Metabolomics and Semen

Seminal plasma has been the major area of focus for all the metabolomic studies of male infertility. It consists of proteins, amino acids, enzymes, fructose and other carbohydrates, lipids and major minerals and trace elements (such as $Zn^{2+}$, $Mg^{2+}$, $Ca^{2+}$, $K^{+}$ and $Na^{+}$) secreted by the testes, epididymis, and accessory sex glands and can be used as potential biomarkers for sperm quality. High levels of tyrosine, and phenylalanine and lower levels of alanine, citrate and GPC, and have been related to oligozoospermia (decreased sperm number in the ejaculate), while reduced levels of metabolites involved in phospholipid (choline), cholesterol, and nucleoside metabolism, as well as the Krebs cycle, have been linked to asthenozoospermia (decreased sperm motility). Furthermore, higher levels of citric acid, choline, D-glucose, tyrosine, alanine, proline, leucine, lysine, myoinositol, lactic acid, threonine, pyruvate, glutamine, valine, and isoleucine have been linked to teratozoospermia (an increase in sperm abnormalities),[36] but still more studies are needed to establish a list of sperm metabolites that can be widely used as biomarkers of male fertility.

Recent meta-analysis has shown that these methods such as near infrared spectroscopy in addition to morphology, do not really improve the live birth rate when compared to embryo selection by morphology alone.[37] According to a recent systematic review, there is no evidence to support the use of metabolomics in clinical practice to improve fertility outcomes.[38]

Also, despite the numerous published articles and their complexity, OMICS techniques have not been employed in IVF to identify good quality sperm. The procedures used to search for proteome or metabolomics fingerprints differ, and reproducible results remain a promise rather than an actuality, with clear diagnostic and/or quality signals still to be discovered.

## CONCLUSION

Despite the vast amount of biomarker data supplied by OMICS, there is still insufficient evidence to link data from all OMICS to better implantation outcomes. OMICS are reshaping our understanding of these complex processes by significantly increasing the identification of new potential biomarkers to characterize viable embryos and providing a large number of key molecules that can be used to help identify the molecular causes of implantation failures and other disorders. The use of next-generation technology in less invasive techniques, together with new complicated and integrative computer analysis, will most likely aid in the adoption of OMICS assays. As a result, OMICS technologies may aid in improving the likelihood of embryo implantation, resulting in much higher pregnancy rates and live birth rate while reducing pregnancy losses.

## REFERENCES

1. Altmäe S, Esteban FJ, Stavreus-Evers A, Simón C, Giudice L, Lessey BA, et al. Guidelines for the design, analysis and interpretation of 'omics' data: focus on human endometrium. Hum Reprod Update. 2014;20(1):12-28.
2. Hernández-Vargas P, Muñoz M, Domínguez F. Identifying biomarkers for predicting successful embryo implantation: applying single to multi-OMICs to improve reproductive outcomes. Hum Reprod Update. 2020;26(2):264-301.
3. Soini S, Ibarreta D, Anastasiadou V, Aymé S, Braga S, Cornel M, et al. The interface between assisted reproductive technologies and genetics: technical, social, ethical and legal issues. Eur J Hum Genet. 2006;14:588-645.
4. Griffin DK, Ogur C. Chromosomal analysis in IVF: just how useful is it? Reproduction. 2018;156(1):F29-F50.
5. Forozan F, Karhu R, Kononen J, Kallioniemi A, Kallioniemi OP. Genome screening by comparative genomic hybridization. Trends Genet. 1997;13(10):405-9.
6. Kirchhoff M, Gerdes T, Rose H, Maahr J, Ottesen AM, Lundsteen C. Detection of chromosomal gains and losses in comparative genomic hybridization analysis based on standard reference intervals. Cytometry. 1998;31(3):163-73.
7. Lichter P, Joos S, Bentz M, Lampel S. 2000 Comparative genomic hybridization: uses and limitations. Semin Hematol. 2000;37:348-57.
8. Wells D, Sherlock JK, Handyside AH, Delhanty JD. Detailed chromosomal and molecular genetic analysis of single cells by whole genome amplification and comparative genomic hybridisation. Nucleic Acid Res. 1999;27:1214-8.
9. Wells D, Escudero T, Levy B, Hirschhorn K, Delhanty JD, Munné S. First clinical application of comparative genomic hybridization and polar body testing for preimplantation genetic diagnosis of aneuploidy. Fertility and Sterility 2002;78:543-9.
10. Knapp M, Stiller M, Meyer M. Generating barcoded libraries for multiplex high-throughput sequencing. Methods Mol Biol. 2012;840:155-70.
11. Maxwell SM, Colls P, Hodes-Wertz B, McCulloh DH, McCaffrey C, Wells D, et al. Why do euploid embryos miscarry? A case-control study comparing the rate of aneuploidy within presumed euploid embryos that resulted in miscarriage or live birth using next-generation sequencing. Fertil Steril. 2016;106(6):1414-1419.e5.
12. Wells D, Kaur K, Grifo J, Glassner M, Taylor JC, Fragouli E et al. Clinical utilisation of a rapid low-pass whole genome sequencing technique for the diagnosis of aneuploidy in human embryos prior to implantation. J Med Genet. 2014;51:553-62.
13. McCallie B, Schoolcraft WB, Katz-Jaffe MG. Aberration of blastocyst microRNA expression is associated with human infertility. Fertil Steril. 2010;93(7):2374-82.
14. Rosenbluth EM, Shelton DN, Wells LM, Sparks AE, Van Voorhis BJ. Human embryos secrete microRNAs into culture media—a potential biomarker for implantation. Fertil Steril. 2014;101(5):1493-500.
15. Seli E, Robert C, Sirard MA. OMICS in assisted reproduction: possibilities and pitfalls. Mol Hum Reprod. 2010;16(8):513-30.
16. Dobson AT, Raja R, Abeyta MJ, Taylor T, Shen S, Haqq C, et al. The unique transcriptome through day 3 of human preimplantation development. Hum Mol Genet. 2004;14:1461-70.
17. Assou S, Boumela I, Haouzi D, Monzo C, Dechaud H, Kadoch IJ, et al. Transcriptome analysis during human trophectoderm specification suggests new roles of metabolic and epigenetic genes. PLoS One. 2012;6:e39306.
18. Yan L, Yang M, Guo H, Yang L, Wu J, Li R, et al. Single-cell RNA-Seq profiling of human preimplantation embryos and embryonic stem cells. Nat Struct Mol Biol. 2013;9:1131-9.
19. Licciardi F, Lhakhang T, Kramer YG, Zhang Y, Heguy A, Tsirigos A. Human blastocysts of normal and abnormal karyotypes display distinct transcriptome profiles. Sci Rep. 2018;1:14906-018-33279-0.
20. Sanchez-Ribas I, Diaz-Gimeno P, Sebastian-Leon P, Mercader A, Quinonero A, Ballesteros A, et al. Transcriptomic behavior of genes associated with chromosome 21 aneuploidies in early embryo development. Fertil Steril. 2019;5:991-1001.e.
21. Andrabi S, Mir J. Omics and ART. In: Laboratory Aspects of IVF and Andrology. New Delhi: Jaypee Brothers Medical Publishers (P) Ltd.; 2008.
22. Ouni E, Vertommen D, Amorim CA. The Human Ovary and Future of Fertility Assessment in the Post-Genome Era. Int J Mol Sci. 2019;20(17):4209.
23. Assou S, Haouzi D, De Vos J, Hamamah S. Human cumulus cells as biomarkers for embryo and pregnancy outcomes. Mol Hum Reprod. 2010;8:531-8.
24. Krisher RL, Schoolcraft WB, Katz-Jaffe MG. Omics as a window to view embryo viability. Fertil Steril. 2015;103(2):333-41.
25. Katz-Jaffe MG, McReynolds S, Gardner DK, Schoolcraft WB. Schoolcraft. The role of proteomics in defining the human embryonic secretome. Mol Hum Reprod. 2009;15(5):271-7.
26. Katz-Jaffe MG, Gardner DK, Schoolcraft WB. Proteomic analysis of individual human embryos to identify novel biomarkers of development and viability. Fertil Steril. 2006a;1:101-10.
27. Domínguez F, Gadea B, Esteban FJ, Horcajadas JA, Pellicer A, Simón C. Comparative protein-profile analysis of implanted versus non-implanted human blastocysts. Hum Reprod. 2008;23(9):1993-2000.
28. Dominguez F, Gadea B, Mercader A, Esteban FJ, Pellicer A, Simón C. Embryologic outcome and secretome profile of implanted blastocysts obtained after coculture in human endometrial epithelial cells versus the sequential system. Fertil Steril. 2010;93(3):774-782.e1.
29. Dominguez F, Meseguer M, Aparicio-Ruiz B, Piqueras P, Quiñonero A, Simón C. New strategy for diagnosing embryo

implantation potential by combining proteomics and time-lapse technologies. Fertil Steril. 2015;104(4):908-14.

30. Kaihola H, Yaldir FG, Bohlin T, Samir R, Hreinsson J, Åkerud H. Levels of caspase-3 and histidine-rich glycoprotein in the embryo secretome as biomarkers of good-quality day-2 embryos and high-quality blastocysts. PLoS One. 2019;14(12):e0226419.
31. Gardner DK, Wale PL. Analysis of metabolism to select viable human embryos for transfer. Fertil Steril. 2013;99(4):1062-72.
32. Uyar A, Seli E. Metabolomic assessment of embryo viability. Semin Reprod Med. 2014;32(2):141-52.
33. Picton HM, Elder K, Houghton FD, Hawkhead JA, Rutherford AJ, Hogg JE, et al. Association between amino acid turnover and chromosome aneuploidy during human preimplantation embryo development in vitro. Mol Hum Reprod 2010;10: 557-69.
34. Marhuenda-Egea FC, Martinez-Sabater E, Gonsalvez-Alvarez R, Lledo B, Ten J, Bernabeu R. A crucial step in assisted reproduction technology: human embryo selection using metabolomic evaluation. Fertil Steril. 2010;2:772-4.
35. Ravisankar S, Hanna CB, Brooks KE, Murphy MJ, Redmayne N, Ryu J, et al.. Metabolomics analysis of follicular fluid coupled with oocyte aspiration reveals importance of glucocorticoids in primate periovulatory follicle competency. Sci Rep. 2021;11(1):6506.
36. Lombó M, Ruiz-Díaz S, Gutiérrez-Adán A, Sánchez-Calabuig MJ. Sperm Metabolomics through Nuclear Magnetic Resonance Spectroscopy. Animals (Basel). 2021;11(6):1669.
37. Vergouw CG, Heymans MW, Hardarson T, Sfontouris IA, Economou KA, Ahlstrom A, et al. No evidence that embryo selection by near-infrared spectroscopy in addition to morphology is able to improve live birth rates: results from an individual patient data meta-analysis. Hum Reprod. 2014;3:455-61.
38. Bracewell-Milnes T, Saso S, Abdalla H, Nikolau D, Norman-Taylor J, Johnson M, Holmes E, Thum MY. Metabolomics as a tool to identify biomarkers to predict and improve outcomes in reproductive medicine: a systematic review. Hum Reprod Update. 2017;6:723-36.

CHAPTER

# 118 Intracytoplasmic Morphologically Selected Sperm Injection, Physiological Intracytoplasmic Sperm Injection, and its Clinical Significance

Mohammed Ashraf C

## INTRODUCTION

The selection of a single spermatozoon, its immobilization, aspiration with a microinjection needle, and injection into the cytoplasm of the oocyte began with the introduction of intracytoplasmic sperm injection (ICSI) in 1992 by Palermo et al.[1] Since then, ICSI is being widely used for the treatment of subfertility and is the treatment of choice for male factor infertility. The primary concern with regard to ICSI is the selection of spermatozoon presenting both motility and normal morphology based on the evaluation of its head, neck, and tail.

In ICSI, the selection of sperm is performed under an overall magnification of 400×, which makes it possible to detect in the living state, most of the sperm anomalies recognized by the conventional basic semen analysis, performed on fixed and stained samples. This magnification only allows the observation of sperms with major morphological defects, while sperms with minor morphological defects go undetected. This poses a major drawback as it affects ICSI outcome.

As a result, spermatozoon that appears to be morphologically normal under this magnification could still have numerous structural abnormalities[2] affecting the development of embryos and implantation rates **(Figs. 1A and B)**.[3]

In the literature, only a few studies have reported that there is no correlation between the percentage of morphologically normal spermatozoon and ICSI outcome.[4,5] This may be attributable to a lack of correspondence between the morphological evaluation of seminal fluid performed on random cells obtained from original semen or from the motile fraction and the real morphological aspect of the single spermatozoon selected for microinjection. Starting from these assumptions, it would therefore seem sufficient to identify at least one single morphologically normal spermatozoon for each oocyte insemination to optimize ICSI outcome.

Studies show that ICSI outcomes are significantly influenced by individual sperm morphology.[6] De Vos and colleagues reported that when individual sperm morphology was assessed at the time of ICSI, it had an effect

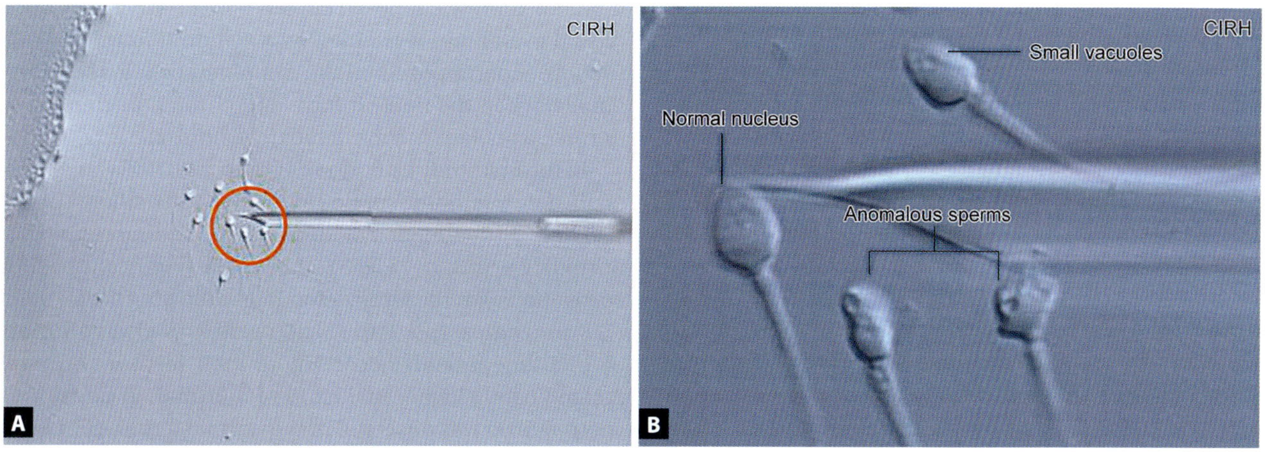


**Figs. 1A and B:** (A) Intracytoplasmic sperm injection (ICSI) at 400×; (B) Intracytoplasmic morphologically selected sperm injection at 8,000×.
*Source:* Adapted from Center for Infertility and Human Reproduction (CIRH). Barcelona, SPAIN.

on the fertilization rate but showed no effects on the embryo development. Implantation rates were lower only when injected with abnormal spermatozoon. This assumption is very important because it can reflect the embryo chromosomal defects of probable paternal origin and was recently confirmed in a shared oocyte model.[3,7,8]

Bartoov et al. in 2002 developed a new method of unstained, realtime, highmagnification motile sperm organelle morphology examination known as MSOME.[2] In MSOME, an inverted light microscope fitted with a high-power Nomarski differential interference contrast optics enhanced by digital imaging is used for achieving a very high magnification of 6,600×. MSOME when used with a micromanipulation system allows for the retrieval of a single motile spermatozoon with a welldefined morphologically normal nucleus to be injected into the oocytes. Since sperms cells are selected based on the morphology, this modified in vitro fertilization (IVF) procedure was named intracytoplasmic morphologically selected sperm injection (IMSI).[9]

## INTRACYTOPLASMIC MORPHOLOGICALLY SELECTED SPERM INJECTION

### Procedure

For semen sample preparation, the density gradient technique is preferred, and the motile sperm fraction was employed for further retrieval based on MSOME. Part of the motile sperm suspension (2–4 μL) is transferred to a 4 μL of a polyvinylpyrrolidone (PVP) medium and placed in a sterile, glassbottomed dish (GWSt1000; Biosoft International, Amsterdam, the Netherlands) covered with mineral oil. Adjustments of sample temperature and PVP concentration were made according to the intensity of sperm motility. When sperm motility was low, the sample temperature was raised to 37°C and no PVP was used, while 6% human serum albumin was added to the recipient droplet.[2] When the sample showed high sperm motility, the suspension temperature was reduced to 20°C, and PVP was added to a final concentration of 8%. In order to gain control of the moving sperms and facilitate their morphological evaluation, Bartoov created a series of small bays, extruding from the rim of the droplets, to block the heads of the motile spermatozoa **(Fig. 2A)**. Microdroplets containing sperm suspensions are subsequently observed under immersion oil under an inverted microscope.[2,9]

### Microscope Equipment

Bartoov used an inverted microscope equipped with Nomarski differential contrast optics, an UplanApo oil/1.35 objective lens, and a 0.55 numerical aperture (NA) condenser lens. This system is coupled with an image capturing high-definition color video camera, with a 0.5 inch, three-chip power holeaccumulation diode chargecoupled device (HAD CCD) containing some 380,000 pixels and a high-definition color video monitor for morphological assessment. The resulting magnification is based on four parameters:

1. Objective magnification 100×
2. Magnification selector 1.5×
3. Video coupler magnification 0.99×
4. Calculated video magnification (CCD × monitor diagonal dimension) 44.45×.

Therefore, total magnification = 100 × 1.5 × 0.99 × 44.45 = 6,600x.[2]

### Motile Sperm Organelle Morphology Examination Criteria for Intracytoplasmic Morphologically Selected Sperm Injection

A spermatozoon selected for IMSI is classified as morphologically normal if it exhibited a normal nucleus as well as an acrosome, a postacrosomal lamina, a neck, and a tail and did not present a cytoplasmic droplet or cytoplasm around the head.[2,9] The subcellular organelles were morphologically classified based on the presence of specific abnormalities, defined according to the arbitrary descriptive approach reported by Bartoov et al., by using transmission and scanning electron microscopy **(Table 1)**. The estimates of transmission electron microscopy suggest that the shape and content of chromatin determine the morphologically normal state of the nucleus. The criterion for the normality of nuclear form was a smooth, symmetric, and oval configuration. The estimates for normal means for length and width were 4.75 ± 2.8 and 3.28 ± 0.20, respectively. When the form presented a variation of two standard deviations in one of the axes (length: ≥5.31 μm or ≤4.19 μm; width >3.7 μm or <2.9 μm), it was classified as abnormal **(Figs. 2A and B)**. For rapid evaluation of the nuclear form, a fixed transparent, celluloid form of a sperm nucleus fitting the criteria was superimposed on the examined cell (chablon construction based on the ASTM E 19512). Similarly, a nuclear form was considered to be abnormal if one or more vacuoles occupied >4% of the nuclear area (visual evaluation was aided by a celluloid form of a large vacuole superimposed on the examined cell, if necessary). Finally, when the nuclear form and chromatin content are normal, a nucleus is considered to be normal.

In the first study by Bartoov's group, MSOME was applied on the leftover motile sperms fraction of 100 random couples seeking ICSI treatment. The mean incidence of morphological normalcy was 3.3% (±0.55), showing a significant positive correlation with the fertilization rates following the standard ICSI procedure ($p < 0.01$). The result was also confirmed by dividing patients according to their fertilization rates. A significantly higher incidence of morphologically normal spermatozoa was observed in the normal fertilization group (>60%, $n = 53$) than in the low fertilization group (<60%, $n = 47$, $p < 0.01$) **(Fig. 3)**.

**TABLE 1:** Specific sperm morphological abnormalities at the subcellular level according to motile sperm organelle morphology examination (MSOME) criteria.

| ***Nucleus*** | | | | | | |
|---|---|---|---|---|---|---|
| ***Shape*** | ***Chromatin content*** | ***Acrosome*** | ***Postacrosomal lamina*** | ***Mitochondria*** | ***Neck*** | ***Tail*** |
| Small oval | Vacuolar area >4% or the entire nuclear area | Lack | Lack | Lack | Abaxial disorder | Lack |
| Large oval | | Partial | Vesiculated | Partial | | Coiled |
| Narrow (<2.9 µm in width) | | Vesiculated | Disorganization | | Cytoplasmic droplet | Broken |
| Wide (>3.7 µm in width) | | | | | | Multi |
| Short (<4.2 µm in width) | | | | | | Short |
| Regional disorder | | | | | | |

*Source:* Adapted with permission from Bartoov et al. (2002).[2]

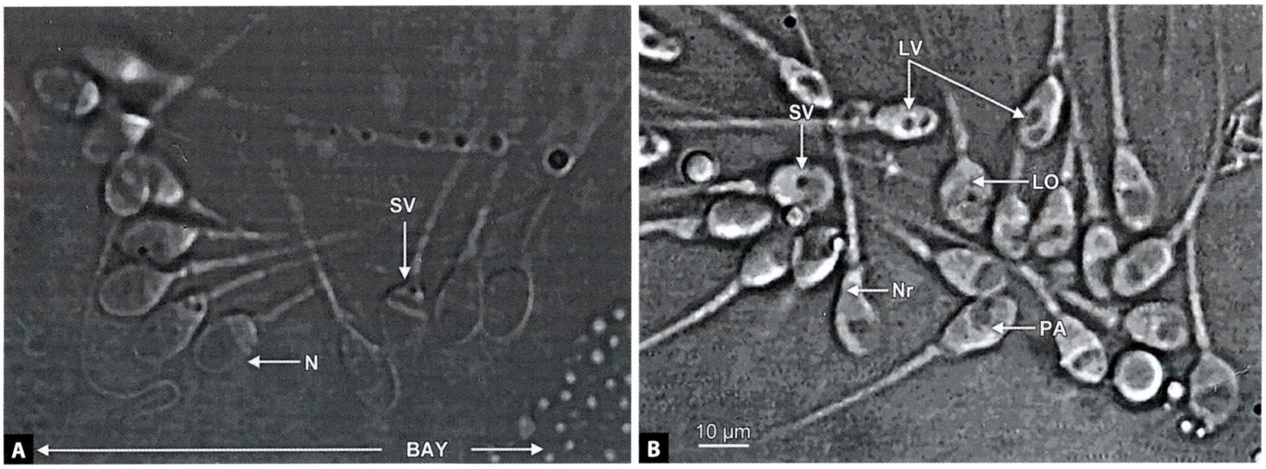


**Figs. 2A and B:** High-power light microscope micrograph of motile sperm (6,500×). The sperm heads were captured in small bays (BAY) extruding from the rim of the droplets.
(LO: large oval sperm cells; LV: large nuclear vacuoles; N: morphologically normal spermatozoa; Nr: spermatozoa with a narrow postacrosomal region; PA: partial acrosome; SV: small nuclear vacuoles)

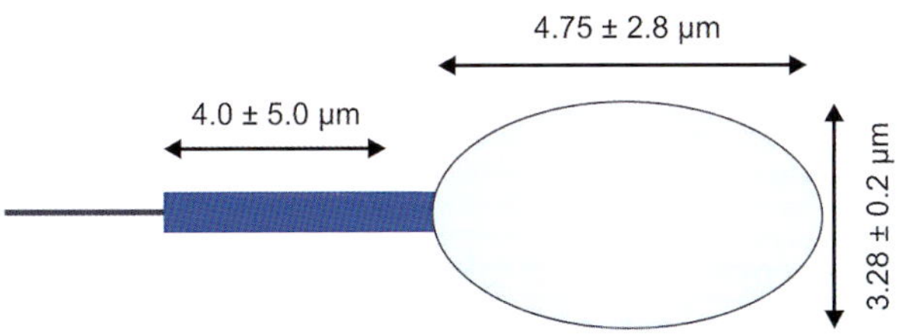


**Fig. 3:** Schematic representation of dimensions of normal spermatozoa according to Bartoov criteria.

The authors demonstrated that among the group of subcellular organelles examined by MSOME, only the morphological normalcy of the sperm nucleus had a positive correlation with fertilization.

## Selection of Vacuole-Free Sperm (Pathological Aspects of Nuclear Vacuoles)

Vacuoles are similar to liquid bubbles observed in the nucleus of a sperm's head. Their presence has been correlated with deoxyribonucleic acid (DNA) anomalies. Vacuole is a sign of molecular defects caused by abnormalities of sperm chromatin packaging and anomalous chromatin remodeling during sperm maturation;[10,11] such defects make the spermatozoa more susceptible to DNA damage. Research shows that the integrity of the chromatin is correlated with the presence or absence of vacuoles in the head of spermatozoa, and defective chromatin compaction makes DNA more susceptible to reactive oxygen species.[12,13] Patients with teratozoospermia index have sperm vacuoles exclusively in the nucleus and are preferentially situated in the anterior part of the sperm head.[14] The chromatin containing large vacuoles was unusually decondensed and showed a high level of immaturity.

## Midpiece Selection

Motile sperm organelle morphology examination allows the detection of midpiece selection and other abnormalities leading to infertility. Ugajin et al. were able to demarcate between a straightshaped and taperingshaped midpiece.[15] The taperingshaped midpiece is a result of aberrant microtubule organization and is thus associated with abnormal centrosomal function,[16] stated that after the nucleus, the centriole plays a vital role in the initiation of the intracytoplasmic fertilization process, as it is responsible for the development of the sperm aster. The dysfunction of centrosomes results in fertilization failure due to the absence of a sperm aster. IMSI allows for the selection of sperms with morphologically straight midpiece where the sperms will have functional centrosomes and therefore increases the rate of fertilization and enhances embryo development post ICSI.

## Vacuoles and Embryo Development (Full Benefit of Intracytoplasmic Morphologically Selected Sperm Injection is Attained with Blastocyst)

The selection of morphologically good-quality spermatozoa by IMSI yields a better embryo quality and higher blastocyst per cycle.[17] The nuclear vacuoles can have a negative impact on human embryo development as the presence of these vacuoles is related to sperm DNA damage. Hence, the embryo development, pregnancy, miscarriage, and malformation are affected by the selected spermatozoa.

Intracytoplasmic morphologically selected sperm injection reduces abortion rates by 50%. Prolonging embryo culture till blastocyst stage (5 days) can serve as a strong diagnostic tool, reflecting genomic activation and providing information on the implantation potential of human embryos.[17,18]

## Clinical Significance of Intracytoplasmic Morphologically Selected Sperm Injection

Many studies report that the morphological quality of the spermatozoa used plays a vital role in the fertilization, implantation, and pregnancy rates in ICSI cycles **(Flowchart 1)**.[6,19]

**Flowchart 1:** Clinical significance of intracytoplasmic morphologically selected sperm injection (IMSI).

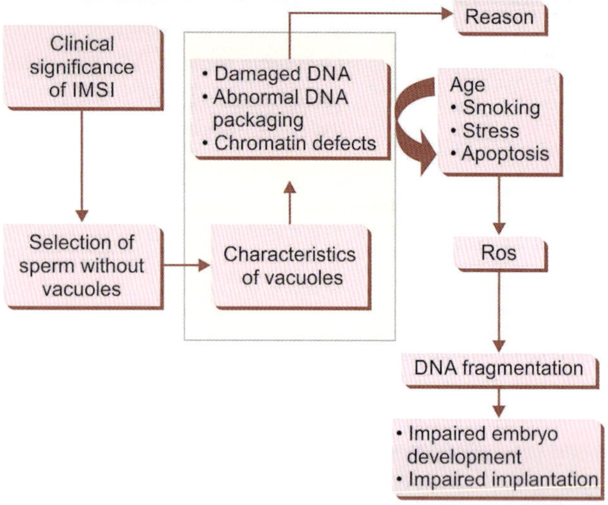


(DNA: deoxyribonucleic acid; ROS: reactive oxygen species)

According to Berkovitz et al., the use of the best ultrastructural morphology sperm in IMSI showed a significant difference in the clinical results over conventional ICSI. The morphological features that had the most detrimental effect on the clinical outcome were the presence of large vacuoles.[20,21]

In a recent metaanalysis comparing ICSI versus IMSI outcome,[22] three studies comprising 357 IMSI cycles and 349 ICSI cycles[9,20,23] were considered. Only the fertilization rate was comparable between the ICSI and IMSI groups (76.7 vs. 75.7%) [odds ratio (OR) 0.95; 95% confidence interval (CI) 0.81–1.11]. The overall results of metaanalysis for topquality embryo (27.7 vs. 41.2%, OR 1.83; 95% CI 1.50–2.24), implantation rate (10.5 vs. 21.9%, OR 1.50–4.95), pregnancy rate (26.6 vs. 47.6%, OR 3.12; 95% CI 1.55–6.26), and miscarriage rate (29 vs. 14.7%, OR 0.42; 95% CI 23–0.78) were all in favor of IMSI.

The weakness of this metaanalysis is the variable study's characteristics. Only one randomized control study was included in this analysis.

In a recent prospective randomized study, 24 a comparison between the clinical outcome of 87 IMSI cycles and 81 ICSI cycles in an unselected infertile population showed that IMSI did not provide any significant improvement in the clinical outcome in comparison with the ICSI cycles. However, the IMSI group showed trends in higher implantation (28.9 vs. 19.5%), clinical pregnancy (54 vs. 44.4%), and live birth rates (43.7 vs. 38.3%). The significantly higher implantation rates, when compared with the ICSI groups (26.9 vs. 15.2%, $p = 0.01$), show that patients with severe male factor infertility benefit from the IMSI procedure.

## Intracytoplasmic Morphologically Selected Sperm Injection for All

Although IMSI is useful in selected patients, routine IMSI for all patients is not shown to be useful.[24,25]

## Intracytoplasmic Morphologically Selected Sperm Injection and Severe Male Factor Infertility

In a prospective randomized trial, the potential of IMSI over ICSI was assessed in the management of 446 couples with severe oligoasthenoteratozoospermia without considering the previous failed attempts. IMSI yielded a significantly higher implantation and pregnancy rates than those for ICSI (17.3 vs. 11.3%, $p = 0.007$ and 39.2 vs. 26.5%, $p = 0.004$, respectively) in cases where patients suffered from severe male factor infertility.[18] In subgroup analysis, the group with at least two previous failed ICSI attempts benefitted from the IMSI procedure in terms of clinical pregnancy rates (29.9 vs. 12.9%, $p = 0.017$). These results are even more valuable when there is restriction in the number of oocytes that were injected.

Spermatozoa showing nuclear normalcy were found to be significantly associated with the lower incidence of aneuploidy in derived embryos, resulting in lower rates of cycle cancellation.[26]

## Intracytoplasmic Morphologically Selected Sperm Injection in Globozoospermia

Globozoospermia is a condition involving premature elimination of acrosomal structures during spermiogenesis. Phospholipase C zeta (PLCζ), which is a decisive factor for the activation of oocytes by inducing $Ca^{2+}$ oscillations, will be absent in most of the globozoospermic cases and in turn results in fertilization failure. Some globozoospermic spermatozoa will have an acrosomal bud that possesses the total amount of PLCζ and is not invariably different from fertile controls, can be detailed with IMSI, and helps to achieve successful oocyte activation and fertilization.[27,28]

## Intracytoplasmic Morphologically Selected Sperm Injection in Previous Intracytoplasmic Sperm Injection Failure Patients

Klement et al. conducted a cohort study to find out the advantage of IMSI versus ICSI in the first assisted reproductive technology (ART) cycle and in consecutive cycles in male factor infertility patients requiring micromanipulation. A total of 1,891 IVF–ICSI and 577 IVF–IMSI cycles were included. The first cycle of IVF treatment showed pregnancy rates of 46 and 47% and delivery rates of 23 versus 30%, respectively. The second cycle following a failed ICSI cycle showed a significant rise in pregnancy and delivery rates in patients that opted an IMSI technique over a second ICSI cycle (56 vs. 38% pregnancy rates and 28 vs. 18% delivery rates). A multivariate analysis showed an approximately threefold increase in the chance for both pregnancy and delivery rates in couples opting IMSI after a failed ICSI attempt.[29]

In a prospective study of 200 couples with at least two prior unsuccessful ICSI, clinical outcomes were evaluated between 100 couples who were assigned to IMSI and 100 couples who were assigned to routine ICSI.[30] There were no significant differences between the two groups with regard to the rate of fertilization, implantation, and pregnancy rate/cycle. However, there is no statistically significant miscarriage rate (IMSI 15.3% vs. ICSI 31.7%), ongoing pregnancy rates (IMSI 22% vs. ICSI 13%), and live birth (IMSI 21% vs. ICSI 12%); the IMSI group showed better clinical outcomes.

## Intracytoplasmic Morphologically Selected Sperm Injection and Sperm DNA Fragmentation

The integrity of DNA is an important factor in the success of human reproduction. It has been clinically proven that the sperm DNA damage has a negative effect on reproductive outcomes. Studies show that the spermatozoa from infertile men possess significantly more DNA damage in comparison with fertile men.

A study by Franco et al.[31] evaluated the amount of DNA fragmentation in 30 unselected patients [by TUNEL (terminal deoxynucleotidyl transferase dUTP nick end labeling) assay] and the prevalence of singlestranded or doublestranded DNA (by acridine orange) in sperm cells with large nuclear vacuoles and in strictly morphologically normal sperms both selected at high magnification (8,400×). A significantly high DNA fragmentation was reported in large nuclear vacuole sperms than in normal sperms (29.1 vs. 15.9%, $p < 0.001$). When compared with normal sperms, the large nuclear vacuole group also showed a significant increase in the amount of single-stranded DNA damage (67.9 vs. 33.1%, $p < 0.001$). Hence with better sperm selection with IMSI, pregnancy outcomes can be improved in semen samples with high sperm DNA fragmentation.

## Intracytoplasmic Morphologically Selected Sperm Injection and Routine Semen Analysis

The correlation between MSOME and much commonly used morphological assessment by Tygerberg criteria was compared[30] by regression analysis of 97 randomly selected semen samples. It was postulated that despite high positive correlation between these two assessments, MSOME provides a much more strict evaluation criterion for sperm morphology since magnification at 6,600× reveals more fine nuclear assessment. In addition, MSOME focuses on motile sperm fraction only, and hence provides information on the fertilization and developmental potential of fraction referred for ART.

## Intracytoplasmic Morphologically Selected Sperm Injection and Prolonged Sperm Manipulation

As IMSI based on MSOME is a time-consuming procedure (average 1–1.5 hours),[10] a study was undertaken to verify whether the prolonged exposure at 37°C could impair the morphological integrity of the sperm nuclei. The morphological normalcy of sperm nuclei was significantly impaired after 2 hours of incubation at 37°C compared with initial rates (4.7 ± 2.8% vs. 6.8 ± 3.5%, $p < 0.01$). A similar detrimental effect was reported for the percentage of sperms with vacuolated nuclei, which was significantly higher than before (80.8 ± 7.2% vs. 75.0 ± 7.6%, $p < 0.01$).

On the other hand, prolonged incubation of sperms at a lower temperature (21°C) did not produce any significant morphological impairment. Hence, an incubation temperature of 21°C is preferred in case of extended sperm manipulation during MSOME.

## PHYSIOLOGICAL INTRACYTOPLASMIC SPERM INJECTION

Physiological intracytoplasmic sperm injection (PICSI) is a technique in which physiologically mature spermatozoa are selected based on their capacity to bind hyaluronic acid **(Fig. 4)**.

Hyaluronan is the primary constituent of cumulus oophorus layer that encloses the human oocyte. It is a biopolymer (polysaccharide) and is found in every human cell. Hyaluronanspecific ligand receptors are present in a mature sperm head that facilitates the sperm to unite to hyaluronan. In comparison, immature sperms do not tend to unite to hyaluronan as they lack these receptors. However, this advancement does not imitate the genomic integrity of the spermatozoa and its aptitude to deliver the best paternal contribution to the zygote.[32]

### Advantages of Physiological Intracytoplasmic Sperm Injection

Selection of sperm based solely on facade and appearance can be flawed as sperms that appear healthy could have chromosomal imperfections. Hyaluronic acid-bound spermatozoa have enhanced morphology and it could reduce the chances of aneuploidies.

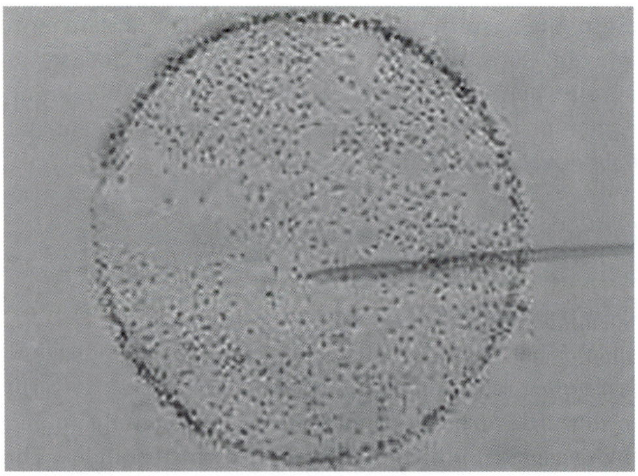

**Fig. 4:** Selection of hyaluronic acid (HA) bound sperms with injection pipette.

### Disadvantages of Physiological Intracytoplasmic Sperm Injection

In case of testicular sperm aspiration (TESA) sample, PICSI cannot be performed as immotile sperms are present and also in cases where occasional sperms are present (sperm counts ≤1 million/mL).

## PHYSIOLOGICAL INTRACYTOPLASMIC MORPHOLOGICALLY SELECTED SPERM INJECTION

Intracytoplasmic morphologically selected sperm injection is a technique that allows the selection of spermatozoa based solely on morphology, wherein highresolution optics and digital analysis are used to reveal morphological abnormalities in the spermatozoa,[33] while in PICSI, the sperm selection is based on the physiological maturity of sperm based on their capacity to bind hyaluronic acid. Wilding et al. in 2012 combined these two techniques and named physiological IMSI (PIMSI).[34]

The application of hyaluronic acid sperm selection techniques and morphological selection of spermatozoa with IMSI are not mutually exclusive. Therefore, they were combined into a new technique termed "PIMSI".

Idiopathic infertility continues to remain a "pathology" that is difficult to treat with ARTs. The main challenge in such cases is the selection of unfragmented DNA from an ejaculate containing high levels of fragmented DNA. In such cases, PIMSI can take a leading role by selecting the matured ones at first followed by performing their morphological assessment.[35]

## KEY POINTS

- Highpower morphological selection of sperms is rather a new technique offering an advanced mode of sperm selection. This becomes more important when the production of supernumerary embryos needs to be overcome for ethical, religious, or legal reasons.
- This procedure which is costly and time consuming has been mainly applied in a selected population of patients.
- The evidence at present shows that patients with previous failed IVF–ICSI cycles, severe male factor patients, and those with high sperm DNA fragmentation may benefit from IMSI compared to conventional ICSI by yielding higher pregnancy rates and lowering miscarriage rates.
- In addition, the PIMSI technique has the potential to be instrumental in treating patients suffering from idiopathic infertility.
- However, there is a need for more prospective randomized studies to confirm and correctly identify the group of patients that could benefit from these methods.

## REFERENCES


1. Palermo G, Joris H, Devroey P, Van Steirteghem AC. Pregnancies after intracytoplasmic injection of single spermatozoon into an oocyte. Lancet. 1992;340:178.
2. Bartoov B, Berkovitz A, Eltes F, Kogosowski A, Menezo Y, Barak Y. Realtime fine morphology of motile human sperm cells is associated with IVFICSI outcome. J Androl. 2002;23:18.
3. Tesarik J. Paternal effects on cell division in the human preimplantation embryo. Reprod Biomed Online. 2005; 10:3705.
4. Nagy ZP, Liu J, Joris H, Verheyen G, Tournaye H, Camus M, et al. The result of intracytoplasmic sperm injection is not related to any of the three basic sperm parameters. Hum Reprod. 1995;10:11239.
5. Svalander P, Jakobsson AH, Forsberg AS, Bengtsson AC, Wikland M. The outcome of intracytoplasmic sperm injection is unrelated to 'strict criteria' sperm morphology. Hum Reprod. 1996;11:101922.
6. De Vos A, Van De Velde H, Joris H, Verheyen G, Devroey P, Van Steirteghem A. Influence of individual sperm morphology on fertilization, embryo morphology, and pregnancy outcome of intracytoplasmic sperm injection. Fertil Steril. 2003;79: 428.
7. Tesarik J, Mendoza C, Greco E. Paternal effects acting during the first cycle of human preimplantation development after ICSI. Hum Reprod. 2002;17:1849.
8. Tesarik J, Greco E, Mendoza C. Late, but not early, paternal effect on human embryo development is related to sperm DNA fragmentation. Hum Reprod. 2004;19:6115.
9. Bartoov B, Berkovitz A, Eltes F, Kogosovsky A, Yagoda A, Lederman H, et al. Pregnancy rates are higher with intracytoplasmic morphologically sperm injection than with conventional intracytoplasmic sperm injection. Fertil Steril. 2003;80:14139.
10. Berkovitz A, Eltes F, Yaari S, Katz N, Barr I, Fishman A, et al. The morphological normalcy of the sperm nucleus and pregnancy rate of intracytoplasmic injection with morphologically selected sperm. Hum Reprod. 2005;20:18590.
11. Hazout A, DumontHassan M, Junca AM, Cohen Bacrie P, Tesarik J. High magnification ICSI overcomes paternal effect resistant to conventional ICSI. Reprod Biomed Online. 2006;12:1925.
12. Garolla A, Fortini D, Menegazzo M, De Toni L, Nicoletti V, Moretti A, et al. Highpower microscopy for selecting spermatozoa for ICSI by physiological status. Reprod Biomed Online. 2008;17:6106.
13. Boitrelle F, Ferfouri F, Petit JM, Segretain D, Tourain C, Bergere M, et al. Large human sperm vacuoles observed in motile spermatozoa under high magnification: nuclear thumbprints linked to failure of chromatin condensation. Hum Reprod. 2011;26:16508.
14. Perdrix A, Travers A, Chelli MH, Escalier D, Do Rego JL, Milazzo JP, et al. Assessment of acrosome and nuclear abnormalities in human spermatozoa with large vacuoles. Hum Reprod. 2011;26:4758.
15. Ugajin T, Terada Y, Hasegawa H, Nabeshima H, Suzuki K, Yaegashi N, et al. The shape of the sperm midpiece in intracytoplasmic morphologically selected sperm injection relates sperm centrosomal function. J Assist Reprod Genet. 2010;27:7581.
16. Van Blerkom J, Davis P. Evolution of the sperm aster after microinjection of isolated human sperm centrosomes into meiotically mature human oocytes. Hum Reprod. 1995;10:217982.
17. Knez K, Zorn B, Tomazevic T, Vrtacnik-Bokal E, Virant-Klun I. The IMSI procedure improves poor embryo development in the same infertile couples with poor semen quality: a comparative prospective randomized study. Reprod Biol Endocrinol. 2011;9:123.
18. Knez K, Tomazevic T, Zorn B, Vrtacnik-Bokal E, Virant-Klun I. Intracytoplasmic morphologically selected sperm injection improves development and quality of preimplantation embryos in teratozoospermia patients. Reprod Biomed Online. 2012;25:16879.
19. Chemes EH, Rawe YV. Sperm pathology: a step beyond descriptive morphology. Origin, characterization and fertility potential of abnormal sperm phenotypes in infertile men. Hum Reprod Update. 2003;9:40528.
20. Berkovitz A, Eltes F, Soffer Y, Zabludovsky N, Beyth Y, Farhi J, et al. ART success and in vivo sperm cell selection depend on the ultramorphological status of spermatozoa. Andrologia. 1999;31:18.
21. Berkovitz A, Eltes F, Lederman H, Peer S, Ellenbogen A, Feldberg B, et al. How to improve IVFICSI outcome by sperm selection. Reprod Biomed Online. 2006;12:6348.
22. Souza Setti A, Ferreira RC, Paes de Almeida Ferreira Braga D, de Cássia Sávio Figueira R, Iaconelli Jr A, Borges Jr E. Intracytoplasmic sperm injection outcome versus intracytoplasmic morphologically selected sperm injection outcome: a metaanalysis. Reprod Biomed Online. 2010;21:4505.
23. Antinori M, Licata E, Dani G, Cerusico F, Versaci C, d'Angelo D, et al. Intracytoplasmic morphologically selected sperm injection: a prospective randomized trial. Reprod Biomed Online. 2008;16:83541.
24. Balaban B, Yakin K, Alatas C, Oktem O, Isiklar A, Urman B. Clinical outcome of intracytoplasmic injection of spermatozoa morphologically selected under high magnification: a prospective randomized study. Reprod Biomed Online. 2011;22:4726.
25. Takeuchi T, Tanka M, Seida K, Oshima S, Nakamura T, Yoshida A. Is morphologically selected sperm injection useful for nonselected patients? Fertil Steril. 2009;92:S83.
26. Figueira Rde C, Braga DP, Setti AS, Iaconelli Jr A, Borges Jr E. Morphological nuclear integrity of sperm cells is associated with preimplantation genetic aneuploidy screening cycle outcomes. Fertil Steril. 2011;95:9003.
27. Gatimel N, Léandri RD, Foliguet B, Bujan L, Parinaud J. Sperm cephalic vacuoles: new arguments for their nonacrosomal origin in two cases of total globozoospermia. Andrology. 2013;1:526.
28. Sermondade N, Hafhouf E, Dupont C, Bechoua S, Palacios C, Eustache F, et al. Successful childbirth after intracytoplasmic morphologically selected sperm injection without assisted oocyte activation in a patient with globozoospermia. Hum Reprod. 2011;26:29449.
29. Klement AH, KorenMorag N, Itsykson P, Berkovitz A. Intracytoplasmic morphologically selected sperm injection versus intracytoplasmic sperm injection: a step toward a clinical algorithm. Fertil Steril. 2013;99(5):12903.

30. Oliveira JB, Cavagna M, Petersen CG, Mauri AL, Massaro FC, Silva LF, et al. Pregnancy outcomes in women with repeated implantation failures after intracytoplasmic morphologically selected sperm injection (IMSI). Reprod Biol Endocrinol. 2011;9:99.
31. Franco Jr JG, Baruffi RL, Mauri AL, Petersen CG, Oliveira JB, Vagnini L. Significance of large nuclear vacuoles in human spermatozoa: implications for ICSI. Reprod Biomed Online. 2008;17:425.
32. Worrilow KC, Huynh HT, Bower JB, Peters AJ, Johnston JB. The clinical impact associated with the use of PICSIderived embryos. Fertil Steril. 2006;86(Suppl 3):S62.
33. Nadalini M, Tarozzi N, Distratis V, Scaravelli G, Borini A. Impact of intracytoplasmic morphologically selected sperm injection on assisted reproduction outcome: a review. Reprod Biomed Online. 2009;19:4555.
34. Wilding M, Coppola G, Fabozzi G, Scotto Di Frega A, Di Matteo L, Dale B. Physiological IMSI (pIMSI) improves results obtained with IMSI in patients with idiopathic infertility. Reprod Syst Sex Disord. 2012;S3:001.
35. Petersen CG, Massaro FC, Mauri AL, Oliveira JB, Baruffi RL, Franco Jr JG. Efficacy of hyaluronic acid binding assay in selecting motile spermatozoa with normal morphology at high magnification. Reprod Biol Endocrinol. 2010;8:149.

CHAPTER 119

# Microfluidics in Assisted Reproductive Technology

*José María de los Santos, Thamara Viloria, Ana Cobo, Josep Lluís Romero, Marcos Meseguer*

## INTRODUCTION

In the last 30 years, human-assisted reproductive technology (ART) has profoundly changed. It is now a scientific field where novel research works continuously emerge, and it is becoming an exciting area to investigate and work in. Since the first in vitro fertilization (IVF) birth,[1] IVF cycles exceed 600,000/year and are performed in more than 50 countries.[2] Despite novel techniques and procedures, such as sperm isolation,[3] intracytoplasmic sperm injection (ICSI),[4] thawed embryo transfer,[5] optimal culture conditions assessment,[6] preimplantation genetic diagnosis (PGD),[7] oocyte vitrification,[8] and timelapse embryo quality assessment,[9] having improved from the very beginning, there are not many approaches that mimic in vivo conditions such as female genital tract and physiological changes. Indeed, the most commonly used culture system is microdrop medium culture with oil overlay in Petri dishes. Perhaps, for this reason, in vitro human embryo culture is inefficient. Although many efforts have been made to improve culture media and optimal microenvironment, physics parameters have not been considered in the majority of these studies. Moreover, the incubators, dishes and plates, and other devices currently used in human IVF have been rescued from cell culture procedures and have not been designed specifically for this objective. Microfluidics chip devices may be a new approach to solve this problem and might replace conventional human embryo culture in microdrops in the future.

At the beginning, microfluidic systems appeared as miniaturized devices designed for chemistry analyses and certain molecular biology procedures and were later used as cell culture platforms. However, some studies showed that it is possible to use them as an alternative to conventional ART; basically, these include sperm isolation, oocyte decumulation, IVF, embryo culture, and even microdevices in all the earlier steps.

Although microdrop culture allows autocrine factors retention around the embryo, it does not provide mechanical stimulation. The main property whereby a microfluidic system is advantageous as compared to conventional culture platforms is its behavior at the microscopic level. Turbulent fluid flow is usually observed on a normal environment scale; therefore, stream of fluid is unpredictable. However, if the physics parameters (density, viscosity, and velocity) are adequate and the microfluidic device is produced to take them into account, laminar fluid flow can be achieved. In this way, it is foreseeable to track a particle through it. Thereby, a continuous interface between different density fluids can be achieved by acting as an ideal surface to exchange gases, growth factors, and even cell isolation. The introduction of microfluidics into gamete or embryo culture systems is a change of paradigm as gametes or embryos stay in the same place throughout the process, while the culture media surrounding them can change continuously, thus minimizing harm to them, such as temperature or pH oscillation, osmolarity changes, shear stress, and preserving microenvironments around gametes or embryos.

Furthermore, there are some disadvantages involved due to excessive flow rate and the washing of autocrine or paracrine factors released for embryos, shear stress, osmolarity changes for culture media evaporation, etc. For this reason, it is very important to achieve a correct flow pattern, the complete refreshing or recirculation of the culture media, and the cell surface interactions required to correctly handle these microfluidic devices, which can be responsible for earlier unsuccessful experiences with such platforms.[10-12] Furthermore as regards culture media composition, efforts must be made because, nowadays, these culture media are designed for microdrop static culture systems. Thus, a new composition (subtracts, hormones, and growth factors) is required to improve those results. Currently, these platforms aim to operate along wide-ranging times with no manipulation, automatic fluid flow, and culture media control for each embryo development step (as with gravity-driven flow, syringe pump, and piezo-Braille pin actuation). An ultimate aim is to employ a system that is capable of combining the aforementioned qualities and which is, at the same time, able to use a video timelapse system for morphokinetics embryo assessment.

The objective of this chapter is to explain the different areas of ART where microfluidic devices have been used. Moreover, the authors attempt to summarize their design, results, and possibilities for future human ART use. They pay attention to those studies which they believe are the most interesting and didactic for students.

## MANUFACTURING MICROFLUIDIC DEVICES

Although a wide range of materials to construct micro-devices, including microfluidic platforms, have been used, plastic polymer platforms are currently the best option because they are easy to handle and are cheaper to produce as compared with other materials.[13] Specifically, the use of polydimethylsiloxane (PDMS) became the first option because its physical properties render it suitable for rapid prototyping and aqueous applications, and its use is compatible with biological systems. PDMS is nontoxic, chemically inert, colorless, and allows gas exchange. A commonly used microfluidic fabrication technique is polymer casting, also known as soft lithography or replica molding. Briefly, the steps to be taken are: (1) Casting a PDMS mixture on a silicon master, (2) curing by heat (65°C/2 h) and demolding PDMS, (3) bonding ($O_2$ plasma/30 s), and (4) adding glass slides and placing connectors for inlet and outlet ports.[13] Moreover, PDMS platforms have been tested to assess potential harm to mammalian and human gametes and embryos. These studies found no significant differences as compared with traditional culture performed by microdrops systems.[14-16]

However, there are certain restricting PDMS properties such as deformation, evaporation, leaching, hydrophobic recovery, and absorption that discourage its use in cell culture and ART, at least at naïve status.[17] For this reason, different PDMS pretreatments have been developed to solve these problems. On the other hand, bypassing the previous inconveniences, some authors argue thermoplastics as the solution. One of the most interesting examples is polystyrene (PS), widely used for cell culture and ART. The PS handicaps include mold fabrication, hot embossing, thermal bonding, and inlet ports/outlet port creation, raising final production costs.[17] Some efforts have been made to reduce these inconveniences, and currently, there are some procedures able to have the best things of both options making PS platforms and devices of an efficient manner.[18]

## SPERM ISOLATION

Nowadays, two sperm isolation techniques, swim up and density gradient separation,[19] are used. However, there are studies that report deoxyribonucleic acid (DNA) damage and reactive oxygen species (ROS) release by these procedures.[20] Some attempts have been made to replace them with microfluidics prototypes, but we focus on what most interests us.[16] This microfluidic device is formed by two inlet ports and two outlet ports which, in turn, form one area with two parallel laminar flow streams. A gravity-driven pump generates fluid flow. It places the sample in the first inlet port, and it places fresh culture media in the second inlet port. Therefore, an interface appears between the two flows, which only allows particles to pass by diffusion or by active movement such as motile sperm. In this way, the first outlet port obtains debris, round cells, and nonmotile sperm, while the second port acquires motile sperm **(Fig. 1)**. To test this microfluidic platform, unprocessed human semen, which was artificially enriched with debris and round cells, was placed in the first inlet port (44% of sperm motility and an approximate 10/1 round cells/sperm ratio). As a result,

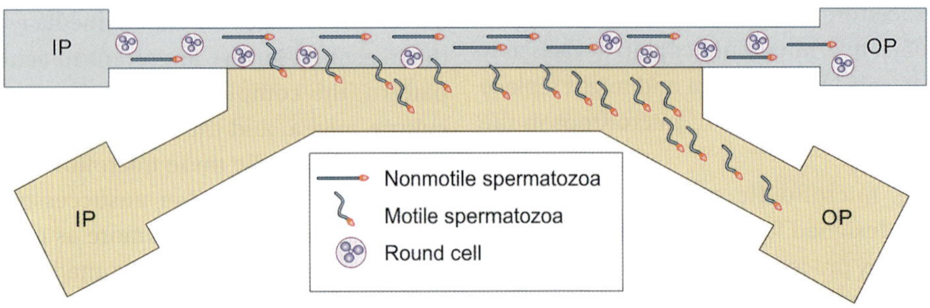


**Fig. 1:** Model showing a microfluidic device that is formed by two inlet ports and two outlet ports. It places the sample in the first inlet port (upper port, at left), and it places fresh culture media in the second inlet port (lower port, at left). A gravity-driven pump generates fluid flow. Motile sperm are able to swim between parallel laminar flow streams interface. In the first outlet port (upper port, at right), debris, round cells, and nonmotile sperm are obtained and in the second outlet port (lower port, at right), motile sperm is acquired. Model is not at a real scale. (IP: inlet port; OP: outlet port)

the sperm motility in the second outlet port was increased to 98%, and the round cells/sperm ratio was lowered to 1/33. Therefore, this novel device can act as a sperm isolation alternative because, at the same time, it was able to achieve both increased morphology and decreased debris/round cells. Nevertheless, its main limitation was its low volume processing at a rate of 20–40 μL/h. Although ICSI does not need total semen sample processing because the total sperm cell required for microinjection is low, we can consider that this device needs to be improved to be an alternative to other techniques.

## OOCYTES DENUDATION

Inevitably, the oocytes employed to perform conventional IVF or ICSI must be denuded. Basically, the oocytes retrieved after ovum pickup are cultured for around 4 hours. If ICSI is performed, oocytes are denuded to assess maturity and are microinjected as soon as possible.

Following conventional IVF, oocytes must be denuded at around 18 hours postinsemination to assess fertilization success. In any case, denudation implies stress to oocytes, so this is carried out by gentle repeated aspiration through several glass or plastic pipettes to mechanically remove cumulus and corona radiata cells. To reduce such stress, some microfluidics devices have been designed. Some experiences have been performed in bovine oocytes rendering good results.[15] These oocytes were placed on this platform 22 hours after conventional IVF by a standard pipetting procedure. The oocytes placed in the inlet port flow along the microchannel, and they consecutively pass through the contrition-conditioning areas. Then systematically, cumulus and corona radiata cells were trapped or aspirated by constricted microchannels or twin microchannels placed at a 90° angle to each other **(Figs. 2A to C)**. As a result, 90% of these zygotes were successfully denuded, and the mean time taken was only 20 s/oocyte. Moreover, these oocytes were apparently not injured because subsequent embryo development was not affected.

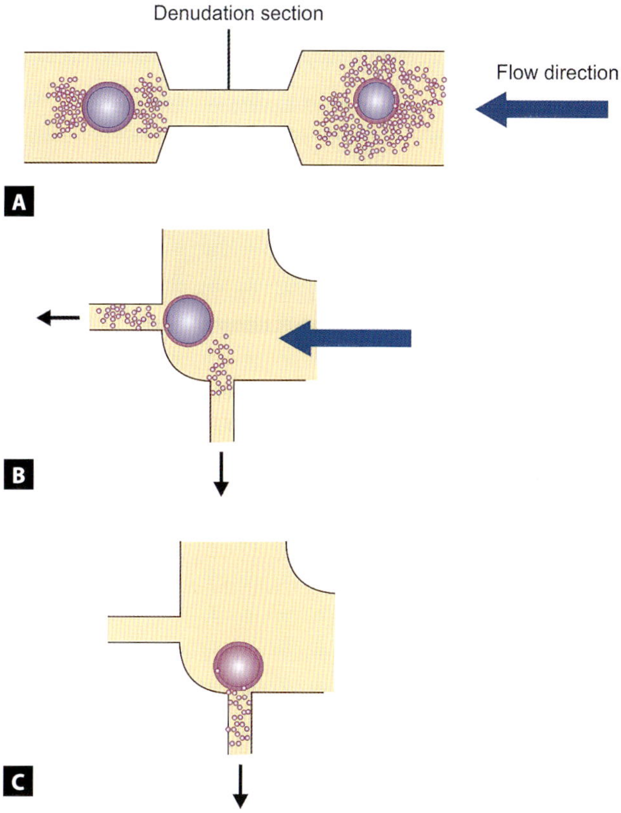


**Figs. 2A to C:** Model presenting a microfluidic platform for oocyte denuding. The oocyte placed in the inlet port (not shown in the figure) flows along the microchannel and it is denuded by the action of contrition-conditioning areas (A) or aspiration by twin microchannels placed at a 90° angle to each other (B and C). Model is not at real scale.

## IN VITRO FERTILIZATION

Conventional IVF is an easy procedure because if the sperm parameters are good, it is necessary to only adjust the sperm concentration correctly and then perform the insemination. Microdrops in Petri dishes and well-plate platforms with an oil overlay are widely used. The sperm concentration used in human IVF is around $1 \times 10^5$ motile sperm/mL, but total motile sperm depends on the total volume used. Thus, if we use 50 μL drops, the ratio is 5,000, this being the total number of motile sperm per oocyte. Thanks to this "easy-to-use" procedure, no drastic changes take place at all. However, is it the best microenvironment for oocyte integrity and future embryo competence. Many sources can produce ROS, such as oocyte or sperm metabolism, granulosa or corona radiata cells, and culture media.[21] ROS accumulation occurs during the insemination period because sperm and oocytes were coincubated for around 18 hours until fertilization assessment. In fact, DNA damage[22] and high ROS levels on the fertilization day were related to low pregnancy rates when conventional IVF was performed.[23] When performing conventional IVF, possible solutions for this problem can include a reduced coincubation time[24] or the use of microfluidics platforms as they offer certain advantages as compared with traditional systems (e.g., reduced total motile sperm required and diminished polyspermic zygotes formation).

One of these platforms consists in a funnel inlet port for media and gametes.[14] A microchannel (500 μm wide × 180 μm high) allows continuous media and sperm flow, retains oocytes, and at the same time avoids possible harm from oocyte deformation. Negative pressure and a gravity-driven pump acting by silicon tubes from the outlet port generate the fluid flow. To perform this IVF test, mice-denuded oocytes and capacitated sperm were used. Oocytes were pipetted to the inlet port, and flow was transported and

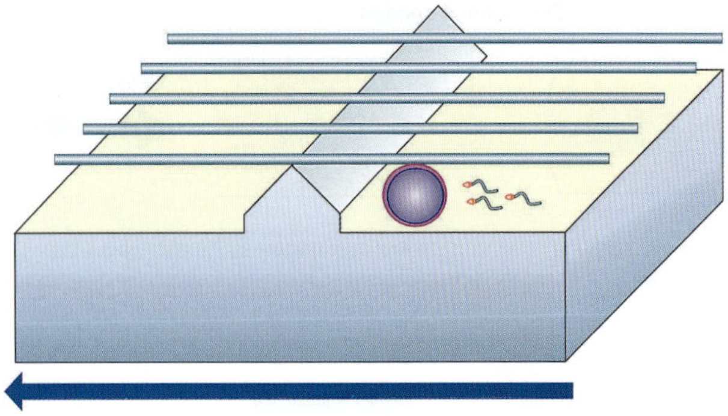


**Fig. 3:** This platform consists in a funnel inlet port for culture media and gametes. Negative pressure and gravity-driven pump acting by silicon tubes from the outlet port generate the fluid flow. Oocytes are pipetted to the inlet port (not shown in the figure), and the flow transports and retains them at the microchannel gate (as shown in the figure). Sperm is also loaded in the same inlet port and flows to oocytes along the microchannel. Static coincubation lapses are carried out to improve the interaction with them. Model is not at real scale.

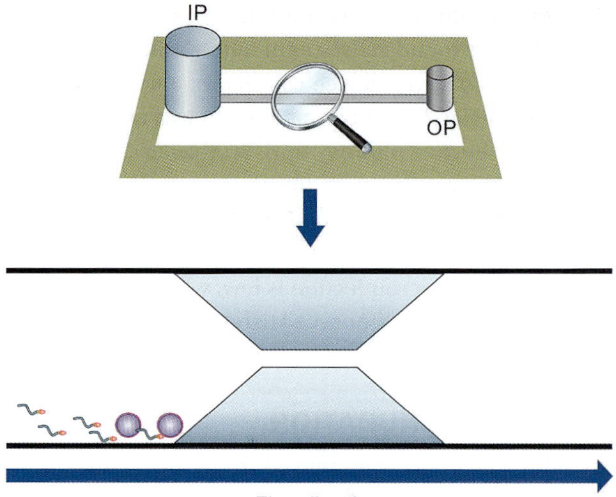


**Fig. 4:** Device consists in two opposite glass reservoirs, the inlet funnel port and the outlet port (upper picture). A microchannel is combined with them to allow sperm and oocytes' flow by a gravity-driven pump. Oocytes are located in the middle of the microchannel to be stopped by a constricted area. Capacitated sperm are placed in the inlet port and are carried to the trapped oocytes. Model is not at a real scale. (IP: inlet port; OP: outlet port)

retained at the microchannel gate **(Fig. 3)**. Sperm was also loaded in the same inlet port, the flow to oocytes goes along the microchannel (the total media volume used was 50 μL), and static coincubation lapses were carried out to improve the interaction with them. Conventional IVF in center-well Petri dishes was used as the negative control (the total media volume used was 500 μL). Moreover, to assess the potential harm of PDMS to oocytes or sperm, parallel conventional IVF was done with this material present, and no significant differences in the respective fertilization rates (42% without PDMS vs. 41% with PDMS) were observed. However, the fertilization rate in conventional IVF center-well Petri dishes using a standard sperm concentration ($1 \times 10^6$ sperm $mL^{-1}$) was higher than in the microfluidic device (43 vs. 12%, respectively). Interestingly, the microfluidic platform proves the best option to achieve better fertilization rates when the sperm concentration lowers, showing a plateau when concentrations between $8 \times 10^4$ sperm $mL^{-1}$ (10% conventional IVF vs. 27.1% microfluidics conventional IVF, respectively) and $2 \times 10^4$ sperm $mL^{-1}$ (10% conventional IVF vs. 27.4% microfluidics, respectively) were used. Knowledge of this phenomenon is interesting mainly for microdevice improvement and for future use in human IVF. Thus, it can offer possibilities to perform IVF to patients who can currently choose only ICSI because a decreasing volume with a constant sperm concentration reduces the total number of sperm required to carry it out.

Another problem encountered when using conventional IVF is polyspermic zygote formation[25] because it can achieve low polyspermic formation rates for microfluidics platforms as compared with conventional IVF.[26] For this study, porcine-capacitated sperm and in vitro matured denuded oocytes were used. Basically, the inlet funnel port and the outlet port device consist in two opposite glass reservoirs (10 × 10 mm). A microchannel (100 mm wide × 250 μm tall × 38 μm long) is combined with them to allow sperm flow by a gravity-driven pump, and at the same time, oocytes are located in the middle of the microchannel to be stopped by a constricted area. In this way, the microchannel allows sperm flow and mimics the oviduct tract. Oocytes were pipetted to the inlet funnel port, dropped to the channel, and rolled into the constricted area **(Fig. 4)**. During this time, 200 μm of capacitated sperm ($6 \times 10^5$ sperm $mL^{-1}$) were placed in the inlet port and were carried to the trapped oocytes by a gravity-driven flow to be mixed with 200 μL of fertilization medium in the microchannel. As a negative control, conventional IVF was performed by microdrop in Petri dishes with an oil overlay by adding 50 μL of the same sperm solution ($6 \times 10^5$ sperm $mL^{-1}$) to 50 μL of the fertilization medium drops. Therefore, the final concentration in both systems was $3 \times 10^5$ sperm $mL^{-1}$. When comparing 10 or 15 oocytes inseminated at the same time in both experiments, the results obtained were similar. The sperm penetration rate was comparable (96% microdrop vs. 88% microfluidics; 97% microdrop vs. 87% microfluidics), but the monospermic rate increased significantly when the microfluidic system was employed (22% microdrop vs. 55% microfluidics; 22% microdrop vs. 63% microfluidics) and gave a comparable male pronucleus formation rate (78% microdrop vs. 82% microfluidics; 80% microdrop vs. 73% microfluidics). Moreover, the mean sperm in the penetrated oocytes was significantly higher in the microdrop than in the microfluidic system (6.47 sperm/oocyte in microdrop vs.

2.03 sperm/oocytes in microfluidics; 7.39 sperm/oocyte in microdrop vs. 1.66 sperm/oocytes in microfluidics). Thus, this microfluidic system allows comparable penetration and male pronucleus formation rates, but significantly reduces polyspermy when performing an IVF with porcine oocytes. Likewise, the physical microfluidic system parameters can be responsible for these results because presence of flow can change the behavior and dynamics of the sperm around the oocytes. Moreover, oocytes can be stimulated by fluid flow, and a tridimensional microenvironment can simulate an in vivo oviductal tract architecture.

## EMBRYO CULTURE

We focus on one of the devices, presented as IVFLab 6, which uses microfluidics in an automated cell culture device for IVF **(Figs. 5A and B)**. The medium is automatically controlled to a flow rate of up to 20 μL/h, and two types of media can be used, which were automatically administered. Fresh medium is added to each well and waste products are removed. The flow conditions in the form of a shear strain rate and the local concentration of the new medium after 10 seconds of flow are presented in **Figures 6A to D**. The simulation is based on a hydrodynamic flow difference of 2 mm. **Figures 6A and B** illustrate the gentle conditions in relation to shear stress. By assuming that cells are placed in the middle and at the bottom of the well (level –2 mm, at the bottom of the yellow lines), the shear strain rates influencing cells are very low. **Figures 6C and D** show the local new medium concentrations (dimensionless). The graphs indicate the isosurface plots of different concentration levels and demonstrate how changing the medium in the wells is performed. The medium enters the wells along the least flow resistance path, meaning that the main stream is transported in and out through the channels, and that the transport which is perpendicular to the flow direction is a combination of diffusion transport and a slower drag flow. **Figure 6D** depicts the concentration plots for an imaginary axis in the middle of the well from the bottom (–2 mm) to the top (1.5 mm).

It is clear that the highest concentration is rapidly reached at the level of the channels. The transport to the bottom of the well links mainly to the diffusion process. As seen in **Figures 6A and C**, cells are placed in small wells; hence, there is a risk of high shear stress conditions and of reduced washing out of autocrine substances. When culturing cells to the blastocyst stage, many protocols facilitate the use of two different types of medium. The conventional way of changing the medium involves preparing a different Petri dish containing the new medium and then transferring embryos to the new dish by pipette. Moving embryos from one dish to another can prove harmful because cells are exposed to physical stress and changes from one medium to another are abrupt. **Figures 7A and B** show a computational fluid dynamics (CFD) simulation of the flow condition in a 200 μL pipette when manually changing the medium. It is assumed that it takes the user 2 seconds to fill the pipette, which results in a flow rate of 100 μL/s. The velocity field **(Fig. 7A)** and the shear strain rate field and a graph plot for the shear strain rate of 1 mm behind the inlet opening across the diameter **(Fig. 7B)** are presented. The highest velocities are reached at the smallest diameter close to the tip opening. Hence, the lowest shear strain rates are found in the center of the pipette. Yet, if we continue to compare the above levels reached, the rates are still about five times higher with the pipette.

Our research group tested this device (manuscript is still being actively written), analyzing 223 embryos from microdrops group and 234 from microfluidics dish, and we have observed that those who had optimal development on days 2 and 3, according to embryo culture dish, were statistically comparable (day 2: 56.9 vs. 52.56%; day 3: 57.14 vs. 55.45%, respectively). Optimal blastocyst quality

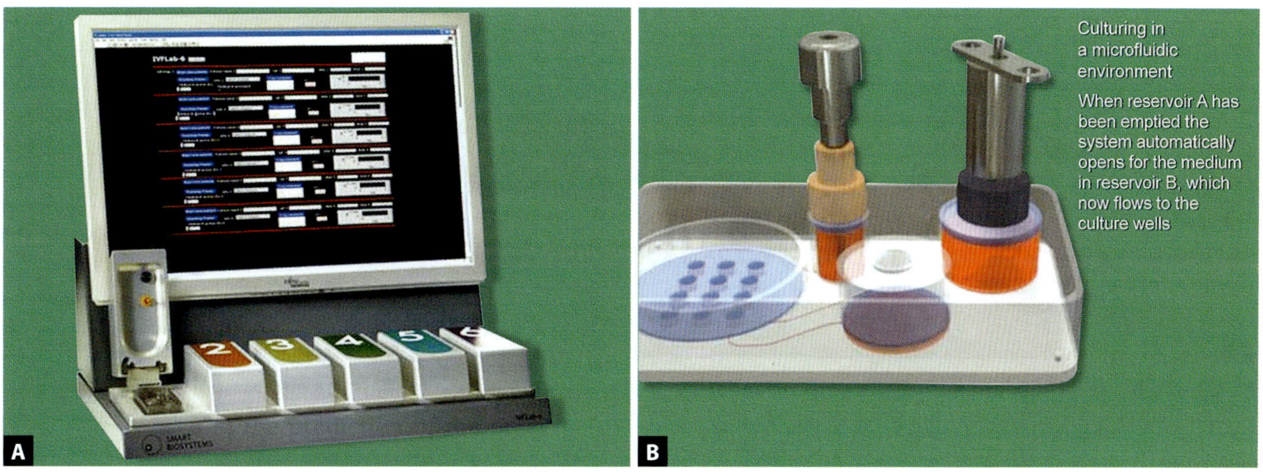


**Figs. 5A and B:** (A) Incubation chambers and software screen; (B) Microfluidic culture plate and culture media changing procedure model.

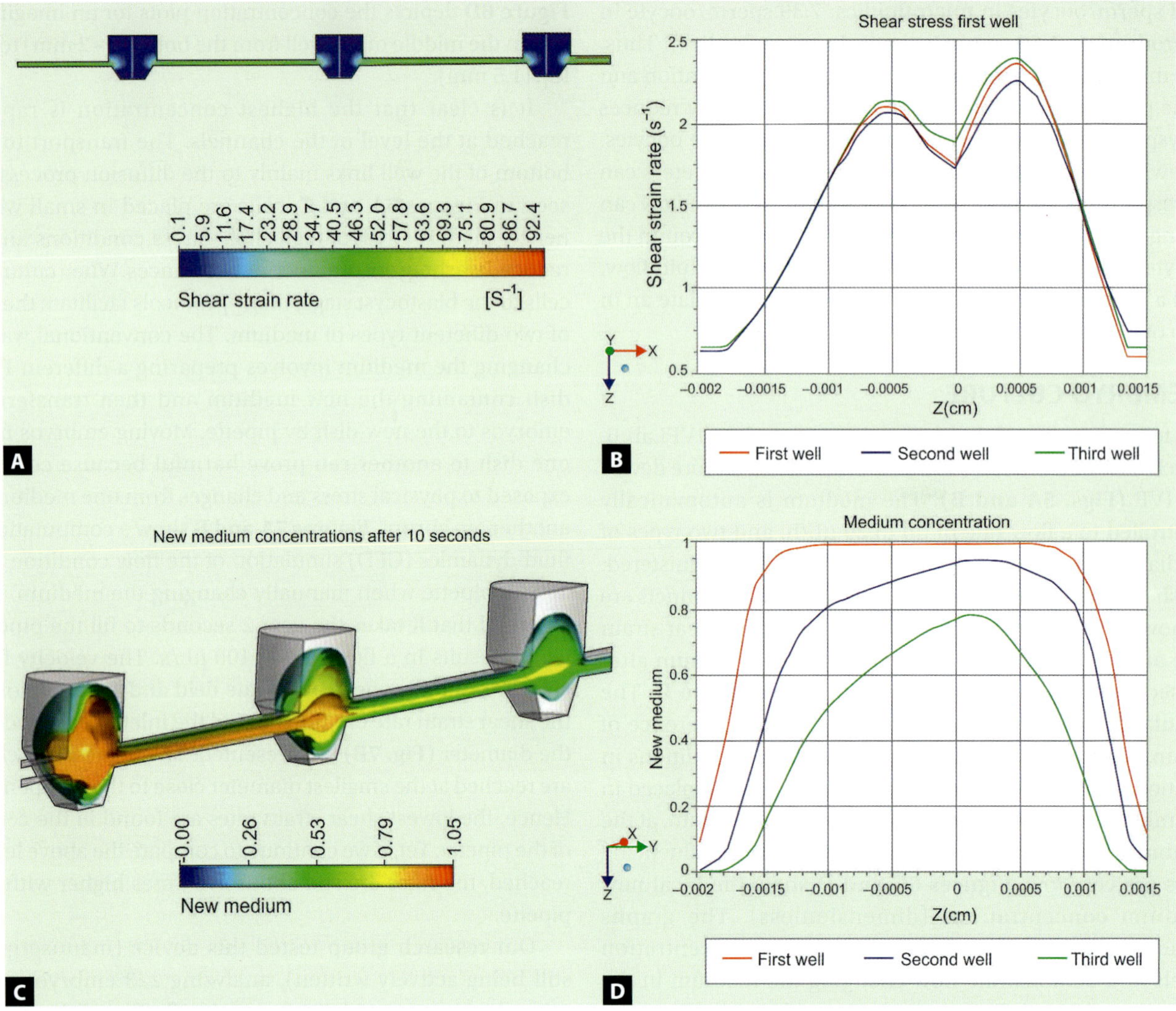


**Figs. 6A to D:** (A and B) the gentle conditions in relation to shear stress. By assuming that cells are placed in the middle and at the bottom of the well, the shear strain rates influencing cells are very low; (C and D) The local new medium concentrations. The graphs indicate the isosurface plots of different concentration levels. The medium enters the wells along the least flow resistance path, meaning that the main stream is transported in and out through the channels; (D) The concentration plots for an imaginary axis in the middle of the well from the bottom to the top. It is clear that the highest concentration is rapidly reached at the level of the channels. The transport to the bottom of the well links mainly to the diffusion process. Cells are placed in small wells; hence, there is a risk of high shear stress conditions and of reduced washing out of autocrine substances.

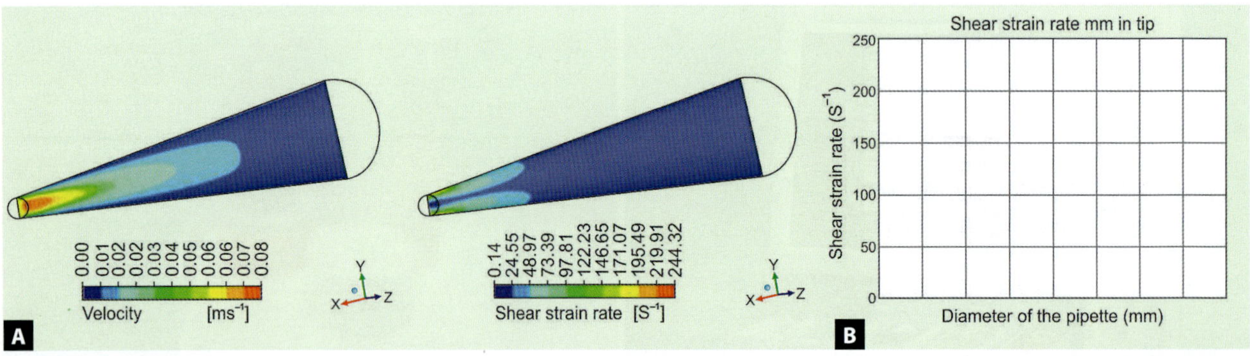


**Figs. 7A and B:** Computational fluid dynamics (CFD) simulation of the flow condition in a 200 μL pipette when manually changing the medium. The velocity field (A), and the shear strain rate field and a graph plot for the shear strain rate of 1 mm behind the inlet opening across the diameter (B) are presented. The highest velocities are reached at the smallest diameter close to the tip opening. Hence, the lowest shear strain rates are found in the center of the pipette. The rates are still about five times higher with the pipette than those observed in this platform.

according to embryo culture dish was significantly improved on day 5: 33.5 vs. 42.31% ($p < 0.05$) and similar in day 6: 29.03 vs. 31.51%,. However, implantation rates (IRs) were not significantly different between both systems in both groups (64.7 vs. 44.4%; $p = 0.199$).[27]

Another platform we can attempt to do embryo culture and automatic medium changing is described below.[28] In this microfluidic device, zygotes or embryos are cultured in microfunnels. Culture media changes are achieved by pump computer-controlled piezoelectric movable pins on a commercial braille display. The pump controls the fresh media flow from the inlet port to the culture funnels and to the outlet port. Moreover, a computer simulation analysis was performed to analyze fluid flow, shear stress, biomolecules retention, and microchannel dimension. Thus, two parameters were used to ensure an optimum flow rate. First, the epidermal growth factor (EGF) was employed as a beneficial factor model, and ammonia was employed as a waste molecule to calculate the mass production rate. Second, by means of two beneficial factors such as EGF and insulin-like growth factor1 (IGF1), the diffusion coefficient flow rate was calculated, defined as the volume with ligands which are accessible for receptor binding on an embryo. The microchannel dimensions were 1.5 mm long × 1 mm wide × 0.11 mm high, and the microfunnel dimensions were 0.25 mm bottom radius × 1.77 mm top radius × 2.63 mm high **(Fig. 8)**. Mice zygotes were used; female mice were placed with male mice overnight.

If mating occurred, presumptive zygotes were retrieved and isolated from the oviduct, and were finally decumulated. Three options to culture these zygotes were randomly chosen and performed: (1) Microdrop culture in Petri dishes with overlay oil, (2) culture in the microfluidic chip device with no fluid flow, and (3) culture in the microfluidic chip device with a fluid flow. All the platforms were placed in the same incubator and cultured under the same culture conditions. Embryo development was assessed at 96 hours of culture using two parameters: First, blastocyst morphology; second, the total cell number of each blastocyst by staining them with Hoechst 33342. As a result, blastocyst development was improved under dynamic microfunnel culture conditions. Therefore, the best hatching or hatched blastocyst formation rate was observed in the microfunnel-pulsatile model as compared with the microfunnel-static control and microdrop control (71, 23, and 31%, respectively) ($p < 0.01$). Likewise, the mean total cell blastocyst number was significantly higher for the microfunnel-pulsatile model if compared with the microfunnel-static control and microdrop control (109 ± 5, 60 ± 3, and 67 ± 3, respectively) ($p < 0.01$). It is noteworthy that the total cell blastocyst number was related in a time-dependent manner by improving blastocyst development when at least half the embryonic development of embryos or blastocyst was performed under dynamic flow conditions. All the previous results were consistent with the following because the blastocyst culture done with the microfunnel-pulsatile model offered the best IR ($p < 0.05$). Furthermore, normal pregnancy or development parameters were observed when they were transferred to the uterus. Based on these results, the authors claim that this microfluidic platform seems a very good model given the results obtained, which ensure that dynamic culture can enhance embryo development, and can improve the microenvironment as it retains the beneficial factor and washes waste molecules. Moreover, it should be taken into account that flow can break the gradients formed around gametes or embryos and can help the exchange of gases or metabolites. Finally, the physical stimulation due to the media flow can act on them.

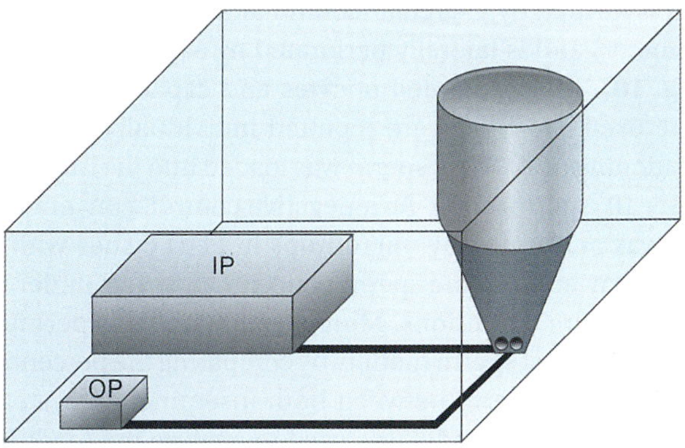


**Fig. 8:** In this microfluidic device, zygotes or embryos are cultured in microfunnels. Culture media changes are achieved by pump computer-controlled piezoelectric movable pins on a commercial braille display. The pump controls the fresh media flow from the inlet port to the culture funnels and to the outlet port. Model is not at real scale. (IP: inlet port; OP: outlet port)

## INTEGRATED PLATFORMS

### In Vitro Fertilization, Oocyte Positioning, Sperm Screening, Fertilization, Medium Replacement, and Embryo Culture by Microfluidics

Currently, there are very few microfluidic platforms that integrate all the IVF process steps. However, to achieve this goal, a research group is currently testing two microfluidic prototypes. The obtained design and results are promising. We now go on to look at how both experiments can prove to be the best attempt to integrate each step of the IVF process, oocyte positioning, sperm screening, fertilization, medium replacement, and embryo culture.

This first integrated microfluidic platform is described as follows.[29] A computational model for fluid flow analyses was performed to design it. Mice-denuded oocytes and capacitated sperm were utilized. A microchannel connects the inlet port and the outlet port which, in the middle, transforms into a microwell array area where oocytes/zygotes/embryos are positioned during insemination or

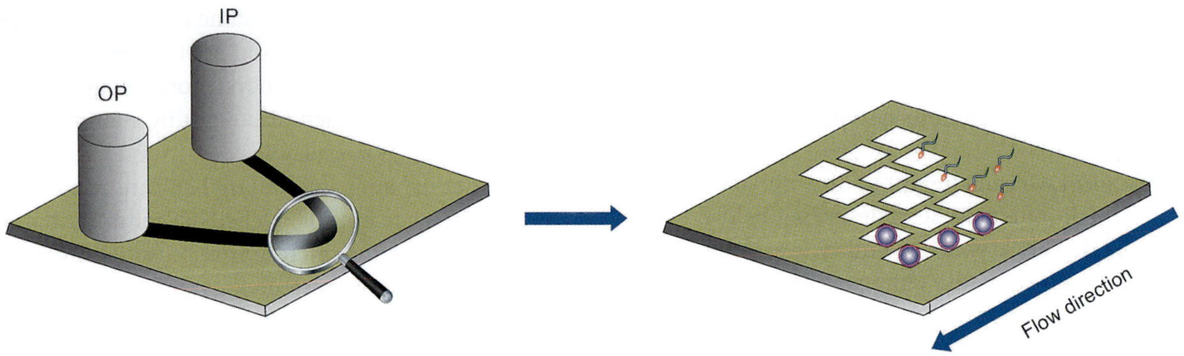


**Fig. 9:** A microchannel connects the inlet port and the outlet port which, in the middle, transforms into a microwell array area where oocytes/zygotes/embryos are positioned during insemination or fertilization and the culture process (at left). Thus, in the same place, fertilization occurs and embryo development becomes continuous (at right). Model is not at real scale.
(IP: inlet port; OP: outlet port)

fertilization and culture process. Thus, in the same place, fertilization occurs and embryo development becomes continuous. Microchannel dimensions were 1 mm wide × 200 µm deep. The microwell array area dimensions were 10 mm long × 3 mm wide **(Fig. 9)**. To assess how well the microwell performs to trap debris and to retain oocytes, several microwell depths were tested (50, 100, 150, and 200 µm). Therefore, after the culture media, the prefilling device was used, and oocytes or dead sperm samples were placed into the inlet port. The negative pressure-driven flow was achieved by a syringe pump connected to the outlet port to control flow culture media velocity. Consequently, the 50 µm and 100 mm depths did not allow high washing-out velocities to be observed when culture media or sperm were loaded in the inlet port. However, no significant difference was found between 150 and 200 µm when testing the debris trapping capacity, and the first size was unable to retain oocytes inside the microwell when velocity increased substantially.

Finally, the best size was 200 µm because it exhibited the best debris trapping capacity and it also retained oocytes at the fastest medium perfusion velocities. After completing these test trials, the IVF process was performed. For insemination purposes, a standard sperm concentration was used ($1 \times 10^6$ sperm $mL^{-1}$) in both the microdrop system and the microfluidic device. Denuded oocytes were pipetted to the inlet port and placed inside the microwells array area by a gravity-driven flow generated by medium aspiration in the outlet port. After performing single oocyte positioning, sperm was added to the inlet port and was transported to the array area by the same gravity-driven flow, where fertilization is to occur later. As a negative control, conventional IVF was performed by microdrops in Petri dishes with an oil overlay at the same sperm concentration and under the same culture conditions. Fertilization assessment was done at 9 hours postinsemination by checking for the presence of two pronuclei. To perform an extended embryo culture, the media of two ports were depleted and changed for suitable fresh media. Embryo development was checked after 14, 48, 72, and 92 hours postinsemination. Finally, at 104 hours, an individual pickup of the obtained blastocysts was done and stained by Hoechst 33342 to assess normal development. As a result, the fertilization rate in both the microdrop system and the microfluidic device did not show a significant difference (71 vs. 69%, respectively). Similarly, embryo development was not affected by the microfluidics culture. Thus, two-cell, four-cell, morula, and the blastocyst formation rate were similar with no significant differences being found.

The second novel platform shares the same goals but improves the design of the previous prototype.[30] This platform has three regions: (1) Sperm inlet ports, (2) motility screening microchannel, and (3) an area for oocyte positioning. Four sperm inlet ports (4 mm diameter × 5 mm depth) surround the area of central oocyte positioning (6 mm diameter × 5 mm deep) and are connected by four microchannels (1.5 mm width × 9 mm length × 80 mm deep). At the bottom of the area for oocyte positioning, a 4 × 4 array structure allows to position oocytes individually, as well as their insemination and culture. For this purpose, each array unit is formed by a circular columnar structure (200 µm in diameter) and is laterally perforated by eight gaps (50 µm) **(Fig. 10)**. Mice-denuded oocytes and capacitated sperm were used. Oocytes were pipetted individually into each positioning unit. Then, sperm was loaded into the inlet ports ($2.5 \times 10^4$ sperm/port). As a negative control, conventional IVF was performed by microdrops in Petri dishes with an oil overlay at the same sperm concentration and under the same culture conditions. Moreover, a parallel experiment was done to test sperm motility by comparing the percentage of the motile sperm between both insemination systems. A computational model was used to analyze the medium's behavior and to adjust medium replacement. The mineral oil and culture media of the four ports were removed and changed in accordance with the suitable culture conditions.

To track embryo development, an assessment was done every 24-hour postinsemination. The obtained blastocysts

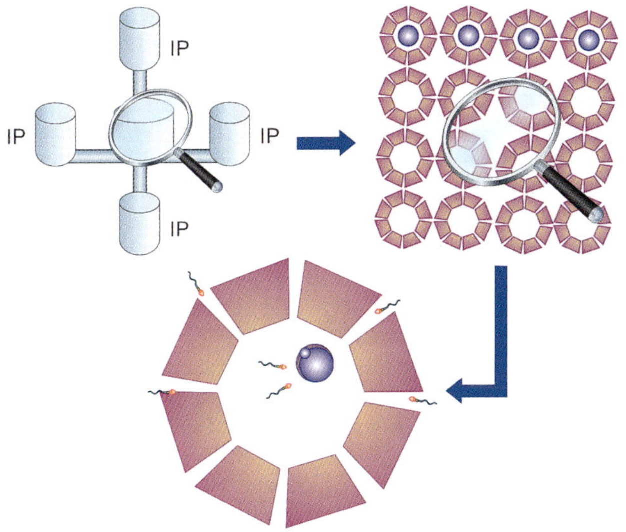


**Fig. 10:** This platform has three regions: (1) Sperm inlet ports, (2) motility screening microchannel, and (3) an area for oocyte positioning (upper picture, at left). Four sperm inlet ports surround the area of central oocyte positioning and are connected by four microchannels. At the bottom, the area for oocyte positioning allows to position oocytes individually, as well as their insemination and culture (upper picture, at right). Each array unit is formed by a circular columnar structure and is laterally perforated by eight gaps (lower picture). Model is not at real scale.
(IP: inlet port; OP: outlet port)

were Hoechst 33342 stained to assess normal development and the total cell number.

As a result, and in relation to sperm motility screening, the sperm motility rate in the central well device was significantly higher than the control group until 6 hours postload, when both rates were similar. The comparable cleavage rate (two-cell embryo formation) was observed between this microfluidic device and the conventional microdrop culture (64 vs. 61%, respectively). Likewise, the formation rate of four-cell embryos, morula and blastocyst, in accordance with the formation rate of the two-cell embryo, showed no significant differences. Finally, in situ fluorescent staining was done to assess the total cell number of obtained blastocysts, and no significant differences between the microfluidic device and the conventional microdrop culture (50.0 vs. 50.7, respectively) were observed.

In short, these two experiments provide similar results for the different platforms because they actually share many concepts and designs. They show similar conventional IVF and embryo development rates, and combine some daily IVF laboratory routine steps in the same platform.

## MICROFLUIDICS FOR AUTOMATED VITRIFICATION

Another assisted reproduction area that may benefit from automation is oocytes and embryo cryopreservation.

Addition of cryoprotectants can be automated by microfluidity, and even vitrification can be either controlled or done simultaneously, particularly in the light of the recent progress made in vitrification techniques, which have become the most extended procedure for oocyte and embryo vitrification.[31]

In order to optimize cryopreservation protocols, microfluidic technology can be applied to minimize osmotic effects and to improve outcomes. A computer-controlled multichannel microfluidics device has been developed to systematically mix cryoprotectant agents and to produce smoother osmotic changes.

In fact, this researching group has comparable results compared with Cryotop method, the current manual "gold standard". This automated method is named Gavi and it allows automatic equilibration steps necessary for successful oocyte/zygote/embryo vitrification. Thus, for mouse zygotes, warming recovery rates were 97% using Gavi and 100% using Cryotop, and achieving the same rate of fully hatched blastocyst (43 and 57%, respectively, by D5 and D6). Warming recovery rates for mouse blastocysts were 99% in both methods, being 54% vitrified by Cryotop and 50% by Gavi, able to arrive at the fully hatched blastocyst stage 48 hours later. In the same way, results with mouse blastocysts showed 99% warming recovery rate for both methods and fully hatched blastocyst rate comparable between them. Finally, results with human blastocysts were similar, showing 100% of recovery rate and comparable rates for different blastocyst stage formations 24 and 48 hours later.[32] Apparently, this procedure is less time-consuming and offers minimal interembryologist variability for oocyte and embryo cryopreservation.[33]

## KEY POINTS

- New technologies and approaches have been emerging since the last few years, changing our concept about ART. They are an exciting discovery that helped us to imagine so many different IVF laboratories in only few years. However, in the day-to-day life, we witness the difficulties that we face to change established concepts. Some reasons such as state regulatory laws, company's policy, ethical and research commission supervision, high cost, clinical ineffectiveness of novel culture platforms, and, obviously, the own embryologist's opposition are stopping these emerging methods. Even so, satisfactory experiences in humans show the way forward. Thus, embryologists, engineers, and researchers working as a multidisciplinary team aim to solve the challenges imposed by design, manufacturing, and daily use and work towards improvements of new platforms and devices.
- Currently, our vision of the introduction of microfluidic technology in ART is rather like a big jigsaw puzzle

with few connecting pieces. However, pieces will gradually join and we can imagine the future, IVF laboratories becoming a lab on a chip. Therefore, it is perfectly conceivable that future microfluidic devices with video timelapse systems can replace current IVF platforms. Moreover, microfluidic platform outlet ports could be connected to "omics" analyzers able to asses implantation and development potential of each cultured embryo without invasive assessments. Hence, the embryologist's tasks will possibly change in the future due to continuous gamete/embryo handling and culture, and the combination with automatic embryo assessment by timelapse video microscopy. New tasks should be clinically managed by the embryologists in these new IVF labs, such as surveillance of automated procedures, quality control assessment, and improving technology/scientific background, and they should do active research with the embryological data generated by these novel devices and platforms.

## REFERENCES


1. Steptoe PC, Edwards RG. Birth after the reimplantation of a human embryo. Lancet. 1978;2(8085):366.
2. International Committee for Monitoring Assisted Reproductive Technology, de Mouzon J, Lancaster P, Nygren KG, Sullivan E, Zegers-Hochschild F, et al. World collaborative report on assisted reproductive technology, 2002. Hum Reprod. 2009;24(9):2310-20.
3. Mortimer D. Sperm recovery techniques to maximize fertilizing capacity. Reprod Fertil Dev. 1994;6(1):25-31.
4. Palermo G, Joris H, Devroey P, Van Steirteghem AC. Pregnancies after intracytoplasmic injection of single spermatozoon into an oocyte. Lancet. 1992;340(8810):17-8.
5. Trounson A, Leeton J, Besanko M, Wood C, Conti A. Pregnancy established in an infertile patient after transfer of a donated embryo fertilised in vitro. Br Med J (Clin Res Ed). 1983;286(6368):835-8.
6. Gardner DK, Lane M. Culture of viable human blastocysts in defined sequential serum-free media. Hum Reprod. 1998;13(Suppl 3):148-59.
7. Handyside AH, Kontogianni EH, Hardy K, Winston RM. Pregnancies from biopsied human preimplantation embryos sexed by Y-specific DNA amplification. Nature. 1990;344(6268):768-70.
8. Cobo A, Diaz C. Clinical application of oocyte vitrification: a systematic review and meta-analysis of randomized controlled trials. Fertil Steril. 2011;96(2):277-85.
9. Meseguer M, Rubio I, Cruz M, Basile N, Marcos J, Requena A. Embryo incubation and selection in a time-lapse monitoring system improves pregnancy outcome compared with a standard incubator: a retrospective cohort study. Fertil Steril. 2012;98(6):1481-9.e10.
10. Lim JM, Reggio BC, Godke RA, Hansel W. Perfusion culture system for bovine embryos: improvement of embryo development by use of bovine oviduct epithelial cells, an antioxidant and polyvinyl alcohol. Reprod Fertil Dev. 1997; 9(4):411-8.
11. Goverde HJ, Peeters RH, Willems PH. The development of a superfusion system for studying intracellular and secretory processes in embryos. In Vitro Cell Dev Biol Anim. 1994;30A(12):819-21.
12. Pruitt JA, Forrest DW, Burghardt RC, Evans JW, Kraemer DC. Viability and ultrastructure of equine embryos following culture in a static or dynamic system. J Reprod Fertil Suppl. 1991;44:405-10.
13. Hatoya S, Sugiyama Y, Torii R, Wijewardana V, Kumagai D, Sugiura K, et al. Effect of co-culturing with embryonic fibroblasts on IVM, IVF and IVC of canine oocytes. Theriogenology. 2006;66(5):1083-90.
14. Suh RS, Zhu X, Phadke N, Ohl DA, Takayama S, Smith GD. IVF within microfluidic channels requires lower total numbers and lower concentrations of sperm. Hum Reprod. 2006;21(2):477-83.
15. Beebe D, Wheeler M, Zeringue H, Walters E, Raty S. Microfluidic technology for assisted reproduction. Theriogenology. 2002;57(1):125-35.
16. Schuster TG, Cho B, Keller LM, Takayama S, Smith GD. Isolation of motile spermatozoa from semen samples using microfluidics. Reprod Biomed Online. 2003;7(1):75-81.
17. Berthier E, Young EWK, Beebe D. Engineers are from PDMS-land, biologists are from polystyrenia. Lab Chip. 2012;12:1224-37.
18. Young EWK, Berthier E, Guckenberger DJ, Sackmann E, Lamers C, Meyvantsson I, et al. Rapid prototyping of arrayed microfluidic systems in polystyrene for cell-based assays. Anal Chem. 2011;83:1408-17.
19. Cittadini E, Albano C, Cimino C, Palermo R. Assisted reproductive technologies in severe male infertility. Acta Eur Fertil. 1992;23(3):123-30.
20. Aitken RJ, Jones KT, Robertson SA. Reactive oxygen species and sperm function—in sickness and in health. J Androl. 2012;33(6):1096-106.
21. Goto Y, Noda Y, Mori T, Nakano M. Increased generation of reactive oxygen species in embryos cultured in vitro. Free Radic Biol Med. 1993;15(1):69-75.
22. Guérin P, El Mouatassim S, Ménézo Y. Oxidative stress and protection against reactive oxygen species in the pre-implantation embryo and its surroundings. Hum Reprod Update. 2001;7(2):175-89.
23. Bedaiwy MA, Falcone T, Mohamed MS, Aleem AA, Sharma RK, Worley SE, et al. Differential growth of human embryos in vitro: role of reactive oxygen species. Fertil Steril. 2004;82(3):593-600.
24. Kattera S, Chen C. Short coincubation of gametes in in vitro fertilization improves implantation and pregnancy rates: a prospective, randomized, controlled study. Fertil Steril. 2003;80(4):1017-21.
25. Coy P, Avilés M. What controls polyspermy in mammals, the oviduct or the oocyte? Biol Rev Camb Philos Soc. 2010;85(3):593-605.
26. Clark SG, Haubert K, Beebe DJ, Ferguson CE, Wheeler MB. Reduction of polyspermic penetration using biomimetic microfluidic technology during in vitro fertilization. Lab Chip. 2005;5(11):1229-32.
27. Viloria T, De Los Santos JM, De Los Santos MJ, et al. Microfluidics Device Applied to Embryo Culture Improves Blastocysts Morphology. Oxford: Oxford University Press;

2014. pp. 175-6. Available from: https://academic.oup.com/humrep/article-pdf/doi/10.1093/humrep/deac107.078/44305959/deac107.078.pdf

28. Heo YS, Cabrera LM, Bormann CL, Shah CT, Takayama S, Smith GD. Dynamic microfunnel culture enhances mouse embryo development and pregnancy rates. Hum Reprod. 2010;25(3):613-22.
29. Han C, Zhang Q, Ma R, Xie L, Qiu T, Wang L, et al. Integration of single oocyte trapping, in vitro fertilization and embryo culture in a microwell-structured microfluidic device. Lab Chip. 2010;10(21):2848-54.
30. Ma R, Xie L, Han C, Su K, Qiu T, Wang L, et al. In vitro fertilization on a single-oocyte positioning system integrated with motile sperm selection and early embryo development. Anal Chem. 2011;83(8):2964-70.
31. Cobo A, Meseguer M, Remohí J, Pellicer A. Use of cryo-banked oocytes in an ovum donation programme: a prospective, randomized, controlled, clinical trial. Hum Reprod. 2010;25(9):2239-46.
32. Roy TK, Brandi S, Tappe NM, Bradley CK, Vom E, Henderson C, et al. Embryo vitrification using a novel semi-automated closed system yields in vitro outcomes equivalent to the manual Cryotop method. Hum Reprod. 2014;29:2431-8.
33. Meng L, Huezo X, Stone BA, Baek K, Ringler G, Marrs RP. Development of a microfluidic device for automated vitrification human embryo. Fertil Steril. 2011;96(Suppl. 3):S207.

CHAPTER

120

# Artificial Intelligence in Assisted Reproductive Technology

*Krishna Chaitanya M, Durga G Rao, Ruchi Narula, Selva Karthick M, Sherin Theresa Mathew*

## INTRODUCTION

Assisted reproductive technology (ART) has existed since 1978 to eliminate natural barriers in fertilization. ART procedures can be described as follows: Oocytes aspirated from ovaries using the surgical procedure and fertilized in vitro using the best sperm selected, and the embryo thus developed is introduced to the uterine cavity.[1] Now, ART has evolved with advanced techniques such as preimplantation genetic testing (PGT), time-lapse embryo monitoring method, and clinically advanced laparoscopic procedures. ART has some practical challenges: 100% success rates are not achieved with in vitro fertilization (IVF) procedures, cannot not eliminate human errors such as sample mismatches and culture mishandling, and complete automation of the process is not yet possible. In comparison with other fields of medicine and other sectors, ART has not seen any drastic improvements and advancements. Artificial intelligence (AI) is one of the methods to eliminate the challenges discussed and to introduce more automation in ART. AI is used in most of our daily activities; the easiest and most common example to understand about AI is the "image to text conversion" application: If the words are written in an unknown language, you can scan them using your mobile phone and translate them to your preferred language. In this chapter, we will discuss the following: (1) General AI infrastructure and currently available AI algorithms for ART practices such as embryo selection, gamete selection, prediction of clinical outcomes in IVF cycles, and advanced embryo monitoring techniques; (2) The reasons why we need a machine touch rather than using human intelligence and its possible limitations and disadvantages; (3) Our predictions in ART using AI were prepared it after consulting experts globally; (4) Lab on a cloud, where patient information is stored electronically and is used for statistics, studies, and machine learning (ML) models. In the current situation, we are not clear whether we can rely on the existing time-consuming process of embryologists/clinicians' decisions to decide upon the treatment type, selection of embryos and gametes, and time of transfers or we really need a machine to tell us the accurate choice and correct predictions for the same. We need to consider what would happen if AI applications took over humans, which then completely manipulates the information and provides us with incorrect predictions. To conclude, AI software needs more training to get very accurate results; it may take some more years and a huge amount of data to evolve.

## ARTIFICIAL INTELLIGENCE ARCHITECTURE AND TOOLS USED IN ASSISTED REPRODUCTIVE TECHNOLOGY

The development of AI applications is a very long process with efficient planning; it needs a large amount of raw data, AI software engineers to write programs, and hardware resources. ML is one of the processes in AI that is mostly used in all medicine-related applications, and it is a mathematical model that analyses patterns in huge random data. A common example of an AI application is a self-driven car, where the algorithm is written to run the vehicle and to manage any outward incidences arising out of a mishap; also, it is programmed to update and learn from the situations regularly. Data collection is the first step in building an AI program. In the case of predicting IVF success rate, we need to feed multiple parameters such as age, medical history, administered drug details, previous live birth, and many others.[2] In the field of medicine, data can be obtained from the following sources: Patients' medical records and cloud-sharing hospital information. Data thus obtained will be segregated and fed to the system (input data) after process modifications. For example, in predicting a good embryo program, the embryo image has to be processed—dragging the image and keeping the embryo at the center, correcting image quality to obtain the best results. When we discuss the programming language, Python is a commonly used language in ML software. To build deep learning neural networks,

**Flowchart 1:** Artificial intelligence (AI) concept in the assisted reproductive technology (ART) field.

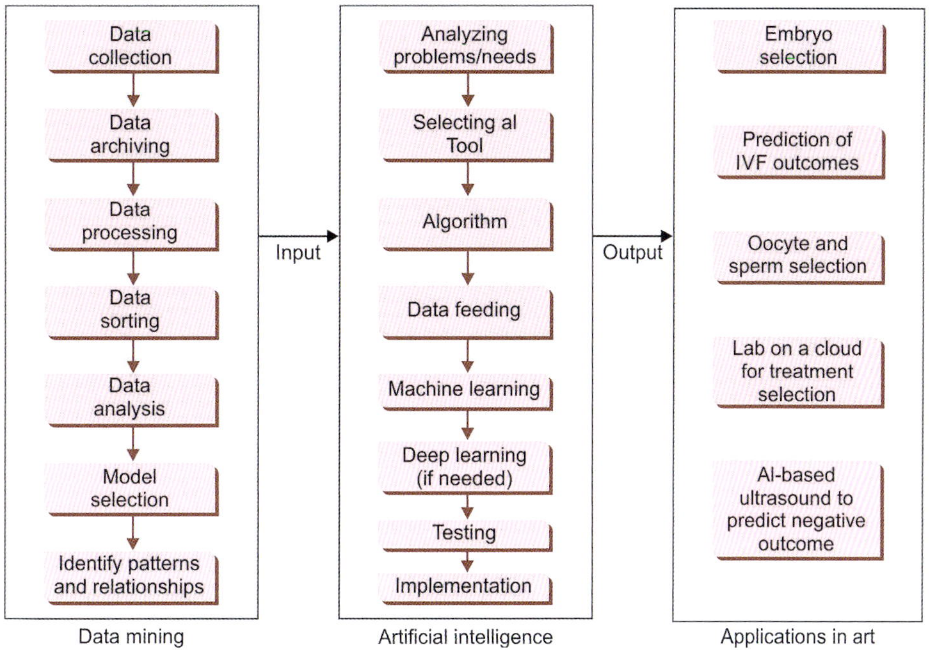


(IVF: in vitro fertilization)

we require a computer microprocessor with sufficient space to run and a graphics card to analyze the images. To implement the algorithm, basically called coding, we need architecture such as TensorFlow, Google's Inception, and Keras neural network library.

Artificial intelligence tools can be widely classified into two methods—supervised and unsupervised learning. In supervised learning, the labeled information predicts the test data, whereas in unsupervised learning, hidden structures in the input data are focused. Supervised learning can be used for image analysis, and unsupervised learning can be used to analyze complex multiple parameters to predict the output. Under supervised learning, commonly used tools are decision tree (DT) and random forest (RF), naïve Bayes classifier (NBS), and support vector machines (SVM). Neural networks and deep learning methods come under unsupervised learning. Based on the input/output, these tools can be generally classified into two types: white- and black-box models. In the white-box model, we can clearly explain the predictions, and in the black-box model, algorithms find patterns without being able to explain their methodology. Each tool has its own algorithms, advantages, and disadvantages. DT and RT have subclasses that have root nodes and decision nodes, and it is a white-box model that can be applied for oocyte cryopreservation and embryo transfer. NBS is a simple algorithm with good accuracy; it is used in the prediction of the outcome of IVF and intracytoplasmic sperm injection (ICSI). SVM is used in complex nonlinear relationships and is currently used for the prediction of the implantation outcome based on transferred embryos. Neural networks and deep learning are used when the problem is having many layers. It is a black-box model and is currently used for the prediction of ART outcomes from multiple parameters **(Flowchart 1)**.[3]

## WHY DO WE NEED A MACHINE TOUCH?

The embryo evaluation and selection at the time of embryo transfer mark the success of the entire IVF process, where an embryologist aims to select the "best" embryo/embryos from the larger cohort of fertilized oocytes. **Figure 1(A)** is grade 3 embryo, which gives live birth, and **Figure 1(B)** is a grade 1 but resulted in a negative pregnancy. It is generally acknowledged that even after embryo selection based on morphology, time-lapse microscopy (TLM), or PGT screening, the implantation rate in humans is difficult to predict. While there has been a vast improvement in the embryo evaluation methods, IVF treatment still remains a gamete-inefficient and embryo-wasting process. The traditional method of morphological assessment for evaluating embryo quality and selecting the best embryo for transfer is a subjective method and leads to inter- and intra-observer variability, resulting in less than optimal IVF success rates. To overcome this factor and increase success rates, it has become a common practice to transfer more than one embryo, leading to a higher risk of multiple pregnancies. We still aim to have methods that enable the selection of both healthy sperm and oocytes and, finally, the selection of

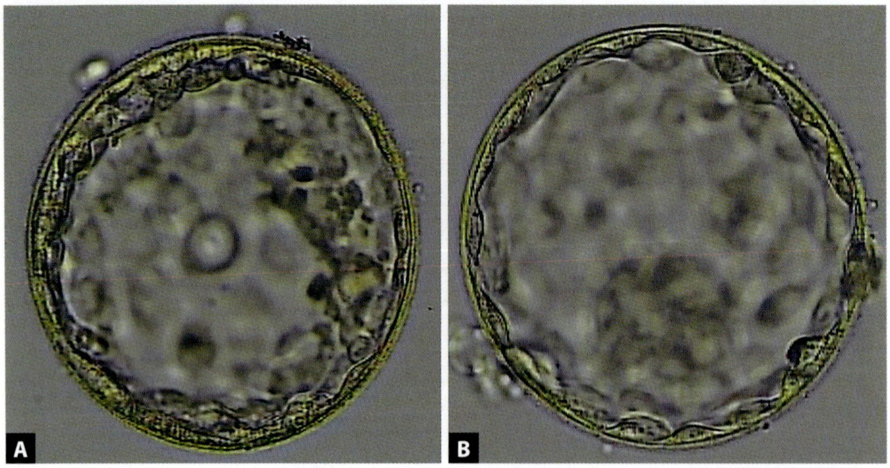

**Figs. 1A and B:** Embryo images. (A) Grade 3 embryo with live birth; (B) Grade 1 embryo result with negative pregnancy.

the best embryos for transfer to optimize the IVF process and gamete efficiency.

Although PGT-A and time-lapse incubators have been introduced to help and increase the chances of live birth, the outcomes still remain less than ideal. The novel noninvasive embryo assessment methods promise to increase IVF efficiency and reduce embryo wastage. AI has long been utilized in other industries and has recently found its place in the field of ART as a noninvasive approach and use of computational applications tools in the IVF laboratory; however, it is just a beginning.

The inclusion of AI in the field of reproductive medicine is highly desirable for many reasons. AI shows good potential in enhancing the embryologist's decision-making ability. AI systems are trained on the vast pool of information and data and can thus make decisions based on facts and supporting data, thus making the decision process reproducible and repeatable versus a human decision which may depend on personnel's experience, training, and emotional states. Manual selection is prone to many types of biases,[4] and the decision is prone to stress, subjectivity, and fatigue; also, AI is smart and eliminates the human element and relies on objective analysis, and can learn to analyze complex patterns with increased resolution while analyzing a greater number of variables in comparison with humans who may not be able to consider multiple variables while taking a decision.[5] Well-trained automated systems can also be used for the training of embryologists on fixed standards. Such automated systems can also help in rapid diagnosis, thereby reducing the time required for evaluation by the embryologists helping them to even evaluate without the need to be physically present in the laboratory.

Artificial intelligence and its application have unlimited potential for development, but ultimately, it should reduce health care costs while improving outcomes, and it should be manageable and feasible without majorly disrupting the IVF laboratory's day-to-day function that strictly relies on morphological criteria for embryo selection. A big question that arises with the adoption of AI in regular IVF laboratory practices is that "Would the traditional manual approach of light microscopy evaluation be totally abandoned or could we simply combine both options?" Ideally, should the final decision be with the embryologist who takes into account the software ranking and the embryo quality as per standard grading techniques? Will AI replace reproductive medicine practitioners and embryologists? All of these are genuine considerations and deserve to be addressed.

Despite the majority of the current research showing that AI can meet or even exceed the performance of experts, AI has not established its role in the world of reproductive medicine, and it is crucial to remember that its role in improving outcomes is limited. Further research is required to prove the application of this approach in routine and its balance with the embryologists' role within the IVF laboratory. Further studies, ideally randomized controlled trials (RCT), are required to identify indicated use of AI. However, the existence of these techniques cannot be overlooked. Possibly, it may prove to be a revolutionary new milestone in the assisted reproduction service.

## RECENT ADVANCES OF ARTIFICIAL INTELLIGENCE IN IN VITRO FERTILIZATION AND ASSISTED REPRODUCTIVE TECHNOLOGY

Artificial intelligence has the potential to soon assist doctors in creating patient-centric treatment regimens, both before and after oocyte collection, and also to reduce the risk of ovarian hyperstimulation syndrome (OHSS) and improve gamete and embryo selection for IVF cycles. The incorporation of this new technology is ideally positioned to improve IVF, predicting an increase in the present static success rate. AI is now being tested and applied in the following ART processes: Live birth prediction prior to IVF, embryo and gamete selection, and treatment selection.

## Gamete Selection and Screening

Conceiving a healthy live baby is the ultimate objective of an IVF cycle. Accurate prediction of IVF cycle outcomes still remains elusive despite several developments in the field of ART. Compared to the relatively limited number of oocytes that are available for selection in a treatment cycle, men mostly have millions of sperm for selection. The current practice of fertilizing all available oocytes limits the use of AI in oocyte selection.

### *Artificial lintelligence Application on Sperm Selection*

We currently use many techniques to select sperms, but the identification of the optimal sperm for ICSI mostly relies on the skill of an embryologist for selecting the best-looking sperm under the inverted microscope without any information regarding its fertility potential. These include microfluidics technology, which uses small fluid streams to sort the best sperms; magnetic-activated cell sorting (MACS), which uses a magnetically charged column that separates apoptotic and nonapoptotic spermatozoa based on the expression of phosphatidylserine; and fluorescence-activated cell sorting (FACS), where fluorescent-labeled cells are sorted based on the scatter from a laser.[6] These sperm-sorting techniques promise to help in the selection of sperms with optimal function from the ejaculate for treatment. Even with the presence of several technologies for sperm sorting, have we reached a point where we can predict the fertilization ability or deoxyribonucleic acid (DNA) integrity of sperm in real time before using it for insemination? Can AI help us to reach this point in the future? Let us look at the advances and developments in the field and come to a conclusion at the end.

Artificial intelligence is already applied in many fertility clinics and research laboratories to improve sperm analysis and selection along with gamete selection and for predicting the outcomes of IVF.[3] AI has been previously applied in semen analyses and has also helped to evaluate sperm morphology.[7,8] It has also been used to measure sperm DNA integrity.[9] A popular sperm analysis method called computer-aided sperm analysis (CASA) integrated a low-level AI ML system for automatic sperm evaluation.[10] Some attempts to apply AI in urology (based on a patient's clinical parameters) have already been reported. AI methods have also been developed to predict the likelihood of sperm extraction in azoospermic patients[11] and to reliably predict the male factor infertility.[12] The impact of lifestyle and environmental factors on fertility rates in men has also been explored using the data-mining methods.[13] The application of AI technologies has gone far ahead with the development of smartphone-based applications for semen analysis as well as sperm viability and DNA integrity.[14,15] CASA vector machine model has been used to classify human sperm into five kinetic classes based on sperm kinetics.[10] Another assay for sperm intracellular pH and sperm membrane potential offers a reliable assessment of sperm capacitation when compared to previous penetration assays. One of such techniques used AI with an assumption that capacitation is an indication of the fertilization potential for which they had introduced a Cap-Score and penetration assay (Androvia, Mountainside, New Jersey, United States).

Another application of AI in the field was pointed out by Gunderson et al. In a study where they used a DT ML to predict success accurately when conventional IVF was considered, they included multiple clinical and demographic variables for each partner, such as sperm intracellular pH, sperm hyperactivated motility, sperm membrane potential, sperm linearity coefficient, sperm lateral head displacement, and sperm curvilinear velocity.[16] The major target for the clinical application of AI in male infertility would be the identification of sperm cells in the microsurgical testicular samples of patients with severe male factor infertility, as identifying these rare sperm cells requires several hours and skills of the embryologists. The idea of developing such a system would require machine training and learning on a massive number of sperm images to correctly differentiate sperm from other types of tissue cells in testicular samples. Most importantly, this system will also need to be rapid and applicable in real time. In 2021, Wu et al. developed a new CASA system, which on testicular sperm extraction utilizes deep learning for near human-level performance.[17] This system helps to automate the identification of sperm in testicular biopsy samples. This study model was benchmarked against embryologists' performance on the detection task. This proposed method has promised to work in real time, but its speed is effectively limited only by the imaging speed of the microscope. The results of this study promise that deep learning-based technologies can improve the efficiency of finding sperm in testicular biopsy samples.

In conclusion, AI techniques for sperm selection that correlate with the fertilization potential and DNA integrity of sperm and, thereby, a successful IVF cycle are limited. Many AI techniques till now have tried to classify sperms based on kinetics, capacitation, and penetration, but none of these have aided in successfully selecting a sperm that can be used in real time for treatment. But all these techniques ultimately yielded sperms that cannot be used for treatment since they get destroyed or wasted. Going ahead, AI can help with newer technologies that help for rapid screening and selection of sperms without inducing cell damage and are usable in real time for treatment.[18] Another target, as discussed above, would be rapid identification and selection of sperms for ICSI in testicular biopsy samples. However, AI is yet to be applied routinely to these sperm-sorting techniques to make the selection faster and smarter.

### *Artificial Intelligence Application on Oocyte Selection*

The female gamete plays a crucial role in determining embryo competence and thus in the success of the IVF treatment. Most of the oocytes retrieved after the ovarian stimulation exhibit one or more types of dysmorphism; thus, finding an ideal oocyte after denudation is rare. There are many extra cytoplasmic anomalies [first polar body (PB), perivitelline space (PVS) size, irregularity of zona pellucida] and abnormal cytoplasmic inclusions [smooth endoplasmic reticulum (SER) centrally located cytoplasmic granulation (CLCG), vacuoles, refractile bodies] noted in the recovered oocytes. It has been speculated that these morphological anomalies, which can be easily identified under light microscopy, may be an indication of the compromised development potential of the oocytes. Rienzi et al. in a retrospective analysis evaluated the influence of different oocyte morphotypes on ICSI outcomes. They also generated an MII oocyte morphologic score (MOMS) capable of predicting the oocyte competence in terms of fertilization potential, pronuclear (PN) morphology, and embryo developmental ability.[19] Several other characteristics correlating with oocyte quality have been identified, such as the composition and amount of accumulated maternal messenger ribonucleic acids (mRNAs), the size of the oocyte and its zona pellucida, its cytoplasmic organization, or the existence of certain specific epigenetic alterations. However, there has never been an agreement on the individual power of these parameters to determine oocyte growth potential, and results are very often incongruous. ML can be used to address this issue since it can automatically identify essential features and consider multiple elements instantly. In both academics and in clinics, the use of computational tools to better characterize an oocyte's developmental potential is thus necessary. Let us go ahead and have an overview of the application of AI and advancements in oocyte selection.

In 2013, in a study by Manna et al., texture analysis of 269 oocyte images was performed, and the corresponding embryo development was tracked. Texture features were used with neural networks to predict the outcome of an IVF cycle.[20] In 2021, Targosz et al. analyzed 71 deep neural network models for semantic oocyte segmentation;[21] they trained their algorithm to classify the oocyte morphological features such as clear cytoplasm, dark cytoplasm, diffuse cytoplasmic granularity, smooth endoplasmic reticulum, vacuoles, first PB, multi-PB, fragmented PB, PVS, zona pellucida, cumulus cells, and the presence of germinal vesicle (GV). In this study, the training accuracy (acc) reached about 85 and 79% for training patterns and for validation, respectively. Kanakasabapathy and colleagues, in 2020, trained a convolutional neural network (CNN) to predict fertilization potential using oocyte images and then identify the oocytes with the highest fertilization potential.[22] A deep CNN was used in 2020 by Dickinson et al. to locate the first extruded PB, which allowed them to distinguish the mature metaphase II (MII) oocytes from metaphase I (MI) and GV stage oocytes. This algorithm also helped to pinpoint the location of the extruded PB, which can help to identify the correct location on the oocyte to inject spermatozoa for ICSI. Unfortunately, the available scoring systems have shown extreme variability regarding their types and methods for individual scoring of investigated features and outcome parameters. Hence, at present, they can only be regarded as diverse approaches to the same strategy, but their comparative evaluation is not possible. Experimental research procedures such as in vitro maturation (IVM) of oocytes, somatic cell nuclear transfer and reprogramming, in vitro gametogenesis (IVG), and others have a good potential to benefit from the introduction of the AI system. A study on the animal model has demonstrated that using an ML pipeline makes it possible to predict oocyte maturation with accuracy between 80 and 90%. Furthermore, scientists also identified two new features, the texture of the zona pellucida and the size of cytoplasmic particles, as good predictors of mouse oocyte maturation potential. They also defined a competence score to rank mouse oocytes by their capacity for maturation. Moreover, it has also shown that the zona pellucida texture could be a good predictor of human oocyte maturation potential and revealed a defect in the cytoplasmic activity in poor-quality oocytes. This ranking could be utilized to augment IVM protocols by identifying the most viable oocytes. Furthermore, the small increase in IVF efficiency in recent studies can mostly be credited to the use of a PolScope microscope for detecting zona retardance and presence, position, and retardance of the spindle, a technique that is used in a limited number of ART facilities around the world. The use of polarized light microscopy for imaging the spindle has been previously investigated, and it has been reported that there are associations between meiotic spindle morphology and oocyte quality. Thus, imaging of meiotic spindles might also provide useful information for selecting high-quality oocytes using AI tools trained on these concepts. In future, it would be interesting if the imaging of mitotic spindles in early embryos could provide additional information to help in identifying aneuploidy in embryos.

At present, comprehensive oocyte morphology scoring is not performed as a routine procedure, the morphological assessment of oocytes currently seems to be informative rather than predictive, and the use of AI for oocyte selection is limited due to the practice of fertilizing all available oocytes. Oocyte selection before insemination may have important benefits in certain situations; for example, in countries with legal restrictions where noninvasive AI methods can be used to evaluate oocytes with the best competency can become an important selection and prediction tool to reduce the number of embryos created and wasted, and thus, it would lead to the overall efficiency of an IVF treatment cycle. Such tools would thus help to restrict supernumerary embryos and also provide patients with counseling over the prognosis of the success of an IVF cycle. Oocyte morphology assessment can be especially useful in oocyte donation cycles where we have restrictions on the number of oocytes to be allotted to a recipient during oocyte freezing for fertility preservation. Finally, objective oocyte scoring can be important in cases of very poor treatment outcomes as a tool for an explanation of results to the patient. Currently, there is a need for more intensive and coordinated research to reach a consensus and exploit fully the predictive potential of morphological examination of the oocytes.

## Embryo Selection

Many studies are performed every year focused on individual variables, yet a clear cause cannot be identified in the majority of IVF failures. With the Istanbul consensus since 2011, the field of clinical embryology has made strides in relation to embryo selection. However, horizontal adoption of a consensus on embryo grading has yet to be achieved to a satisfactory extent and is commonly accepted and practiced, and unfortunately, there are many grading systems. Even with the "Gardner" system of grading, which is used universally, variations and deviations are seen quite commonly, and this subjective method leads to inter- and intra-observer variability, resulting in less optimal IVF success rates. To overcome the failures, it has become a common practice to transfer more than one embryo, resulting in high-risk multiple pregnancies. Even with the introduction of time-lapse incubators and preimplantation genetic testing for aneuploidy (PGT-A), the IVF outcomes remain less than ideal. The utilization of AI has been increasingly tried in the embryology laboratory to help improve IVF outcomes. Many studies investigating the use of AI as an automated and unbiased approach for embryo assessment have been published. Embryo selection is subjective and is based on developmental and morphological characteristics such as the granularity of cytoplasm, the color of cytoplasm, multinucleation, number of blastomeres, degree of fragmentation, size of blastocoel, the timing of cleavage and morphokinetics, roundness of oolemma, thickness of zona and more and already sufficient sets of qualities to judge an embryo have been explored. Numerous experimental methods have been developed to predict the implantation potential and live birth rate from images or videos of the embryos, including morphometric analysis by time-lapse imaging, mathematical-statistical tools, and computer-assisted scoring. AI is already being tried for embryo selection at various stages of development, such as the PN stage, cleavage stage, and blastocyst stage. We are going to discuss the AI application at these stages individually under the following subheadings and thereby try to get answers to some important questions such as, Is AI ready to replace the traditional manual assessment? Can we expect better lab work management with a cut down in time required in labs? Can we predict the euploidy status and development potential of embryos at the early stages of development so as to transfer or freeze at day 2 or day 3 by reducing the chance of epigenetic changes that may be caused by prolonged culture?

### *AI Application on Pronuclear-stage Embryos*

Fertilization checks and embryo quality assessments require manual examination, status recording, and embryo development scoring. Manually scoring the zygotes is labor-intensive and subjective and also requires an embryologist's presence in the lab at the correct timeline. Dimitriadis and colleagues, in 2019, described a CNN that can distinguish between 2PN and non-2PN zygotes at 18 hours post-insemination with >90% accuracy.[23] This system can be used to help embryologists confirm the fertilization assessment of each oocyte and also monitor individual embryologists performing ICSI for advanced quality assurance to improve patient outcomes. Using AI, these predictive features can be incorporated into an embryo selection algorithm. Early parameters of zygotic (cytoplasmic movement) development, analyzed by AI-powered methods, have been shown to be predictive of blastocyst development. Compared to human evaluation and prediction using morphological parameters, AI-based methods using cytoplasmic kinetics showed, on average, 10% higher accuracy.[24] These studies collectively show that the use of AI in PN stage scoring can help in the prediction of blastocyst development and also save the time required for fertilization checks.

### *AI Application on Cleavage-stage Embryos*

Cleavage-stage embryos are generally graded based on three features: Blastomere cell count, percentage of overall cytoplasmic fragmentation, and degree of asymmetry between the cells. These grades are mostly assigned by visual morphology examination and AI technology which is proposed as a solution to these labor constraints and the subjective nature of selection, including morphology and morphokinetic measurements. A deep learning CNN was used by Kanakasabapathy et al. to train and validate embryo assessments on day 3 embryo images based on embryo developmental outcomes observed on day 5 of culture. This algorithm was trained to make expected day 5 developmental predictions such as embryo arrest, morula, early blastocyst, full blastocyst, and high-quality blastocyst. Using a test set of 748 embryos, the accuracy of the algorithm in predicting blastocyst development was 71.9%.[25,26] This was also the first AI-based system to be used to predict the developmental fate of cleavage-stage embryos. Some algorithms used cleavage-stage embryo images with DT methods and statistical analysis of features to determine the implantation potential of cleavage-stage embryos.[27,28] Using CNN, Meyer et al. in 2020 demonstrated the ability of CNN to identify noninvasive markers for detecting genetically abnormal embryos. They classified day 3 cleavage-stage embryo images as aneuploid or euploid with high specificity and were thus able to sufficiently identify 85.5% of aneuploid embryos.[29] Kelly and colleagues used CNN to identify safe regions on a cleavage-stage embryo to perform laser-assisted hatching.[30] These studies collectively show that a variety of AI techniques can be used to extract very important information from cleavage-stage embryos, which may be used for classification, assessment, and ranking, and thus, to aid in clinical decision making. Also, by prediction of the euploidy status and development potential of embryos at day 2 or day 3 itself, prolonged culture can be avoided, thereby reducing the chance of epigenetic changes that may be caused.

### *AI Application on Blastocyst-stage Embryos*

The AI tools available for blastocyst stage assessment have been either trained on time-lapse microscope images or static images of blastocysts.

*AI-based on TLM image analysis:* The advances in time-lapse technologies have led to the development of embryo selection algorithms and the high-powered computer processing to analyze a large set of images along with the combination of some parameters which may be linked to embryonic viability. The first AI-based on time-lapse images developed a predictive algorithm capable of automatically quantifying the duration of cytokinesis and the time between mitoses.[31] This tool was marketed under the name of Early Embryo Viability Assessment (Eeva), the first clinically validated platform that integrates time-lapse, two predictive parameters, and automatic software. In another study, a different approach was used to predict blastocyst development using the TLM data up to D3 of embryo development. Two different AI algorithms were developed: An automatic morphokinetic data model and a TLM embryo image model, with both models having comparable predictive power, and when both were combined, the different weights were used to optimize the blastocyst prediction. More weight was given to the morphokinetic data compared to the image data. When compared to embryologists, the AI model performed better in terms of sensitivity and specificity.[32] In another unique approach in which AI measures the kinetics of blastocyst expansion and correlates it to the outcome, where faster-expanding blastocysts were seen to exhibit higher implantation potential.[33] Bori et al. presented a novel model utilizing AI to predict embryo implantation. The authors were able to make a high implantation prediction by combining AI image analysis and proteomic profile of the spent culture media from the PGT euploid embryo. Using AI image analysis combined with a proteomic profile on spent culture media from the PGT euploid embryo, the authors were able to demonstrate very high implantation prediction. Although the study is preliminary, it demonstrates the power of AI to combine different data points (proteins and morphology).[34]

*AI-based on static image analysis of blastocysts:* An AI deep learning model was studied in 2019 that can evaluate blastocyst quality, and in this AI-based prediction model, the blastocyst expansion followed by inner cell mass (ICM) and trophectoderm (TE) quality were important parameters. The precise time point used for the AI evaluation (at 110 hours) demonstrated the importance of embryo developmental kinetics for embryo prediction.[35] In a 2020 study, a CNN system by Bormann et al. was used to classify blastocysts based on the presence of the cavity and the morphological quality of the ICM and TE.[36] In another algorithm based on implantation outcomes of the images of blastocysts selected by humans for transfer, a blastocyst ranking system called the "blastocyst score" was established, which showed over 50% positive outcomes. The variations seen among the embryologists making decisions on vitrification and embryo biopsy based on standard morphological assessments can be significantly improved by using deep neural networks, according to Bormann et al. in their study.[37,38] Souter et al. in 2019 further demonstrated in their study that a deep learning CNN could be used with 96.3% specificity and 93.7% sensitivity to find which D3 assisted hatched embryos met D5 criteria for TE biopsy and cryopreservation. This validation study was the first to demonstrate that an embryo decision-making algorithm could be successfully applied to embryos that had been breached to promote herniation of TE cells for blastocyst-stage biopsy.[38] Thirumalaraju et al. in 2021 compared the use of eight different architectures to classify blastocyst-stage embryo images captured on a variety of imaging platforms and showed that "Xception" performed best in learning the embryo data and was able to accurately classify blastocysts based on their morphological quality, it could correctly classify >99.5% of the highest quality blastocysts, which is of critical importance, clinically, when identifying embryos suited for transfer.[39] In 2020, Eduardo et al. evaluated KIDScore as an algorithm for morphological assessment and preimplantation genetic testing for aneuploidies (PGT-A) to improve implantation and ongoing pregnancy rates. This algorithm can thus help in enhancing the embryologist's decision making capacity to choose the embryo with the greatest potential.[40] Vermilyea et al., in 2020, presented another study in which they used computer vision image annotation techniques to compose AI (The Life

Whisperer AI), providing a reliable and robust assessment of blastocysts with different types of cameras, microscopes, and focal planes. They concluded that in all these variables, the results suggest that this method of preprocessing and automatic annotation, as well as AI trained in a globally diverse dataset, creates a generalizable AI that is robust to the type of camera and focal configuration, regardless of hardware.[41]

To conclude, as of now, AI has still not reached an accuracy level so as to replace the manual grading completely as there are many doubts on the amount and quality of images the software is trained on. By using AI, it might be possible to strengthen the correlation between blastocyst assessment and outcome in a more objective manner. But we clearly see the benefit of AI only when we have multiple good-quality blastocysts to choose between, and if we have low egg and embryo numbers, then it probably will not be as useful. It will be necessary to perform a comparative prospective study to identify the (dis)agreement in blastocyst selection for transfer between AI models and embryologists. A question needs to be answered by existing AI applications, which have, till now, used both fixed and flexible time-based methods of evaluation because blastocyst development is a dynamic process: Should we evaluate and grade blastocysts when they are exhibiting the "best" appearance? Or should we evaluate them at a particular time? Also, the ability of AI blastocyst applications predicted by early developmental versus later developmental events needs to be explored.

## Artificial Intelligence and Screening for Aneuploidy

Embryo euploidy has been an important consideration while selecting embryos for transfer. Although PGT-A has been available since the early 1990s, testing methods have evolved rapidly in terms of the types of chromosome abnormalities that may be identified and in the terms of accuracy that may be expected. PGT-A is a globally performed screening test for embryo euploidy; however, its role as an adjuvant in IVF treatment still remains controversial because the weight of evidence in support of improving delivery rates is still considered questionable. Also, a recent American Society for Reproductive Medicine (ASRM) committee opinion concluded that the effectiveness of PGT-A cannot yet be determined.[42] One serious limitation plaguing preimplantation genetic diagnosis (PGD) studies is the issue of mosaicism. It has been reported that up to 24% of embryos that are diagnosed with PGD may be mosaics.[44] Now, If AI can differentiate "normal" embryos from those that are chromosomally abnormal with higher accuracy and proficiency than the other types of PGT, it promises to reduce costs, miscarriage, and stillbirth rates and will also eliminate the invasive techniques ultimately. In the future, this technology could be valuable for patients who do not wish to subject their embryos to the invasive biopsy procedure or cannot afford PGT-A, and so on.

The various algorithms designed to accurately predict the embryo euploidy are based on the morphokinetical characteristics obtained through TLM.[45] Some algorithms have proposed to divide embryos into categories (low, medium, and high) on the basis of aneuploidy risk in association with the time required from insemination to reaching the blastocyst stage with demonstrated high prediction ability of 97% regarding embryos at high risk of being aneuploid, whereas low-risk embryos presented a 37% probability of aneuploidy.[46,47] However, it should be noted that the sample size in the studies was considerably small (<100 embryos each), highlighting the limitation. Another larger study proposed algorithm based on completely different morphokinetics with the evaluation of earlier stages of embryo development. This algorithm attempts to be statistically more efficient in terms of predicting embryo euploidy with the advantage of enabling embryo transfer on D3.[44] However, the statistical significance of the parameters considered has been argued.[46] Using CNN, Meyer et al. (in 2020) were able to classify D3 cleavage-stage embryo images as aneuploid or euploid with high specificity and thus were able to sufficiently identify 85.5% of aneuploid embryos. These results demonstrate the ability of CNN to identify noninvasive markers for detecting genetically abnormal embryos.[31] Based on AI, CooperGenomics has developed a completely new PGT-A data analysis platform named PGTai which promises to improve the accuracy of PGT-A interpretation and reporting while "removing subjectivity" in interpretation and avoiding reporting transcription errors by using a larger dataset for baseline than other available PGT-A software in use today.[48] Some AI start-ups and products are already claiming significant results, for example, the detection of chromosome 21 aneuploidy (by Life Whisperer and Ovation Fertility), where the companies have announced that it is possible to screen embryos for aneuploidy using AI embryo analysis, instead of aspirating the embryos for genetic testing. But without proper peer review, it is difficult to evaluate any of these claims, and another point to consider is whether we have enough images of aneuploid embryos to build a dataset huge enough to allow AI to detect an anomaly.

As of now, couples who have a large number of embryos available for testing may be able to save money by testing only the embryos with a moderate to high likelihood of genetic defects. Currently, AI is used in IVF laboratories as a tool to prescreen and identify viable embryos with a low likelihood of genetic defects before proceeding with PGT. The available prediction models for embryo euploidy are few, and the published studies indicate that substantial work is still needed before they can be used in ordinary clinical practice. Hence, we may be able to utilize these prediction models in the future to help choose which embryos should undergo PGT-A screening because of their strong negative predictive values, but we are still not at the point where AI can reliably identify an embryo as euploid or aneuploid before transfer.

### Artificial Intelligence in Prediction of Treatment Selection and Success Rate Prediction

In recent years, couples approaching test tube centers have become very common due to their lifestyle and stress levels, but IVF cycles are again a stress factor with their cost, continuous medication, and side effects. Currently, researchers are attempting to predict success rates using multiple parameters. The application of AI to choose treatment types is not much explored, and very little research has been published. Intrauterine insemination (IUI) success rate can be predicted using a neural network model with 71.92% accuracy results.[49] In this study, morphology, total motility, female factors, and underlying factors are fed to predict success rates. Another work predicts IVF success rates using multiple parameters; in their study, they have used 1,456 patient data using NBC and RF.[50] Siristatidis et al. proposed a new model to predict success rate using lifestyle, previous cycle details, the metabolomics profile of each embryo, transcriptomics of the oocyte and endometrium, reactive oxygen species in follicular fluid, micro RNA (miRNA) of the endometrium.[51] In this model, we can predict the clinical outcomes—miscarriage rate and live birth rate. Huang et al.[52] predicted the live birth outcome using a deep learning model from single embryo transfers. Xi et al.[53] developed a hierarchical model to understand the embryo implantation potential in double embryo transfers. Hassan et al. developed a prediction model with the help of multiple ML types using attributes such as antral follicle count, NbreM2, fertilization rate in vitro, follicles on D14, and others.[54] Durairaj et al. claimed 75% accuracy in success rate prediction using the artificial neural network (ANN) model.[55] These models are at the beginning level; many models have to be developed by involving all possible parameters to achieve >90% accuracy.

## CURRENTLY AVAILABLE TOOLS AND APPLICATIONS

The first time-lapse system (TLS) for use in IVF labs was sold in 2008 (Primo Vision™, Vitrolife, Sweden), and today we have a lot of such systems available in the market, such as EmbryoScope and EmbryoScope Plus [Food and Drug Administration (FDA)-authorized, Vitrolife]; Miri (ESCO, Denmark); Geri (ESCO, Denmark) (GeneaBiomedx, Australia). Many experimental approaches, including morphokinetic studies available through the TLS, have been developed to examine the implantation potential and live birth rate of IVF embryos using photos and videos. Advances in TLS technology have resulted in the creation of embryo selection algorithms to address the subjective issues associated with manual scoring, such as blastocyst morphological evaluation and embryo selection.

The FDA-approved Eva test, which is driven by the updated Xtend algorithm (a standard multidimensional, static algorithm), can effectively predict which blastocyst has the better chance to develop into an embryo, based not only on its appearance but also on the combination of this new algorithm with traditional morphology grading attained by the embryologist and could actively promote Eset. KIDScore, also known as the implantation data score, is another time-lapse DT-based technique that includes morphokinetic characteristics as well as cell counts. The KIDScore algorithm outperformed the ALPHA/European Society of Human Reproduction and Embryology (ESHRE) rating system in terms of blastocyst development and quality prediction. A new version of the KIDScore contains a D5 decision support tool (KIDScore D5) that can only be used in culture systems with certain oxygen conditions. However, no consensus on these findings and the advantages associated with them has yet been published. Due to its relatively recent emergence and availability for only 2 years, the KIDScore has not been studied to the same level as Eeva. An Australia-based company, Life Whisperer, claims to have evaluated the embryo quality using AI so as to increase the success of implantation by 50% over manual grading by morphology alone. They use a database of embryo images, each with the embryologist assigned morphological grade, along with genetic screening results and pregnancy outcome data to train its AI system. It is a web-based decision tool with instant reporting where we simply upload pictures of the embryos and receive a scoring in real time. This company has also recently announced its ability to screen for aneuploidy. Another AI tool, "iDAScore," which integrates time-lapse monitoring and AI-based embryo evaluation in one workflow, is currently being tested in an international multicenter RCT. More recently, an AI, called Stork, was trained on over 12,000 images and eventually achieved a 97% accuracy rate for identifying healthy embryos that might produce a viable pregnancy and poor-quality embryos that might not.

Despite several studies which support the use of AI in embryo selection, there are also large number of excellent reviews which demonstrate that there is not enough data to differentiate between TLS and traditional incubation in cases of live delivery, miscarriage, stillbirth, or clinical pregnancy. As always, when applying new technologies, it is important that they are validated and should be used as supportive tools rather than a replacement for humans until we are confident that they operate in a reliable and safe manner. To this end, properly designed RCT are the way forward. AI comes with the "black box" problem, this behavior of AI is something that even the engineers who create these AI fail to explain, and as a result, there is a significant amount of inadvertent bias connected with AI. Private companies are eager to sell their products in the market; these products currently available in the market are often without peer review, which in contrast to AI projects developed through research where the reviewers have full access to the source code, and the AI under development undergoes extensive peer review. It is crucial that the use of smart tools should not compromise the safety and efficiency of the clinic.

## LAB ON A CLOUD

For two decades, the field of medicine has completely digitalized its documents, archiving patient records electronically, and information is stored on a cloud server. Electronic medical record (EMR) reduces our time and helps to conveniently retrieve the data wherever and whenever possible when provided with a suitable system to access and good internet connection. Lab on cloud is much used in research studies, where we can get numerous patient information within a short time. To build an AI model in ART, Lab on a cloud becomes an important and necessary tool to teach algorithms. Individual ART clinics have their own software to store their data, and it would be much appreciated if all this information is shared in a common platform so that we can develop a prediction model with more accuracy as the data will be huge. We propose in the future, all the national and international registries could initiate to archive data in a general linear form that is easy to access for the research.

## POSSIBLE LIMITATIONS

Although AI has shown promising results, its use currently has certain limitations. Premature adoption of models without considering its limitations may be associated with risks in clinical practice. One such underlying reason behind the risks involved in wide-ranging applications is the fact that different IVF laboratories follow different practices, employ different criteria, and select embryos on different grounds, using different cutoff values. All users must be educated on how to evaluate AI system results and also to be aware of the limitations regarding validation procedures and the conditions of the model.

### Reasons to Interpret Reproduction Artificial Intelligence Studies with Caution

- *Unbalanced data/intrinsic bias:* AI algorithms are trained on a specific set of data, and it performs their function based on that data only. Hence, when the training set is highly unbalanced, the model is prone to intrinsic bias; thus, the description of the algorithm should include the actions taken to avoid such bias.[56,57] It is very important that the IVF scientific community reaches a consensus on the algorithm's use and value as a prognostic tool in the IVF laboratory.
- *Lack of generalizability assessment:* Reproductive treatments at different clinical setups can vary widely. Ideally, an AI-based algorithm should be tested for generalizability across multiple clinics around the world and should include a wide spectrum of sample types available in clinical practice. However, the majority of the studies published to date have AI-based algorithms trained using data from a single clinic or with very narrow inclusion criteria (e.g., a single type of incubators, specific brand of culture media, category of patients, age group, study on only day 5 blastocysts), limiting their applicability in other conditions. An AI model's performance, to a large extent, is related to the quality of the database it was trained on. For example, on the type of images the AI model was trained on, suppose for training the images used were of day 3 embryos which were obtained after ICSI. Will this model be generalizable to images taken on day 3 or day 3.5? Will it be accurate for IVF-inseminated oocytes? Will it be applicable when different culture media are used? Hence, the clinic should access an AI system only if that was trained under conditions similar to those in the clinic where it would be implemented. A quality assurance test should be performed before the model is used in real cases. To date, there have been no prospective studies published in which the performance of an AI model is compared with standard clinical decisions, and the use of a universally commonly accepted, more evidence-based efficient algorithm remains the goal.
- *Sample size:* By nature, AI algorithms should be trained on large databases because a small sample size can compromise the model's performance and introduce overconfidence.[58] The creation of an efficient program would require a learning set consisting of a vast number of IVF cycles and an equally large testing dataset with known implantation data and pregnancy outcomes. If the training data sample size is small, the sample diversity is insufficient, or the ratio among samples is not balanced, this could lead to bias in the model regarding monitoring and learning, which would further result in the low generalization of the models with poor practical application effects.[59]
- *Controversy on its efficiency:* Even though there is an active ongoing controversy regarding the use and clinical efficacy of these systems,[23,60-62] advanced imaging techniques such as TLS have already obtained a significant market share of IVF-laboratories in the United States.[63] Other research subscribes to the view that the data on the merits of time-lapse services is yet insufficient to justify the device's and consumables' associated costs or

the major adjustments that must be made to IVF's usual operations. TLM-based embryo grading failed to make a statistically significant difference in enhancing clinical pregnancy or ongoing pregnancy rates when compared to regular embryo grading methods.[62] However, several validation studies revealed varying prediction capacities; hence, external validation on a large sample is required prior to the reproduction, acceptance, and horizontal application of the proposed models in order to identify the models' strengths and flaws.

- *Limited performance metrics reported:* Algorithms designed for AI, which are used in assisted reproduction, are largely classification systems that tell us whether a biological sample has a poor or good prognosis. Two most common metrics used to assess these classifiers are accuracy and area under the curve, but with these two metrics alone, a reader cannot execute a deeper performance analysis. Hence, other tests should be performed before the technology is implemented into daily practice.
- *High cost:* This technology is not widely used in clinics worldwide, and its cost initially seems to be remarkably high and can put an additional burden on the patients.
- *Increased workload:* This may come at the cost of increased workload (e.g., increased annotations) and may require the need for specific training on using this type of equipment.
- *Ethical issues:* Many patients will not allow or give consent to the uploading of their medical data online for intelligent analysis, as they would consider this as a threat to their privacy.
- *Images quality-related issues:* The transfer learning (TL) algorithms are mostly trained on high-quality image data. Different laboratory setups may have the provision of microscopes with cameras, and thus images range from low resolution to high resolution. The question is, would it be possible to train an AI system on high-resolution images and apply it to low-resolution images or vice versa? Also, a single image cannot be used to evaluate the dynamic process of embryo development or events, such as blastocoel collapse, which can potentially interfere with the assessment. Moreover, it is unclear how AI will perform with data it has never "seen before".
- *Need of RCTs:* Furthermore, before an AI model's clinical application, quality assurance should always be considered whenever a model is introduced into a new setting for the first time. This is in contrast to the complex logistics required for an RCT and the long time it takes from design and recruitment until publication. In other words, a 2-year RCT project could end up demonstrating that a 2.5-year-old version of an AI/ML model is good; by that time, the same ML model is already in its third or fourth version/update.[64,65]

## FUTURE ASPECTS

Artificial intelligence will predominantly occupy the ART field; here are some possible predictions:

- Complete ART treatment planned using AI, based on their diagnosis and history, whether the patient can undergo IVF, ICSI, PGT, or IUI.
- Most accurate prediction model to check the pregnancy outcomes before undergoing the IVF treatment cycle.
- Exact uterine implantation time predicted by AI system.
- Proper embryo selection protocol to provide high success pregnancy rates.
- AI-based embryo culture system to prevent degeneration by addressing changes in any chemical, metabolites, and gaseous exchange parameters such as glucose, calcium, lactose, pH, $pO_2$, $pCO_2$, sodium, zinc, and others.
- Evaluation of embryo without embryologist presence. Prediction models can be improved if patient information is shared globally on a common platform.
- Extended blast cultures can be cut down if we can predict the embryo with a good success rate in implantation and live birth occurrence; by this, we could prevent epigenetic damage.

To pick the most morphologically normal sperm, software such as intracytoplasmic morphologically selected sperm injection (IMSI) and motile sperm organelle morphology examination (MSOME) are already available. CASA is a type of software that is frequently used for sperm analysis. Automated machines are being used routinely for embryo vitrification. The use of well-calibrated AI algorithms in ART will improve the efficiency with which sperms and oocytes are picked for IVF, which will, in turn, increase clinically achieved pregnancy rates. In the future, AI algorithms will aid clinicians in automating, systematizing, and improving IVF outcomes.

## CONCLUSION

The use of AI in ART is steadily growing, and in the future, it may be possible to use AI and machine language to incorporate and analyze, all IVF-cycle-associated data from various clinics treating infertility, so as to significantly improve reproductive outcomes in infertile couples. However, at present, despite being around for a decade, advanced imaging techniques such as TLM have failed to earn the trust of embryologists, who strongly believe that the TLS is more of a curiosity but not a requirement. AI has not yet established a stronghold in the world of reproductive medicine, as it still has to prove its use in improving reproductive outcomes.

Despite all these hurdles, in the near future, AI is poised to boost and appreciably improve the present stagnant success rates, which have plagued fertility clinics for over a decade.

## REFERENCES


1. Amjad S, Rehman R. Assisted reproductive techniques. Subfertility: Recent Advances for Management and Prevention. Elsevier; 2020. pp. 185-97 [Chapter 12].
2. Venket G, AI-Nasser R, Jerkovic S, Craft I. Prediction of success in IVF treatments using neural networks. Fertil Steril. 2004;82:S215.
3. Wang R, Pan W, Jin L, Li Y, Geng Y, Gao C, et al. Artificial intelligence in reproductive medicine. Reproduction. 2019;158(4):R139-54.
4. Phillips-Wren G, Adya M. Decision making under stress: the role of information overload, time pressure, complexity, and uncertainty. J Decis Syst. 2020;29:213-25.
5. Wang S, Summers RM. Machine learning and radiology. Med Image Anal. 2012;16:933-51.
6. Mangum CL, Patel DP, Jafek AR, Samuel R, Jenkins TG, Aston KI, et al. Towards a better testicular sperm extraction: novel sperm sorting technologies for non-motile sperm extracted by microdissection TESE. Transl Androl Urol. 2020; 9:S206-14.
7. Agarwal A, Henkel R, Huang CC, Lee MS. Automation of human semen analysis using a novel artificial intelligence optical microscopic technology. Andrologia. 2019;51:e13440.
8. Javadi S, Mirroshandel SA. A novel deep learning method for automatic assessment of human sperm images. Comput Biol Med. 2019;109:182-94.
9. McCallum C, Riordon J, Wang Y, Kong T, You JB, Sanner S, et al. Deep learning-based selection of human sperm with high DNA integrity. Commun Biol. 2019;2:250.
10. Goodson SG, White S, Stevans AM, Bhat S, Kao CY, Jaworski S, et al. CASAnova: a multiclass support vector machine model for the classification of human sperm motility patterns. Biol Reprod. 2017;97:698-708.
11. Zeadna A, Khateeb N, Rokach L, Lior Y, Har-Vardi I, Harlev A, et al. Prediction of sperm extraction in non-obstructive azoospermia patients: a machine-learning perspective. Hum Reprod. 2020;35:1505-14.
12. Chu KY, Nassau DE, Arora H, Lokeshwar SD, Madhusoodanan V, Ramasamy R. Artificial intelligence in reproductive urology. Curr Urol Rep. 2019;20:52.
13. Sahoo AJ, Kumar Y. Seminal quality prediction using data mining methods. Technol Health Care. 2014;22:531-45.
14. Kanakasabapathy M, Thirumalaraju P, Yogesh V, Natarajan V, Bormann CL, Bhowmick P, et al. Automated smartphone-based system for semen assessment through the hyaluronic binding assay. Fertil Steril. 2017;108:E74.
15. Dimitriadis I, Bormann CL, Kanakasabapathy MK, Thirumalaraju P, Kandula H, Yogesh V, et al. Automated smartphone-based system for measuring sperm viability, DNA fragmentation, and hyaluronic binding assay score. PLoS One. 2019;14:e0212562.
16. Gunderson SJ, Puga Molina LC, Spies N, Balestrini PA, Buffone MG, Jungheim ES, et al. Machine-learning algorithm incorporating capacitated sperm intracellular pH predicts conventional in vitro fertilization success in normospermic patients. Fertil Steril. 2021;115:930-9.
17. Wu DJ, Badamjav O, Reddy VV, Eisenberg M, Behr B. A preliminary study of sperm identification in microdissection testicular sperm extraction samples with deep convolutional neural networks. Asian J Androl. 2021;23(2):135-9.
18. Agarwal A, Henkel R, Huang CC, Lee MS. Automation of human semen analysis using a novel artificial intelligence optical microscopic technology. Andrologia. 2019;51:e13440.
19. Rienzi L, Ubaldi FM, Iacobelli M, Minasi MG, Romano S, Ferrero S, et al. Significance of metaphase II human oocyte morphology on ICSI outcome. Fertil Steril. 2008;90:1692-700.
20. Manna C, Nanni L, Lumini A, Pappalardo S. Artificial intelligence techniques for embryo and oocyte classification. Reprod Biomed Online. 2013;26:42-9.
21. Targosz A, Przystałka P, Wiaderkiewicz R, Mrugacz G. Semantic segmentation of human oocyte images using deep neural networks. Biomed Eng Online. 2021;20:40.
22. Bormann CL, Kanakasabapathy MK, Thirumalaraju P, Gupta R, Pooniwala R, Kandula H, et al. Performance of a deep learning based neural network in the selection of human blastocysts for implantation. Elife. 2020;9:e55301.
23. Dimitriadis I, Bormann CL, Kanakasabapathy MK, Thirumalaraju P, Gupta R, Pooniwala R, et al. Deep convolutional neural networks (CNN) for assessment and selection of normally fertilized human embryos. Fertil Steril. 2019; 112:e272.
24. Coticchio G, Fiorentino G, Nicora G, Sciajno R, Cavalera F, Bellazzi R, et al. Cytoplasmic movements of the early human embryo: imaging and artificial intelligence to predict blastocyst development. Reprod Biomed Online. 2021;42:521-8.
25. Bortoletto P, Kanakasabapathy MK, Thirumalaraju P, Gupta R, Pooniwala R, Souter I, et al. Predicting blastocyst formation of day 3 embryos using a convolutional neural network (CNN): a machine learning approach. Fertil Steril. 2019;112:e272-3.
26. Kanakasabapathy MK, Thirumalaraju P, Bormann CL, Gupta R, Pooniwala R, Kandula H, et al. Deep learning mediated single time-point image-based prediction of embryo developmental outcome at the cleavage stage. ArXiv. 2020;08346:5-21.
27. Carrasco B, Arroyo G, Gil Y, Gómez MJ, Rodríguez I, Barri PN, et al. Selecting embryos with the highest implantation potential using data mining and decision tree based on classical embryo morphology and morphokinetics. J Assist Reprod Genet. 2017;34:983-90.
28. Wang LH, Fu ZX, Ye SZ, Ke DG. Pattern recognition of IVF's early embryo images based on support vector machines and texture features. Int J Eng Trends Technol. 2018;66:7-11.
29. Kelly N, Bormann CL, Dickinson J, Meyer AD, Kanakasabapathy MK, Thirumalaraju P, et al. Future of automation: use of deep convolutional neural networks (CNN) to identify precise location to perform laser assisted hatching on human cleavage stage embryos. Fertil Steril. 2020;114:E144.
30. Wong CC, Loewke KE, Bossert NL, Behr B, De Jonge CJ, Baer TM, et al. Non-invasive imaging of human embryos before embryonic genome activation predicts development to the blastocyst stage. Nat Biotechnol. 2010;28:1115-21.
31. Meyer A, Dickinson J, Kelly N, Kandula H, Kanakasabapathy M, Thirumalaraju P, et al. Can deep convolutional neural network (CNN) be used as a non-invasive method to replace preimplantation genetic testing for aneuploidy (PGT-A). Hum Reprod. 2020;35:1238.
32. Liao S, Pan W, Dai WQ, Jin L, Huang G, Wang R, et al. Development of a dynamic diagnosis grading system for infertility using machine learning. JAMA Netw Open. 2020; 3:e2023654.
33. Huang TTF, Kosasa T, Walker B, Arnett C, Huang CTF, Yin C, et al. Application of a deep learning neural network for the analysis of human blastocyst expansion from defined time-lapse image files. Reprod Biomed Online. 2021;42:1075-85.
34. Bori L, Paya E, Alegre L, Viloria TA, Remohi JA, Naranjo V, et al. Novel and conventional embryo parameters as input data for artificial neural networks: an artificial intelligence model applied for prediction of the implantation potential. Fertil Steril. 2020;114:1232-41.

35. Khosravi P, Kazemi E, Zhan Q, Malmsten JE, Toschi M, Zisimopoulos P, et al. Deep learning enables robust assessment and selection of human blastocysts after in vitro fertilization. NPJ Digit Med. 2019;2:21.
36. Bormann CL, Kanakasabapathy MK, Thirumalaraju P, Gupta R, Pooniwala R, Kandula H, Hariton E, Souter I, Dimitriadis I, Ramirez LB, Curchoe CL, Swain J, Boehnlein LM, Shafiee H. Performance of a deep learning based neural network in the selection of human blastocysts for implantation. eLife 2020; 9: e55301. doi:10.7554/eLife.55301.
37. Bormann CL, Thirumalaraju P, Kanakasabapathy MK, Kandula H, Souter I, Dimitriadis I, Gupta R, Pooniwala R, Shafiee H. Consistency and objectivity of automated embryo assessments using deep neural networks. Fertil Steril. 2020; 113:781-87.
38. Souter I, Vagios S, Sacha C, Kanakasabapathy MK, Thirumalaraju P, Bormann CL, et al. Validation of a deep convolutional neural network trained to assess whether an embryo meets criteria for biopsy/cryopreservation using a test set of PGT embryos. Hum Reprod. 2020;35:1257-8.
39. Thirumalaraju P, Kanakasabapathy MK, Bormann CL, Gupta R, Pooniwala R, Kandula H, Souter I, Dimitriadis I, Shafiee H. Evaluation of deep convolutional neural networks in classifying human embryo images based on their morphological quality. Heliyon. 2021;7:E06298.
40. Gazzo E, Peña F, Valdéz F, Chung A, Bonomini C, Ascenzo M, et al. The Kidscore D5 algorithm as an additional tool to morphological assessment and PGT-A in embryo selection: a time-lapse study. JBRA Assist Reprod. 2020;24:55-60.
41. VerMilyea M, Hall JMM, Diakiw SM, Johnston A, Nguyen T, Perugini D, et al. Development of an artificial intelligence-based assessment model for prediction of embryo viability using static images captured by optical light microscopy during IVF. Hum Reprod. 2020;35:770-84.
42. Practice Committees of the American Society for Reproductive Medicine and the Society for Assisted Reproductive Technology. The use of preimplantation genetic testing for aneuploidy (PGT-A): a committee opinion. Fertil Steril. 2018;109:429-36.
43. Curchoe CL, Bormann CL. Artificial intelligence and machine learning for human reproduction and embryology presented at ASRM and ESHRE 2018. J Assist Reprod Genet. 2019;36:591-600.
44. Mastenbroek S, Twisk M, van der Veen F, Repping S. Preimplantation genetic screening: a systematic review and meta-analysis of RCTs. Hum Reprod Update. 2011;17:454-66.
45. Campbell A, Fishel S, Bowman N, Duffy S, Sedler M, Thornton S. Retrospective analysis of outcomes after IVF using an aneuploidy risk model derived from time-lapse imaging without PGS. Reprod Biomed Online. 2013;27:140-6.
46. Simopoulou M, Sfakianoudis K, Maziotis E, Antoniou N, Rapani A, Anifandis G, et al. Are computational applications the "crystal ball" in the IVF laboratory? The evolution from mathematics to artificial intelligence. J Assist Reprod Genet. 2018;35:1545-57.
47. Basile N, Nogales Mdel C, Bronet F, Florensa M, Riqueiros M, Rodrigo L, et al. Increasing the probability of selecting chromosomally normal embryos by time-lapse morphokinetics analysis. Fertil Steril. 2014;101:699-704.
48. Campbell A, Fishel S, Bowman N, Duffy S, Sedler M, Hickman CF. Modelling a risk classification of aneuploidy in human embryos using non-invasive morphokinetics. Reprod Biomed Online. 2013;26:477-85.
49. Sene AA, Zandieh Z, Sofaei M, Torshizi HM, Sheibani K. Using artificial intelligence to predict the intrauterine insemination success rate among infertile couples. Middle East Fertil Soc J. 2021;26:46.
50. Güvenir HA, Misirli G, Dilbaz S, Ozdegirmenci O, Demir B, Dilbaz B. Estimating the chance of success in IVF treatment using a ranking algorithm. Med Biol Eng Comput. 2015; 53:911-20.
51. Siristatidis C, Stavros S, Drakeley A, Bettocchi S, Pouliakis A, Drakakis P, et al. Omics and artificial intelligence to improve in vitro fertilization (IVF) success: a proposed protocol. Diagnostics (Basel). 2021;11:743.
52. Huang B, Zheng S, Ma B, Yang Y, Zhang S, Jin L. Using deep learning to predict the outcome of live birth from more than 10,000 embryo data. BMC Pregnancy Childbirth. 2022;22:36.
53. Xi Q, Yang Q, Wang M, Huang B, Zhang B, Li Z, et al. Individualized embryo selection strategy developed by stacking machine learning model for better in vitro fertilization outcomes: an application study. Reprod Biol Endocrinol. 2021;19:53.
54. Hassan MR, Al-Insaif S, Hossain MI, Kamruzzaman J. A machine learning approach for prediction of pregnancy outcome following IVF treatment. Neural Comput Appl. 2018;32:2283-97.
55. Durairaj M, Thamilselvan P. Applications of artificial neural network for IVF data analysis and prediction. J Eng Comput Appl Sci. 2013;2:11-5.
56. Adams NM, Hand DJ. Comparing classifiers when the misallocation costs are uncertain. Pattern Recognit. 1999; 32:1139-47.
57. Drummond C, Holte RC. Cost curves: an improved method for visualizing classifier performance. Mach Learn. 2006;65:95-130.
58. Vabalas A, Gowen E, Poliakoff E, Casson AJ. Machine learning algorithm validation with a limited sample size. PLoS One. 2019;14:e0224365.
59. Zheng X, Fu X, Wang K, Wang M. Deep neural networks for human microRNA precursor detection. BMC Bioinformatics. 2020;21:17.
60. Kirkegaard K, Campbell A, Agerholm I, Bentin-Ley U, Gabrielsen A, Kirk J, et al. Limitations of a time-lapse blastocyst prediction model: a large multicentre outcome analysis. Reprod Biomed Online. 2014;29:156-8.
61. Racowsky C, Kovacs P, Martins WP. A critical appraisal of time-lapse imaging for embryo selection: where are we and where do we need to go? J Assist Reprod Genet. 2015;32:1025-30.
62. Chen M, Wei S, Hu J, Yuan J, Liu F. Does time-lapse imaging have favorable results for embryo incubation and selection compared with conventional methods in clinical in vitro fertilization? A meta-analysis and systematic review of randomized controlled trials. PLoS One. 2017;12:e0178720.
63. Dolinko AV, Farland LV, Kaser DJ, Missmer SA, Racowsky C. National survey on use of time-lapse imaging systems in IVF laboratories. J Assist Reprod Genet. 2017;34:1167-72.
64. Sanson-Fisher RW, Bonevski B, Green LW, D'Este C. Limitations of the randomized controlled trial in evaluating population-based health interventions. Am J Prev Med. 2007;33:155-61.
65. Nichol AD, Bailey M, Cooper DJ, POLAR, EPO Investigators. Challenging issues in randomised controlled trials. Injury. 2010;41(Suppl 1):S20-3.

SECTION

# 17 Laboratory Management

CHAPTER 121

# Setting-up an ART Laboratory

*R Suchindra, Anuja Kamath*

## INTRODUCTION

Over the last few decades, the services provide by an assisted-reproductive technology (ART) clinic have evolved. The types of treatment offered by an in vitro fertilization (IVF) clinic, today, include procedures like intrauterine insemination (IUI), IVF, intracytoplasmic sperm injection (ICSI), other micromanipulation techniques, cryopreservation, and preimplantation genetic diagnosis (PGD). The ART laboratory is the place where gametes, i.e., oocytes and sperms are handled to form an embryo. This requires a sterile, stable, and nontoxic environment. Therefore, it is very critical to setup an optimum ART laboratory. The infrastructure, equipment, and the design depend on the number and the type of ART cycles performed in the clinic.

## LAYOUT OF AN ART LABORATORY

The layout of an ART laboratory is described in **Figure 1**.

*A basic ART laboratory should have:*

- A fully equipped operation theater (OT) for ovum pickup (OPU), embryo transfer (ET), and for surgical sperm retrievals [percutaneous epididymal sperm aspiration (PESA)/testicular sperm aspiration (TESA)/testicular sperm extraction (TESE), etc.].
- The embryology laboratory is like the *sanctum sanctorum*, the heart of the ART clinic and it should be located adjacent to the OT. The laboratory should have restricted access, and a pass window should be provided on the wall, which is shared between the OT and the embryology laboratory. The follicular fluid aspirated during OPU is passed to the embryology laboratory through the pass box, this minimizes the door opening and helps prevent the entry of outside air.
- Andrology laboratory for semen analysis and semen preparation should be located next to embryology laboratory. It should also have a semen collection room adjacent to it with a closed pass box on the wall common to andrology and collection room. This is to facilitate the transfer of samples from the collection room to the laboratory, minimizing the movement from the laboratory.
- Cryopreservation materials like liquid nitrogen, and stored samples container should be kept in a room adjacent to the embryology laboratory.
- Carbon dioxide and nitrogen cylinders used for the incubators should be kept in a separate area outside the laboratory creating a gas bank, from which gas should be supplied to the incubators through piped gas lines. This will prevent the interference in embryology laboratory, caused by the movement of the cylinders while changing them. An inline-activated charcoal (CODA) and high-efficiency particulate air (HEPA) filter should be always provided to filter out the volatile gas and particulate matter.
- IVF culture media should always be kept in a refrigerator, which should be exclusively used for embryology.
- Scrub area should be located at a convenient place.
- There should be a recovery room for patients, which can be used for preparation as well as post procedure.
- Changing rooms with toilets should be planned well.

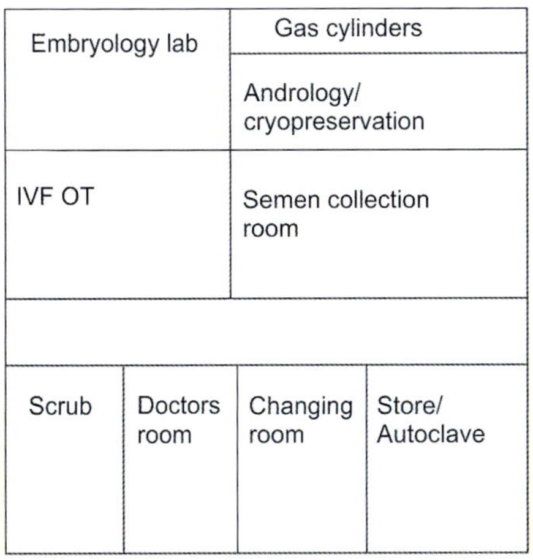


**Fig. 1:** Layout of an assisted-reproductive technology laboratory. (IVF: in vitro fertilization; OT: operation theater).

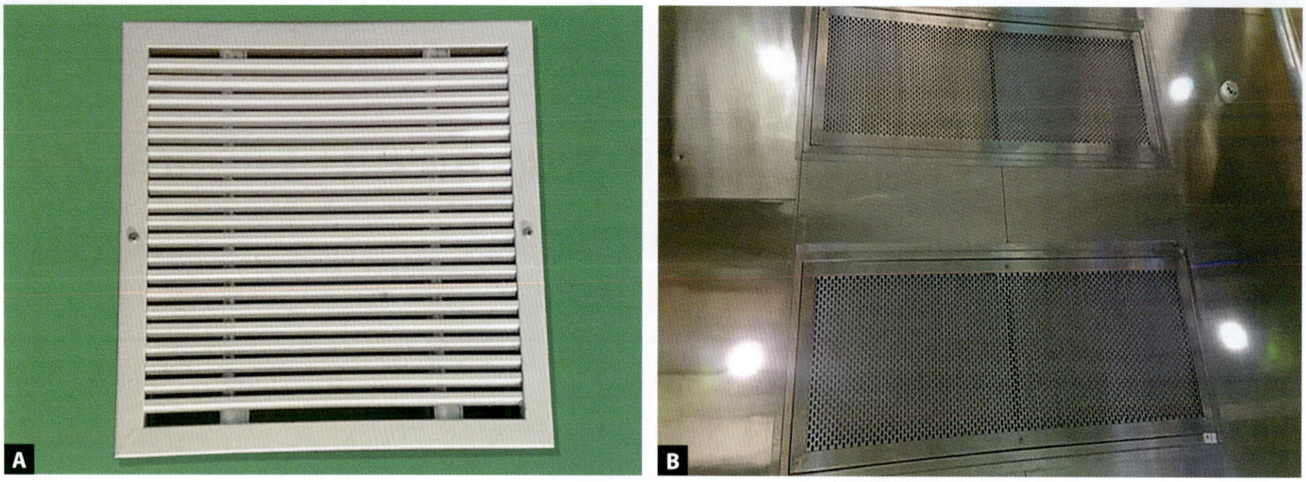

**Figs. 2A and B:** Heating, ventilation, and air-conditioning system.

- Stores for embryology consumables should be separate from others.
- Staff room, counseling room, and discussion rooms should also be planned accordingly.

## INFRASTRUCTURE FOR NEW LABORATORY SET-UP

### Site Suitability and Basic Design

The location of the building in which the IVF laboratory is to be set up is very important. Attention should be paid to possible sources of chemical and particulate pollution, e.g., foundries, petroleum processing units, vehicle garages etc. The IVF laboratory should have a supply of HEPA -filtered air similar to that of an operating theater.

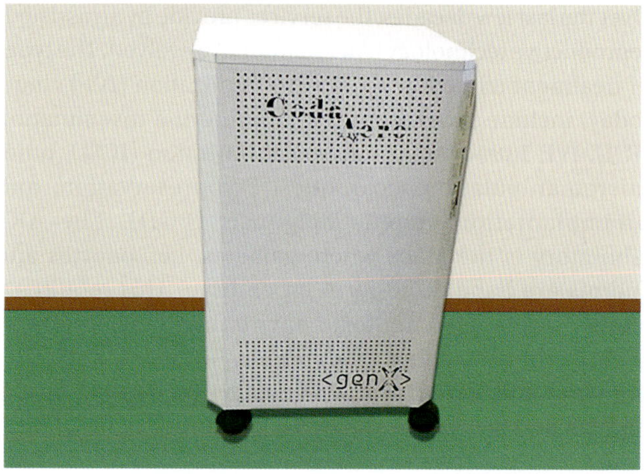


**Fig. 3:** Coda mini tower as stand-alone.

### Air Quality

- Particulates: Ideally should be less than 352,000 particles larger than 0.5–10 μm per $m^3$
- Micro-organisms: ideally should be less than 10 cfu/$m^3$ and less than 2 spores/$m^3$ "at rest".
- VOC: Ideally total VOCs should be less than 500 μg/$m^3$ (~400–800 ppb total VOC); aldehydes should be less than 5 μg/$m^3$.
- Air changes: Ideally 15 total air changes per hour (ACH), including three fresh air changes per hour (20% outside air)
- Positive Pressure: The ideal target is +38 to +50 Pa in the IVF laboratory (minimum recommended is at least +30 Pa).
- Temperature: Temperature in the IVF laboratory should be regulated by the HVAC system (**Figs. 2A and B**). The HVAC comprises of heating, ventilation, and air-conditioning. The temperature should be maintained in the range of 20–24°C (depending on region).[1]
- Humidity: The relative room humidity (RH) should be between 40 and 45%. Higher humidity helps growth of contamination like molds, while lower humidity may cause discomfort to the laboratory personnel, and also can cause higher evaporation of media during dish preparation, which may consequently affect osmolarity of the culture medium and be detrimental to the embryo quality **(Fig. 3)**.[2]
- General design and construction criteria
  - The IVF laboratory should be equipped with a dedicated AHU to prevent contamination of the cleanroom air with air from adjoining places. The HVAC system must run constantly, not just during working hours.
  - The fresh air inlet should be located away from sources of obnoxious fumes and it can be further prefiltered to increase the functional life of the filter systems.
  - The HVAC system should be incorporated with activated carbon or potassium permanganate filter for elimination of VOCs
  - The HVAC system should be equipped to provide adequate warming or cooling of incoming fresh air depending on the local climatic conditions.

- The HVAC system should also be able to totally isolate the laboratory air from the outside air, in case of emergencies like local construction works, repairs of the road works, which can generate high VOCs.
- Air supply vents should be placed in the ceiling and outlet return ducts should be placed close to the floor level.
- HEPA filters should be placed in a central position to avoid difficult access during their cleaning and maintenance.
- Ideally, pressure sensors should be installed on the side of the doorway to the IVF laboratory. This pressure gauge should display differential pressure.
- The exterior walls of the IVF laboratory should be a complete wall from the concrete floor to the roof with no perforations present on the wall
- The ceiling must be constructed with solid material like plasterboard, gypsum board, etc. Essential access panels should have air-tight, silicone gaskets.
- Light fittings must be air-tight, designed for cleanrooms and should be air tight.
- All electrical, gas, and data outputs should be sealed to prevent air loss through them.
- Doors must be tight-fitting with bottom "sweeps" and perimeter seals (top and edges). The view panels, if any, should also be installed using gaskets to make them air-tight.
- Pass boxes should be air-tight to preserve room positive air pressure.
- Construction materials: For walls steel modular panels or plasterboard coated with zero VOC paint or antimicrobial wall paper can be used. Floors can be covered with vinyl with impervious sealed joints. The floor of area where cryopreservation procedures will take place should be made of nonthermally fragile material like stainless-steel tread plate.
- Non-porous materials like epoxy, Corian, and Granite should be used for counter tops.
- Furniture like cabinets (under and over benches) should be powder-coated metal or stainless steel.
- Use of manufactured wood products and polish is not recommended, as they have all been demonstrated to be embryotoxic.

## "Burn In" of an IVF Laboratory

- A newly constructed or renovated IVF laboratory will have a compromised air quality, due to the VOCs and other contaminants released from construction materials like paint.
- "Burn In" of an IVF involves increasing the laboratory temperature by 10–15°C and also increasing the air cycles for better ventilation, for at least 2–4 weeks before its operation.
- This facilitates offgassing from various building materials and also facilitates lowering of the VOCs.
- A final check of the air quality and VOCs should be done before commencing the work.

## Equipment

The equipment for an embryology laboratory depends on the number of cycles and the type of procedures offered by the clinic. The equipment can be classified into essential and optional.

- Essential equipment:
  - The integrated workstation (laminar air flow)
  - $CO_2$ incubator or box incubator
  - Trigas incubator or bench-top incubator
  - Micromanipulator with inverted microscope
  - Centrifuge
  - Makler chamber
  - Cryopreservation equipment (cryocans).
- Optional equipment:
  - Intracytoplasmic morphologically selected sperm injection (IMSI)
  - Laser
  - Timelapse imaging or embryoscope.

### *The Integrated Workstation or Laminar Air Flow*

- The workstation should have a temperaturecontroled floor, maintained at 37°C. Temperature maintenance is of utmost importance for the spindle integrity in oocytes and also likely for normal fertilization and subsequent embryo development **(Fig. 4)**.[7]
- Also it should be equipped with a stereo zoom microscope (**Figs. 5A and B**), 10× or 15× magnifications for screening of oocytes, denudation, and then visualizing the embryos.

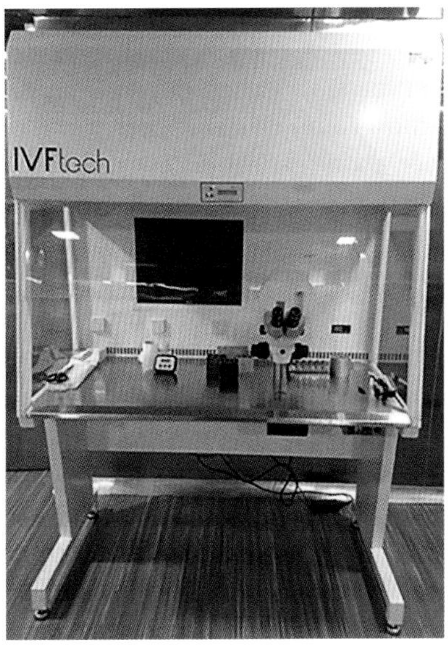


**Fig. 4:** In vitro fertilization workstation with laminar air flow.

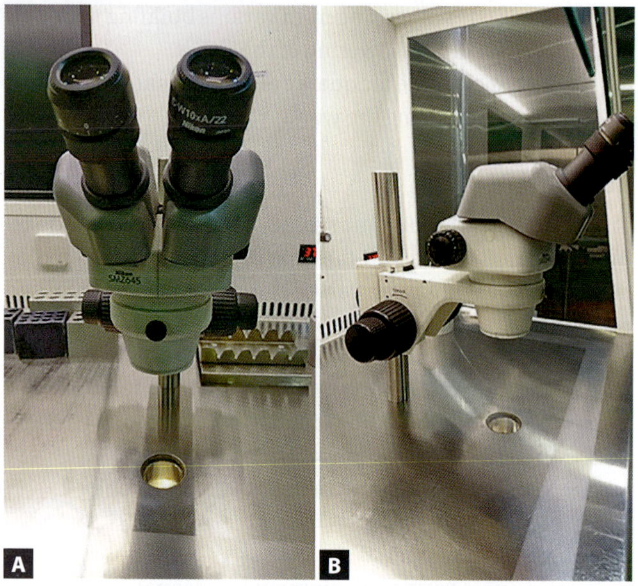

**Figs. 5A and B:** Stereozoom microscope.

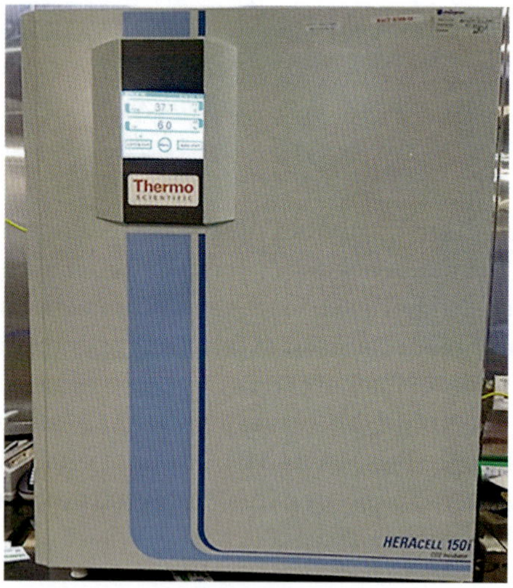


**Fig. 6:** Box type $CO_2$ incubator (Heracell).

- The size of the workstation depends on the workload, 3*2 is the most common size.
- Turbulence pattern of the flow differs in horizontal and vertical laminar flow, therefore a vertical flow is preferred.[8]
- Ideally two workstations are required, one for sperm preparation and another one for preparing culture dishes, screening and grading of oocytes and embryos, and loading embryos into catheters for transfer.

### $CO_2$ Incubator or Box Incubator

- $CO_2$ incubators provide optimum environment for the culture of embryos **(Fig. 6)**.
- These are used to incubate media, holding the oocytes after screening, for semen preparation, and to hold embryos before ET.
- The box incubators usually control concentration of one gas, i.e., $CO_2$. The concentration of $CO_2$ depends on the bicarbonate concentration in the culture media.
- The door of the incubator is also heated, so as to maintain the temperature inside, and also facilitate quick recovery of temperature after closing the door. Also there will be a gas tight door inside, which prevents the gas leak. Preferably incubator with more chambers should be preferred as the recovery of temperature and pH will be faster.
- The incubators should be equipped with infrared sensors for $CO_2$ monitoring.
- Medical grade $CO_2$ should be provided and should pass through inline filters, to eliminate all contaminants present in the gas.
- The incubator should be equipped with failure alarm, and also there should be provision to install independent probes, remote alarm system, and uninterrupted power supply (UPS).
- "Burn in" of the incubators before starting the operations is necessary, absence of "burn in" of incubators before use resulted in stress to embryos possibly via induction of VOCs thus producing a significant difference in the ART outcome.[9]

### Tri-gas Incubator or Benchtop Incubator

- A benchtop incubator combine optimal embryo growth conditions due to individual chambers and also have advanced user control (**Figs. 7A and B**). They minimize the pH and temperature fluctuations.
- $O_2$ concentrations can be reduced to 5%, the reduced $O_2$ tension in the gas mixture closely mimics physiological circumstances[10] and minimizes oxidative stress to the embryos that may arise at 20% $O_2$.[11,12]
- Embryos cultured in a 5% $O_2$ environment consistently resulted in higher rates of implantation and live births when compared with rates among women whose embryos were cultured in an atmospheric $O_2$ environment.
- They may require a premix gas, e.g., MINC, Planar, or there might be integrated gas mixing unit in the incubator, e.g., K System, ESCO.

### Micromanipulator with Inverted Microscope

- Micromanipulator is an integrated system with inverted microscope, used for micromanipulation of oocytes with sperm, also known as ICSI **(Fig. 8)**.
- The inverted microscope is used for detailed examination of oocytes and embryos. Interference optics such as Hoffman and Nomarski are preferable as they permit the best measure of detail and depth.

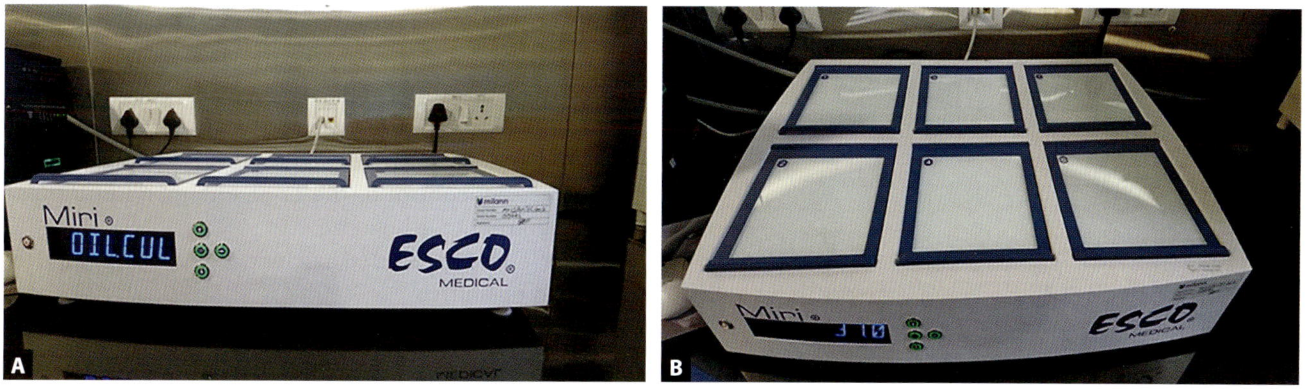


**Figs. 7A and B:** Benchtop incubator.

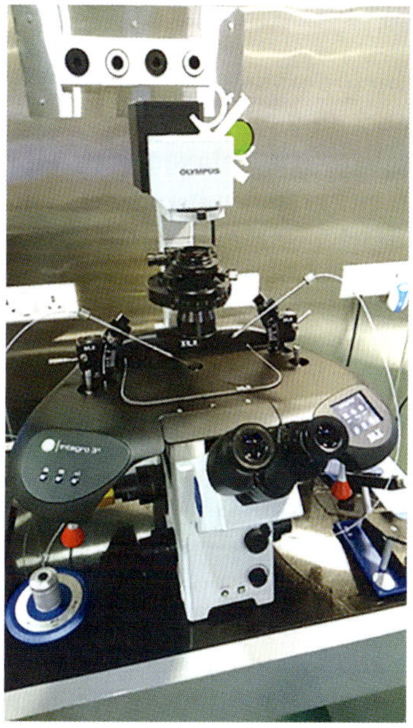

**Fig. 8:** Micromanipulator.

- The manipulator is equipped with a stage heater to maintain temperature in culture dishes during ICSI, pronuclear check, embryo development check, LAH, and biopsy for preimplantation genetic screening or PGD.
- Rigorous thermal control produced by a heating system stabilized spindles and increased fertilization, embryo development, and clinical pregnancy rates achieved after ICSI.[13]
- The inverted microscope should be equipped with a *still camera and/or video camera and monitor*, to capture images which can be analyzed after returning the gametes to the incubator. It also helps in training new embryologist and allows placement of still photos in patient file.
- *Micromanipulator* should be equipped with microtool holders for bilateral micromanipulation, suction or injection, and biopsy device.[14]
- A micromanipulator should be placed on an antivibration table.

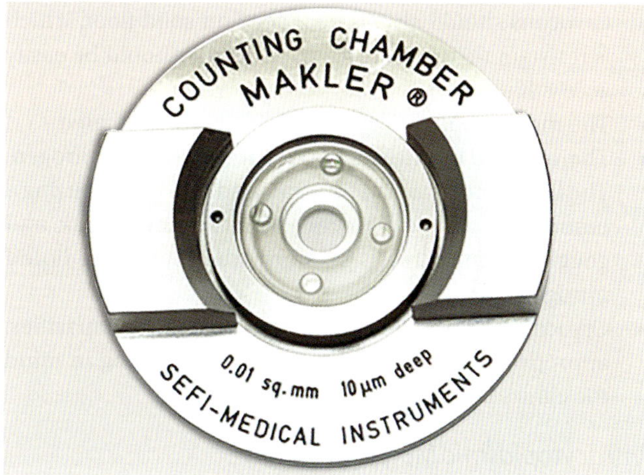


**Fig. 9:** Makler chamber.

### *Centrifuge*

- Centrifuges are required for sperm preparation.
- Swing-out rotor centrifuges are preferred as they have a gentler effect on separated particles.
- The relative centrifugal field should not go beyond 800 g as this may cause accidental damage to the sperm.

### *Makler Chamber*

- The *Makler counting chamber* is a simpletouse device for rapid and accurate sperm count, motility, and morphology evaluation from undiluted specimen **(Fig. 9)**.
- The chamber is composed of two parts:
  1. The *lower part has a metal base* and two handles. In the center of the base there is a flat disc made of optical flat glass on which the sample is placed.
  2. The *upper part is the cover glass* encircled with a metal ring. At the center of its lower surface there is a 1 mm$^2$ grid, subdivided into 100 squares, each one of 0.1 × 0.1 mm.
- When the cover glass is placed on the four tips, the space bounded in a row of 10 squares is exactly

onemillionth of mL. Therefore, the number of sperm heads in 10 squares indicates their concentration in million/mL.

- The depth of 10 microns eliminates blurring and allows sperm to move freely. The applied sample is observed in one focal plane.

### Cryopreservation

- A separate room or an area in the laboratory, earmarked for cryostorage is essential.
- There should be enough space, and the growth of the clinic in future years should also be taken into consideration while ordering the cryogenic equipment also known as cryocans.
- Cryocans should always be placed on solid floor, which is resistant to liquid nitrogen; each tank should be easily accessible.
- The room should be safely and efficiently ventilated.
- There should be one storage can, to store liquid nitrogen. The liquid nitrogen can be dispensed into dewars using a pump. Appropriate protective gear like gown, mask, and goggles should always be worn when handling liquid nitrogen.
- Cryocans are available in different makes and capacities, appropriate ones should be procured keeping in mind the clinics load of cases **(Fig. 10)**.

### Intracytoplasmic Morphologically Selected Sperm Injection

- Intracytoplasmic morphologically selected sperm injection is a variation of ICSI using higher magnification of 6600× **(Fig. 11)**.
- IMSI is used to study the sperm head in detail and look for abnormal head, vacuolation, and acrosome abnormalities.
- IMSI is configured of an inverted microscope with Nomarski optics, with video zoom and digital imaging system.

### Laser

- The laser system is made up of a laser objective, which generates and releases the required energy in the form of laser shots allowing the zona pellucida to be dissolved.
- It comprises a software, which provides to the operator a precisely control of the laser energy output, pulse duration, and the hole size.
- Laser is used for assisted hatching, zona thinning, and for biopsy of embryo.

### Embryoscope

- The embryoscope is an incubator that maintains the necessary physiological conditions required by a living embryo while they are in the IVF laboratory (**Figs. 12A and B**).
- It has an incorporated timelapse system that has a camera that continuously captures images and records them as a video of the embryonic development.
- This system allows the embryologist to monitor embryo cell divisions while the embryos are still in the incubator and we can carry out a study of the development of the embryos.

### Electronic Witnessing System

- Electronic Witnessing System (EWS) is a modern day tool in the ART Laboratory.
- It acts as a double witnessing system for Embryologists.
- It provides complete electronic traceability and minimizes potential mix ups.
- An EWS uses radio frequency identification tags (RFID) for tracking and recording patients' information and the biological samples during the ART procedures.
- The EWS monitors each and every instance wherein the gametes or embryos are shifted from one dish to the next and ensures that only one patient can be worked on at one time. Monitoring is constant, so an identity check can never be overlooked.

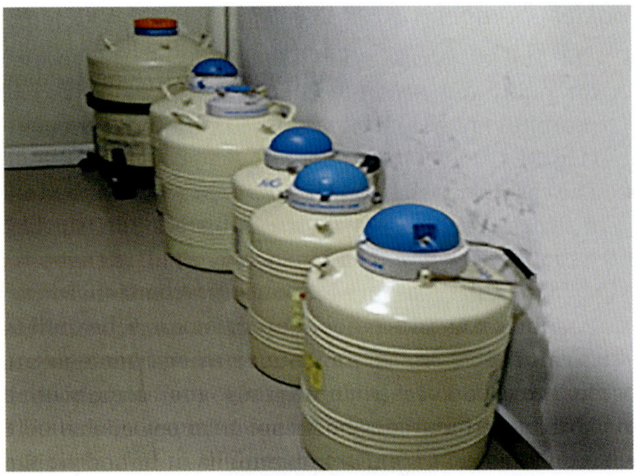

**Fig. 10:** Cryocans.

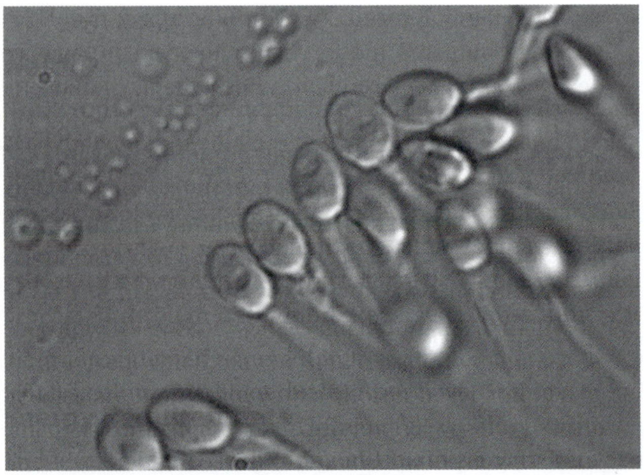

**Fig. 11:** Intracytoplasmic morphologically selected sperm injection.

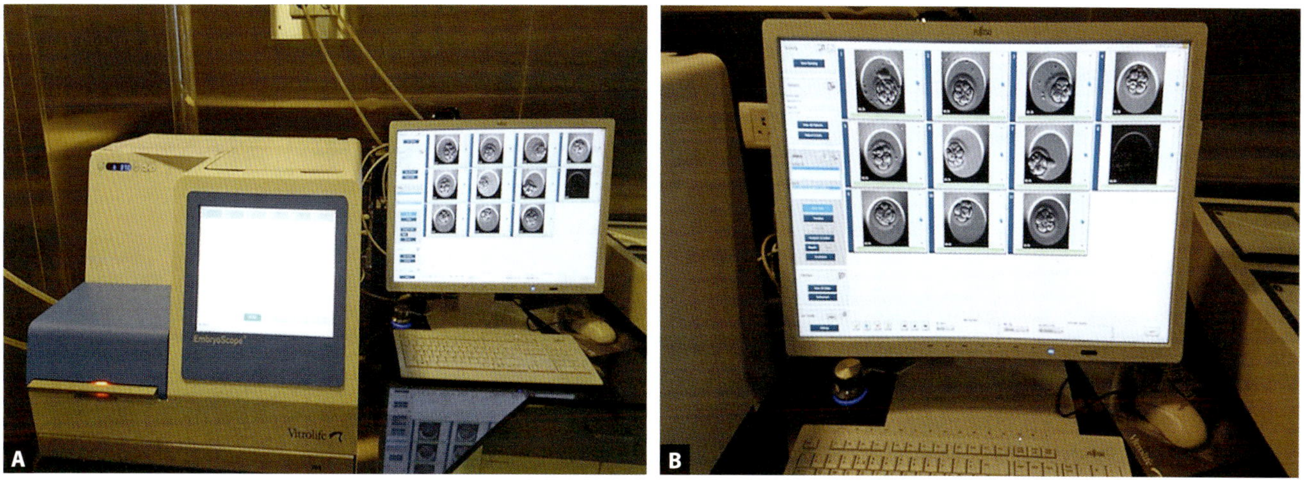


**Figs. 12A and B:** Embryoscope.

## KEY NOTES

Careful Planning of the design, facilities, equipment, and layout is required for dedicated, focused, and uninterrupted concentration while working in an ART laboratory. Also equally important are the personnel who are trained and professional and can carry out the required procedures with proficiency. This maintains high pregnancy rates despite multifactorial variables. Thus, it is important to provide the IVF laboratory with the "best" technology available to produce top quality embryos, develop best methods to select best embryos, and develop optimized cryopreservation procedure.

## REFERENCES

1. Panizzo R (2010). Air pollution linked to lower IVF success. Progress Educational rust [online]. Available from: http://www.bionews.org.uk/ page_58675.asp.
2. Forman M, Polanski V, Horvath P, Gilligan A, Rieger D. Reductions in volatile organic compounds, aldehydes, and particulate air contaminants in an IVF laboratory by centralized and standalone air filtration systems. Fertil Steril. 2004;82(2):S324.
3. Cohen J, Gilligan A, Esposito W, Schimmel T, Dale B. Ambient air and its potential effects on conception in vitro. Hum Reprod. 1997;12(8):1742-9.
4. Cohen J, Gilligan A, Willadsen S. Culture and quality control of embryos. Hum Reprod. 1998;13(Suppl 3):137-44.
5. Hall J, Gilligan A, Schimmel T, Cecchi M, Cohen J. The origin, effects and control of air pollution in laboratories used for human embryo culture. Hum Reprod. 1998;13(Suppl 4): 146-55.
6. Boone WR, Johnson JE, Locke AJ. Crane MM, Price TM. Control of air quality in an assisted reproductive technology laboratory. Fertil Steril. 1999;71(1):150-4.
7. Wang WH, Meng L, Hackett RJ, Odenbourg R, Keefe DL. Limited recovery of meiotic spindles in living human oocytes after cooling rewarming observed using polarized light microscopy. Hum Reprod. 2001;16(11):2374-8.
8. Avis KE, Levchuk JW. Special considerations in the use of vertical laminarflow workbenches. Am J Hosp Pharm. 1984;41(1):81-7.
9. Singh S, Chakraborty P, Goswami SK, Chattopadhyay R, Chakravarty B. The impact of "burning in" of incubators before initiating assisted repro ductive cycles—a comparative study. Fertil Steril. 2015;104(3):e189.
10. Fischer B, Bavister BD. Oxygen tension in oviduct and uterus of rhesus monkeys, hamsters and rabbits. J Reprod Fertil. 1993;99(2):673-9.
11. Thompson JG, Simpson AC, Pugh PA, Donnelly PE, Tervit HR. Effects of oxygen concentration on in vitro development of preimplantation sheep and cattle embryos. J Reprod Fertil. 1990;89(2):573-8.
12. Noda Y, Goto Y, Umaoka Y, Shiotani M, Nakayama T, Mori T. Culture of human embryos in alpha modification of Eagle's medium under low oxygen tension and low illumination. Fertil Steril. 1994;62(5):1022-7.
13. Wang WH, Meng L, Hackett RJ, Oldenbourg R, Keefe DL. Rigorous thermal control during intracytoplasmic sperm injection stabilizes the meiotic spindle and improves fertilization and pregnancy rates. Fertil Steril. 2002;77(6):1274-7.
14. Cohen J. Zona pellucida micromanipulation and consequences for embryonic development and implantation. In: Cohen J, Malter HF, Talansky BE, Grito J (Eds). Micromanipulation of Human Gametes and Embryos. New York: Raven Press;1992.

CHAPTER

# 122 Quality Control in IVF Laboratory

*Sanjay Shukla*

## INTRODUCTION

Last four decades have witnessed substantial growth in the field of assisted reproduction techniques (ART). Despite all the improvements in the field, ART success rate still remains relatively limited.

The organizational structure of an ART center is complex and multidisciplinary. It comprises medicos, laboratory staff, nursing and paramedics, management office, accounts department, and other support staff. Deficiency or poor performance of any element of this complex structure affects the overall performance of the entire organization and in turn emasculates the efforts to achieve high levels of success.

The Cairo consensus guidelines on IVF culture conditions reiterate the fact that everything in the IVF laboratory influences the outcome.[1] Thus, everything including infrastructure, designing, equipment, culture media, disposables and consumables, laboratory personnel and other staff, processes and procedures, needs to be "perfect" for proper functioning of the laboratory.[1]

In today's time, most of the in vitro fertilization (IVF) laboratories world over are equipped with excellent quality instruments designed to serve specific needs of human clinical embryology, however, only few IVF labs are able to produce consistently better results than the others.[2]

The clinical embryology laboratory's work goes beyond the role of other clinical or diagnostic laboratories and this needs to be understood that procuring good quality equipment or designing modular laboratories or using fancy gadgets only cannot translate into high success rates but the implementation of a total quality management (TQM) is needed to ensure consistency and reproducibility of results.[3,4]

## WHAT IS QUALITY?

In different areas, quality can be defined differently. However, in generalized term it means "the degree of excellence". In medicine, it can be defined as the *duty of care* and is often considered as equivalent to the *best practice.*[5]

It is the responsibility of IVF laboratory to not only comply to the regulatory standards but also to provide quality services to the patients in a safe, effective and satisfying manner.[6]

Professional societies such as European Society of Human Reproduction and Embryology (ESHRE), Association of Clinical Embryologists (ACE) and American Society for Reproductive Medicine (ASRM) have prepared guidelines to standardize the functioning of infertility clinics.[7-14] Similarly, Indian Council of Medical Research (ICMR) has also come up with a National Guidelines for Accreditation, Supervision and Regulation of ART Clinics in India.[15] Indian Society of Assisted Reproduction (ISAR) conducted a consensus meeting (2021) of experts and compiled a set of recommendations to standardize the ethical and safe practices of assisted reproductive technology in the country.[16]

In some countries, ART centers and IVF laboratories are regulated by law. Recently, India has also passed and implemented the long awaited Assisted Reproductive Technology (Regulation) Act and Surrogacy (Regulation) Act.[17,18] The enforcing government machinery like State Boards and Appropriate Authorities are yet to be formed in all the states of the country. The rules and regulations have also been released through subsequent Gazette notifications. However, these guidelines describe only the minimum requirement and recommendations for IVF clinics.[15] Quality control program is left to the discretion and understanding of the individual laboratories.

## QUALITY MANAGEMENT

In author's opinion, quality management (QM) is quality assurance (QA) by quality control (QC) and quality improvement (QI). This means, ensuring consistent "quality" by controlling each and every process, equipment, personnel and materials used in an IVF laboratory in a definite manner without deviations and then implementing strategies to improve further.[19]

This chapter is focused at the QC in human clinical embryology laboratory.

## QUALITY CONTROL

Quality control program in an IVF laboratory required to keep a check on the quality and performance of all the products, equipment, processes and the people working at different levels in the laboratory.[20,21] Measures to control the quality of air and environment of the laboratory are of paramount importance.[22,23]

A special attention is needed on the selection of equipment/devices used for QC measures. All the devices used for this purpose must be certified, calibrated and suitable for the measurement. Not only that, the person performing these QC checks must be properly trained and must possess adequate technical knowledge of the process. The QC activities performed by any person must also be reviewed periodically by appropriate authorities.[13]

This comprehensive QC program is necessary to ensure that every component of laboratory is functioning properly.

The QC program of a successful IVF laboratory must include the following points described here.[24]

### Standard Operating Protocols

Every IVF laboratory requires detailed, well documented, well defined and user-friendly standard operating protocols (SOPs). SOPs must include stepwise details of the scientific or technical procedures, monitoring techniques with methodology of the equipment used, laboratory cleaning and maintenance, etc. The frequency of all the monitoring measures must be decided by the workload of the laboratory. Every laboratory should establish and define the acceptable "range" of measures of activities and performance of all its constituents and these must clearly be mentioned in the SOPs. SOPs must also include corrective measures or actions required in case of any deviation from these predefined "ranges."[7,8,25]

A system to religiously follow the SOPs must be inculcated in every staff member and they must understand the importance of the type of work being carried out in the laboratory. The QC records should be available to the review committee. Proactive review of the QC record may help supervisors to identify possible problems or risks to take preventive measures.[5,26]

### Quality Control of Laboratory Environment

Although, it is a part of laboratory designing, IVF laboratory environment deserves a special mention here as it is the first thing to start a QC program.

Modern day IVF laboratories are designed as per ISO 8 or ISO 7 cleanroom standards.[27] The air delivered in the laboratories is high efficiency particulate air (HEPA) or ultra-low penetration air (ULPA) filtered to reduce the particulate matter. This air is circulated in such a fashion that a constant positive air pressure is maintained inside the laboratory to minimize the entry of outside air. Further, volatile organic compounds (VOCs) and chemical toxicants have serious negative effect on fertilization and embryo development. Therefore, suitable VOC filters are recommended in addition to HEPA or ULPA filters.[23]

Air quality can be monitored by particle counters and microbial testing. Regular maintenance and changing of air filters should be done. It must be kept in mind that in the absence of regular maintenance, the air filtration system may itself become a source of contamination and could even be more detrimental.[9,22,23]

Volatile organic compounds can also be monitored and various VOC monitors are available commercially. The limitation of most of the VOC monitors is that they can detect only few toxicants and that too in the range of parts per million (ppm) only.[9,23]

The personnel working in the laboratory are a major source of particulate and microbial contamination. Therefore, the traffic inside laboratory should be restricted to minimum. The staff must enter the laboratory after donning proper clothing, cap and masks.[9,22,23]

Use of toxic disinfectants and cleaning agents must be avoided and safer alternatives must be used for cleaning and disinfection.

The ambience of IVF laboratory is usually kept cold and dry. Higher temperature and humidity favor microbial growth. Also, important equipment such as warmers and incubators function well when the ambient temperature remains around 7°C less than the set values. Thus, recommended temperature for an IVF laboratory is below 25°C and relative humidity (RH) between 35% and 50%. RH <35% not only causes discomfort to the people working in the laboratory but also promotes static electricity.[27,28]

The location of the incubators, workstations and laminar air flow (LAF) hoods should never be in front of or under the direct air drag from AC or heating, ventilation and air-conditioning (HVAC) inlets to avoid temperature fluctuations.

Room thermometers and hygrometers should be installed to monitor ambient temperature and RH and the record of the readings must be maintained.

### Quality Control of Equipment

Temperature of equipment, such as incubators, heated stages of microscopes, test tube warmers, LAF hoods, dry baths and water baths should be monitored daily. Refrigerators used to keep media should also be monitored on a daily basis.

This monitoring must be independent of the inbuilt display of the equipment itself and must be done by a certified and calibrated thermometer. In case of any disparity in the readings of the equipment and calibrated thermometer, authorized service engineer should be called to get the calibration done and display of the equipment set accordingly.[27-29]

There are a variety of thermometers or probes available commercially to serve this purpose. To monitor the inside temperature of large incubators, test tube warmers, dry bath or water bath and even refrigerators, a thermometer can be placed in an oil filled test tube. Specially designed probes attached to electronic devices can be used to monitor the temperature of heated surface of LAF and benchtop incubators.[27-29]

Gas supply and RH in the incubators need to be monitored daily too. Media manufacturers recommend specific $CO_2$ concentration to achieve the desired pH in that particular medium. Also, same $CO_2$ concentration at different sea levels gives different pH to the same medium. Therefore, more and more laboratories are now preferring to monitor pH of the medium equilibrated in the incubator. Like temperature, gas concentration in the incubators and pH in the medium can be measured by various devices. Proper humidity is essential to avoid evaporation of media and consequent osmolality changes.[27-29]

Laboratories which are using triple gas mixture must ask the supplier to provide certificate of the desired concentration of mixed gases for every cylinder. Inline gas filters adsorb and filter many impurities from the gas supplied to incubators hence, recommended. Such filters must be replaced timely with new filters as recommended by the manufacturers.[28-30]

Incubators must be cleaned, sterilized and water must be changed as per the laboratory's policy and workload. This needs to be understood that the gas censors in the traditional box type incubators do have an expiry. Over the time these may need to change.

Other equipment such as micromanipulators, microscopes, media and gamete handling pipettes, LAF, etc., should be cleaned and serviced regularly as recommended by manufacturer. Regular maintenance of equipment is required for proper functioning.

Gas levels in the supply cylinders must be monitored and recorded daily. Backup gas supplies should be available on site. Similarly, liquid nitrogen ($LN_2$) levels in the cryotanks must be monitored and recorded regularly. A log of $LN_2$ top-ups and refills must be maintained.

It is recommended to install external audible alarms for incubators as well as for cryotanks. These alarms must be tested and mock drills for adverse events must be carried out regularly to ensure that system is working properly.[5,25]

## Quality Control of Culture Media

Culture media preparation demands very stringent quality control and precision. In present days' human IVF, most of the laboratories use commercially available culture media to avoid variations and technical problems that may arise in preparing comparatively smaller volumes in-house.

Laboratories using these media should control the way they store, handle and use the media. In countries such as India, where the temperature is high throughout the year in most parts of the country, transportation of culture media poses a great challenge. Perfect cold chain must be maintained throughout the transit and once the media have reached, these must be delivered to the laboratory without delay.[27-29,31,32]

Manufacturers' instructions must be followed for proper usage and the expired media bottles must be discarded immediately. Every batch of new medium must be observed for any visible contamination, change of color, turbidity and bottle leakage. Before using in a clinical case, every new batch must also be checked for pH after equilibration in the incubators.[27-29]

Buffers that contain HEPES or MOPS are designed to work outside the incubators hence, do not need $CO_2$ equilibration. Keeping them in $CO_2$ incubators may cause pH change and could be detrimental for gametes and embryos.

Culture dishes should be prepared quickly to avoid osmolality changes. It is especially important when droplets or microdroplets are being prepared. Oil overlaying is recommended. Peroxidation of oil could cause serious harm to eggs and embryos. Therefore, oil bottles must not be kept for long and once opened should be consumed as quickly as possible.[23,29]

## Quality Control of Consumables or Disposables

Plastic ware and other consumables which come in contact with the gametes and embryos in IVF laboratory need to be off-gassed before use. Many of the plastic wares are sterilized by ethylene oxide (ETO).[33,34] The manufacturers keep them in special ventilated areas for off-gassing as a standard protocol before they are released for customer use. Still, it is recommended to let the residual toxic gas flush away by keeping them in a well aerated area in IVF facility before they are brought to the laboratory for clinical use.

The plastics themselves are a source of VOCs therefore the material should be selected which are nontoxic and intended for use in an IVF laboratory.[27]

Many large laboratories perform their own QC tests such as Mouse Embryo Assays (MEA), limulus amebocyte lysate test (LAL) and Sperm Survival or Sperm Motility Assay to test the suitability of contact material as well as culture media before use.[35] Small laboratories can at least do simple sperm motility test of any new batch against the previously tested and used regular consumables.[8,25,36,37]

## Quality Control of Laboratory Personnel

Proficiency testing of all laboratory personnel should be done regularly. Those who perform poorly, must be given an opportunity to go through a refresher training and learning to improve upon their performance. Those who perform well should also be encouraged to attend seminars/trainings/conferences to keep themselves updated with the newer technological advancements in the field. Strict actions may also be taken against someone who repeatedly fails to improve.[25]

Sufficient staffing is the key to reduce workload related errors and helps better performance.[25,32]

### Quality Control to Avoid Mix-ups and Errors in the Laboratory

The IVF laboratories have a great responsibility to avoid mix-ups of the sample and gametes in view of serious legal, social, and financial consequences associated with ART procedures. Utmost attention is required to perform IVF laboratory procedures.[5,8,38-40]

Proper labeling of each and every sample, container or culture dishes or tubes with patients name and unique IDs must be done and double checked throughout the procedures. A witnessing system is a *must* in every laboratory for every step a gamete or biological sample is being handled. The operator and the witness must sign all the papers and records of the procedures done by them. Further, many laboratories are now adapting electronic witnessing systems to minimize human errors.[5,39-41]

A culture of error and incidents reporting must be developed in the laboratories. It is the responsibility of the directors and supervisor to build a trust among the staff members so that any incident or error is religiously reported and recorded. The root cause analysis (RCA) helps the laboratories minimize the likelihood of recurrence of such incidents in future. Also, an emergency plan should also be prepared in case of emergencies, natural disasters such as floods, earthquakes, storms, etc. To deal with all such situations a team of experts should be made that includes not only laboratory supervisors or directors and senior members but also clinicians, engineers, fire experts and even legal consultants who have expertise and experience of troubleshooting and capable of taking appropriate actions.[5]

A hierarchy of authority and responsibilities must be clearly defined in the structural organization to address any issues in the ART center.[25]

Adequate power back-up system should also be installed and regular validation of functioning must be done.

### Key Performance Indicators for Quality Control

Vienna consensus meeting of renowned scientists from ESHRE and Alpha has produced a comprehensive document for key performance indicators (KPI) for IVF laboratory setups. These KPIs should be considered as the true reflection of the quality of an IVF laboratory.[38]

Alpha scientists also prepared another consensus document defining KPIs for cryopreservation of oocytes and embryos. This document describes minimum performance levels, basic competency and benchmark values for 14 KPIs.[42]

Based on the recommendations of various guidelines and consensus documents, every laboratory should set its own set of KPIs and regular evaluation of the laboratory performance of KPIs should be done and all the efforts should be done to improve and meet the set benchmarks.[38,42-43]

## DISASTER MANAGEMENT

In vitro fertilization laboratory is a high complexity laboratory, involving handling of human gametes and embryos and performing sensitive procedures. Thus, in the event of a disaster, these laboratories are prone to suffer not only the disruption of services but also serious harm and damage; sometimes irreparable.[44] Disasters can be natural or man-made. Some natural disasters are common round the globe while some others could be location and area specific.[5,44]

Therefore, it is pragmatic to include disaster and risk management in the quality control program. A proactive approach to disaster and risk management is to prepare a risk-register.[5,44-46] Every laboratory should enlist potential risks or disasters that can be anticipated or that usually occur or that already have happened. This register in turn helps in developing emergency plans to deal with different types of extreme situations.[44]

The ongoing COVID-19 pandemic has taught us the importance of emergency planning and preparedness.[47,48] Several guidelines and directives were issued by different professional bodies to help fellow practitioners to safeguard their patients and the staff.[48-51] Safer approaches and procedures for sanitization and decontamination of the IVF laboratories were proposed and adopted.[47-51]

## CONCLUSION

Quality control or quality management is a continuous process. Initially, it may appear cumbersome, once implemented properly, it becomes a habit. Self-motivation to apply the QC measures is the key to success. Laboratories that succeed to implement QC system are the ones that achieve consistent and dependable results.[2]

Since, the QC guidelines or standards or not uniform and not so well defined, following ISO 9001 2000 standards and getting accredited has been in practice by many ART centers. Recent version of ISO standards—ISO 15189 2002 is a more advanced version and may be adapted and followed by IVF laboratories.[52-54]

Moreover, government regulations, media coverage and public concern has led to recognize the need of implementing a TQM as the field of reproductive medicine has developed remarkably over few years. Most often, only IVF laboratory is considered to have QC in place however, it is just a part of complex structure of whole ART program and desired results can only be achieved when the organization integrates a TQM system.

## REFERENCES


1. 'There is only one thing that is truly important in an IVF laboratory: everything' Cairo Consensus Guidelines on IVF Culture Conditions. Reprod BioMed Online. 2020;40:33-60.
2. Van Vooris BJ, Thomas M, Surrey ES, Sparks A. What do consistently high performing in vitro fertilization programs in the US do? Fertil Steril. 2010;94:1346-9.
3. Packard T. TQM and organizational development. 1996.
4. Schoolcraft WB, Surrey ES, Gardner DK. Embryo transfer: techniques and variables affecting success. Fertil Steril 2001; 76(5): 863-9.
5. Mortimer D, Mortimer ST. Quality and Risk Management in the IVF Laboratory, 2nd edition. Cambridge: Cambridge University Press; 2015.
6. Boiso I, Veiga A, Edwards RG. Fundamentals of human embryonic growth in vitro and selection of high-quality embryos for transfer. Reprod BioMed Online. 2002;5:328-50.
7. Association of Clinical Embryologists (1996). Accreditation standards and guidelines for IVF laboratories. Bengaluru: ACE; 1996.
8. Committee of the Special Interest Group on Embryology. ESHRE guidelines for good practice in IVF laboratories. Hum Reprod. 2000;15:2241-6.
9. European Foundation for Quality Management. EFQM Excellence Model. 1992.
10. Nygreen KG, Andersen AN. Assisted reproductive technology in Europe, 1999. Results generated from European registers by ESHRE. Hum Reprod. 2002;17:3260-74.
11. Land JA, Evers JL. Risks and complications in assisted reproduction techniques: report of an ESHRE consensus meeting. Hum Reprod. 2003;18:455-7.
12. Magli MC, Van den Abbeel E, Lundin K, Royere D, Van der Elst J. Revised guidelines for good practice in IVF laboratories. Hum Reprod. 2008;23(6):1253-62.
13. Society of ART and American Society for Reproductive Medicine. Assisted reproductive technology in the United States: 1999 results generated from the American Society for Reproductive Medicine/Society for Assisted Reproductive Technology Registry. Fertil Steril. 2002;78:918-31.
14. Gianaroli L, Plachot M, Van Kooij R, Al-Hasani S, Dawson K, DeVos A, et al. Guidelines for good practice in IVF laboratories. Hum Reprod. 2000;15:2241-6.
15. Indian Council of Medical Research. National Guidelines for Accreditation, Supervision and Regulation of ART Clinics in India. New Delhi: ICMR;2005.
16. Talwar P, Kannan P, Singh P, Malhotra J, Malhotra K, Kumar Y, et al. ISAR consensus guidelines on safety and ethical practices in in vitro fertilization clinics. J Hum Reprod Sci. 2021;14(5):48.
17. Ministry of Law and Justice. The Assisted Reproductive Technology (Regulation) Act, 2021. New Delhi: Ministry of Law and Justice, Govt of India: 2021.
18. Ministry of Law and Justice. The Surrogacy (Regulation) Act, 2021. New Delhi: Ministry of Law & Justice, Govt of India; 2021.
19. Balaban B, Urman B. Embryo culture as a diagnostic tool. Reprod BioMed Online. 2003;7(6):671-82.
20. Van Royen E, Mangelschots K, Neubaurg D, Valkenburg M, Van de Meerssche M, Ryckaert G, et al. Characterization of a top quality embryo, a step towards single-embryo transfer. Hum Reprod. 1999;14:2345-9.
21. Wiemer K, Anderson A, Weikert L. Quality control in the IVF laboratory. In: Gardner DK, Weissman A, Shoham C, Howles CM (Eds). Textbook of Assisted Reproductive Techniques: Laboratory and Clinical Perspectives. London: Martin Dunitz; 2001. pp. 27-33.
22. Cohen J, Gilligan A, Esposito W, Schimmel T, Dale B. Ambient air and its potential effects on conception in vitro. Hum Reprod. 1997;12:1742-9.
23. Esteves SC, Bento FC. Implementation of cleanroom technology in reproductive laboratories: the question is not why but how. Reprod BioMed Online. 2016;32:9-11.
24. Alper M, Brinsden P, Fisher R, Wikland M. Is your IVF programme good? Hum Reprod. 2002;17(1):8-10.
25. Practice Committee of the American Society for Reproductive Medicine, Practice Committee of the Society for Assisted Reproductive Technology. Revised guidelines for human embryology and andrology laboratories. Fertil Steril. 2008;90(5):S49-59.
26. Kastrop P. Quality management in the ART laboratory. Reprod BioMed Online. 2003;7:691-4.
27. Janssen R, Guns J. Quality Contro: maintaining stability in the laboratory. In: Gardner DK, Weissman A, Howles CM, Shoham Z. (Eds). Textbook of Assisted Reproductive Techniques, Laboratory Perspectives 5th edition. New York: CRC Press, 2017.
28. Boone WR, Higdon III HL, Johnson JE. Quality management issues in the assisted reproduction laboratory. J Reprod Stem Cell Biotechnol. 2010;1:30-107.
29. Martin KL. Quality Assurance and Quality Control in the In Vitro Fertilization Laboratory. In: Gardner DK (Ed). In vitro fertilization: A practical approach. London: Informa Healthcare; 2007. pp. 365-80.
30. Mayer J, Jones E, Dowling-Lacey D, Nehchiri F, Muasher SJ, Gibbons WE, et al. Total quality improvement in the IVF laboratory: choosing indicators of quality. Reprod BioMed Online. 2003;7:192-6.
31. Mansour R, Aboulghar M. Optimizing the embryo transfer technique. Hum Reprod. 2002;171149-53.
32. McCulloh DH. Quality control: maintaining stability in the laboratory. In: Gardner DK, Weissman A, Howles CM, Shoham Z (Eds). Textbook of Assisted Reproductive Techniques. 3rd edition. London: Taylor and Francis; 2009. pp. 9-25.
33. Schiewe MC, Schmidt PM, Bush M, Wildt DE. Toxicity potential of absorbed/retained ethylene oxide residues in culture dishes on embryos development in vitro. J Anim Sci. 1985;60:1610-9.
34. Ackerman S, Swanson R, Stokes G, Veeck L. Culture of preimplantation mouse embryos as a quality control assay for human in vitro fertilization. Gamete Res.1984;9(2):145-52.
35. Parinaud J, Reme J, Monrozies X, Favrin S, Sarramon MF, Pontonnier G. Mouse system quality control is necessary before the use of new material for *in vitro* fertilization and embryo transfer. J In Vitro Fert Embryo Transf. 1987;4:56-8.

36. Bertheussen K, Holst N, Forsdahl F, Høie KE. A new cell culture assay for quality control in IVF. Hum Reprod. 1989;4:531-5.
37. Franco J, Mauri A, Petersen C, Baruffi RL, Campos MS, Oliveira JB. Efficacy of the sperm survival test for the prediction of oocytes fertilization in culture. Hum Reprod. 1993;8:916-8.
38. ESHRE Special Interest Group of Embryology and Alpha Scientists in Reproductive Medicine. The Vienna consensus: Report of an expert meeting on the development of ART laboratory performance indicators. Reprod BioMed Online. 2017;35:495-510.
39. Thornhill AR, Brunetti XO, Bird S, Benett K, Rios LM, Taylor J. Reducing human error in IVF with electronic witnessing. Fertil Steril 2011;96(3):S179.
40. Van Kooij RJ, Peeters MF, Te Velde ER. Quality control and quality assurance in IVF. Twins of mixed races: consequences for Dutch IVF laboratories. Hum Reprod. 1997;12:2585-7.
41. Wikland, M, Sjöblom C. The application of quality systems in ART programs. Mol Cell Endocrinol. 2000;166:3-7.
42. The Alpha consensus meeting on cryopreservation key performance indicators and benchmarks: proceedings of an expert meeting. Reprod Biomed Online. 2012;25:146-67.
43. Franco Jr JG, Petersen CG, Mauri AL, Vagnini LD, Renzi A, Petersen B, et al. Key performance indicators score (KPIs-score) based on clinical and laboratorial parameters can establish benchmarks for internal quality control in an ART program. JBRA Assist Reprod. 2017;21(2):61-6.
44. Bormann CL, Lewis EI. Risk and Disaster Management for the IVF Laboratory. In: Fleming SD, Varghese AC (Eds). Organization and Management of IVF Units. New York: Springer International Publishing; 2016. pp. 71-83.
45. Development of an emergency plan for in vitro fertilization programs: a committee opinion. Fertil Steril. 2021;115: 870-3.
46. Reproductive Technology Accreditation Committee (RTAC). Technical Bulletin 9: Disaster Management. Fertili Soc Aust. 2016.
47. Hickman C, Rogers S, Huang G, MacArthur S, Meseguer M, Nogueira D, et al. Managing the IVF laboratory during a pandemic: international perspectives from laboratory managers. Reprod Biomed Online. 2020;4:141-50.
48. American Society of Reproductive Medicine. Patient management and clinical recommendations during coronavirus (COVID-19) pandemic. Washington, DC: ASRM: 2020.
49. British Fertility Society/Association of Reproductive and Clinical Scientists. Guidance for the care of fertility patients during the Coronavirus COVID 19 Pandemic. London: British Fertility Society; 2020.
50. Veiga A, Gianaroli L, Ory S, Horton M, Feinberg E, Penzias A. Assisted reproduction and COVID-19: A joint statement of ASRM, ESHRE and IFFS. Fertil Steril. 2020;114:484-5.
51. Prasad S, Trivedi P, Malhotra N, Patil M, Swaminathan D, Shukla S, et al. Joint IFS-ISAR-ACE Recommendations on Resuming/Opening up Assisted Reproductive Technology Services. J Hum Reprod Sci. 2020;13(2):82-8.
52. ISO 15189 2002 Medical laboratories – particular requirements for quality and competence. Geneva: International Organization for Standardization; 2002.
53. ISO 17025 2000 General requirements for the competence of testing and calibration laboratories. Geneva: International Organization for Standardization; 2000.
54. ISO 9001 2000 Quality management systems – requirements. Geneva: International Organization for Standardization; 2000.

CHAPTER 123

# Embryo Culture Systems

*Goral Gandhi*

## INTRODUCTION

Human embryos are metabolically dynamic and their nutritional requirements change from day-to-day and from stage-to-stage. The embryos are grown in culture systems that mimic in vivo conditions. In vitro culture of human embryos was first successfully carried out by Dr John Rock in 1944.[1] Recent advances have resulted in the development of more physiological and effective culture media capable of maintaining the viability of the developing embryo. Suboptimal culture conditions may lead to impaired embryo development and a decrease in resultant implantation and pregnancy rates.[2] Therefore, improved embryo culture systems will enhance the overall success rates of assisted reproductive technologies (ART). The main objective of any in vitro fertilization (IVF) program is to generate viable embryo that is capable of efficaciously implanting in the uterus and giving rise to a healthy baby. Nowadays, embryologists have the option of selecting different culture media. The day of the embryo transfer also varies from day 2 till day 5 or day 6. The culture system includes culture media, culture oil, type of culture, disposables, and the air quality.

This chapter aims to discuss the various constituents of the culture system. At the end of the chapter, the readers should be able to decide on a culture system that facilitates optimal embryo development.

## CULTURE MEDIA

In the early days of ART, the main energy sources in the culture media were glucose, lactate, and pyruvate. The buffered salt solution was supplemented with these compounds. Later on, the culture media were supplemented with serum albumin as the source of amino acids.[3]

Albumin is an important protein constituent for embryo development. Fatty acids play a major role in early embryo metabolism required for membrane synthesis. They are mainly bound to albumin but some albumins are heavily contaminated with lipid peroxides which are highly embryo toxic. Recombinant human serum albumin (HSA) is available as equivalent medium support since 2002.

In 1985, Quinn, et al., developed a media named human tubal fluid (HTF). The HTF resembled the composition of the fluids in human fallopian tubes.[4,5] HTF consisted of a salt solution supplemented with whole serum or serum albumin. This media was widely used to grow embryos till the day 3 stage.[6]

It is important to understand the physiology and metabolic needs of any cell type in order to culture it successfully in the laboratory. A number of physiological changes occur in the human embryo during the preimplantation period as it undergoes successive stages of development.

Several individual components go into making a majority of the embryo culture media. Till the 8-cell stage, the embryo development is still under maternal control and the developing embryos have pyruvate lactate preference for its energy requirements. After the 8-cell stage, the embryos move toward a glucose-based metabolism once the embryonic genome has been activated which then supports their growth up to the blastocyst stage.

The ART media needs to provide hydration ions, nutrients, and also waste products dilutants.

### Water

Water is the basic foundation for culture media. The water used for culture media has to be highly purified and of high quality. From past many years, there has been progression in processing of water to be used for culture media preparation. In 1963, Brinster used deionized water whereas Whitten used distilled water in 1971 from deionized tap. Later, water processed through a Millipore Reverse Osmosis unit was used.[7,8]

### Energy Requirements

The levels of glucose, lactate, and pyruvate vary between the oviduct, uterus as well as within the cycle.[9] The preimplantation embryo is thus subjected to a diverse gradient of carbohydrates during the course of its development. Literature suggests that lactate is required for the embryo development after the 2-cell stage and glucose is required after the 8-cell stage.[10] The media used for early stages of development thus consist of pyruvate. After the 8-cell stage, the glucose intake is increased.[11] However, in a phosphate buffer medium which does not have amino acids, high levels of glucose lead to embryo arrest at the 8-cell stage. The addition of amino acids, Ethylene Diamine Tetraacetic Acid (EDTA) and vitamins to the culture medium minimizes the harmful effects of glucose. This explains the delicate balance of interactions amongst the media constituents. This also emphasizes the disastrous effects of using simple salt solutions as culture media. The key is the inclusion of pyruvate and exclusion of glucose at the early developmental stages. This will prevent developmental block at the 8-cell stage. This will also aid in the production of more trophectoderm cells.[12,13]

## Amino Acids

Amino acids are without doubt the most important constituents of culture media. The studies evaluating the composition of fallopian tube fluid shave revealed that they contain high levels of some amino acids such as taurine and glutamine. This led to the belief that these amino acids must be playing a significant role in embryo development.[14-16] As the embryo progresses in development, its requirement of amino acids seems to be changing.

The nonessential amino acids (NEAA) and glutamine are present in high concentration in the oviduct fluid during the cleavage stage. NEAA are used for protein metabolism and pyruvate and lactate are used as energy sources by the cleavage stage embryos. The inner cell mass (ICM) needs essential amino acids for development.[17] A variety of advantages of amino acids are observed in the embryo development.

## Chelators—Ethylenediamine Tetraacetic Acid

The beneficial effects of the divalent cation EDTA were first reported by Ambruzak, et al., over 20 years ago.[18] The positive effect of EDTA is limited to the cleavage stage embryos. EDTA is shown to reduce the ICM of human embryos past the cleavage stage and also negatively affect the fetal development.[19-22] A reason for this biphasic effect of EDTA is the inhibitory role that it plays in the glycolysis pathway by inhibiting cytosolic kinases during the cleavage stage of the embryos. However, in contrast to the cleavage stage embryos, the ICM uses glycolysis as its main energy producing pathway and the presence of EDTA has an adverse effect on the ICM growth and the subsequent fetal development.

## Macromolecules

The IVF culture media used to be supplemented by human serum, even though in vivo, the embryo is not exposed to serum.[19,23] However, some harmful effects on embryo development have been attributed to the addition of serum. These harmful effects include morphological changes, early blastulation and disturbances in energy metabolism.[24,25] There were many drawbacks associated with the use of serum. Since all batches of serum would vary in composition, there was no standardization of the culture medium.[26] Due to these disadvantages associated with whole serum, the media was supplemented with HSA instead of whole serum.[27,28] Albumin has a lot of benefits on embryo development and is abundantly found in the reproductive tract of the female.[27] Albumin also helps in in vitro handling of the gametes. It avoids the embryos from sticking to the bottom of the culture dishes due to its effect on the surface tension.[29,30] Hyaluronan is another molecule that is found in the tract as well as used increasingly in the culture media.[31] Hyaluronan is said to increase implantation as well as aid in the survival of embryos after cryopreservation.[32-34]

## Antibiotics

The presence of numerous components in the embryo culture medium makes it susceptible to bacterial contamination. Use of antibiotics in the culture medium prevents this. Penicillin (B-lactam; 100 U/mL), gentamycin (aminoglycoside; 50 µg/mL), and streptomycin (aminoglycoside; 100 µg/mL) are commonly used antibiotics in culture media.[35,36]

## Protein Supplement

In early days, 10% heat inactivated patient serum or fetal cord blood serum was used to supplement the media but it was becoming difficult with increase in number of cycles. To overcome this burden of logistics of collecting and preparing maternal serum the use of pooled donor sera was started but this resulted in an episode of hepatitis B cross contamination.

Twenty-four women conceived following IVF treatment but suffered acute hepatitis B infection, five pregnancies aborted spontaneously, and remaining 19 led to birth of 24 children but the episode confirmed that the use of poorly screened human serum in IVF is unacceptable.[37]

Working without albumin has been attempted but protein or similar macromolecule (polyvinyl alcohol or hyaluronate) is required for IVF for many reasons.[37,38]

- *Sperm capacitation:* Albumin acts as sterol acceptor molecule in media.
- *Handling:* Prevents embryos and sperm from sticking to pipettes, dishes, or tubes.
- Proteins act as peptide and lipid carriers.

Recombinant HSA is used in the medium as a source from 2002. Human serum contains approximately 4.5% albumin

(45 mg/mL). An addition of 10% HSA provides albumin of 4.5% concentration.[39]

## MEDIA SYSTEMS

An ideal culture system simulates in vivo microenvironment for human gametes. Defining and designing an ideal culture system is a herculean task because the detailed composition of in vivo environment of the gametes is not clear. Selection of proper culture system is one of the key factors, which can influence the development of embryos in vitro. Other factors influencing are $CO_2$-$O_2$ level and number of incubator chamber.

### Sequential Culture Media System

Back to nature is the principle for the sequential media systems. In this system, the media constituents vary as per the developmental stage of the embryos, based on the natural environment of the reproductive tract.[40,41] The embryo has the ability to control its ionic gradients and can self-regulate its internal environment. The preimplantation period of the embryo can be categorized into two phases with respect to the embryo physiology: pre-and postcompaction.[41] Classification of the preimplantation period is essential while considering alterations to media formulations. It is also important to consider activation period of the embryonic genome.[41]

There has been a remarkable rise in usage of sequential culture media wherein for initial 3 days one medium is used and for next 2 days another medium is used which supports morula, compaction, and blastocyst development.[42] The glucose and other energy substrate levels are modified in the latter media along with altering concentration of amino acids, chelators, etc.[10,17,19] Embryos at the early stage needs pyruvate and lactate in higher concentrations and glucose at lower levels. This ratio reverses at the blastocyst stage, with higher glucose requirement.[11] Since the composition of oviduct fluid varies from uterine, two different medium are used so as to imitate in vivo conditions of embryo. This also facilitates elimination of harmful by-products, such as ammonia, and to ensure adequate supply of substrates replenishing of media is involved in the method **(Table 1)**.[43]

### Monoculture Media System

The principle of monoculture media system is to let the embryo decide its needs during development and differentiation.[44] This culture medium has a mixture of all required components.[10] In this media system, the entire components essential for the embryo development is provided. This system hence does not need the media to be replenished daily. Therefore, during the development of embryo till blastocyst a single formulation is used. The embryo will utilize the required components, whose concentrations are optimum and will adapt to the medium.[10,40,44,45] The response of embryos to different permutation and concentration of constituents can also be analyzed. The best media in monoculture media system is the one with combination of components with defined concentrations providing a maximum response.[10]

### Coculture System

The system of adding different cell types to the culture medium is called coculture system.[46] The oviduct is the natural site of early embryo development. Coculture mimics the oviduct environment in vivo which provides developmental support to the embryos.[47]

Embryo coculture endeavors to perk up the cleavage and blastulation rate, reduced fragmentation, with good implantation rates.[48-50] Maternal serum or protein substitutes are often used to supplement the media.[47] Coculture helps in cases of poor quality embryo with low implantation rate and in cases where in spite of obtaining good quality embryos, implantation failure occurs.[51,52] Oviductal cells in coculture have shown to provide a better support because of their varied ability to produce embryotrophic factors.[53,54] In coculture apart from oviductal cells, endometrial cells, granulose cells, and vero cells can also be used.[55] In practice, presently only homologous endometrial cell coculture is used.[56]

### Open and Closed System

Overlay of oil protects media droplets and has been an important part of human IVF culture since 1960s. Closed system consists of microdroplets of culture media which is then covered with liquid paraffin oil so as to maintain the

**TABLE 1:** Media systems: culture, monoculture, and sequential culture systems.

| *Culture systems* | *Monoculture systems* | *Sequential culture systems* | |
|---|---|---|---|
| Days | Day 1–Day 6 | Day 1–Day 3 | Day 4–Day 6 |
| NEAA | ✓ | ✓ | ✓ |
| EAA | ✓ | ✓ | ✓ |
| Glucose | ✓ | Reduced | Elevated |
| Pyruvate | ✓ | ✓ | ✓ |
| Lactate | ✓ | ✓ | ✓ |
| EDTA | ✓ | ✓ | ✓ |

(EAA: essential amino acid; EDTA: ethylene-diamine-tetra-acetic acid; NEAA: nonessential amino acids)

osmolarity, pH, and temperature of the media.[57] The open system consists of culture media in sterile multiwell plates without the oil overlay. The main difference between both types of systems is the volumes of media required. Larger volumes (0.5–2 mL/dish) are needed in the open system and the closed system, involves comparatively smaller volumes of the media (25–100 μL/drop).

There is a risk of rapid fluctuations in temperature and pH with the open systems. The closed system with its microdroplet culture has a better fertilization rate mainly due to the homogenous distribution of sperms in the culture medium.[58]

## CULTURE CONDITIONS

Several culture conditions are reviewed here, each of them directly affecting the media performance.

### Osmolality

The osmolality of human fallopian tube fluid is >360 mOsmol.[59] The osmolality of the culture media is kept around 300 mOsmol. Osmolality higher than this is harmful for the embryo development.[36] Amino acids added to the culture media become organic osmolytes. They protect the embryos against hypertonicity as well as aid in the growth and development of embryos.[36,60,61]

### pH

If pH is permitted to drift outside of an optimized working range of 7.2–7.4, this may place "stress" on gametes or embryos. The pH of the media is affected by its constituents.[62] Cleavage stage embryos are cultured at a slightly lower pH whereas the advanced stage blastocysts are cultured at a slightly higher pH.[63,64] It is advisable to keep the $CO_2$ concentration between 5 and 6% as this will help to maintain the optimal pH of the bicarbonate buffer media.[65]

While using $CO_2$/bicarbonate, it is important not to expose the culture dish in the external environment to prevent changes in the pH. When the gametes need manipulation outside the incubator, as while performing intracytoplasmic sperm injection (ICSI), media buffered with 20 mM HEPES or MOPS can be used together with 5 mM bicarbonate.[66] An overlay of oil also prevents increase in pH due to loss of $CO_2$.

### Temperature

Exposure of embryos and oocytes to low temperatures is detrimental to their microtubules thus risking aneuploidy in resulting embryos.[67] High temperatures (39°C) can also disrupt the microtubule organization. Exposure to suboptimal temperatures also affects transmembrane transport and metabolism and slows down the embryo development. It is essential to maintain the temperature at 37°C.[67]

### Light

The effect of exposure of visible light on the growth of embryos in vitro has been studied. In human IVF, low light setting is preferred. Exposure of the embryos to light should be kept at a minimum.[68]

## MEDIA STORAGE AND EQUILIBRATION

Culture media mimics the natural environment of the female reproductive tract. Most of the components of commercially available media are labile and hence have restricted shelf life. Media is thus prone to deterioration during storage.[69] Storage and handling of culture media is thus very crucial to successful in vitro embryo development.

The most labile components in a culture media known are amino acids and vitamins. Vitamins are light sensitive and are preferably stored in dark bottles so as to minimize exposure to light. Amino acids are comparatively stable in solution at 4°C. However, they break down and release ammonium when kept at 37°C. Ammonium is known to have deleterious effect on the embryo development.[70] Hence, it is of utmost importance not to incubate media for long before use.

During the entire culture period, all media need to be equilibrated for temperature and pH for minimum 4–6 hours prior to use. It is a common practice to incubate the media at 37°C for an overnight period.[69] The composition of the media must be taken into consideration as incubation in certain types of media has been found to initiate a depletion of glutathione (GSH) content of oocyte.

The equilibration time to acquire optimum temperature and pH should be asserted by validation.

The temperature and pH fluctuation causes many problems such as precipitation of $CaCO_3$, which makes media alkaline. Pyruvate present in media tends to become acidic and converts to pyruvic acid which will polymerize and decompose. The glutamine decomposition produces ammonium ions ($NH^+$) at 37°C it decomposes at 10%/day whereas when stored at 4°C it takes 9 days for the same.

### Oil Equilibration

An overlay of equilibrated oil confers specific advantages to enhance culture conditions. Oil forms a physical barrier between the culture medium droplets and the external environment carrying air borne particles or pathogens. It also helps in maintaining the pH, temperature and osmolality of the medium by preventing evaporation of the media.[58,71]

## INCUBATORS

The incubators are special chambers used for the growth of the developing embryos. Incubators are designed to maintain a controlled temperature, humidity, osmolality, pH level as well as gas content as per the requirement of the growing embryos. The embryos spend most of their in vitro time inside the stable atmosphere of the incubator. This makes the incubator undoubtedly one of the most important equipment in any IVF laboratory.

Human embryos are generally cultured at 37°C with a 5–7% Cor concentration. The oxygen concentration is either reduced or not reduced. Many different types of incubators are now available in the market for specific use for IVF. These include water jacket incubators, drawer incubators, benchtop incubators, and the latest time-lapse incubators.[72] The main differences in these incubators are the ways in which temperature, pH, gas content, and humidity are maintained. There are many studies comparing different types of incubators, however, most studies have concluded that the type of incubators does not have any effect on the embryo development or the success rates.[73-75] The atmosphere inside the incubator has to be maintained perfectly and a robust quality control program needs to be in place to ensure optimal incubator performance. The number of incubators in a laboratory needs to be decided based on daily and annual number of cycles. A lot of planning needs to go regarding allotment of dishes to incubators, so that there is minimum opening of incubator doors.

## AIR PURIFICATION UNIT

The quality of air in the laboratory is of utmost importance when it comes to embryo culture. Ambient air in an IVF laboratory may consist of various components such as volatile organic compounds (VOCs), perfumes, deodorants, microbes as well as odors coming from the external environment. All these components have a negative effect on the in vitro development of the embryos.[73,76,77] VOCs are shown to have a negative impact on embryos in a way that they attach directly to the deoxyribonucleic acid (DNA) and terminate growth of embryos during embryonic development.[78] Episodes of air pollution in an IVF laboratory has been shown to cause fragmentation of the human sperm DNA.[79,80] Embryo culture and subsequent ART success rates are thus compromised in a poor air quality environment.

It is, thus, of great importance to set up proper air cleaning systems. Removal of these airborne pathogens, however, requires an advanced air handling system/air-handling unit (AHU). The air purification unit must be affordable, effective, quiet and should have the ability to filter VOCs, hydrocarbon pollutants, chemical air contaminants, and other chemically active compounds.[81,82] Creating a stable environment for embryo culture ensures embryo viability which in turn supports favorable pregnancy outcome. Some of the filters used in a number of air handling units are activated carbon filters and high efficiency particulate air (HEPA) filter. Outside air that enters the unit can be filtered using activated carbon filters which have the ability to remove hydrocarbon pollutants. HEPA filters, on the other hand, can filter out particulate pollutants as small as 0.3 µm.

## QUALITY CONTROL

Establishing a successful IVF laboratory essentially requires the incorporation of an appropriate quality control system.[83] Quality control procedures in an IVF laboratory mainly involve fine tuning of the existing protocols, so as to achieve optimum embryo development and desirable pregnancy rates.[84] Quality control should not only be limited to the culture media used, but also the gases and all the other supplies used in a regular IVF procedure. Temperature, pH, and osmolality are some of the important physical conditions that require regular monitoring and documentation as part of the quality control protocols.

## EPIGENETIC CHANGES

The time period of a few weeks before conception till fertilization, cleavage, and preimplantation embryonic development has greatly increased possibilities of epigenetic changes.[85,86] There are many studies showing evidence of this.

It has also been shown that adult diseases have their origins in the conditions around the early stages of development.[87,88] Animal studies have also supported this association between preimplantation development and diseases in adults.[89] Just as in vivo, in vitro culture can also induce epigenetic changes.[85,90] Millions of babies born through IVF worldwide have shown that there not many adverse effects of IVF, however, we must bear in mind that the first baby born through IVF, Louise Brown is still only 43 in the year 2022. Any possible causes of alarm in later years of adulthood are yet to be explored.

## CONCLUSION

There are many parameters that should be kept in mind in order to maintain the optimal conditions for both gamete and embryo development in an IVF laboratory. In vitro, cells and embryos are exposed to different stress situations that must be minimized. Therefore, a routine control at different levels needs to be performed, so that the environment in the laboratory is adapted to resemble the reproductive tract and the intrauterine conditions.

A detailed attention must be paid to not only the selection of culture media but the designing of the entire of culture system. Creation of viable embryos is dependent as much on the environment of the IVF laboratory as on the constituents of the culture media. Finally, we must remember that no culture system in the world can be as good as the mother's womb. We should also pay attention to the emerging evidence of epigenetic changes during the periconception and preimplantation period. It is our duty as reproductive scientists to take care of the human eggs and embryos to the best of our ability, to create embryos with highest implantation potential that turn into human beings with a healthy life.

## MULTIPLE CHOICE QUESTIONS

1. The combination of which amino acid and EDTA gives rise to optimum blastocysts?
   a. Glycine b. Lysine
   c. Glutamine d. Taurine
2. What is the function of EDTA in embryo culture media?
   a. Vitamins
   b. Hyaluronan
   c. Promotes production of reactive oxygen species
   d. Suppresses the production of reactive oxygen species
3. Which one of the following statements is false?
   a. Exposure of embryos and oocytes to low temperatures is detrimental to their microtubules thus risking aneuploidy in resulting embryos.
   b. Amino acids in embryo culture media are comparatively stable in solution at 25°C, but they release ammonium at 37°C.
   c. The blastocysts are cultured at a higher pH than the cleavage stage embryos.
   d. The osmolality of human fallopian tube fluid is more than 360 mOsmol.
4. At what stage of development does the EMP cycle of the embryo gets fully functional?
   a. Blastocyst stage b. 4-cell stage
   c. 8-cell stage d. 16-cell stage
5. Serum has the following reaction on culture of embryos:
   a. Perturbation in ultrastructure
   b. Changes in energy metabolism
   c. Premature blastulation
   d. All of the above
6. Embryo culture media was first developed to grow __________ embryos.
   a. Rabbit b. Mouse
   c. Hamster d. Bovine
7. What is the major source of energy for cleavage stage embryos?
   a. Glucose b. Pyruvate
   c. Lactate d. Sucrose
8. Which antibiotic inhibits peptidoglycan synthesis?
   a. Gentamycin b. Penicillin
   c. Streptomycin d. All of the above
9. What should be osmotic pressure of embryo culture media?
   a. 250–300 mOsmol
   b. 350–400 mOsmol
   c. 200–250 mOsmol
   d. 300–350 mOsmol
10. In coculture system which cells have the ability to produce embryotrophic factors?
    a. Vero cells b. Granulosa cells
    c. Endometrial cells d. Oviductal cells

## REFERENCES


1. Menkin MF, Rock J. In vitro fertilization and cleavage of human ovarian eggs. Science. 1944;100(2588):105-7.
2. Bowman P, McLaren A. Cleavage rate of mouse embryos in vivo and in vitro. J Embryol Exp Morphol. 1970;24:203-7.
3. Quinn P, Pool T. Development of modern culture media. In: Fleming S, Cooke S (Eds). Textbook of Assisted Reproduction for Scientists in Reproductive Technology. Fremantle: Vivid Publishing; 2009.
4. Tank P, Malhotra N, Malhotra N. History of human assisted reproductive technology. In: Malhotra J, Tank J, Haththotuwa R (Eds). Handbook of managing fertility. New Delhi: Jaypee Brothers Medical Publishers (P) Ltd.; 2012.
5. Quinn P. Culture systems: sequential. Methods Mol Biol. 2012;912:211-30.
6. Guota S. Media in ART. In: Talwar P (Ed). Manual of assisted reproductive technologies and clinical embryology. New Delhi: Jaypee Brothers Medical Publishers; 2012.
7. Quinn P. Culture Media, Solutions and Systems in ART. United Kingdom: Cambridge University Press; 2014.
8. Quinn P, Kerin JF, Warnes GM. Improved pregnancy rate in human in vitro fertilization with the use of a medium based on the composition of human tubal fluid. Fertil Steril. 1985;44(4):493-8.
9. Leese HJ, Hooper MA, Edwards RG, Ashwood-Smith MJ. Uptake of pyruvate by early human embryos determined by a noninvasive technique. Hum Reprod. 1986;1(3):181-2.
10. Summers MC, Biggers JD. Chemically defined media and the culture of mammalian preimplantation embryos: historical perspective and current issues. Hum Reprod Update. 2003;9(6):557-82.
11. Leese HJ, Conaghan J, Martin KL, Hardy K. Early embryo metabolism. Bioessays. 1993;15(4):259-64.
12. Gardner D, Lane M. Embryo culture. In: Gardner DK, Weissman A, Howles CM, Shoham Z (Eds). Textbook of Assisted Reproductive Techniques, 2nd edition. United Kingdom: Martin Duntiz Ltd; 2001.
13. Conaghan J, Handyside AH, Winston RM, Leese HA. Effects of pyruvate and glucose on the development of human preimplantation embryos in vitro. Soc Reprod Fertil. 1993;99:87-95.
14. Miller JG, Schultz GA. Amino acid content of preimplantation rabbit embryos and fluids of the reproductive tract. Biol Reprod. 1987;36:125-9.
15. Casslen BG. Free amino acids in human uterine fluid. Possible role of high taurine concentration. J Reprod Med. 1987;32:181-4.
16. Leese HJ, Aldridge S, Jeffries KS. The movement of amino acids into rabbit fluid. J Reprod Fertil. 1979;56:623-6.
17. Lane M, Gardner DK. Differential regulation of mouse embryo development and viability by amino acids. J Reprod Fertil. 1997;109:153-64.
18. Abramczuk J, Solter D, Koprowski H. The beneficial effect of EDTA on development of mouse one-cell embryos in

chemically defined medium. Philadelphia: Elsevier; 1977. pp. 378-83.
19. Gardner DK, Lane M. Embryo culture systems. In: Gardner DK, Trounson A (Eds). Handbook of In Vitro Fertilization. New York: CRC Press; 1999.
20. Gardner DK, Lane M. Alleviation of the "2 cell block" and development to the blastocyst of CFI mouse embryos: role of amino acids, EDTA and physical parameters. Hum Reprod. 1996;11:2703-12.
21. Gardner DK, Lane MW, Lane M. EDTA stimulates cleavage stage bovine embryo development in culture but inhibits blastocyst development and differentiation. Mol Reprod Devel. 2000;57:256-61.
22. Hoshi M, Toyoda Y. Effect of EDTA on the pre-implantation development of mouse embryos fertilized in vitro. Jpn J Zootech Sci. 1985;56:931-7.
23. Bavister BD. Culture of preimplantation mammalian embryos: facts and artifacts. Hum Reprod Update. 1995;1(2):91-148.
24. Gardiner CS, Reed DJ. Status of glutathione during oxidant-induced oxidative stress in the preimplantation mouse embryo. Biol Reprod. 1994;51:1307-14.
25. Thompson JG, Gardner DK, Pugh PA, McMillan WH, Tervit HR. Lamb birth weight is affected by culture system utilized during in vitro pre-elongation development of ovine embryos. Biol Reprod. 1995;53(6):1385-91.
26. Maurer HR. Towards serum-free, chemically defined media for mammalian cell culture. In: Freshney RI (Ed). Animal Cell Culture: A Practical Approach. Oxford: Oxford University Press; 1992.
27. Meintjes M. Media composition: macromolecules and embryo growth. Methods Mol Biol. 2012;912:107-27.
28. Meintjes M, Chatilis SJ, Ward DC, Douglas JD, Rodriguez AJ, Guerami AR, et al. A randomized control study of human serum albumin and serum substitute supplements as protein supplements for IVF culture and the effect on live birth rates. Hum Reprod. 2009;24(4):782-9.
29. Gardner DK. Dissection of culture media for embryos: the most important and less important components and characteristics. Reprod Fertil. 2008;20(1):9-18.
30. Bungum M, Bungum L, Humaidan P, Yding Andersen C. Day 3 versus day 5 embryo transfer: a prospective randomized study. Reprod Biomed Online. 2003;7(1):98-104.
31. Biggers JD, McGinnis LK, Lawitts JA. Enhanced effect of glycyl-L-glutamine mouse preimplantation embryos in vitro. Reprod Biomed Online. 2004;9(1):59-69.
32. Stojkovic M, Kölle S, Peinl S, Stojkovic P, Zakhartchenko V, Thompson JG, et al. Effects of high concentrations of hyaluronan in culture medium on development and survival rates of fresh and frozen-thawed bovine embryos produced in vitro. Reproduction. 2002;124(1):141-53.
33. Lane M, Maybach JM, Hooper K, Hasler JF, Gardner DK. Cryo-survival and development of bovine blastocysts are enhanced by culture with recombinant albumin and hyaluronan. Mol Reprod Dev. 2003;64(1):70-8.
34. Bontekoe S, Blake D, Heineman MJ, Blake D. Adherence compounds in embryo transfer media for assisted reproductive technologies. Cochrane Database Syst Rev. 2010;(7):CD007421.
35. Lemeire K, Van Merris V, Cortvrindt R. The antibiotic streptomycin assessed in a battery of in vitro tests for reproductive toxicology. Toxicol in vitro. 2007;21:1348-53.
36. Borland RM, Biggers JD, Lechene CP, Taymor ML. Elemental composition of fluid in the human Fallopian tube. J Reprod Fertil. 1980;58:479-826.
37. Ali J, Shahata MA, Al-Natsha SD. Formulation of protein free medium for human assisted reproduction. Hum Reprod. 2000;15(1):145-56.
38. Ali J. Generation of viable human embryos in a protein-free embryo culture medium enhances clinical pregnancy rate and prevents disease transmission in assisted reproduction. Middle East Fertility Soc J. 2004;9(2):118-127.
39. Bungun M, Humaidan P, Bungum L. Recombinant human albumin as protein source in culture media used for IVF: a prospective randomized study. Reprod Biomed Online. 2002;4(3):233-6.
40. Biggers JD, Summers MC. Choosing a culture medium: making informed choices. Fertil Steril. 2008;90(3):473-83.
41. Biggers JD, McGinnis LK. Evidence that glucose is not always an inhibitor of mouse preimplantation development in vitro. Hum Reprod. 2001;16:153-63.
42. Gardner DK, Lane M. Culture and selection of viable blastocysts: a feasible proposition for human IVF? Hum Reprod Update. 1997;3:367-82.
43. Brinster RL. A method for in vitro cultivation of mouse ova from the two cell to blastocyst. Exp Cell Res. 1963;32:205-7.
44. Van Os, Verdoux H, Maurice-Tison S, Gay B, Liraud F, Salamon R, et al. Self-reported psychosis-like symptoms and the continuum of psychosis. Soc Psychiatry Psychiatr Epidemiol. 1999;34(9):459-63.
45. Bigger JD. Thoughts on embryo culture conditions. Reprod Biomed Online. 2001;4:30-8.
46. Ledger W, Tan SL, Bahathiq A. The Fallopian tube in infertility and IVF practice, 1st edition. United Kingdom: Cambridge University Press; 2010.
47. Bongso A, Fong CY, Ng SC, Montag M, Tok V, Sathananthan AH, et al. Micromanipulation and possible new approaches to help the severe male-factor patient. J Assist Reprod Genet. 1992;9(3):191-6.
48. Wiemer KE, Garrisi J, Steuerwald N, Alikani M, Reing AM, Ferrara TA, et al. Beneficial aspects of coculture with assisted hatching when applied to multiple failure in vitro fertilization patients. Hum Reprod. 1996;11:2429-33.
49. Daniel EE, Lucien P, Posey VA, Paton DM. A functional analysis of the myogenic control systems of the human Fallopian tube. Am J Obstet Gynecol. 1975;15(121):1046-53.
50. Daniel EE, Posey VA, Paton DM. A structural analysis of the myogenic control systems of the human Fallopian tube. Am J Obstet Gynecol. 1975;15(121):1054-6.
51. Brundin J. Pharmacology of the oviduct. In: Hafez ES, Blandau RJ (Eds). The mammalian oviduct. Chicago: University of Chicago Press; 1969.
52. Talo A, Pulkkinen MO. Electrical activity in the human oviduct during the menstrual cycle. Am J Obstet Gynecol. 1982;142(2):135-47.
53. Reinecke M. Neurotensin in the human Fallopian tube: Immunohistochemical localization and effects of synthetic neurotensin on motor activity in vitro. Neurosci Lett. 1987; 73(3):220-4.

54. Yeung WS, Xu JS, Lee CK. The oviduct and preimplantation embryo development. Reprod Med Rev. 2002;10:21-44.
55. Xu JS, Cheung TM, Chan ST, Ho PC, Yeung WS. Temporal effect of human oviductal cell and its derived embryotropic factors on mouse embryo development. Biol Reprod. 2001;65:1481-8.
56. Bahatik A, Stewart RL, Wells M, Moore HD, Pacey AA, Ledger WL. Production of activiness by the human endosalpings. J Clin Endo Meta. 2002;87:5283-9.
57. Halbert SA, Tam PY, Blandau RJ. Egg transport in rabbit oviduct: The roles of cilia and muscles. Science. 1976; 191(4321):1052-3.
58. Johnson CA, Hofmann GE, Scott RT. The use of oil overlay for in vitro fertilization and culture. Assisted Reprod Rev. 1994;4:198-201.
59. Marianowski P, Szymusik I, Grzechocinska B, Cyganek A. The comparison of two different embryo culture methods in the course of in vitro fertilization program. Folia Histochem Cytobiol. 2007;45:S115-7.
60. Biggers JD, Lawitts JA, Lechene CP. The protective action of betaine on the deleterious effects of NaCl on preimplantation mouse embryos in vitro. Mol Reprod Dev. 1993;34:380-90.
61. Van Winkel LJ, Haghighat N, Campione AL. Glycine protects preimplantation mouse conceptuses from a detrimental effect on development of the inorganic ions in oviductal fluid. J Exp Zool. 1990;253:215-9.
62. Ho Y, Wiggelsworth K, Eppig IJ, Schultz RM. Preimplantation development of mouse embryos in KSOM: augmentation by amino acids and analysis of gene expression. Mol Reprod Dev. 1995;41:232-8.
63. Bavister BD, McKiernan SH. Regulation of hamster embryo development in vitro by amino acids. In: Bavister BD (Ed). Preimplantation Embryo Development. New York: Springer Verlag; 1993.
64. Edwards LE, Williams DA, Gardner DK. Intracellular pH of the mouse preimplantation embryo: amino acids act as buffers of intracellular pH. Hum Reprod. 1998;13:3441-8.
65. Edwards LJ, Williams DA, Gardner DK. Intracellular pH of the preimplantation mouse embryo: effects of extracellular pH and weak acids. Mol Reprod Dev. 1998;50:434-42.
66. Jackson KV, Racowsky C. Embryo culture techniques. In: Carrell DT, Peterson CM (Eds). Reproductive endocrinology and infertility. New York: Springer; 2010.
67. Good NE, Winget GD, Winter W. Hydrogen ion buffers for biological research. Biochemistry. 1996;5:467-77.
68. Menezes J. Embryo culture systems. In: Nair MS (Ed). Insights into infertility management. New Delhi: Jaypee Brothers Medical Publishers (P) Ltd.; 2012.
69. Noda Y, Goto Y, Umaoka Y, Shiotani M, Nakayama T, Mori T. Culture of human embryos in alpha modification of Eagle's medium under low oxygen tension and low illumination. Fertil Steril. 1994;62(7):1022-7.
70. Elder K, Dale B. In vitro fertilization, 3rd edition. United Kingdom: Cambridge University Press; 2011.
71. Gardner DK, Lane M. Amino acids and ammonium regulate mouse embryo development in culture. Biol Reprod. 1993; 48:377-85.
72. Swain JE. Decisions for the IVF laboratory: comparative analysis of embryo culture incubators. Reprod Biomed Online. 2014;28(5):535-547.
73. Kovacs G. How to improve your ART success rates. United Kingdom: Cambridge University Press; 2011.
74. Fujiwara M, Takahashi K, Izuno M, Duan YR, Kazono M, Kimura F, et al. Effect of microenvironment maintenance on embryo culture after in-vitro fertilization: comparison of top-load mini incubator and conventional front-load incubator. J Assist Reprod Genet. 2007;24(1):5-9.
75. Fawzy M, AbdelRahman MY, Zidan MH, Duan YR, Kazono M, Kimura F, et al. Humid versus dry incubator: a prospective, randomized, controlled trial. Fertil Steril. 2017;108(2):277-83.
76. Brown SK. Chamber assessment of formaldehyde and VOC emissions from wood-based panels. Indoor Air. 1999;9:209-15.
77. Cohen J, Gilligan A, Esposito W, Schimmel T, Dale B. Ambient air and its potential effects on conception in vitro. Hum Reprod. 1997;12:1742-9.
78. Hall J, Gilligan A, Schimmel T, Cecchi M, Cohen J. The origin, effects and control of air pollution in laboratories used for human embryo culture. Hum Reprod. 1998;13:146-55.
79. Ritz B, Wilhelm M. Ambient air pollution and adverse birth outcomes: methodologic issues in an emerging. Field Basic Clin Pharmacol Toxicol. 2008;102(2):182-90.
80. Dadvand P, Rankin J, Rushton S, Pless-Mulloli T. Association between maternal exposure to ambient air pollution and congenital heart disease: a register-based spatiotemporal analysis. Am J Epidemiol. 2011;173(2):171-82.
81. Rubes J, Selevan SG, Evenson DP, Zudova D, Vozdova M, Zudova Z, et al. Episodic air pollution is associated with increased DNA fragmentation in human sperm without other changes in semen quality. Hum Reprod. 2005;20(10):2776-83.
82. Chang JC, Fortmann R, Roache N, Lao HC. Evaluation of low-VOC latex paints. Indoor Air. 1999;9:253-8.
83. Elder K, Dale B. In vitro fertilization, 2nd edition. United Kingdom: Cambridge University Press; 2000.
84. Sharma L, Tarchala S, Nakagawa J, Perry J, Rawlins R. Next Generation Quality Control in the IVF Laboratory Using data loggers to monitor real time incubator temperature. Chicago. Illinois: Rush Center for Advanced Reproductive Care; 2010.
85. El Hajj, Haaf T. Epigenetic disturbances in vitro cultured gametes and embryos: implications for human assisted reproduction. Fertil Steril. 2013;99:632-41.
86. Steegers-Theunissen RP, Twigt J, Pestinger V, Sinclair KD. The periconceptional period, reproduction and long-term health of offspring: the importance of one-carbon metabolism. Hum Reprod Update. 2013;19(6):640-55.
87. Barker DJ. The intrauterine origins of cardiovascular disease. Acta Paediatr Suppl. 1993;82 (39):93-9.
88. Barker DJP. The developmental origins of adult disease. Eur J Epidemiol. 2003;18:733-6.
89. Langley-Evans SC. Developmental programming of health and disease. Proc Nutr Soc. 2006;65(1):97-105.
90. Grace KS, Sinclair KD. Assisted reproductive technology, epigenetics, and long-term health: a developmental time bomb still ticking. Semin Reprod Med. 2009;27(5):409-16.

CHAPTER

# 124 Micromanipulators

*Mir Jaffar, Syed Waseem Andrabi, Veena Gangaraju, Mohammed Ashraf C*

## INTRODUCTION

The use of micromanipulator for the manipulation of cells by biologists and physiologists dates back more than a century. It was GI Kite who reported first microinjection of sperm into the oocyte of starfish in 1914.[1] A series of experiments was carried on different species demonstrating major species differences. Ryuzo Yanagimachi demonstrated the development of pronuclei from the hamster oocyte nuclei after microinjection into homologous eggs, and a similar result was observed after injecting freeze-dried human spermatozoa into the hamster egg.[2] These experiments indicated that the membrane fusion of the gametes during natural fertilization can be bypassed during the activation of mammalian oocytes without compromising the normal development. The experiments led a foundation stone to a new technique in clinical embryology. Later many experiments were carried out by cell biologists with subsequent improvements in the technology and methods. Earlier experiments were carried out with the primary intention to record the early events in the oocyte after injecting the sperm.

It was the birth of Louise Brown in 1978 that changed the mind of reproductive biologists to implement the microinjection techniques in the medical field for infertile human couples. This was a milestone to overcome the female infertility with the primary cause of their infertility as tubal block. But later the focus shifted toward infertile men. On the other hand, surgical sperm retrieval techniques came into practice, which gave a new ray of hope to the men to father their own child who could not do so earlier either because of the absence, low count or morphologically abnormal sperms in their ejaculate **(Table 1)**.

The first technique implemented in the clinical field was partial zona dissection (PZD) by Jacques Cohen and colleagues. In this micromechanical technique, a breach is created by a sharp glass micropipette and subsequently the oocyte is placed into a suspension of spermatozoa, assuming the uninterrupted entry of sperm through the slit created by the micromanipulation technique to yield fertilization. Very soon subzonal sperm injection (SUZI) was experimented in which several spermatozoa are injected into the perivitelline space to bypass the vestments of zona pellucida. The practice of SUZI was soon followed by the introduction of intracytoplasmic sperm injection (ICSI) in which a single spermatozoon is injected directly into the ooplasm. ICSI[8] opened new vent for very poor male factor infertility. In conjugation with other methods like percutaneous epididymal sperm aspiration (PESA) and testicular sperm aspiration (TESA), ICSI became "the technique" for azoospermia. Assisted hatching (AH) for embryos with thick zona, blastomere biopsy for preimplantation genetic diagnosis (PGD), cytoplasmic transfer to overcome the inherent defect in oocyte, were the other methods to improve the success rate of human assisted conception.

## MICROMANIPULATOR

A micromanipulator is a device which is used to physically manipulate the microscopic structures under a high magnification, where a level of precision of movement is necessary which cannot be achieved by the unaided human hand. Micromanipulator in assisted reproduction is meant for microscopic handling of human gametes such as holding,

**TABLE 1:** Landmarks of micromanipulation in assisted reproductive techniques.

| *Technique* | *Reference* |
|---|---|
| Zona drilling (ZD)[3] | Gordon and Talansky (1986) |
| Partial zona dissection (PZD)[4] | Cohen et al. (1988) |
| Subzonal sperm injection (SUZI)[5] | Ng et al. (1988) |
| Assisted hatching (AH)[6] | Cohen et al. (1991) |
| Preimplantation genetic diagnosis (PGD)[7] | Handyside et al. (1990) |
| Intracytoplasmic sperm injection (ICSI)[8] | Palermo et al. (1992) |

injection, drilling, and aspiration of oocyte, sperm or embryo with very precised movements under microscope.

## Features Desirable in a Micromanipulator

- *Single control:* Single control is typically attained by operating the single joystick, which gives the operator the flexibility to travel in X-, Y-, and Z-axis without changing the hand from the control unit.
- *Variable sensitivity of control:* It is extremely useful to be able to vary the sensitivity of control with different magnification objectives. If it cannot be done, it may be found that work under low powers is too slow, as it may take a long time to traverse the field typically during alignment of microtools prior to the procedure and too fast and jerky when working under high power magnification, especially during the actual manipulation of the gametes.
- *Freedom from play/backlash:* It is essential that the microtool holder (receiver unit) should respond to the control unit without any delay, and that there should not be any further movement or creep on sudden removal of the hand from the control unit.
- *Freedom from vibration:* The dampening of vibration to the maximum possible limit is essential during microinjection. It can be achieved by (1) massive construction; (2) clamping the micromanipulator and microscope to a common heavy weight metallic base plate; (3) remote control; and (4) flexible tubing connection between the control unit and drive unit (microtool holding unit).
- *Rapid centration:* This function is highly desirable and convenient for the operator like in Eppendorf the prefixed operating placement of the microtool can be brought back with one click and in IntegraTi [Research instruments (RI)] the "home function" delivers the function after aligning the microtool in the space under the spacer object.
- *Three-dimensional movements:* The instrument should offer three-dimensional movements and the movement should take place in the same direction as the hand, so that there should be no apparent reversal of the movement under the microscope giving the operator better control.

Different types of manipulators have been developed by different manufacturing companies from time to time with subsequent improvements with each model. Although the commercial models are different but the basic principle is same among all: Scale down of movement from "macroscale to microscale" with the highest possible precision and convenience, which avoids the possible damage to the oocyte. This can be achieved by mechanically, hydraulically, and electronically depending on the manufacturing company. But the combination of any of the two gives more convenience to the operator. The commercially available micromanipulators used in assisted reproductive techniques (ARTs) include:

- Research instruments (IntegraTi, UK): Mechanical
- Narishige (Japan): Hydraulic and electronic
- Eppendorf (Germany): Electronic
- S-Corporation (Japan): Hydraulic.

Micromanipulation of gametes was initially performed with mechanical manipulators followed by hydraulic micromanipulator with single axis device and they were in use for a long time, which were later upgraded by three-axis hydraulic and electronic micromanipulators after careful evaluation of different possibilities (Narishige, Japan). The combination of both hydraulic and electrical incorporated in one instrument turned to be more promising.

## Micromanipulation Systems

Broadly, a micromanipulator system comprises a "controller unit" containing one or more manual controls, and a "drive unit" (receiver unit) containing the microtool holder, which is observed under high magnification optical lens of microscope. Since the cells to be manipulated can be observed only if magnified several times, which is possible only under the microscope. Unaided human hands cannot manipulate the microscopic cells with the extreme precision so a micromanipulator is needed to attain such a manipulation control to handle such delicate cells like oocytes. Micromanipulators of any choice can be built on any inverted microscope, generally with 4×, 10×, 20×, and 40× objectives. Two types of contrast systems are employed in the microscope: (1) Hoffman modulation contrast optics to visualize the cells on plastic petri dishes and (2) Nomarski optics uses polarized light and can be used to visualize the cells on glass petri dishes (PolScope). Inverted microscopes are available from different companies like Nikon, Olympus, Leica and Zeiss. Apart from inverted microscope and micromanipulator, the micromanipulation system also needs microtools to manipulate the gametes. Two types of microtools are used in ICSI procedure:

1. Holding pipettes to manipulate and stabilize the oocyte with round and fire-polished aperture
   - Outer diameter: 0.080–0.150 mm
   - Inner diameter: 0.018–0.025 mm
2. Injecting pipette with sharp beveled tip to immobilize, aspirate and inject the oocyte with sperm with minimal damage
   - Outer diameter: 0.0068–0.0078 mm
   - Inner diameter: 0.0048–0.0056 mm.

Generally, both the microtools are bent to an angle of approximately 30° at the distal end to facilitate smooth movements on the dish. Different diameters and shapes of the pipettes are used for different procedures like PGD, PZD, AH, etc.

## Narishige Micromanipulator

Most commonly used micromanipulator in the field of embryology is by Narishige brand (Narishige Company Limited, Tokyo, Japan) **(Fig. 1)**.

Narishige comes with both hydraulic as well as motorized micromanipulators installed in one instrument itself. Motorized is used for coarse adjustments and the hydraulic for fine adjustments and manipulations, which is most important function of any micromanipulator for successful results. Like any other micromanipulator, this manipulator also exists of two main parts, namely the control unit and the drive unit.

The control unit consists of a heavy weight metal plate on which is mounted the control unit system, which can be locked and unlocked to hold and release the parts from the metallic plate by turning the magnetic control knobs. The parts of the control unit used for manipulation are the hanging joystick, which can work in both X-axis as well as Y-axis travel. The joystick has a distal rotating knob, which controls Z-axis travel. All the knobs are kept at neutral before starting the alignment or when not in use to maintain the precision and life of the instrument. On the whole the hanging joystick controls all the required moments but with very limited freedom and speed, so this set of control system is used for final fine movements like when actually manipulating the gametes. Normally, the right-hand dominant embryologists prefer the injecting pipette control unit on the right-hand side and the holding on the left-hand side for their convenience. This hydraulic unit also has three rotating knobs on the upper side, which controls movements in only two axis (X and Y). This unit is connected to the drive unit mounted on the microscope by three flexible oil contained tubings. The rotation of any knob or any movement of the joystick creates a pressure in the oil containing tubings, which is translated in the form of micromovement in the drive unit.

The second control unit of Narishige is motorized with an upright joystick mounted on either the separate metallic plate or on the same as on hydraulic. It controls movements in X-, Y-, and Z-axis with different speeds as desired. It can be slanted either toward laterally on both sides or forward and backward to translate the same direction movements in the drive unit. It has two press buttons (blue and red) on the top to control Z-axis movements. The speed of the movements can be made fast by pressing a front press button on the same joystick or by turning the speed knob placed just in front of the joystick mounted on the metallic base plate. Normally, this unit is used for coarse adjustments and a backup for the hydraulic unit especially the hanging joystick to regain it in the middle before starting the actual procedure of ICSI or even during the procedure when the joystick loses the freedom.

The second part of the Narishige manipulator is the drive unit mounted on the coarse manipulator and connected with the control unit by three flexible, noncompressible and inelastic tubings filled with light mineral oil. The tool holder can be fixed in the universal joint that is mounted in the drive unit. The movement of the control unit causes the compression in the oil contained in the tubes, which is transferred to the small pistons fixed in the universal joint and causes the movement in the microtool holder to move according to the movement of the control unit. The movement in the drive unit is in proportion to the amplitude and speed executed on the joystick or other control knobs. This direct and proportional transfer of movement from control unit to the drive unit gives a feeling of direct control, which gives confidence to the operator.

The Narishige TAKANOME MTK-1 four-axis hanging joystick oil hydraulic micromanipulator system is a new generation micromanipulator **(Fig. 2)**. With a large retraction range of 50 mm, the MTK-1 fulfills multiple functions

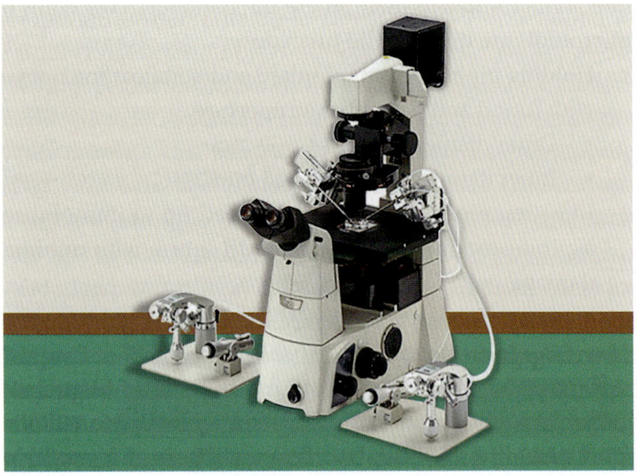

**Fig. 1:** Narishige micromanipulator unit incorporated to Nikon microscope.

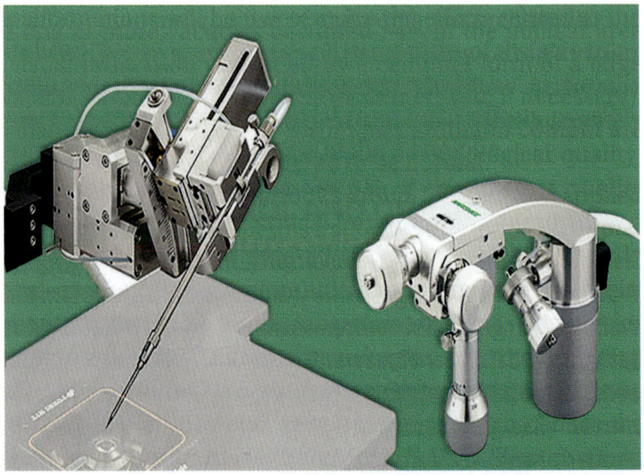

**Fig. 2:** Four-axis hanging joystick oil hydraulic micromanipulator (MTK-1).

in a single unit, eliminating the need for a separate coarse manipulator **(Fig. 3)**. Additionally, this upgraded version includes an innovative design that allows the user to change the pipette angle while keeping the needle tip in the center of the field of view, making angle adjustment a very easy **(Figs. 4A and B)**. One can easily switch the pipette from its "home" position to its "working" position, resulting in a significant reduction in the probability of pipette breakage and save the time by not having to reposition the injection holder each time you change pipettes **(Figs. 5A and B)**.

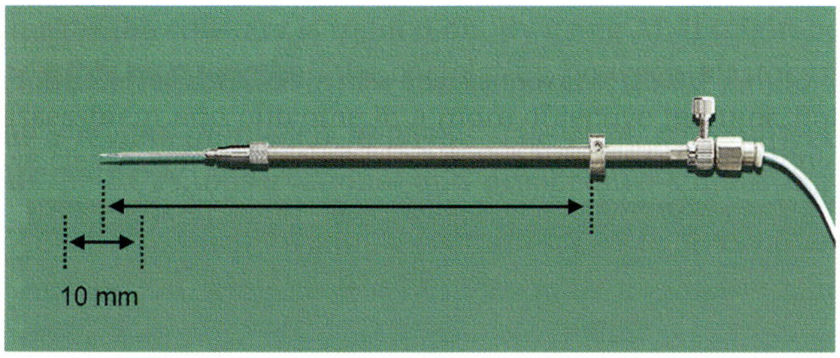


**Fig. 3:** Easy attachment of a pipette.

## *Alignment of Microtools*

It is always advisable to check the proper functioning of the micromanipulator well in advance of any ICSI procedure to ensure that the machine is in good working condition. Proper alignment of the microtool before starting the injection procedure is crucial for successful ICSI.

First of all, all the alignments of the drive unit as well as control units are brought to the neutral position. The drive unit has scale marked on the universal joint. All the three scales on the universal joint are brought to zero with the help of motorized joystick, preferably by keeping the speed knob to the highest or front speed button pressed to gain the neutral position very quickly. Make sure while doing this the hydraulic control system is already placed in neutral position to enjoy the maximum freedom of movement during the actual procedure. If the rotating knobs over the joystick are kept to any extremes then movement of joystick will not cause respective movement to the microtools. Check all the tubings for any traction which may hamper the smoothness of the movement. This setting is same on both the sides.

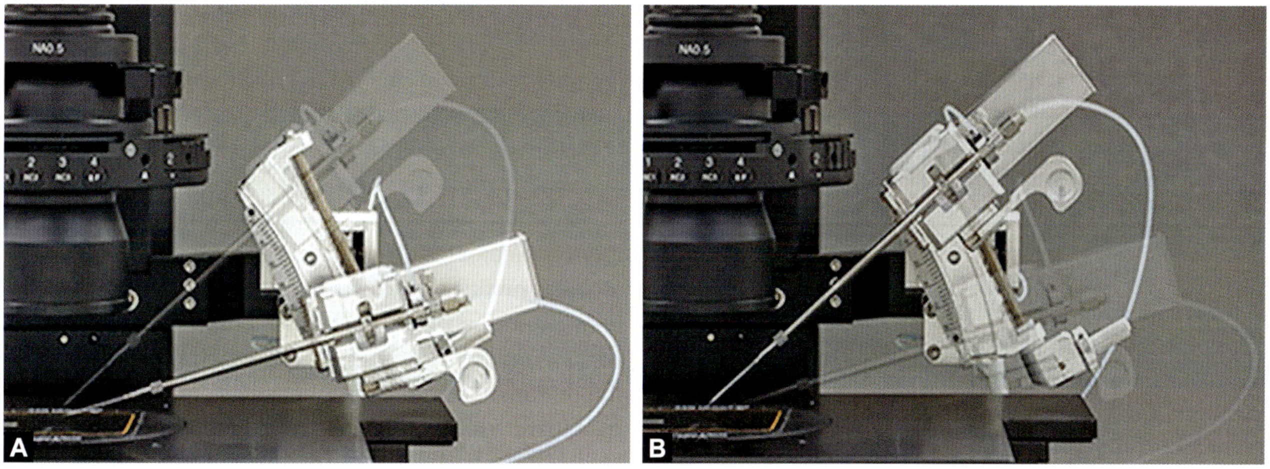


**Figs. 4A and B:** Pipette angle adjustment centered at the tip to stay in view. (A) 15°; (B) 40°.

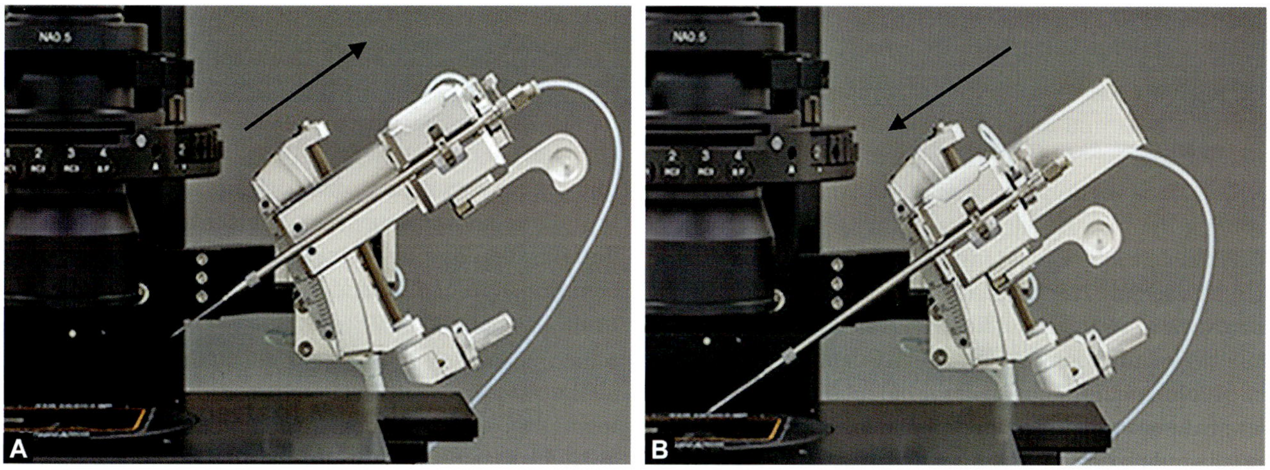


**Figs. 5A and B:** Simple and reliable motion from home to working position.

Once all the scales are set to the neutral position, the oil syringe (IM-11-2, Narishige) is checked for proper oil loading without any air bubbles, neither in the syringe nor in the tubings, connecting the syringe to the respective tool holder. If enough oil is not loaded in the syringe, then one must load prewarmed (37°C) light mineral oil in it. Narishige has two options of oil loading, one is either directly at the tip of the syringe with a BD syringe connected to a three-way valve which can be rotated to open the desired channel marked by an arrow and sign "OFF" on the valve. The other way to load the oil is by dipping the tip of the tool holder inside a round bottom tube containing oil with the "pipette tightening screw" loose.

After loading with oil and getting the oil syringe as well as control unit of the holding pipette to the neutral position (middle), microtools are fitted into the microtool holder preferably with the injecting one on the right-hand side and the holding one on the left-hand side or as desired. Make sure to discard few drops of oil before fitting the micropipette (injecting or holding) into their respective holders to avoid any air bubble formation inside the pipette, which may seriously hamper the sensitivity of the injecting pipette while aspiration of sperm and injection of the oocyte with the spermatozoa. Gently push the pipettes past the sealing rings inside the tool holder. No attempt should be made to take pipette "in and out" rather it should be done with one go to avoid the formation of air bubbles. Set the microscope to 20x or 40x objective, the tip of which serves as the pointer close to the warm stage, so that pipettes can be aligned just over the tip of the objective with direct visualization. Mark an ICSI dish with a marker or scratch with a hypodermic needle and focus under the lowest objective by using both coarse and fine adjustments available on both the sides of the microscope. Next place the microtool holder back in the universal joint and tighten the respective screw after placing the tip of the pipette very close to the tip of the inverted objective visible over the transparent heating plate stage. Rotate the pipette by holding the distal screw on the pipette holder in such a way that the tip is pointed upward. Get both holding as well as injecting pipette tips very close to each other right over the tip of the objective used as a pointer. Now turn the objective to 4× and focus under the microscope first the holding pipette because it is easier to focus compared to the injecting pipette because of its bigger diameter. While focusing the pipette the hydraulic adjustments are kept at neutral position constantly until the actual injecting procedure starts. Pipette alignment is done with motorized adjustments first then later fine adjustments can be assisted with the help of hydraulic control unit. Once both the pipettes are properly aligned the marked empty dish used for the alignment is replaced with the ICSI dish proper loaded with the gametes by gently lifting the whole microscope. Injecting microtool is slowly lowered in polyvinylpyrrolidone (PVP) through mineral oil to allow priming of mictotool with PVP for better control. To check the proper angle of the injecting pipette, an attempt to immobilize a spermatozoa, is done with not more than two attempts, till a proper angle is found which yields easy immobilization of sperms. Once both the pipettes can be visualized and moved without any dragging sensation, that must be considered the proper angle. Immobilization, loading of sperm and injection of oocyte is done under higher magnification (20× or 40×) preferably with the help of hydraulic joystick.

## Research Instruments (Integra 3)

Micromanipulator RI (TDU500, Cornwall, UK) has been manufacturing the mechanical micromanipulators since 1964. In the early 1990s, following the successful application of ICSI to the human gametes, RI modified their manipulators with number of user-friendly features and precisely controlled heated plates with two touch screen displays for temperature control (TDU500, IntegraTi). The current version of the Integra is known as Integra 3. A special objective of 4x spacer allowes the micropipette to be adjusted 16 mm above the petri dish to avoid the advertent pipette breakage during the alignment of the pipettes. After focusing in the mid-air (16 mm above the dish), the pipette could be dropped down without any chance of breaking it and this function was referred as a "home function".

Another feature added was tool holder angle adjustment indicators for more accurate alignment for a range of micropipettes with various degrees of bend between the tip and the shank. It allows the user to make very fine adjustments to the angle of the micropipette without the tip ever moving out of focus, ensuring that the micropipette is slightly "toe-down" during sperm immobilization and horizontal during injection. For PGD, RI has developed a unique double tool holder, which offers independent movement of both micropipettes **(Fig. 6)**.

Later they introduced three heated plates over the working stage, middle, left and right, each having independent control. In integra 3 an extra heating blower is given which blows the warm air at the bottom of the dish through the aperture in the middle of the glass heating stage. Apart from this, a fourth extra channel is also given, which can be used to connect an external heating plate or if any of the three channels does not function then the fourth one can be connected as a backup option. All four heating plates can be controlled independently with the settings set on the touch-screen display.

Like Narishige, RI also has a control unit and a drive unit. In control unit, it has two levers, one protruding upright over the stage on both sides and one hanging joystick underneath the stage exactly opposite to the upper one. The

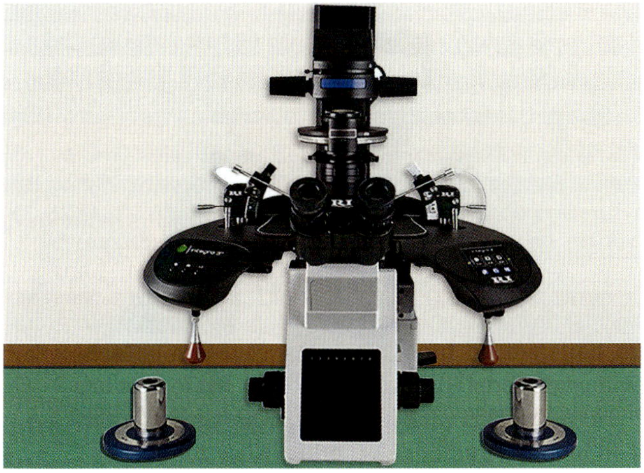

**Fig. 6:** Integra 3 micromanipulator incorporated to Nikon microscope showing the PL30 tool holder and touch screen display.

upper protruding one is for coarse adjustments, which gives freedom in only X- and Y-axis. While the lower hanging lever (joystick) is for fine movements and gives freedom in X-, Y-, and Z-axis.

The drive unit (tool holder) is very simple with marvelous functions. It has a special lever on the outer side of the tool holders to focus the pipette in the mid-air by lifting it up and once focused can be dropped down exactly over the surface of the petri dish. Also the tool holder has a single screw for angle adjustment to set the pipette to the desired angle or as per the angle of the pipette provided with different angles.

### *Alignment of Microtools*

Alignment of microtools in IntegraTi is very simple with minimal chances of breaking the pipette. Like in any other micromanipulator, oil syringe and its tubings should be checked for proper oil filling without any air bubbles. In this equipment, oil loading can be done only through PL30 microtool holder unlike Narishige where one can directly load the oil in the syringe. Once oil filling is done, make sure both the control levers are kept in the neutral position with the desired angle already preset. Both the levers can be seen in the neutral position except the fine control rotating knob on the hanging lever for Z-axis movement. In order to avoid running out of travel mid-procedure, it is recommended to set its travel of movement at the midpoint, which can be done by turning the knob to either of the extreme till it stops and then mark on the knob to count the total number of turnings. Typically, this knob can turn 24 (±2) rounds, so it is easy to calculate to turn back the knob to the middle (12 turns) to ensure its neutral position. In the latest version (Integra 3), the turning status can be seen on the display given.

Discard few droplets of oil from the syringe in an upright position, without wiping it fit the microtool (pipette) in the tool holder till one senses the hard end feel with one go, unlike Narishige where the operator has to go few millimeters beyond after feeling the pipette passing through the rubber ring. Repeated in and out will create air bubbles in the pipette and affect the sensitivity of the aspiration. The holding micropipette usually come with air controlled so does not need oil filling. Fix the micropipettes to their respective tool holders. Once the micropipettes are fitted, clip them back into their respective holders. Using the 4x objective lens the ICSI dish is focused like in any other microscope. Once the mark or scratch on the inner side of the dish is focused, turn the objective to 4x spacer. With outer levers still raised, the micropipettes are brought closer to each other by turning the knobs placed over the tool holder till the tip of the microtools illuminates.

The micropipettes have to be fitted, aligned and equilibrated before starting the ICSI procedure. Since the holding pipette is much bigger than the injection pipette, it can be used as a guide for positioning and equilibrating. Align the injecting pipette close to the holding pipette by directly visualizing the microtools. After focusing both the microtools, now it is safe to bring down the tool holders to the dish by using the home function. Now ICSI dish can be placed by just lifting and dropping the tool holder with the help of respective lever on the tool holder (home function). Briefly touch the tips of both pipettes in oil, and then in medium (ideally PVP), which gives better control because of its high viscosity, so that the ends fill by capillary action. The alignment in the horizontal plane has to be done with great care. Both the pipettes should be aligned flat on the bottom of the dish.

## Microinjectors

### *Screw-actuated Syringe*

The screw-actuated syringe (SAS) is for air-assisted microinjection and aspiration incorporated on a heavy circular base, which provides a good stability to the unit. It provides sensitive control with an extremely low dead-air volume of 10 mL capacity. When required they can generate high aspiration and pressure. Positive and negative pressure is created by turning the metal colored actuator screw control incorporated on top of the syringe. On top of the syringe, a release button is provided to overcome the equilibration problems by pressing the release button once the microinjection needle is taken underneath the medium for rapid equilibration. These are the only air syringes suitable for air injection of the sperm, eliminating the need for oil. The syringe is connected to the PAR21 microtool holder by hard yet flexible polythene tubing. For those who prefer to use an oil microinjector, RI provides the option with micrometer-actuated sealed oil syringe (SOS) mounted upon a heavy metallic base **(Fig. 7)**.

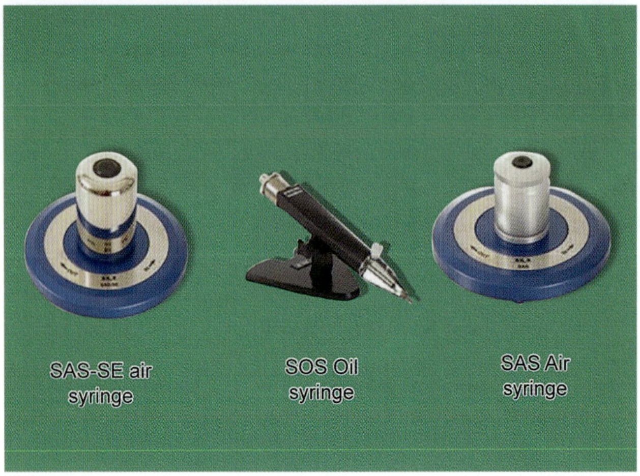


**Fig. 7:** Examples of air and oil syringes of research instruments (RI) micromanipulator.

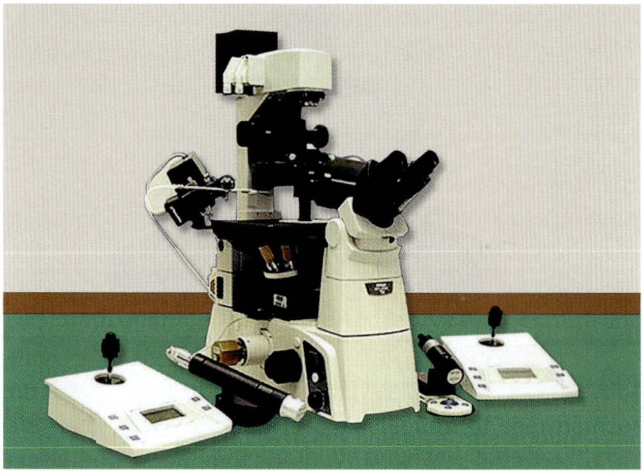

**Fig. 8:** Eppendorf micromanipulator unit incorporated to Nikon microscope showing motor module unit, control board and oil syringes.

### *Stage Heating*

The Integra 3 incorporated with three independently controlled heated surfaces that are accurately calibrated to within 0.05°C of the set point. It also provides one extra heating channel for external device adjacent to the manipulator like stereo dissecting microscope if required. The combination of the warm inserted stage and the warm blower provides the most accurate heated system available to maintain the temperature of additional petri dishes.

### *Mechanical Stage*

The Integra 3 is supplied as standard with dynamic voltage scaling (DVS) variable reduction mechanical stage incorporated with stainless steel stage plate. The DVS offers both X and Y positioning from a single hanging lever just underneath the stage on the right-hand side, enabling quick and precise positioning of the cells. Each turn of the stage control moves the stainless steel stage plate 28 mm in either the X or Y plane, with total 40 mm travel.

## Eppendorf Micromanipulator

The company was founded by two German scientists in Hamburg-Eppendorf University Hospital after World War II. To repair the broken instruments, a workshop was conducted under the supervision of both the scientists. The team of doctors and scientists who participated succeeded in repairing many devices and also invented the new ones out of these damaged instruments.

The Eppendorf micromanipulator **(Fig. 8)** is also motorized/electronic one like Narishige but the advantage of the Eppendorf micromanipulator is that movement of the joystick is sensed by the microprocessor and certain preferred positions can be saved in its inbuilt memory, so that they can be recalled at any time as desired. This particular function of Eppendorf makes it outstanding compared to the other commercial micromanipulators.

The Eppendorf micromanipulator is composed of mainly motor module unit and control board.

### *Motor Module Unit*

The motor module unit can be fixed on any microscope but typically it is fixed on both sides of the microscope, especially for micromanipulation of gametes, so that they can be fitted with commercially available microtools close to the operating petri dishes. The whole motor unit can be rotated in and out of the stage to create the space for the replacement of petri dishes or while fixing the microtools without losing the exact original place. It consists of two main parts attached to each other through a straight guide fixed with a screw and a wire. One part of it plays Y- and Z-axis movements (Y/Z module) and the other part plays only X-axis movements (X module).

### *Control Board*

It consists of two control boards placed on either side of the microscope on the table away from the microscope **(Fig. 9)**. Both the control boards are connected to the motor module unit by flexible electrical wires. The control board contains following features:

- An upright joystick protruding in the middle of the board, which contains a button on the top of the joystick. It enables the user to move in all the planes (X, Y, and Z) in a desired speed according to the preset speed settings. The joystick can also be disabled by pressing and holding the top button on the joystick, which gives the operator the freedom of replacing the joystick to the desired position without any movement in the microtools. One of the main advantages of the manipulator is that it can save certain positions and limit certain movements,

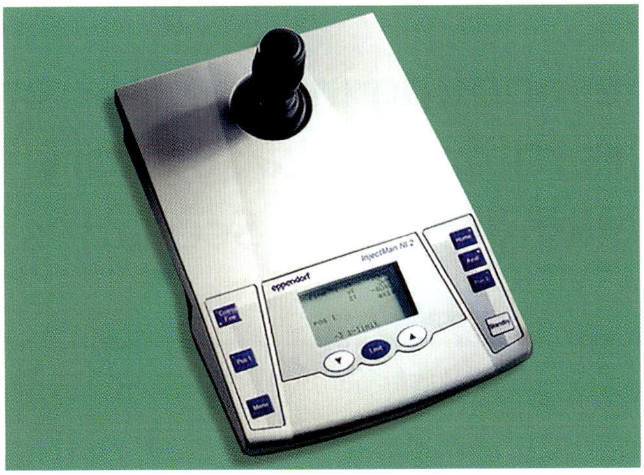

**Fig. 9:** Control board of Eppendorf micromanipulator.

which might break the micropipette. Once a working alignment is attained, it can be saved, so that after every procedure it can be regained back by pressing the home button with just one click. This feature is found only in Eppendorf micromanipulator.

- A multifunctional keypad, which can be used for different functions to feed the microprocessor to save particular alignment and adjust or limit the speed.
- A light-emitting diode (LED) display on the upper side, which displays the axis coordinated and the options chosen.

## CONCLUSION

New developments in microscopy and the need of manipulating the cells have brought a renewal of interest in methods of micromanipulation. While human hand can be very deft and may be capable of surprisingly well controlled movements but when it comes to handling microtools or living cells under high magnification, a micromanipulator is an incredible invention, which provides the solution beyond certain unaided human limits. The micromanipulators work in such a limited environment that a minor tremor or muscle contraction could be devastating for manipulating the living cells. However, we must not forget that the first baby born through ICSI procedure was in 1992, which is still immature to conclude its long-term consequences because of lack of data. Since ICSI is also routinely being performed for normozoospermic male couples, when conventional in vitro fertilization (IVF) yields similar outcomes, it should be restricted only for the couples with severe male factor infertility.

## REFERENCES


1. Lillie FR. Studies of fertilization. VI. The mechanism of fertilization in arbacia. J Exp Zool. 1914;16:523-90.
2. Yanagimachi R. Gamete manipulation for development: new methods for conception. Reprod Fertil Dev. 2001;13(1):3-14.
3. Gordon JW, Talansky BE. Assisted fertilization by zona drilling; a mouse model for correction of oligospermia. J Exp Zool. 1986;239:347-54.
4. Cohen J, Malter H, Fehilly C, Wright G, Elsner C, Kort H, et al. Implantation of embryos after partial opening of oocyte zona pellucida to facilitate sperm penetration. Lancet. 1988;2:162.
5. Ng SC, Bongso A, Ratnam SS, Sathananthan H, Chan CL, Wong PC, et al. Pregnancy after transfer of multiple sperm under the zona. Lancet. 1988;2:790.
6. Cohen J. Assisted hatching of human embryos. J In Vitro Fert Embryo Transf. 1991;8(4):179-90.
7. Handyside AH, Kontogianni EH, Hardy K, Winston RM. Pregnancies from biopsied human preimplantation embryos sexed by Y-specific DNA amplification. Nature. 1990;344:768-70.
8. Palermo G, Joris H, Devroey P, Van Steirteghem AC. Pregnancies after intracytoplasmic injection of single spermatozoon into an oocyte. Lancet. 1992;340:17-8.

CHAPTER 125

# Troubleshooting in the In Vitro Fertilization Laboratory: Challenging Case Scenarios

*Varsha Samson Roy, Sangita Sharma*

## INTRODUCTION

The laboratory processes are understood to be well designed, protocols standardized for the respective laboratory, operator involvement well defined, and observation of even the smallest of details mandatory. With so much precision into how, what, when, and where, we do not expect the laboratory to face adverse scenarios frequently. Over the years, a lot of understanding, acceptance, and conformance to quality management has made assisted reproductive technologies (ARTs) more proficient.

The basic principle of quality management is based on the cycle of plan-do-check-act **(Fig. 1)**.

Before performing a procedure, the in vitro fertilization (IVF) laboratory needs to plan how to do it. A well-written standard operating procedure (SOP), written in a manner that is easily understood, easily accessible, and does not assume the operator to "know it", becomes mandatory. Proper documentation is the key to troubleshooting. Inadequate or improper documentation may not provide the required information to identify the probable factors contributing toward the adverse outcomes. Corrective measures can only be implemented once the causative factor is identified. Unfortunately, it may not be a single but multiple factors contributing, namely clinical, procedural, patient factors, operator, and culture conditions.

Hence, troubleshooting requires the involvement of both the clinician and the laboratory personnel.

The basic physiology behind the event should be well understood by the clinicians and embryologists. A deviation from what is normal can only be identified and addressed only with an adequate understanding of the normal.

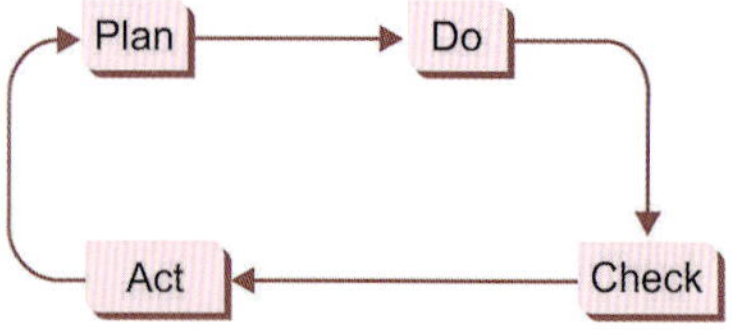


**Fig. 1:** Plan-do-check-act cycle.

As per the guidelines for good practices in IVF laboratory,[1] quality requirements cover the organization, management, personnel, equipment and materials, facilities/premises, documentation, records, and quality review.

Troubleshooting should target the following aspects on a broader scale as discussed here.

## LABORATORY QUALITY MANAGEMENT PROGRAM

Quality management includes quality control (QC), quality assurance (QA), and quality improvement (QI). A total quality management (TQM) for the ART clinic includes not only quality management but also system management and risk management.

A validated, written, authorized, signed instruction for each process (SOP), addressing every small detail, is mandatory. There should not be any scope for assumption. The SOP should be regularly updated and the operators should be informed and trained on the changes before implementing.

Identification and traceability of the patient, their biological materials, and records are extremely crucial Corrective action to keep procedures under conformity and risk assessment analysis for all procedures should be done. A protocol for management of adverse events should also be in place.

Every laboratory should determine its own key performance indicators (KPIs) and the critical level. Data relevant to that should be collected and evaluated at regular intervals. For batch IVF, some part of the data [e.g., fertilization rate, cleavage rate, embryo utilization, blastulation rate, cryosurvival in frozen embryo transfer (FET) cycles] can be evaluated immediately after the ongoing cycle and before the resumption of the next batch.

Internal quality control (IQC) and external quality assurance (EQA) programs are highly recommended.

## EQUIPMENT

Quality control of lab equipment involves (1) design qualification (DQ), (2) installation qualification (IQ), and (3) operational qualification (OQ). This also includes periodic equipment calibration, disinfection, service, and maintenance. A log book for maintenance/repair and breakdown of each equipment will help decide on the continuity or replacement of the equipment.

Critical equipment such as incubators, microscopes, manipulators, freezing machines, and computers should be on uninterruptible power supply (UPS) backup. All the essential equipment should be in appropriate numbers to the workload. This is most crucial for incubators to prevent frequent openings, which are detrimental to embryo development.

Consumables should be off-gassed prior to use to reduce the volatile organic compound (VOC) burden.

## AIR QUALITY AND CULTURE CONDITIONS

Studies by Cohen[2,3] have shown that air quality impacts embryo quality. Improving the air quality improves the ART success by increasing the pregnancy rates and reducing miscarriage rates.[4]

Manipulation of gametes and embryos in vitro should be performed under controlled environment. Laboratory air should be subjected to high-efficiency particulate air (HEPA) filtration system and should be low on VOC.

The gametes and embryos should be manipulated and cultured under appropriate $CO_2$ concentration, temperature, and pH for the best outcomes.

Culturing embryos under low $O_2$ tension has shown to reduce the stress, improve blastulation rate in pregnancy, and implantation rate.[5,6]

Accepted ranges for parameters (e.g., temperatures, $CO_2$ concentration, pH) should be determined and recorded at regular intervals with calibrated instruments.

## DISPOSABLES AND MEDIA

Media and consumables designed for use in human ART and of embryo culture grade should be used. Commercially available media and disposables are tested for quality, using stringent QC assays in compliance of the regulations. It is important to ensure that the cold chain for media is maintained from the manufacturing unit through the shipment to the doorstep of the laboratory. Package integrity and appropriate certificates complying to the QC tests should be available with the distributor and a copy of the same should be retained with the laboratory. The media and oil should be stored and used as per the manufacturer's instructions. Media, once uncapped, should be consumed at the earliest, prior to the expiry date.

Other factors such as culture droplet size, group or individual culture, and oil overlay are also known to influence the embryo development.

## OPERATOR SKILLS

Operator skill and culture conditions are crucial to the IVF laboratories' performance. It is important to define the responsibilities and ensure that all personnel are qualified and competent to handle the particular procedure.

Operator performance should be accessed regularly to ensure competence, compliance, and consistency. These can be done by accessing the individual's KPIs and direct observation of procedural skills (DOPS). They should be provided assistance in improving and upgrading their skills.

In a study by Dessolle et al., the first 50 vitrification warming cycles of trainees were analyzed on the basis of embryo wastage and survival. The results suggested that after 35–45 procedures, the individuals achieved proficiency as per the set standard by the investigators.[7] Most of the procedures do have a learning curve and embryologists should handle procedures under supervision till they achieve proficiency in the particular procedure.

## PROCEDURAL ASPECTS

Appropriate consents for the procedures to be performed should be obtained after adequate couple counseling and verified by both the clinical and the laboratory staff. A system should be in place to ensure patient identity and sample identification is done at appropriate steps and by appropriate people.

During the follicular scans done at the time of controlled ovarian stimulation (COS), a mention should be made about the ovarian accessibility, presence of endometriomas, hydrosalpinges, or other ovarian cysts.

The records of the patient, including the ultrasound images, should be seen by the clinician before commencing the procedure.

Oocyte retrieval is a very sensitive procedure. There should be standard SOPs for it, which should be followed by all the clinicians in the particular unit. A checklist should include the inquiry about the final oocyte maturation trigger. Consents should be checked not only by the staff nurse, but also by the clinician himself as troubleshooting can take place not only in the IVF laboratory or operation theater but also in a courtroom. The clinician should have undergone a structured training program, with a minimum of 20 (a minority may require up to 50) oocyte retrievals done under supervision to achieve the required proficiency.[8] During the follicular scans done at the time of COS, a mention should be made about the ovarian accessibility, presence of endometriomas, hydrosalpinges, or other ovarian cysts. The records of the patient, including the ultrasound images, should be seen by the clinician before commencing the procedure. It is needless to emphasize the importance of confirming the patient identity and communicating it to the embryologist. Depth of anesthesia should be adequate to make the patient comfortable and to help in retrieving the maximum number of oocyte-cumulus complexes (OCCs). In case of arrival of a new lot (batch) of oocyte retrieval sets or embryo transfer catheters in the center, their expiry dates, QC assays, and packaging should be checked like any other consumables and media, and the lot number recorded separately. As the OCCs are highly sensitive to any sudden change in temperature and pH, the oocyte retrieval set, test tubes, and 3-(*N*-morpholino) propanesulfonic acid (MOPS)/4-(2-hydroxyethyl)-1-piperazineethanesulfonic acid (HEPES) buffered media should all be prewarmed. The test tube warmers and holders should have a digital display of temperature, and its record should be maintained. An external thermometer should be used to check the accuracy of the temperature displayed. It is of utmost importance to hand over the OCCs to the embryologist as quickly as possible, while minimizing any change in the temperature. The efficacy of the procedure in terms of the number and quality of OCCs retrieved depends on the integrity of the circuit, negative suction pressure, laminar or turbulent flow of the follicular fluid, velocity of the flow, sharpness and thickness (gauge) of the aspiration needle, length of the tubing, experience of the clinician, depth of anesthesia,, and accessibility of the ovaries.

Simultaneous communication between the clinician and the embryologist is crucial to ensure proper retrieval of OCCs in the follicular fluid reaching the laboratory. After the procedure, the oocyte recovery rate should be documented in relation to the larger (>17 mm) follicles mentioned in the follicular scan reports. Any gross discrepancy should be mentioned and audited.

Every IVF laboratory should have an emergency backup plan. There should be uninterrupted power supply to the ultrasound machine and the suction apparatus for uninterrupted functioning during the procedure. An extra suction pump is ideal, but it might be a costlier issue. At least, facilities for manual aspiration of the follicles should be there, although the negative pressure generated this way is uncontrolled and sometimes might be detrimental to the OCCs.

## PATIENT FACTORS

Complete evaluation of a couple before starting an ART cycle is very important. There should be a complete history taking and proper examination. All the previous records should be studied and relevant history/findings should be documented in a systematic manner. Every center should have a complete pro forma designed to document relevant history, examination, investigations, imaging reports, findings of endoscopic procedures if done earlier and any related treatment taken in past. Having such information helps in maintaining uniformity in the presence of more than one clinician in the unit. Moreover, the record-keeping becomes easier for any future reference. Such data can also be stored electronically for simpler handling.

### Documentation of Previous In Vitro Fertilization Cycles

A detailed history of any treatment taken in the past for infertility is important, including IVF or intrauterine insemination (IUI) cycles. Effort should be made to gather information about the protocols used, types and doses of gonadotropins given, evidence of ovulation (IUI cycle), number of oocytes retrieved (IVF cycle), and endometrial thickness during insemination/embryo transfer. Any adverse events such as failure to retrieve oocytes or premature/postmature oocytes, poor or failed fertilization, low and poor quality of the embryos complications such as ovarian hyperstimulation syndrome (OHSS) should be documented. Other relevant information, such as stage of embryos transferred and cryopreservation details, should also be sought.

Apart from the ovarian response, it is equally important to check for the endometrial thickness and pattern achieved in past. Finally, the outcome of the previous cycles, namely, successful/unsuccessful cycle, biochemical pregnancy, blighted ovum, missed abortion, or an uneventful pregnancy, completes the list.

Each and every aspect is important and can give us a clue to avoid troubleshooting situations by taking prior precautions, making changes in the protocols or drugs used, getting any further investigations, or endoscopic procedures done if required, before the commencement of the next cycle.

This detailed evaluation and record-keeping also help us in prognostication of the further cycles.

### Documentation of the Current In Vitro Fertilization Cycle

All investigations done, including the hormonal assays and transvaginal scans, should be documented in charts or pro formas made for this purpose. The protocol decided, type and dose of gonadotropins given and the ovarian response to it in terms of number of larger follicles and serum estradiol levels if done, should be mentioned, along with all the details of the oocytes retrieved and embryos formed, as mentioned earlier also (vide supra). Any coincidental finding during the COS such as an endometrial polyp or a hydrosalpinx should be noted separately. Any correction in a problematic situation in future cannot be done without a retrospection of the cycle details.

Certain patient factors are known to be associated with lower pregnancy rates and poorer outcomes of an ART cycle. The most important ones being:[9]

- Higher age of the patient
- Poor ovarian reserve
- Unexplained long-standing infertility
- Recurrent implantation failures in past
- Persistent suboptimal endometrium[10]
- Severe oligoasthenoteratozoospermia (OAT)[11]
- Obesity
- Smoking, alcohol, and caffeine consumption.

## CLINICAL ASPECTS

Apart from the laboratory aspects and culture conditions, clinical aspects can be equally responsible for a problematic situation during an IVF cycle.[12]

Gonadotropins and gonadotropin-releasing hormone (GnRH) analogs have become an essential part of an IVF/ART program. Production and purification of gonadotropins have to undergo stringent QC assessment, thus ensuring a pure product of high quality. As these preparations are highly temperature sensitive, it is of utmost importance to ensure the maintenance of cold chain from the manufacturer to the IVF center via the distributors. It is equally important to sensitize the patients about the importance of cold chain while they carry the gonadotropin preparations from the center and keep it with them before finally injecting. A person should be made responsible for receiving, proper storage, and record-keeping of the gonadotropins and GnRH analogs. Every new batch which is received at the center should be documented, the batch number should be mentioned, expiry dates checked, and cold chain ensured.

There should be a dedicated staff nurse or a counselor who would make the patients understand the doses of the injectable, their reconstitution, administration, adjusting, and administering the doses with pens. Any misunderstanding of the doses or wrong administration can have significant effects on the final outcome.

Monitoring of the ovarian response by a transvaginal scan is very crucial and preferably should be done by the same person. Over or underestimation of the number and size of follicles before the final oocyte maturation trigger can lead to retrieval of premature or postmature oocytes.

The final oocyte maturation trigger [human chorionic gonadotropin (hCG) or GnRH agonist] is the most crucial in terms of adhering to the exact timing and proper administration. It is one of the single most important factors responsible for the oocyte yield with regard to quantity and maturity. The patient should be given clear written instructions about the dose, timing, date, and route of administration. On the day of oocyte retrieval, the checklist should include asking about the date and timing of the injection taken. Some centers routinely perform a urinary hCG testing with a urine pregnancy kit before oocyte collection, while others get serum β-hCG levels done on the next morning of the trigger, and still others rely on their embryologist mentioning about the presence or absence of the OCCs in the given initial tubes with follicular fluid after aspiration.

## CHALLENGING SCENARIOS

### Oocyte Retrieval

Prior to starting aspiration, the complete circuit of the aspiration pump connected to the tubing of the aspiration needle should be checked. This is done to ensure the integrity of the circuit and adequate buildup of the required pressure, which is around 90–120 mm Hg for conventional IVF cases. Oocyte retrieval is usually done using a 17-gauge single-lumen needle. Thinner needles with smaller diameters (20 gauge) significantly prolong the operating time but are associated with lesser postoperative pain without affecting the oocyte yield.[13] As the thinner needles are less stiff, they can bend and may cause technical difficulties, especially in deep-seated ovaries.[14] Flushing of the follicles with a double-lumen needle has been found to be associated with longer procedural time and need of more anesthetic agent without any significant difference in the oocytes retrieved, fertilization, or pregnancy rates when compared with direct aspiration with a single-lumen needle.[15]

Aspiration of culture media into the tubing should be done to rinse the tubing and needle prior to penetrating the follicles. This also helps in removing the dead space of the needle and the tubing and allows a uniform laminar flow as turbulent flow can damage the OCC.[14]

#### *Failure to Aspirate a Follicle/Failure to Build up Adequate Negative Pressure*

In case of failure to generate negative suction pressure, ensure the functioning of the suction pump, power supply to it, check the digital pressures displayed, confirm the needle is inside the follicle, any break/interruption in the circuit should be looked for, e.g., cracked tubes, loose caps of the tubes or kinks and bends in the tubing. Slight rotation of the needle might be helpful if the bevel of the needle tip is blocked by the adjacent follicular wall. Once all this has been ruled out, a blocked needle can be a possibility due to a blood clot or tissue blocking the tip or the lumen. The emergency button, present in some aspiration pumps, can be pressed, which generates sudden high negative pressures to dislodge any clot, or the needle can be withdrawn and flushed with media.

#### *No Oocytes Obtained/Less than Anticipated Number Obtained*

At times if the patient has been triggered earlier when the follicles are still smaller, the OCCs are immature with very few layers of granulosa cells. This makes identification difficult, especially if the embryologist is not consciously "looking" for the OCCs. This is also the scenario in in vitro maturation (IVM) cycles wherein cell strainers or filters have to be used for faster OCC identification.[16]

Sometimes, in spite of normal ovarian response on ultrasound and normal follicular steroidogenesis, there is a complete failure to retrieve any OCC. This so-called "empty follicle syndrome (EFS)" can be false EFS or genuine EFS.[17] The reported incidence varies from 0.45 to 7% of the IVF cycles in different studies[18] and most of the cases are sporadic.[19] The false EFS is due to a fault in the administration of the final oocyte maturation trigger in terms of dose, time, date, or administration of the injection.[20] Good communication between embryologist and the clinician during oocyte retrieval is crucial. In case of failure to find any OCC in the initial few tubes with follicular fluid, the serum hCG levels or urinary hCG should be checked, although there is no consensus on the threshold of circulating hCG levels to define an adequate trigger. HCG values ranging from 5 to 160 IU/L after about 36 hours from the hCG administration have been reported as the concentration threshold by different groups.[21,22] Some authors have even reported checking hCG in the follicular fluid.[23] However, a positive test cannot exclude incomplete administration of the injection or any wrong timing of it. In case of a negative hCG test, the oocyte maturation trigger should be given and oocyte retrieval planned after 36 hours of it. There can be reduced in vivo biological activity of some batches of commercially available hCG, especially in cases of urinary products.[18] Thus, it is important to document any change in the batch entering the center. Other causes of false EFS can be incomplete aspiration of the follicles or defects in the aspiration circuit such as too low suction pressures, which might be missed during the procedure.

Nowadays, with increasing use of antagonist protocol for COS and GnRH agonist trigger to minimize the incidence of OHSS, testing for hCG holds no relevance in such cycles. In such cases with GnRH agonist trigger, serum luteinizing hormone (LH) and progesterone level testing have been proposed, but the exact thresholds are yet to be established. Some investigators have indicated an LH circulating level of 15 IU/L as the cutoff value.[24]

The true or the genuine EFS is failure to retrieve oocytes in spite of a correctly and timely administered trigger (hCG or GnRH agonist). This is associated with older age, prolonged infertility, poor ovarian reserve, and poor responsiveness to gonadotropins during ovarian stimulation (indicating dysfunctional folliculogenesis).[25]

The pathophysiology of genuine EFS is still poorly understood, but probably there is a role of specific genetic factors. These patients are predisposed to abnormal folliculogenesis and precocious atresia of the OCCs as seen by the increased expression of some proapoptotic genes and a significant reduction in transcripts whose products are responsible for normal follicular growth.[26] Cases have been reported where after a second bolus of hCG, adequate number of OCCs were retrieved after 24 hours (i.e., much later to the initial hCG trigger), indicating partial and slow response of the follicle to hCG, thus requiring an extended time for complete follicular maturation.[27,28] Meniru and Craft[27] suggested that there could be a delayed detachment of OCC from the follicular wall following hCG injection.

The molecular mechanism(s) underlying the slow or insufficient follicular response to LH/hCG receptor stimulus is not yet understood but could involve the receptor sensitivity itself or the efficiency of postreceptor signal transducing pathways.[29] Still, there are different kinds of patients who do not respond even to a second bolus of hCG, in whom mutations have been identified in the gene encoding for the LH/hCG receptor.[30]

Recurrence of EFS increases with age, 24% recurrence rate in 35–39 years age group and 57% for those over 40 years have been reported.[31]

Thus, the different strategies to prevent EFS in the subsequent IVF cycles are: Changing the batch of hCG[32,33] using recombinant hCG,[34] changing the protocol to antagonist with a GnRH agonist trigger,[35] administering a dual trigger with hCG and GnRH agonist[23] increasing the interval between the trigger and oocyte retrieval.[28]

### *Only Immature Oocytes Obtained*

Retrieval of only immature oocytes can happen if the aspiration is done too early after the oocyte maturation trigger (<34 hours). This can be due to the wrong timing of the trigger, which is not reported to the center by the patient on the day of oocyte retrieval. Therefore, it is important to make the patient understand the importance of the correct timing of the trigger. Overestimation of the size of the follicles on ultrasound before the trigger can also be a reason. The pathophysiology of such a condition (all immature oocytes retrieved) is at times same as that of an EFS, both being different presentations of the same etiology. This is further explained by a few cases which were initially thought to be genuine EFS, but on more careful examination of the follicular fluid with strainers, few immature OCCs were found.[36] Prognosis in subsequent cycles depends on the underlying cause. If the trigger was correctly administered on the right time, then it could be due to genetic predisposition to partial and slow response to hCG. The immature oocytes should be followed and any signs of IVM should be considered as a good prognostic factor. Delayed aspiration (>36 hours) after the oocyte maturation trigger should be planned in the subsequent cycle.

### *Follicular Aspirates are too Bloody*

Aspirating smaller diameter follicles as in cases of IVM usually end up with bloody aspirates. In these cases, the follicular walls are thick and penetrating them requires force and at times multiple punctures. Aspiration needles which are being reused cause difficulty in penetrating the ovarian tissue due to blunting of the tip on repeated washing. Hence, aspiration needles should not be reused. The embryologist should make the utmost attempts to get rid of any blood clot in the OCCs as they are known to be toxic to the gamete and can retard embryo development. If the blood clot with OCCs is used for IVF insemination, they can also increase the reactive oxygen species (ROS) production. Hence, cutting the part of the granulose cells that are embedded in the blood clot with an insulin needle should be attempted prior to inseminating or even culturing these OCCs further till denuding or inseminating.

## Poor Oocyte Quality

Sometimes poor oocyte quality is seen, the reasons of which can be intrinsic or extrinsic. It can be found in women with higher age, poor ovarian reserve, long-standing unexplained infertility, polycystic ovarian syndrome, and endometriosis. Environmental changes and psychological stress are also reasons for poor quality oocytes due to the high ROS generated in ovaries.[37] A particular batch of urinary human menopausal gonadotropin (hMG) or hCG might have higher protein impurities or lower bioavailability, thus resulting in poor quality oocytes. Repeated problem in a few patients, especially during a batch IVF, should alert us toward a drug-related issue. Poor oocyte quality may indicate chromosomally abnormal oocytes, which may be associated with low fertilization rates, poor embryo grades, lower implantation and pregnancy rates, and higher miscarriage rates.[38]

## Semen Quality

### *Unable to Produce Semen on Day of Oocyte Pickup*

Unexpected ejaculation failures for the first time can occur on the day of retrieval due to stress and anxiety or "uninviting surroundings".[39] Ideally, all the patients going through the procedure of oocyte retrieval should have adequate frozen semen sample as backup. The number of samples to be frozen per individual depends on the semen quality and the number of oocytes expected. The first line of management should always be reassurance, irrespective of availability or nonavailability of a frozen backup. Counsel the patient and ask him to try another attempt after 30–60 minutes of break. In the meanwhile, the frozen sample (if available) can be thawed and kept ready. Prescription of sildenafil citrate 50 mg followed by an attempt to ejaculate 30–40 minutes later. Other methods of getting sperms in case of anejaculation are penile vibratory stimulation (PVS), prostate massage, and electroejaculation. Electroejaculation is usually reserved for spinal cord injury cases where even PVS fails as it requires general anesthesia, special equipment, and expertise. Surgical sperm retrieval can be the last resort.

In case of failure of all these methods, the patient should be offered oocyte vitrification. The results of vitrified oocytes are best when they are vitrified within 1–2 hours of retrieval; hence, timely decisions will optimize the outcomes even in challenging scenarios.

### *Semen Sample with Pus Cells/Debris/Infected*

Chances of bacterial contaminations seem to be more in males who require female partner assistance for collection. In cases of contamination reported during the routine semen analysis, an andrologist's opinion and adequate antibiotic treatment to the sensitive organism should be considered. Pus cells are most common in patients with chronic prostatitis/urethritis. On the day of oocyte retrieval, semen samples with presence of debris/pus/contamination are best treated with gradient method of semen processing. Density gradient followed by wash and swim-up significantly reduced the risk of transmission in human immunodeficiency virus (HIV)-discordant couples regardless of viral suppression in the male partner.[40]

## Fertilization Issues

Fertilization rates in the range of 70–80% are achieved by both conventional IVF insemination and/or intracytoplasmic sperm injection (ICSI). To combat fertilization failure, many laboratories subject the oocytes to ICSI without good evidence in its favor. Approximately 30% of the oocytes fail to fertilize with ICSI[41] and total fertilization failure (TFF) occurs in 2–3% of the cases.[42]

Poor or TFF can be anticipated in severe male factor infertility (severe OAT, immotile sperms, globozoospermia, nonviable sperms), poor oocyte quality, and low oocyte numbers (≤3 oocytes).

Some metaphase II (MII) oocytes although may appear meiotically mature in displaying extrusion of the first polar body, they may not have achieved the complete degree of cytoplasmic maturity. These oocytes may actually be lacking essential maternal factors required for subsequent fertilization, pro-nucleus (PN) formation, and embryo development. Thus, visualization of the oocytes does not give us the complete picture of oocyte maturity.

In aberrant phospholipase C zeta (PLCζ) expression, abnormal chromatin, centrosome dysfunction, and lack of sperm aster formation affect the ability of the sperm to contribute successfully toward normal fertilization.

To understand fertilization failure, the sperm-oocyte interactions are crucial especially in IVF. To understand the causes of fertilization failure in IVF and ICSI, the process of fertilization can be divided into pre-sperm interaction (cumulus cell interaction, sperm-oocyte binding and penetration, and sperm oocyte fusion) and post-sperm penetration events (oocyte activation, sperm decondensation, and PN formation). The pre-sperm penetration events are bypassed by ICSI.

In poor or TFF with IVF, the factors contributing could be semen parameters (count, motility, and morphology), contaminated sample, sperm processing method, and final insemination count. Thick zona pellucida and immature oocyte can contribute toward these adverse outcomes. Finally, the inseminating technique—too low sperm count and more oocytes, suboptimal culture conditions, frequent openings of the incubator doors, and contamination of the culture media or oil.

Intracytoplasmic sperm injection requires single sperm, which is injected directly into the ooplasm. Hence, the pre-sperm penetration events, the sperm count, and zona abnormalities are least contributory to the failure. However, procedural aspects such as too gentle injection, which prevent oocyte activation, poor sperm selection, too harsh technique of injection leading to oocyte degeneration especially in a compromised oocyte, and expulsion of the injected sperm can adversely affect the fertilization. There is a learning curve associated with micromanipulation, which will vary in individuals and a beginner should be supervised and evaluated for the same before assigning him independent case handling. Prolonged exposure of the oocyte, temperature of the heated plate during denuding and microinjection, and the culture conditions, which also include the laboratory air quality, can affect the outcome.

Artificial oocyte activation can be beneficial in patients with history of TFF or low fertilization (<30%) in the previous cycle.[43] Different methods have been proposed and used to increase calcium oscillations and thereby increasing intracellular calcium ion concentration, which sets in a cascade of events, leading to better fertilization rates:

- Treatment with calcium ionophores, e.g., ionomycin or calcimycin A23187[44]
- Treatment with strontium chloride[45]
- Mechanical methods such as vigorous aspiration of cytoplasm and a different position of the pipette tip when ejecting sperm in the oocyte[46]
- Injection of human recombinant PLCζ into oocytes[47]
- Electric and piezoelectric stimulation of oocytes.[48]

A recent systematic review and meta-analysis indicated that using calcium ionophore to activate oocytes was beneficial for couples with poor fertilization rates following ICSI.[49] Although, the limitation of this systematic review is that there were only 5 randomized controlled trials (RCTs) and the rest 17 studies were observational studies.

Abnormal fertilization (multiple PN) in IVF could be due to high insemination count. The inability of the oocyte to release the second polar body can also cause abnormal fertilization both in IVF and ICSI. The oocyte deficiencies are more common in women of advanced maternal age, poor oocyte quality, postmature oocytes, and giant oocytes.

## Embryo Quality

### *Poor Embryo Quality/Increased Fragmentation*

Embryo quality is a strong determining factor for the success rates of IVF programs. Fragmentations of variable degrees are observed in about 75% of human embryos produced in vitro[50] and have also been observed in in vivo embryos,[2] though in vitro culture conditions affect embryo quality. In vitro culture conditions that can affect embryo quality are inadequate media and oil equilibration and media pH, frequent incubator openings, and poor laboratory air quality with increased VOC. Similarly, the gas in the incubator should be filtered by attaching an inline filter. Oocytes fertilized by IVF insemination may be exposed to high ROS due to the exposure to dead sperm and cumulus cells, especially if long duration of insemination is followed. Hence, these zygotes should be transferred to a fresh culture dish. Oil overlay prevents rapid and drastic change in pH and temperature and hence preferred over open cultures, especially if using microdroplet culture. To prevent change in media pH and temperature, overexposure of the embryos should be prevented. During dish preparation, embryo monitoring and transferring, the embryologist needs to be conscious of the time factor. Maternal oocyte cytoplasmic factors also play a critical role in early embryo development. These maternal factors include cell-death regulatory elements, stress-response proteins, and mitochondrial content. It may originate from multiple cellular defects altering the cytoskeletal organization.[51] In the group of patients who exhibit embryo fragmentation in repeated IVF attempts, it has been postulated that deficiencies in some maternal factors, such as stress-response factors, might have a role.[52] Embryo fragmentation is also known to be increased in chromosomally abnormal embryos.[53]

Thus, in order to overcome the stress imposed by sub optimal culture conditions, embryos have to be able to synthesize essential compounds not provided by the medium and adapt to conditions imposed by the artificial environment.[54]

Fragmentation rate has been associated with chromosomal abnormalities. Chromosome abnormalities increase from 50–60% in nonfragmented embryos to 70–90% in embryos with >35% fragmentation.[55,56]

Embryo viability is severely compromised when fragmentation exceeds 50%.[57] The early miscarriage rate is also significantly increased when fragmentation is >20% of the volume in 4-cell embryos.[58]

The live birth rate (LBR) increases when high-quality embryos are obtained.[57] Extended cultures until blastocyst stage poses its own limitations due to high risk of developmental arrest partly due to inherent poor embryo status but also the suboptimal culture conditions.

### *Slow Cleavage Rate and Embryo Arrest*

Delayed embryo development and/or embryo arrest could be related to the poor sperm or oocyte quality. It is known that the impact of the male gamete on the embryo development is evident after day 3 and results in poor blastulation. Though not all but aneuploidy embryos also exhibit poor blastocyst formation rate and undergo embryo arrest during extended culture. Suboptimal culture conditions and contamination of the cultures can be detrimental to early embryo development.

## Troubleshooting in Cryopreservation

The most common issues related to embryo cryopreservation are poor embryo survival post warming and poor pregnancy rates in FET cycles.

Prefreezing embryo selection plays an extremely important role in the outcome of the freezing program. This is irrespective of the method used for freezing. Freezing poor quality embryos or oocytes does not improve or alter its potential to implant.

Today most of the clinics use the vitrification method. In this procedure, the crucial factors determining success are rapid cooling rates (15,000–30,000°C/min). To achieve this, higher concentrations of cryoprotectants are used. Thus, timing of exposure to these cryoprotectants, equilibration of the freeze and warming media, and temperature at which they are used become crucial. The manufacturer's instructions have to be followed for optimum results. Selection of the correct device for vitrification is important since it also determines the loading volume. Vitrification is also called "the minimal volume" method. The loading volume is crucial to obtain high rates of cooling. Thus, lesser the volume loaded higher the cooling rate and better the embryo survival. The loading volume should be <1 μL. This procedure too has a learning curve, and the skill and timing of the operator affects the outcome. For oocyte vitrification, the denuded oocytes should be frozen within 1–2 hours of retrieval and they should be injected 1 hour post warming for fertilization.

The factors affecting vitrification are:

- Type and concentration of cryoprotectant agent
- Temperature of vitrification solution at exposure
- Length and time of exposure to the final cryoprotective additive (CPA) before plunging into liquid nitrogen ($LN_2$)
- Loading volume on the device
- Device used
- Technical proficiency of the embryologists
- Quality of the cells to be vitrified
- Device used for vitrification
- Risk of recrystallization during warming.

The American Society for Reproductive Medicine (ASRM) has published the practical recommendations to optimize patient outcomes with oocyte and embryo vitrification. KPIs of rapid-cooling vitrification success are also defined for the TQM program of vitrification.[59]

## Outcome

### *Poor Pregnancy Rate in Spite of Good Embryos Transferred*

Repeated implantation failure (RIF) can be due to multiple reasons. Apart from the embryonic factors, which have been discussed separately, other factors contributing could be anatomic, endometrial, thrombophilia, immunological factors, and male factor. There can be other reasons such as presence of hydrosalpinges, the correction of which (salpingectomy) would significantly improve the implantation rates.[33,60] Each factor has to be looked into carefully before any further IVF cycle. A hysteroscopy is highly recommended in RIF. Intrauterine lesions such as small endometrial polyps or flimsy adhesions, which can be missed on an ultrasound, can be directly visualized and corrected during hysteroscopy.[61] Moreover, even if no abnormality is detected during hysteroscopy, pregnancy rates are still found to improve after the procedure in the subsequent IVF cycles.[62] An element of fibrosis or decreased endometrial vascularity due to previous curettages and/or infections can also be responsible for suboptimal endometrium leading to RIF. In such cases, different therapies have been reported with conflicting results, e.g., aspirin, vitamin E, pentoxifylline, sildenafil, granulocyte colony-stimulating factor (G-CSF), endometrial scratch, high-dose estrogen, and recently stem cell therapy in form of platelet-rich plasma.[63-66]

Contribution of the sperm is also to be kept in mind. For RIF, deoxyribonucleic acid (DNA) fragmentation index (DFI) of the semen should be checked. This can be high even with normal semen parameters. In case of high DFI, intracytoplasmic morphologically selected sperm injection (IMSI) or surgical sperm retrieval can be considered.[67-69]

There is no definitive proven management for thrombophilia or immunological factors which might improve the implantation rates, but many are being used, namely, low molecular weight heparin (LMWH), aspirin, intravenous immunoglobulin (IVIg), etc.

Naturally displaced window of implantation (WOI) has been found to have a role in RIF in some patients, for which endometrial receptivity array (ERA) is recommended and a personalized embryo transfer can improve the reproductive outcome in the subsequent cycles.[70] Further evidence is however required before its role in improving implantation rates can be established beyond doubt.[71] Blastocyst culture[72,73] and laser-assisted hatching[33] have shown improvement in pregnancy rates in RIF. Preimplantation genetic testing of embryos for aneuploidies (PGT-A) by array comparative genomic hybridization (array CGH) earlier and now by next-generation sequencing (NGS) at blastocyst stage has also shown improvement in clinical pregnancy rates in couples with RIF.[74,75] Although PGT-A increases the LBR per embryo transfer, it decreases the time taken to get pregnant, but it comes with a cost of many embryo transfers being cancelled in the absence of a euploid blastocyst. Dealing with the blastocysts having mosaicism is another challenge, and yet another disadvantage is the higher cost of the cycle with PGT-A.[76] These findings need to be further validated by well-designed RCT.

Apart from the viability of the embryo and the endometrial receptivity, the pregnancy and implantation rates are also influenced by a third variable, the embryo transfer procedure technique. The clinician should be well-trained in the procedure; there should be clear SOPs. Patients with particular anatomic defects such as presence of a false passage, acute anteversion/retroversion of the uterus, and cervical stenosis, have to be dealt with very carefully with good skill and expertise in order to improve the pregnancy rates. A systematic review of literature was done and guidelines were published regarding how to perform embryo transfer, based on whether the interventions demonstrated a benefit or not in improving the pregnancy rates.[77]

### *High Biochemical Pregnancy Rate*

Biochemical/chemical pregnancy is defined as one where in spite of a "positive" β-hCG test, the pregnancy fails to progress to the point of ultrasound confirmation.[78]

Biochemical pregnancies are considered to be very common in natural spontaneous conceptions, being as high as about 40–50%. But nearly half of these biochemical pregnancies are usually not detected as in most of the instances, the woman does not even miss her periods.[79]

In patients undergoing an ART cycle, due to time-bound testing of the β-hCG levels in serum and the availability of ultrasensitive pregnancy tests, many biochemical pregnancies are discovered, which would have otherwise gone undetected. Recently, a comparison of biochemical pregnancy rates was reported between women who underwent IVF and fertile controls who conceived spontaneously.[80] Both fresh and frozen transfers were included and were found to have comparable biochemical pregnancy rates (13.8 vs. 14.4%, $p = 0.82$). In spite of the use of gonadotropins for COS in fresh cycles and the use of estradiol and progesterone in the FET cycles, which are all thought to alter the gene expression of endometrium, surprisingly the biochemical pregnancy rates were significantly lower in ART cycles when compared to fertile controls with natural conceptions (13.8 vs. 18%, $p = 0.01$). Selection of better embryos for transfer in IVF cycles was probably thought to be one of the reasons.

This further shows that the detection of chemical pregnancies might be apparently higher in ART cycles, but actually, the spontaneous conceptions also have a high pro portion of such pregnancies, which go unrecognized.

Different reasons for biochemical pregnancies have been proposed, including aneuploidy embryos, suboptimal culture conditions, and suboptimal endometrium.[78] Some have found a higher incidence in older women, while others have failed to see any such correlation with age.[81,82]

However, a biochemical pregnancy means that at least an embryo reached blastocyst stage and is finally implanted in the endometrium.

Thus, pregnancy rates in subsequent IVF cycles are better in women who have had a biochemical pregnancy as compared to those who had a negative pregnancy test.[51] In case of high biochemical pregnancy rates in an IVF laboratory, both the embryo and the endometrium need a reevaluation. Everything which might affect the embryo should be looked into, namely, batch of gonadotropins, media, consumables, air quality, and other aspects of the IVF laboratory. Three-dimensional (3D) scans, Doppler for subendometrial blood flows, and hysteroscopy are used for the endometrial evaluation.

## KEY POINTS

- Every batch, every laboratory, every patient, and every professional involved is a variable. To add to these, the culture conditions and air quality, which in spite of stringent controls, can always be challenging.
- Every ART clinic will go through ups and downs in their success rates though most of the times with the implementation or introduction of new variables. However, it is not always that we would be able to identify the causative factor.
- A proper documentation, adherence to QC measures, and follow through of the SOPs can prevent most of these challenges.
- Troubleshooting is a team effort which should be undertaken with the clinical, nursing, biomedical, and the laboratory personnel on board.

## REFERENCES

1. European Society of Human Reproduction and Embryology. (2015). The revised guidelines for good practice in IVF laboratories. [online] Available from: https://www.eshre.eu/Guidelines-and-Legal/Guidelines/Revised-guidelines-for-good-practice-in-IVF-laboratories-(2015).aspx. [Last accessed March, 2018].

2. Buster JE, Bustillo M, Rodi IA, Cohen SW, Hamilton M, Simon JA, et al. Biologic and morphologic development of donated human ova recovered by nonsurgical uterine lavage. Am J Obstet Gynecol. 1985;153:211-7.
3. Cohen J, Gilligan A, Esposito W, Schimmel T, Dale B. Ambient air and its potential effects on conception in vitro. Hum Reprod. 1997;12:1742-9.
4. Esteves SC, Gomes AP, Verza Jr S. Control of air pollution in assisted reproductive technology laboratory and adjacent areas improves embryo formation, cleavage and pregnancy rates and decreases abortion rate: comparison between a class 100 (ISO 5) and a class 1.000 (ISO 6) cleanroom for micromanipulation and embryo culture. Fertil Steril. 2004;82:S259-60.
5. Meintjes M, Chantilis SJ, Douglas JD, Rodriguez AJ, Guerami AR, Bookout DM, et al. A controlled randomized trial evaluating the effect of lowered incubator oxygen tension on live births in a predominantly blastocyst transfer program. Hum Reprod. 2009;24(2):300-7.
6. Waldenström U, Engström A, Hellberg D, Nilsson S. Low-oxygen compared with high-oxygen atmosphere in blastocyst culture, a prospective randomized study. Fertil Steril. 2009;91(6):2461-5.
7. Dessolle L, Biau DJ, de Larouzière V, Ravel C, Antoine JM, Daraï E, et al. Learning curve of vitrification assessed by cumulative summation test for learning curve (LC-CUSUM). Fertil Steril. 2009;92(3):943-5.
8. Goldman KN, Moon KS, Yauger BJ, Payson MD, Segars JH, Stegmann BJ. Proficiency in oocyte retrieval: how many procedures are necessary for training? Fertil Steril. 2011;95(7):2279-82.
9. National Institute for Health and Clinical Excellence. (2013). Fertility problems: assessment and treatment. [online] Available from https://www.nice.org.uk/guidance/cg156. [Last accessed March, 2018].
10. Wu Y, Gao X, Lu X, Xi J, Jiang S, Sun Y, et al. Endometrial thickness affects the outcome of in vitro fertilization and embryo transfer in normal responders after GnRH antagonist administration. Reprod Biol Endocrinol. 2014;12:96.
11. Hashimoto H, Ishikawa T, Goto S, Kokeguchi S, Fujisawa M, Shiotani M. The effects of severity of oligozoospermia on intracytoplasmic sperm injection (ICSI) cycle outcome. Syst Biol Reprod Med. 2010;56:91-5.
12. Olofsson JI, Banker MR, Sjoblom LP. Quality management systems for your in vitro fertilization clinic's laboratory: why bother? J Hum Reprod Sci. 2013;6(1):3-8.
13. Kushnir VA, Kim A, Gleicher N, Barad DH. A pilot trial of large versus small diameter needles for oocyte retrieval. Reprod Biol Endocrinol. 2013;11:22.
14. Wdowiak A, Wdowiak E, Bojar I. Improving the safety of the embryo and the patient during in vitro fertilization procedures. Wideochir Inne Tech Maloinwazyjne. 2016; 11(3):137-43.
15. Levy G, Hill MJ, Ramirez CI, Correa L, Ryan ME, DeCherney AH, et al. The use of follicle flushing during oocyte retrieval in assisted reproductive technologies: a systematic review and meta-analysis. Hum Reprod. 2012;27(8):2373-9.
16. Son WY, Tan SL. Laboratory and embryological aspects of hCG-primed in vitro maturation cycles for patients with polycystic ovaries. Hum Reprod Update. 2010;16:675-89.
17. Quintans CJ, Donaldson MJ, Blanco LA, Pasqualini RS. Empty follicle syndrome due to human errors: its occurrence in an in-vitro fertilization programme. Hum Reprod. 1998;13:2703-5.
18. Zegers-Hochschild F, Fernández E, Mackenna A, Fabres C, Altieri E, Lopez T. The empty follicle syndrome: a pharmaceutical industry syndrome. Hum Reprod. 1995;10:2262-5.
19. Peñarrubia J, Balasch J, Fábregues F, Creus M, Cívico S, Vanrell JA. Recurrent empty follicle syndrome successfully treated with recombinant human chorionic gonadotrophin. Hum Reprod. 1999;14:1703-6.
20. Stevenson TL, Lashen H. Empty follicle syndrome: the reality of a controversial syndrome, a systematic review. Fertil Steril. 2008;90:691-8.
21. Blazquez A, Guillén JJ, Colomé C, Coll O, Vassena R, Vernaeve V. Empty follicle syndrome prevalence and management in oocyte donors. Hum Reprod. 2014;29:2221-7.
22. Madani T, Jahangiri N. Empty follicle syndrome: the possible cause of occurrence. Oman Med J. 2015;30:417-20.
23. Deepika K, Rathore S, Garg N, Rao K. Empty follicle syndrome: successful pregnancy following dual trigger. J Hum Reprod Sci. 2015;8:170-4.
24. Kummer NE, Feinn RS, Griffin DW, Nulsen JC, Benadiva CA, Engmann LL. Predicting successful induction of oocyte maturation after gonadotropin-releasing hormone agonist (GnRHa) trigger. Hum Reprod. 2013;28:152-9.
25. Baum M, Machtinger R, Yerushalmi GM, Maman E, Seidman DS, Dor J, et al. Recurrence of empty follicle syndrome with stimulated IVF cycles. Gynecol Endocrinol. 2012;28:293-5.
26. Inan MS, Al-Hassan S, Ozand P, Coskun S. Transcriptional profiling of granulosa cells from a patient with recurrent empty follicle syndrome. Reprod Biomed Online. 2006;13:481-91.
27. Meniru GI, Craft IL. Evidence from a salvaged treatment cycle supports an aetiology for the empty follicle syndrome that is related to terminal follicular developmental events. Hum Reprod. 1997;12(11):2385-7.
28. Hassan HA, Saleh HA, Khalil O, Baghdady I, Ismaiel I. Double oocyte aspiration may be a solution for empty follicle syndrome: case report. Fertil Steril. 1998;69:138-9.
29. Revelli A, Carosso A, Grassi G, Gennarelli G, Canosa S, Benedetto C. Empty follicle syndrome revisited: definition, incidence, aetiology, early diagnosis and treatment. Reprod Biomed Online. 2017;35:132-8.
30. Yariz KO, Walsh T, Uzak A, Spiliopoulos M, Duman D, Onalan G, et al. Inherited mutation of the luteinizing hormone/choriogonadotropin receptor (LHCGR) in empty follicle syndrome. Fertil Steril. 2011;96:125-30.
31. Zreik TG, Garcia-Velasco JA, Vergara TM, Arici A, Olive D, Jones EE. Empty follicle syndrome: evidence for recurrence. Hum Reprod. 2000;15(5):999-1002.
32. Ndukwe G, Thornton S, Fishel S, Dowell K, Aloum M, Green S. Curing empty follicle syndrome. Hum Reprod. 1997;12:21-3.
33. Practice Committee of the Society for Assisted Reproductive Technology, Practice Committee of the American Society for Reproductive Medicine. The role of assisted hatching in in vitro fertilization: a review of the literature. A Committee opinion. Fertil Steril. 2008;90(5 Suppl.):S196-8.
34. Driscoll GL, Tyler JP, Hangan JT, Fisher PR, Birdsall MA, Knight DC. A prospective, randomized, controlled, double-blind, double-dummy comparison of recombinant and urinary HCG

for inducing oocyte maturation and follicular luteinization in ovarian stimulation. Hum Reprod. 2000;15:1305-10.
35. Khalaf Y, Amin Y, Anderson H. Inappropriate timing of hCG administration: an avoidable cause of empty follicle syndrome in in-vitro fertilization. Middle East Fertil Soc J. 1999;4:254-6.
36. Vutyavanich T, Piromlertamorn W, Ellis J. Immature oocytes in "apparent empty follicle syndrome": a case report. Case Rep Med. 2010;2010:367505.
37. Prasad S, Tiwari M, Pandey AN, Shrivastav TG, Chaube SK. Impact of stress on oocyte quality and reproductive outcome. J Biomed Sci. 2016;23:36.
38. Alvarez Sedó C, Miguens M, Andreucci S, Ortiz N, Lorenzi D, Papier S, et al. Correlation between cytoplasmic oocyte maturation and chromosomal aneuploidies—impact on fertilization, embryo quality and pregnancy. JBRA Assist Reprod. 2015;19(2):59-65.
39. Okohue JE, Ikimalo JI, Onuha SO. Ejaculation failure on the day of oocyte retrieval for IVF: a report of five cases. Middle East Fertil Soc J. 2011;16:159-62.
40. Zafer M, Horvath H, Mmeje O, van der Poel S, Semprini AE, Rutherford G, et al. Effectiveness of semen washing to prevent HIV transmission and assist pregnancy in HIV-discordant couples: a systematic review and meta-analysis. Fertil Steril. 2016;105(3):645-55.
41. Payne D, Flaherty SP, Jeffrey R, Warnes GM, Matthews CD. Successful treatment of severe male factor infertility in 100 consecutive cycles using intracytoplasmic sperm injection. Hum Reprod. 1994;9:2051-7.
42. Mahutte NG, Arici A. Failed fertilization: is it predictable? Curr Opin Obstet Gynecol. 2003;15:211-8.
43. Montag M, Köster M, van der Ven K, Bohlen U, van der Ven H. The benefit of artificial oocyte activation is dependent on the fertilization rate in a previous treatment cycle. Reprod Biomed Online. 2012;24:521-6.
44. Lv M, Zhang D, He X, Chen B, Li Q, Ding D, et al. Artificial oocyte activation to improve reproductive outcomes in couples with various causes of infertility: a retrospective cohort study. Reprod Biomed Online. 2020;40(4):501-9.
45. Fawzy M, Emad M, Mahran A, Sabry M, Fetih AN, Abdelghafar H, et al. Artificial oocyte activation with SrCl2 or calcimycin after ICSI improves clinical and embryological outcomes compared with ICSI alone: results of a randomized clinical trial. Hum Reprod. 2018;33(9):1636-44.
46. Ebner T, Moser M, Sommergruber M, Jesacher K, Tews G. Complete oocyte activation failure after ICSI can be overcome by a modified injection technique. Hum Reprod. 2004;19(8):1837-41.
47. Yoon SY, Eum JH, Lee JE, Lee HC, Kim YS, Han JE, et al. Recombinant human phospholipase C zeta 1 induces intracellular calcium oscillations and oocyte activation in mouse and human oocytes. Hum Reprod. 2012;27(6):1768-80.
48. Mansour R, Fahmy I, Tawab NA, Kamal A, El-Demery Y, Aboulghar M, et al. Electrical activation of oocytes after intracytoplasmic sperm injection: a controlled randomized study. Fertil Steril. 2009;91(1):133-9.
49. Shan Y, Zhao H, Zhao D, Wang J, Cui Y, Bao H. Assisted oocyte activation with calcium ionophore improves pregnancy outcomes and offspring safety in infertile patients: a systematic review and meta-analysis. Front Physiol. 2022;12:751905.
50. Hardy K. Apoptosis in the human embryo. Rev Reprod. 1999;4:125-34.
51. Levy T, Dicker D, Ashkenazi J, Feldberg D, Shelef M, Goldman JA. The prognostic value and significance of preclinical abortions in in vitro fertilization-embryo transfer programs. Fertil Steril. 1991;56(1): 71-4.
52. Sermondade N, Delarouzière V, Ravel C, Berthaut I, Verstraete L, Mathieu E, et al. Characterization of a recurrent poor-quality embryo morphology phenotype and zygote transfer as a rescue strategy. Reprod Biomed Online. 2012; 24:403-9.
53. Antczak M, Van Blerkom J. Temporal and spatial aspects of fragmentation in early human embryos: possible effects on developmental competence and association with the differential elimination of regulatory proteins from polarized domains. Hum Reprod. 1999;14:429-47.
54. Biggers JD. Reflections on the culture of the preimplantation embryo. Int J Dev Biol. 1998;42:879-84.
55. Magli MC, Gianaroli L, Ferrareti AP. Chromosomal abnormalities in embryos. Mol Cell Endocrinol. 2001;183(Suppl. 1): S29-34.
56. Munné S, Sandalinas M, Cohen J. Chromosome abnormalities in human embryos. In: Gardner DK, Weissman A, Howles CM, Shoham Z (Eds). Textbook of Assisted Reproductive Techniques: Laboratory and Clinical Perspectives. London: Martin Dunitz; 2001. pp. 297-318.
57. Ziebe S, Petersen K, Lindenberg S, Andersen AG, Gabrielsen A, Andersen AN. Embryo morphology or cleavage stage: how to select the best embryos for transfer after in-vitro fertilization. Hum Reprod. 1997;12:1545-9.
58. Fauque P, Lèandri R, Merlet F, Juillard JC, Epelboin S, Guibert J, et al. Pregnancy outcome and live birth after IVF and ICSI according to embryo quality. J Assist Reprod Genet. 2007;24:159-65.
59. Practice Committees of the American Society for Reproductive Medicine and Society of Reproductive Biologists and Technologists. A review of best practices of rapid-cooling vitrification for oocytes and embryos: a committee opinion. Fertil Steril. 2021;115:305-10.
60. Practice Committee of American Society for Reproductive Medicine in collaboration with Society of Reproductive Surgeons. Salpingectomy for hydrosalpinx prior to in vitro fertilization. Fertil Steril. 2008;90:S66-8.
61. Cenksoy P, Ficicioglu C, Yıldırım G, Yesiladali M. Hysteroscopic findings in women with recurrent IVF failures and the effect of correction of hysteroscopic findings on subsequent pregnancy rates. Arch Gynecol Obstet. 2013;287(2):357-60.
62. Demirol A, Gurgan T. Effect of treatment of intrauterine pathologies with office hysteroscopy in patients with recurrent IVF failure. Reprod Biomed Online. 2004;8:590-4.
63. Barad DH, Yu Y, Kushnir VA, Shohat-Tal A, Lazzaroni E, Lee HJ, et al. A randomized clinical trial of endometrial perfusion with granulocyte colony-stimulating factor in in vitro fertilization cycles: impact on endometrial thickness and clinical pregnancy rates. Fertil Steril. 2014;101:710-5.
64. Gleicher N, Kim A, Michaeli T, Lee HJ, Shohat-Tal A, Lazzaroni E, et al. A pilot cohort study of granulocyte colony-stimulating factor in the treatment of unresponsive thin endometrium resistant to standard therapies. Hum Reprod. 2013;28:172-7.

65. Lebovitz O, Orvieto R. Treating patients with "thin" endometrium—an ongoing challenge. Gynecol Endocrinol. 2014; 30:409-14.
66. Zadehmodarres S, Salehpour S, Saharkhiz N, Nazari L. Treatment of thin endometrium with autologous platelet-rich plasma: a pilot study. JBRA Assist Reprod. 2017;21(1):54-6.
67. Balaban B, Yakin K, Alatas C, Oktem O, Isiklar A, Urman B. Clinical outcome of intracytoplasmic injection of spermatozoa morphologically selected under high magnification: a prospective randomized study. Reprod Biomed Online. 2011;22:472-6.
68. Souza Setti A, Ferreira RC, Paes de Almeida Ferreira Braga D, de Cássia Sávio Figueira R, Iaconelli Jr A, Borges Jr E. Intracytoplasmic sperm injection outcome versus intracytoplasmic morphologically selected sperm injection outcome: a meta-analysis. Reprod Biomed Online. 2010;21:450-5.
69. Wilding M, Coppola G, di Matteo L, Palagiano A, Fusco E, Dale B. Intracytoplasmic injection of morphologically selected spermatozoa (IMSI) improves outcome after assisted reproduction by deselecting physiologically poor quality spermatozoa. J Assist Reprod Genet. 2011;28:253-62.
70. Mahajan N. Endometrial receptivity array: clinical application. J Hum Reprod Sci. 2015;8(3):121-9.
71. Ben Rafael Z. Endometrial receptivity analysis (ERA) test: an unproven technology. Hum Reprod Open. 2021;2021(2): hoab010.
72. Guerif F, Bidault R, Gasnier O, Couet ML, Gervereau O, Lansac J, et al. Efficacy of blastocyst transfer after implantation failure. Reprod Biomed Online. 2004;9:630-6.
73. Levitas E, Lunenfeld E, Har-Vardi I, Albotiano S, Sonin Y, Hackmon-Ram R, et al. Blastocyst-stage embryo transfer in patients who failed to conceive in three or more day 2-3 embryo transfer cycles: a prospective, randomized study. Fertil Steril. 2004;81:567-71.
74. Greco E, Bono S, Ruberti A, Lobascio AM, Greco P, Biricik A, et al. Comparative genomic hybridization selection of blastocysts for repeated implantation failure treatment: a pilot study. Biomed Res Int. 2014;2014:457913.
75. Tong J, Niu Y, Wan A, Zhang T. Next-generation sequencing (NGS)-based preimplantation genetic testing for aneuploidy (PGT-A) of trophectoderm biopsy for recurrent implantation failure (RIF) patients: a retrospective study. Reprod Sci. 2021;28(7):1923-9.
76. Practice Committee and Genetic Counseling Professional Group (GCPG) of the American Society for Reproductive Medicine. Clinical management of mosaic results from preimplantation genetic testing for aneuploidy (PGT-A) of blastocysts: a committee opinion. Fertil Steril. 2020;114: 246-54.
77. Practice Committee of the American Society for Reproductive Medicine, Practice Committee of the American Society for Reproductive Medicine. Performing the embryo transfer: a guideline. Fertil Steril. 2017;107:882-96.
78. Annan JJ, Gudi A, Bhide P, Shah A, Homburg R. Biochemical pregnancy during assisted conception: a little bit pregnant. J Clin Med Res. 2013;5(4):269-74.
79. Schreiber CA, Sammel M, Hillier SL, Barnhart KT. A little bit pregnant: modeling how the accurate detection of pregnancy can improve HIV prevention trials. Am J Epidemiol. 2009; 169(4):515-21.
80. Zeadna A, Son WY, Moon JH, Dahan MH. A comparison of biochemical pregnancy rates between women who underwent IVF and fertile controls who conceived spontaneously. Hum Reprod. 2015;30(4):783-8.
81. Dickey RP, Olar TT, Taylor SN, Curole DN, Harrigill K. Relationship of biochemical pregnancy to pre-ovulatory endometrial thickness and pattern in patients undergoing ovulation induction. Hum Reprod. 1993;8(2):327-30.
82. Salumets A, Suikkari AM, Mäkinen S, Karro H, Roos A, Tuuri T. Frozen embryo transfers: implications of clinical and embryological factors on the pregnancy outcome. Hum Reprod. 2006;21(9):2368-74.

CHAPTER

# 126 Quality Management in Assisted Reproductive Technology Clinics

*Gautham T Pranesh*

## PRINCIPLES OF QUALITY MANAGEMENT

Quality in healthcare systems refers to the ability of being able to achieve conformance consistently to the requirements of patients and healthcare providers are the users of the services. "Total quality management" provides a management philosophy and process for development of systems that improve the quality of work across all areas. This encompasses a view that healthcare organizations are composed of a set of interlinked repetitive processes that aim at achieving optimal outcomes for patients. The quality management systems provide a framework to support the identification of issues or problems within processes and empower employees to resolve them to ensure consistent and sustainable delivery of optimal outcomes. Establishing such systems within an organization requires a commitment to quality by the management and resources including manpower, time, and money which contribute to the costs quality. The costs of quality conformance also may lead to advantages such as cost reduction and competitive advantages for organizations by reducing wastage, improving efficiency, and adding value to customers. Examples of the potential costs and benefits of quality are provided in **Table 1**.

## DEVELOPING A QUALITY MANAGEMENT SYSTEM IN ASSISTED REPRODUCTIVE TECHNOLOGY CLINIC

In the last five decades after the first successful in vitro fertilization (IVF), understanding of assisted reproductive techniques has improved increasing success rates and outcomes. As a result, the body of scientific evidence has established best practice guidelines and standards. Organizations may adopt one or more of standards for development of a quality management system. A quality management system is a framework of business processes within an organization focused on providing reliable, efficient, and consistent services to customers and ensuring compliance to regulations. Such systems include several elements such as organizational goals, objectives, policies, procedures, and documents to monitor the effectiveness of implementation, structured in a hierarchical manner **(Fig. 1)**. Standard definitions of elements within quality management systems are provided in **Table 2**.

Organizations must strategically select appropriate quality standards and regulations that may be applicable in their operational environment. Establishing an effective quality management system requires organizations to align policies, processes, and practices to meet the requirements of these quality standards and regulations to achieve desirable outcomes. Policy directives are expressed from the top management in the form of a quality policy which is documented and communicated across the organization. Individual clinical and nonclinical departments within an organization such as embryology, andrology, nursing, clinical, operations, billing, etc., establish written standard operating procedures (SOPs) for key business and technical processes. SOPs are written documents which provide step by step instructions to help individuals to carry out tasks

**TABLE 1:** Concept of cost of quality.

| *Quality costs* | *Type of costs* | *Examples* |
|---|---|---|
| Costs of prevention | Conformance costs | Cost of equipment maintenance, infrastructure for quality systems, calibration, and maintenance |
| Costs of appraisal | Conformance costs | Cost of establishing periodic checks and an audit process |
| Costs of internal failure | Costs of nonconformance | Cost of rework and wastage of media, reagents, etc. |
| Costs of external failure | Costs of nonconformance | Cost of patient complaint resolution, patient dissatisfaction with services, and litigation risk |

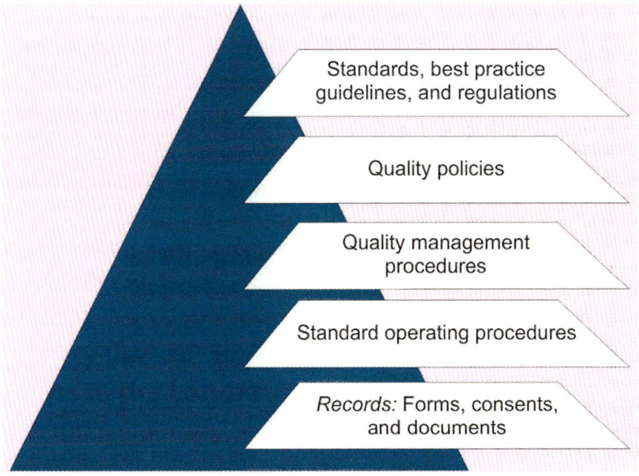


**Fig. 1:** Structure of quality management systems in an organization.

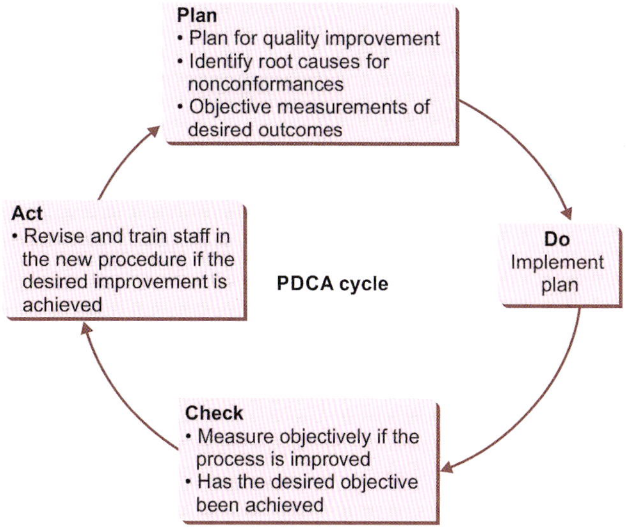


**Fig. 2:** Plan-do-check-act (PDCA) cycle for continuous quality improvement.

**TABLE 2:** Standard definitions in quality management systems.

| *Terms* | *Definition* |
|---|---|
| Accreditation | A procedure by which an authoritative body gives formal recognition that an organization is competent to carry out specific tasks (ISO 15189:2012) |
| Nonconformity | Nonfulfillment of a requirement in the quality management system (ISO 9000:2005) |
| Quality | Degree to which a set of inherent characteristics fulfill requirements (ISO 9000:2005) |
| Quality management system (QMS) | Management system to direct and control an organization with regard to quality (ISO 9000:2005) |
| Quality policy | Overall intentions and direction of a laboratory related to quality as formally expressed by the laboratory management (ISO 9000:2005) |
| Quality indicator | Measure of a degree to which a set of characteristics fulfill requirements |
| Validation | Confirmation, through the provision of objective evidence, that the requirements for a specific intended use or application has been fulfilled (ISO 9000:2005) |
| Verification | Confirmation, through the provision of objective evidence, that specified requirements have been fulfilled |

in a consistent and correct manner. Implementation of SOPs is ensured through appropriate data records that are created during the tasks, which may be reviewed or audited periodically.

Standard operating procedures must be comprehensive and prepared by individuals who are proficient in the tasks being performed. Training and compliance to such written procedures is critical to ensure consistency in the tasks performed, standardization across operators, regulatory compliance, clarity in communication, reduction in errors, and help to retain the knowledge created within an organization.

## MAINTAINING ONGOING COMPLIANCE TO A QUALITY MANAGEMENT SYSTEM

Once a quality management system is established in an organization, maintaining compliance, and ensuring continual improvements are the next objective. Assessment of compliance and ongoing modifications for quality management systems based on evidence is a continuous process. Typical methods used to evaluate compliance include periodic review of records, review of documentation of procedures, records and nonconformances, and audits by internal or external groups. Reviews of processes can be performed by supervisors using an ask-observe-review model. This involves asking staff questions to evaluate their understanding on procedures and policies, observing staff when they are performing tasks and review of records, and documents to evaluate availability of standardized procedures and compliance to the same.

Continual improvements in the quality management system are initiated using repetitive iterations of the plan-do-check-act cycle **(Fig. 2)**. The management can appoint a "project team" with a mandate to review internal processes and identify areas for improvement. The team is empowered to use a structured methodology for review of processes within the organization. The methodology employed must:

- Carefully define conformance desired within a process.
- Accurately describe the nonconformances observed.
- Establish the baseline measures for process performance and conformance.
- Identify the root cause for nonconformances within the process.
- Establish an effective plan for correction and prevention of such nonconformance.
- Verify that the established plan provides desired conformance on implementation.

- Standardize the solution for routine implementation of the improved process.
- Establish metrics to ensure ongoing control and effective monitoring of the process.

Key performance indicators or quality indicators must be established to objectively measure outcomes of critical processes. Measures such as oocyte retrieval rate, fertilization rate, lysis rate, cleavage rate, freeze-thaw survival rates, blastocyst conversion rate, clinical pregnancy rate, and live-birth rates are examples of such indicators in an assisted reproductive technology (ART) setting. Benchmarks for such indicators may be set by the laboratory management and are usually derived based on acceptable consensus across clinical settings. Clinics and laboratories must periodically review quality indicators and initiate root cause analysis of problems, corrective, and preventive actions when required.

## ACCREDITATION, CERTIFICATION, AND LICENSING REQUIREMENTS FOR ASSISTED REPRODUCTIVE TECHNOLOGY CLINICS

Several countries have developed frameworks to regulate assisted reproductive techniques **(Table 3)**. Quality systems may be aligned by the process of accreditation or certification to one or more of these standards.

The process of certification involves an assessment by a third party to verify that the processes for an operational quality management system are adequate within an organization. Laboratories participating in accreditation programs the quality management systems evaluated, by third party accreditation providers to ensure that the system delivers the intended quality of results.

Organizations operating in regulated environments must comply with the local and national laws. Compliance to regulatory requirements may be enforced through licensing procedures **(Table 4)**.

## KEY ELEMENTS OF A QUALITY MANAGEMENT SYSTEM

Accreditation programs oriented toward ART clinics are focused toward laboratory quality. Such programs broadly mandate standard requirements in areas such as systems for management, qualifications, experience and proficiency requirements for staff, technical requirements for embryology and andrology laboratory processes, validation and maintenance of laboratory equipment, systems for management of IT systems, and requirements for safety. International quality standards such as ISO further breakdown these requirements into numbered sections **(Box 1)**.

**TABLE 3:** Quality standards and accreditation standards.

| *Standards* | *Scope of quality management* |
|---|---|
| ISO 9001:2008 | • General guideline on quality management<br>• Focus primarily on best practices in general management systems, equipment selection and maintenance, and personnel management |
| ISO 17025:2005 | Guideline specific to testing and calibration laboratories—Developed on the basis on ISO 9001 standards; focus on general management and technical management in laboratories. Covers aspects of validation, quality control, and quality assurance |
| ISO 15189:2012 | Guideline specific to medical testing laboratories—Developed on the base of ISO 17025 standards; focus on clinical need and outcomes in addition to general and technical management guidelines |
| Joint Commission International (JCI) | Standards specific for healthcare organizations—JCI is an organization that develops healthcare standards with a focus on patient safety and quality. The organization is based out of USA with a reach in over 90 countries |
| Clinical and Laboratory Standards Institute (CLSI) | Nonprofit organization which develops standards and guidelines focused toward laboratory quality |
| GMP/GLP | These guidelines provide minimum requirements that a pharmaceutical or a food product manufacturer must meet to assure that the products are of high quality and do not pose any risk to the consumer or public |
| College of American Pathologists (CAP) | • IVF laboratories must comply with the requirements of the Clinical Laboratories Improvement Act (CLIA) of 1988<br>• Standards and accreditation program specific to embryology, andrology, and tissue cryopreservation. The program is developed jointly with the American Society for Reproductive Medicine (ASRM). The accreditation complies with the CLIA requirements. |

(GLP: good laboratory practice; GMP: good manufacturing practice; IVF: in vitro fertilization)

**TABLE 4:** List of region-wise standards globally for quality management in assisted reproductive technology.

| ***Regions*** | ***Local and regional regulations and licensing requirements*** |
|---|---|
| Asia and Middle East | • *India:* ICMR guidelines, registration is not mandated by the government http://icmr.nic.in/art/art_clinics.htm<br>• *UAE:* IVF centers are governed and licensed by the health authority<br>• *Japan:* Japanese Gynecology Society guidelines for IVF<br>• *Singapore:* Licensing mandated by the Ministry of Health<br>• *China:* Guidelines by Ministry of Health for providing approvals to IVF clinics in the respective province |
| North America | • College of American Pathologists (CAP) in association with American Society for Reproductive Medicine (ASRM) provides an accreditation program for fertility centers in the US http://www.cap.org/web/home/lab/accreditation/reproductive-accreditation-program?_afrLoop=101173589932947#!%40%40%3F_afrLoop%3D101173589932947%26_adf.ctrl-state%3D3oyhhwjha_17<br>• The Society for Assisted Reproductive Technologies (SARTs) covers over 90% of the IVF clinics in the United States. SART is involved in publishing outcomes, quality assurance, participation in patient advocacy and interaction with regulators, and establishment of best practice guidelines http://www.sart.org/patients/what-is-sart/ |
| South America | The Red Latinoamericana de Reproducción Asistida (RED—Latin American Network of Assisted Reproduction) is a scientific and educational institution, which brings together >90% of the centers engaged in assisted reproduction techniques in Latin America http://redlara.com/aa_ingles/default.asp |
| Europe | • IVF laboratories are governed by European Union Tissues and Cells Directive (EUTCD), a legal framework published as a document under the European Union's Public Health Program. The document focuses on patient safety with an objective of preventing transmission of infectious diseases and prevention of inadvertent exchange of gametes or embryos<br>• The European Society of Human Reproduction and Embryology (ESHRE) has provided a position statement and guideline on the EUTCD. "ESHRE guidelines for good practice in IVF laboratories" is complementary to the EUTCD bringing a focus on best practices to improve clinical outcomes<br>• Human Fertilization and Embryology Authority (HEFA) licensing authority in UK |
| Australia | IVF clinics are licensed by Reproductive Technology Accreditation Committee (RTAC) |

(ICMR: Indian Council of Medical Research; IVF: in vitro fertilization)

**BOX 1:** Section titles for management and technical requirements as per ISO 15189:2012 international standard.

*Management requirements:*
- Organization and management responsibility
- Quality management system
- Document control
- Service agreements
- Examination by referral laboratories
- External services and supplies
- Advisory services
- Resolution of complaints
- Identification and control of nonconformities
- Corrective action
- Preventive action
- Continual improvement
- Control of records
- Evaluation and audits
- Management review

*Technical requirements:*
- Personnel
- Accommodation and environmental conditions
- Laboratory equipment, reagents, and consumables
- Pre-examination process
- Examination process
- Ensuring quality of examination results
- Postexamination process
- Reporting of results
- Release of results
- Laboratory information management

## GUIDELINES FOR GOOD PRACTICE IN IN VITRO FERTILIZATION LABORATORIES

The European Society of Human Reproduction and Embryology (ESHRE) guideline group in 2015 published the revised guidelines for good practice in IVF laboratories, a comprehensive document based on current clinical evidence and practice. These recommendations, although not intended as a quality standard, provide a framework to establish quality requirements in ART clinics. The guideline provides suggestions to aid quality and clinical decisions across 11 areas summarized here in **Table 5**.

### Assisted Reproductive Technology Act, 2021 and Its Implication on Quality Management Systems

In India the regulatory framework for assisted reproductive techniques was published in the Assisted Reproductive Technologies Act, 2021. The act prescribes a regulatory framework where clinics and banks offering services in the realm of assisted reproductive techniques need to demonstrate a minimum standard of compliance to the requirements of the act. This has an implication on quality management system wherein clinics must ensure written policies, SOPs, and records to establish the manner

**TABLE 5:** Guideline provides suggestions to aid quality and clinical decisions.

| ***Key areas for quality management*** | ***Summarized recommendations*** |
|---|---|
| 1. Staffing and direction | • The guideline suggests that two qualified embryologists are available for every 150 procedures including retrievals and transfers must be provided<br>• Laboratory director for embryology must have appropriately recognized qualifications (MSc, MD, or PhD), expertise and experience (a minimum of 6 years) in the field of embryology. It is preferable that the laboratory director has completed a certification in embryology in addition to the earlier requirements<br>• Roles and responsibilities of laboratory director, laboratory supervisor, and clinical embryologists are specified in the document<br>• The human resources planning within an organization must enable performance of tasks in a timely manner, adequate backup for staff, ensure patient safety, and provide quality service |
| 2. Quality management | • The clinical embryologist is responsible for implementation of the quality management system in the laboratory. The components of such a quality management system include:<br>– Availability of a comprehensive set of written, validated, and authorized standard operating procedures and evidence of training on the same<br>– Processes ensuring traceability of measuring equipment's to standards<br>– Processes ensuring unique identity of all patients and traceability of their reproductive cells and tissues<br>– Processes to confirm the quality of reagents and consumables before use in the clinic<br>– Processes to ensure appropriate maintenance of equipment including periodic servicing and calibration<br>– Processes to identify, correct, and prevent nonconformities<br>– Processes to collect, record, and review key performance indicators (quality metrics)<br>– Processes to audit, review, and ensure continual compliance and improvement in quality management systems<br>– Analysis of risks and plans for risk mitigation<br>– Periodic review of technical competence, compliance to the management system, and consistency through evaluation, proficiency testing, and training<br>– Processes for internal quality control in critical processes and participation in external quality assurance programs<br>– Processes for statistical evaluation and review of clinical performance on a periodic basis<br>– Processes for periodic review of the quality management system (annual review is recommended) |
| 3. Laboratory safety | *Laboratory design and air quality:*<br>• ART laboratory must be situated adjacent to the operating room performing the oocyte retrieval and transfer procedures<br>• Materials used within the laboratory must be appropriate for clean room use, minimize release of volatile organic compounds, and not embryo toxic<br>• Access to the ART laboratory must be restricted to authorized personnel only<br>• Facilities for changing and hand wash must be available for use before entry into the ART laboratory<br>• The laboratory must have a clean access for personnel and material entry<br>• Incompatible activities such as handling or storage of toxic reagents, cleaners, and sterilization materials must be separate from the laboratory<br>• The laboratory air quality must be subjected to high efficiency particulate air (HEPA) and VOC control<br>• The laboratory must maintain a positive air pressure when compared to the surrounding environment to prevent contamination<br>• Tissue and cell processing procedures must be done in a good manufacturing practice (GMP) grade D environment at a minimum (grade A environment ideal)<br>• The laboratory must have sufficient environmental lighting and air conditioning with controlled humidity and temperature<br>*Laboratory equipment:*<br>• Gas cylinders must be placed outside the laboratory premises with automatic changeover systems and adequate backup. The use of inline HEPA and VOC filters where possible is recommended<br>• Equipment must be validated for performance and to ensure its fitness at the time of installation Performance of an equipment must be verified by calibrated instruments wherever applicable. Records of calibration, maintenance, and repair must be maintained within the laboratory<br>• The laboratory must define acceptable ranges for all measured parameters (e.g., temperature, humidity, etc.). Records of actual measurements must be evaluated against defined ranges. Corrective actions must be initiated if the values are found to be out of range<br>• Critical equipment such as cryostorage tanks and incubators must be continuously monitored for failure and equipped with alarm systems<br>• Power failure alarm systems and backup power must be available for all critical equipment |

*Contd...*

*Contd...*

| ***Key areas for quality management*** | ***Summarized recommendations*** |
|---|---|
| | • The laboratory must have adequate and appropriate equipment to manage the number of procedures within a clinic<br>• Equipment must be kept clean and operational. Malfunctioning equipment must be labeled as "out of use". Instruction and troubleshooting manuals must be available for all critical equipment<br>*Cryopreservation facilities and materials:*<br>• Cryopreservation facilities must be located close to the ART laboratory. The facility must have adequate ventilation with low oxygen alarms for safety<br>• The laboratory must have processes for continuously monitoring cryostorage units. Alarm systems to detect low levels of liquid nitrogen or temperature failures must be incorporated<br>• The laboratory must have a documented process and train staff in handling of liquid nitrogen. Personal protection devices (PPDs) such as glasses, apron, and cryogloves must be used when handling liquid nitrogen<br>*Infectious agents:*<br>• Staff must be vaccinated against hepatitis B. Staff must be trained in use of personal protective devices and handling biological samples<br>• Patients must be screened for infectious diseases as per local regulations<br>• The laboratory must have processes for handling biomedical waste, decontamination, and response to needlestick injuries<br>• Screening results for infectious diseases must be obtained in advance whenever biological materials are imported into a laboratory from another clinic<br>*Protective measures:*<br>• The laboratory must treat all biological material as potentially infectious. The staff must be trained in universal precautions and adopt safe practices within the laboratory |
| 4. Identification of patients and traceability of their reproductive cells | The clinic and laboratory must have processes to insure accurate identification of patients and their reproductive cells. Such processes must include:<br>• Generation of a unique identification code for each patient<br>• Generation of a unique code for each treatment cycle<br>• Clear and permanent labeling of all devices containing biological material<br>• Direct identification of the patient and verification of the unique identifier at all critical steps. A minimum of two identifiers (example: name and date of birth) must be used to generate a unique identifier<br>• A policy to ensure that biological material from different patients is not processed in the same area at the same time to avoid misidentification and sample mix up<br>• Organization of incubators and cryostorage systems to ensure easy access and identification of biological materials<br>• A witness system with double checks to maintain the chain of custody during critical steps involving movement of biological materials<br>• A system for unique coding and identification of nonpartner gametes<br>• A system for verification of identity and conformity of samples, records, and storage devices imported or shipped out of a clinic<br>The clinic must maintain the following records to ensure compliance with earlier processes:<br>• Date and time of each manipulation and movement with the identity of operators and witnesses<br>• Training records as evidence of mandatory training of staff on traceability procedures |
| 5. Consumables | • The laboratory must use media and consumables that are fit for purpose and embryo culture grade. The laboratory must have a process to verify packing integrity, appropriate delivery conditions, and records of quality control testing for each batch of media or consumable used<br>• Reagents, media, and consumables must be used before expiry. The size of packaging must be appropriately selected to minimize contamination. Single use disposable consumables must be used wherever possible<br>• Media and consumables must be stored under appropriate conditions as indicated by the manufacturer<br>• The laboratory must have an appropriate inventory management system including details of batch number, date of entry, and expiry date for stock management<br>• The laboratory must perform a risk assessment to ensure that all consumables and media are easily identified to avoid misuse |
| 6. Handling of biological material | The clinic and the laboratory must have processes for biological materials ensuring:<br>• Safe handling under laminar flow hoods using aseptic precautions<br>• Maintenance of appropriate temperature, pH, and osmolality during culture and handling<br>• Minimal exposure to light, radiation, or toxic substances<br>• Appropriate preparation of buffered media<br>• Maintenance of chain of custody and traceability to the source of origin at all times |

*Contd...*

*Contd...*

| *Key areas for quality management* | *Summarized recommendations* |
|---|---|
| 7. Oocyte retrieval | The clinic and the laboratory must have processes to:<br>• Mandatorily check identity of a patient before oocyte retrieval<br>• Prevent prolonged exposure to follicular fluid and minimize the time between oocyte retrieval and culture.<br>• Maintain oocytes at 37°C using prewarmed media<br>• Check follicular aspirates for oocytes using a stereomicroscope with 8–60X magnification and a heated stage<br>The clinic and the laboratory must have records which:<br>• Document the time of retrieval, the operator, and the number of oocytes retrieved |
| 8. Sperm preparation | The clinic and laboratory must have standard procedures to ensure proper sperm preparation. This includes documented processes for:<br>• Providing instructions to patients for collection of semen samples<br>• Obtaining a backup sample in anticipation of possible difficulties in sperm collection on the day of oocyte retrieval<br>• Correct labeling and correct identification of sample containers and patients<br>• Analysis and preparation of semen samples<br>• Semen preparation in case of patients diagnosed with blood borne viruses<br>• Alternative sperm retrieval procedures when patients are found to be azoospermic<br>The laboratory or clinic would need to maintain the following records in a manner that is traceable to the patient:<br>• Records for sperm collection must include the type of container used, time and place of collection, time between collection, analysis and preparation, use of medications, fever during previous months and completeness, and volume of ejaculate collection<br>• Records for sperm preparation including sample origin, preparation method, pre and postsperm preparation parameters, and dilution, if applicable |
| 9. Insemination of oocytes | The clinic and laboratory must have appropriately documented procedures for insemination of oocytes by conventional IVF or ICSI<br>The laboratory must have established processes for the following in cases of conventional IVF or ICSI:<br>• Use of appropriate sperm concentration for IVF procedure<br>• Use of appropriate immobilization and sperm selection techniques in case if ICSI<br>• Selection of sperm preparation medium and methods which is compatible with the oocyte culture system<br>• Verification of patient identity and traceability of the oocytes and sperms before the procedure<br>• Validated procedure for conventional IVF and ICSI<br>The laboratory must maintain records traceable to patients including data on the time of insemination, the operator, and concentration of progressively motile sperm for conventional IVF. Details of the injection start times and end time must be noted in the case of ICSI |
| 10. Scoring for fertilization | The clinic and laboratory must have procedures to verify the presence of pronuclei and polar bodies 16–18 hours postinsemination. The clinic must document its procedures to discard more than or equal to three PN or less than or equal to one PN oocytes |
| 11. Embryo culture and transfer | The clinic and laboratory must have documents and implement processes for:<br>• Maintaining chain of custody and verification of identity during the process of culture and transfer<br>• The use of a standardized culture system including media and culture conditions<br>• Extended culture for blastocysts<br>• Standardized embryo scoring for cleavage stage embryos and blastocyst<br>• Selection for embryos for transfer<br>• Management of supernumerary embryos<br>The clinic and laboratory must maintain records for:<br>• Embryo quality assessment including the name of the operators, date and time of assessment, and the embryo morphological characteristics<br>• Transfer procedure including the date and time of embryo transfer, name of the operator, name of the practitioner performing the transfer, number of embryos transferred, developmental stage and quality of the embryos at the time of transfer, the type of catheter used, fate of supernumerary embryos, and details of the procedure such as retained embryos or blood in the catheter |
| 12. Cryopreservation | The clinic and laboratory must have processes for cryopreservation of gametes, embryos, and tissues. Such procedures include:<br>• Instructions for selection of cryopreservation approaches according to the type of biological materials<br>• Measures to minimize the risk of transmission of infective diseases<br>• Instructions for clear and permanent labeling of cryodevices |

*Contd...*

*Contd...*

| *Key areas for quality management* | *Summarized recommendations* |
|---|---|
| | • Methods for periodic evaluation of inventory in the cryobank with cross references to storage records<br>• Methods for establishing patient identity before storage and retrieval<br>• Systems to store and handle cryopreserved biological material under safe and appropriate environmental conditions<br>The clinic and laboratory must maintain the following records traceable to patients when storing or handling cryopreserved samples:<br>• Records for cryopreservation including labeling of devices, cryopreservation method, date and time of cryopreservation, operator, details of embryo quality and stage of development, number of oocytes or embryos per device, number of devices per patient, and location of stored samples to ensure traceability<br>• Records for thawing including details of the thawing method, date of thawing, operator, and post-thaw quality of biological sample |
| 13. Emergency plan | The clinic and laboratory must have a tested emergency plan to serve as mitigation in even of exceptional failures of infrastructure or service facilities. Such procedures include:<br>• Communication measures in event of emergency procedures<br>• Systems to ensure redundancy in case of failure of electricity, gas supply, or depletion of liquid nitrogen<br>• Identification of appropriate backup for all critical equipment such as incubators, storage tanks, etc<br>• Measures to backup and store critical medical records identifying ownership and traceability of stored biological material<br>• Regular review and training procedures on the emergency plan<br>• Appropriate arrangements with third party facilities for emergency transfer of gametes or embryos |

(ART: assisted reproductive technology; ICSI: intracytoplasmic sperm injection; IVF: in vitro fertilization; VOC: volatile organic compound)

**TABLE 6:** Internal audit checklist of quality requirements.

| *Checklist requirement (ask questions, observe practices, read policies, procedures, and records)* | *Reference* | *Clause/ section* |
|---|---|---|
| Does the clinic, bank provide facilities and maintain equipment and standards including specialized manpower, physical infrastructure and diagnostic facilities as required by the ART act, 2021 | The Assisted Reproductive Technology (Regulation) Act, 2021 | 15-(4) |
| Has the clinic applied and obtained a valid registration as per the requirements of the above mentioned act? | The Assisted Reproductive Technology (Regulation) Act, 2021 | 15-(3) |
| Has the clinic or bank displayed the registration certificate at a conspicuous place within the facility? | The Assisted Reproductive Technology (Regulation) Act, 2021 | 16-(7) |
| Does the displayed certificate contain the details of validity of such a registration? | The Assisted Reproductive Technology (Regulation) Act, 2021 | 16-(7) |
| Does the clinic and bank have a documented process/procedure to ensure that couple, women and donors are eligible to avail assisted reproductive technology procedures as per the requirements of the act? | The Assisted Reproductive Technology (Regulation) Act, 2021 | 21-(a) |
| Does the clinic have a process/procedure to ensure that donors have been medically tested for the diseases mentioned in the ART act? | The Assisted Reproductive Technology (Regulation) Act, 2021 | 21-(b) |
| Does the clinic have a process/procedure for counselling patients? | The Assisted Reproductive Technology (Regulation) Act, 2021 | 21-(c) |
| Does the process of counselling include documented records as evidence of counselling on:<br>• Implications and the chances of success in ART<br>• Advantages and disadvantages of the prescribed procedure<br>• Cost of the procedure<br>• Medical side effects<br>• Risks involved including the risk of multiple pregnancies<br>• Rights of the unborn child | The Assisted Reproductive Technology (Regulation) Act, 2021 | 21-(c) |
| Does the clinic have policies and procedures in place to ensure confidentiality of information pertaining to treatment of couples, women, and donors? | The Assisted Reproductive Technology (Regulation) Act, 2021 | 21-(d) |

*Contd...*

*Contd...*

| ***Checklist requirement (ask questions, observe practices, read policies, procedures, and records)*** | ***Reference*** | ***Clause/ section*** |
|---|---|---|
| Does the clinic have procedures to make the records available for specific requirements specified in the ART act:<br>• National registry<br>• In a medical emergency<br>• On request of the commissioning couple<br>• By order of a court of competent jurisdiction | The Assisted Reproductive Technology (Regulation) Act, 2021 | 21-(d) |
| Does the clinic have a grievance cell and a procedure to make a complaint before the grievance cell? | The Assisted Reproductive Technology (Regulation) Act, 2021 | 12-(f) |
| Does the clinic have a policy and procedure to provide a discharge certificate to the commissioning couple or women stating the details of the Assisted Reproductive Technology procedure performed? | The Assisted Reproductive Technology (Regulation) Act, 2021 | 21-(h) |
| Is there evidence of such discharge certificates routinely being provided to commissioning couples or women? | The Assisted Reproductive Technology (Regulation) Act, 2021 | 21-(h) |
| Does the clinic maintain records on:<br>• Enrollment of commissioning couples, women and donors<br>• Procedures being undertaken in couples, women and donors<br>• Outcomes of procedures<br>• Complications, if any | The Assisted Reproductive Technology (Regulation) Act, 2021 | 12-(j) |
| Does the clinic have a process/procedure to provide the details in the aforementioned records to the National Registry periodically as prescribed? | The Assisted Reproductive Technology (Regulation) Act, 2021 | 21-(j) |
| Does the clinic have a policy and procedure of obtaining a written informed consent from all parties seeking assisted reproductive procedures? | The Assisted Reproductive Technology (Regulation) Act, 2021 | 22-1-(a) |
| Is there evidence of records indicating the use of a correct and current version of the informed consent? | The Assisted Reproductive Technology (Regulation) Act, 2021 | 22-1-(a) |
| Is there evidence of records indicating completeness of documentation and details on informed consents? | The Assisted Reproductive Technology (Regulation) Act, 2021 | 22-1-(a) |
| Does the clinic have policies and procedures to verify that the donor is insured by the commissioning couple or women before initiating any assisted reproductive procedure? | The Assisted Reproductive Technology (Regulation) Act, 2021 | 22-1-(b) |
| Does the clinic have policies and procedures governing the cryopreservation of human gametes or embryos in event of death or incapacity of any of the parties? | The Assisted Reproductive Technology (Regulation) Act, 2021 | 22-(2) |
| Does the clinic have policies restricting the use of human reproductive material only in any manner other than those permitted by the ART act? | The Assisted Reproductive Technology (Regulation) Act, 2021 | 22-(3) |
| Does the clinic have a policy or procedure on the process to follow when any party in a commissioning couple or women withdraws consent before transfer of human gametes or embryos into the uterus? | The Assisted Reproductive Technology (Regulation) Act, 2021 | 22-(4) |
| Does the clinic maintain ongoing records of all donor oocytes, sperm or embryos, used or unused? | The Assisted Reproductive Technology (Regulation) Act, 2021 | 23-(a) |
| Does the clinic maintain ongoing records of the manner and technique of use of donor oocytes, sperm or embryos? | The assisted reproductive technology (regulation) act, 2021 | 23-(a) |
| Does the clinic maintain ongoing records of progress of the commissioning couple or women? | The Assisted Reproductive Technology (Regulation) Act, 2021 | 23-(b) |
| Does the clinic maintain ongoing records on:<br>• Number of donor sperm or oocytes samples<br>• Number of donors screened<br>• Number of donor samples maintained<br>• Number of donor samples supplied to commissioning couples | The Assisted Reproductive Technology (Regulation) Act, 2021 | 23-(b) |
| Does the clinic have policies, procedures and infrastructure to maintain the aforementioned records for a minimum period of 10 years? | The Assisted Reproductive Technology (Regulation) Act, 2021 | 23-(c) |
| Does the clinic have specific policies governing the maintenance of records in the event of any criminal or other proceedings against the clinic? | The Assisted Reproductive Technology (Regulation) Act, 2021 | 23-(c) |

*Contd...*

*Contd...*

| *Checklist requirement (ask questions, observe practices, read policies, procedures, and records)* | *Reference* | *Clause/ section* |
|---|---|---|
| Does the clinic have policies for handling, maintenance and transfer of records in event of closure to ensure retention for 10 years? | The Assisted Reproductive Technology (Regulation) Act, 2021 | 23-(d) |
| Does the clinic have policies and procedures on oocyte retrieval procedures? | The Assisted Reproductive Technology (Regulation) Act, 2021 | 24-(a) |
| Does the clinic have policies and procedures to ensure that no more than three oocytes or embryos are placed in the uterus during a treatment cycle? | The Assisted Reproductive Technology (Regulation) Act, 2021 | 24-(b) |
| Does the clinic have policies/procedures prohibiting the transfer of gametes derived from more than one man or woman during a single treatment cycle? | The Assisted Reproductive Technology (Regulation) Act, 2021 | 24-(c) |
| Does the clinic have policies/procedures prohibiting the mixing of semen from two individuals for procedures specified under the ART act? | The Assisted Reproductive Technology (Regulation) Act, 2021 | 24-(d) |
| Does the clinic have policies/procedures prohibiting splitting of embryos for twinning to increase the number of available embryos? | The Assisted Reproductive Technology (Regulation) Act, 2021 | 24-(e) |
| Does the clinic have policies/procedures for posthumous collection of gametes? | The Assisted Reproductive Technology (Regulation) Act, 2021 | 24-(f) |
| Does the clinic have policies/procedures prohibiting the use of oocytes derived from a fetus in any process of in-vitro fertilization | The Assisted Reproductive Technology (Regulation) Act, 2021 | 24-(g) |
| Does the clinic have written policies and procedures for the use of pre-implantation genetic testing | The Assisted Reproductive Technology (Regulation) Act, 2021 | 25(1) |
| Does the clinic have policies/procedures prohibiting sex determination or providing a child of a predetermined sex in any manner contravening the requirements of the PCPNDT act, 1994? | The Assisted Reproductive Technology (Regulation) Act, 2021 | 26 |
| Does the clinic have adequate process/procedures and records for storage, identification, security and handling of gametes? | The Assisted Reproductive Technology (Regulation) Act, 2021 | 28-(1) |
| Does the clinic have adequate process/procedures and records for storage, identification, security and handling of embryos? | The Assisted Reproductive Technology (Regulation) Act, 2021 | 28-(1) |
| Does the clinic have policies, procedures and records for storage of gametes and embryos for not >10 years? | The Assisted Reproductive Technology (Regulation) Act, 2021 | 28-(2) |
| Does the clinic have policies, procedures and records for storage of gametes and embryos for a duration of longer than 10 years with permission of the national board in patients with specific medical requirements? | The Assisted Reproductive Technology (Regulation) Act, Rules, June 7 2022 | 13-(b) |
| Does the clinic have policies, procedures and records for disposal of gametes and embryos as per the ART act? | The Assisted Reproductive Technology (Regulation) Act, 2021 | 28-(2) |
| Does the clinic have a policy prohibiting sale, transfer or use of gametes, zygotes or embryos any part thereof or information related thereto to any party other than the commissioning couple within or outside India? | The Assisted Reproductive Technology (Regulation) Act, 2021 | 29 |
| Does the clinic have a policy, procedure and process for the transfer of own gametes or embryos for personal use with the permission of the National Board? | The Assisted Reproductive Technology (Regulation) Act, 2021 | 29 |
| Does the clinic have a policy prohibiting the transfer of human gametes or embryos to any country outside India for research? | The Assisted Reproductive Technology (Regulation) Act, 2021 | 30-(1) |
| Are the staffs recruited in the clinic as per the requirements of "The Assisted Reproductive Technology Act (Regulation) Rules"? | The Assisted Reproductive Technology (Regulation) Act, Rules, June 7 2022 | 4 |
| Does the clinic have the minimum required infrastructure and equipment as per the "The Assisted Reproductive Technology Act (Regulation) Rules" | The Assisted Reproductive Technology (Regulation) Act, Rules, June 7 2022 | 5 |
| Does the clinic have policies, procedures and records that ensure that all unused gametes or embryos shall be preserved by the ART clinic for use on the same recipient? | The Assisted Reproductive Technology (Regulation) Act, Rules, June 7 2022 | 13a |
| Does the clinic have policies, procedures and records that prohibit the use of unused gametes or embryos assigned to recipient to any other couple or woman? | The Assisted Reproductive Technology (Regulation) Act, Rules, June 7 2022 | 13a |
| Does the clinic have adequate policies and procedures to prevent ovarian hyperstimulation in women undergoing controlled ovarian stimulation? | The Assisted Reproductive Technology (Regulation) Act, Rules, June 7 2022 | 13c |

*Contd...*

*Contd...*

| Checklist requirement (ask questions, observe practices, read policies, procedures, and records) | Reference | Clause/ section |
|---|---|---|
| Is the consent form to be signed by a couple or woman in the format specified by "The Assisted Reproductive Technology Act (Regulation) Rules" rule 13(f) (i) Form 6? | The Assisted Reproductive Technology (Regulation) Act, Rules, June 7 2022 | 13(f)(i) |
| Is the format for making complaints to the grievance cell in the format specified by "The Assisted Reproductive Technology Act (Regulation) Rules" rule 11 Form 5? | The Assisted Reproductive Technology (Regulation) Act, Rules, June 7 2022 | 11 |
| Is the format for consent for IUI with husbands semen/sperm in the format specified by "The Assisted Reproductive Technology Act (Regulation) Rules" rule 13(f)(ii) Form 7? | The Assisted Reproductive Technology (Regulation) Act, Rules, June 7 2022 | 13(f)(ii) |
| Is the format for consent for freezing of gametes/sperm/oocytes in the format specified by "The Assisted Reproductive Technology Act (Regulation) Rules" rule 13(f) (v) Form 10? | The Assisted Reproductive Technology (Regulation) Act, Rules, June 7 2022 | 13(f)(v) |
| Is the format for consent for freezing of gametes/Sperm/oocytes and parental consent in the format specified by "The Assisted Reproductive Technology Act (Regulation) Rules" rule 13(f)(vi) Form 11? | The Assisted Reproductive Technology (Regulation) Act, Rules, June 7 2022 | 13(f)(vi) |
| Is the format for consent for Intrauterine Insemination with donor semen in the format specified by "The Assisted Reproductive Technology Act (Regulation) Rules" rule 13(f)(iii) Form 8? | The Assisted Reproductive Technology (Regulation) Act, Rules, June 7 2022 | 13(f)(iii) |
| Is the format for consent for freezing of embryos in the format specified by "The Assisted Reproductive Technology Act (Regulation) Rules" rule 13(f)(iv) Form 9? | The Assisted Reproductive Technology (Regulation) Act, Rules, June 7 2022 | 13(f)(iv) |
| Is the format for consent for oocyte retrieval in the format specified by "The Assisted Reproductive Technology Act (Regulation) Rules" rule 13(f)(vii) Form 12? | The Assisted Reproductive Technology (Regulation) Act, Rules, June 7 2022 | 13(f) (vii) |
| Is the format for consent for the donor of oocytes in the format specified by "The Assisted Reproductive Technology Act (Regulation) Rules" rule 13(f)(viii) Form 12? | The Assisted Reproductive Technology (Regulation) Act, Rules, June 7 2022 | 13(f) (viii) |
| Is the format for consent form for donor of sperm in the format specified by "The Assisted Reproductive Technology Act (Regulation) Rules" rule 13(2)(ii) Form 15? | The Assisted Reproductive Technology (Regulation) Act, Rules, June 7 2022 | 13(2)(ii) |
| Is the format for record of use of donor gametes in the format specified by "The Assisted Reproductive Technology Act (Regulation) Rules" rule 13(2)(i) Form 14? | The Assisted Reproductive Technology (Regulation) Act, Rules, June 7 2022 | 13(2)(i) |

in which they comply to the requirements of the act. Clinics in the coming days may be audited where the records associated with such a quality management process in conjunction with records of training and compliance to such procedures would be required to ensure regulatory compliance. An internal audit checklist of quality requirements to ensure compliance to the act is provided in **Table 6**.

## CONCLUSION

Quality management systems in assisted reproduction clinics help to offer better value, consistency, improve outcomes, maintain regulatory compliance, and enhance efficiency. Organizations must establish their quality management systems based on their size, service objectives and goals.

## KEY POINTS

- Quality management systems aim at standardizing interlinked repetitive processes in healthcare to optimize outcomes.
- Quality management systems are prepared to comply with standards and regulations and are composed of organizational policies, standard operating procedures, and records from top-down.
- Continuous quality management involves continuous monitoring of key performance indicators, non-conformities and risks with appropriate corrective and preventive actions for mitigation.
- Quality management systems may help clinics to maintain ongoing compliance with local or national regulations such as the Assisted Reproductive Technology Act, 2021 in India.